KAPLAN & SAD

Study Guide and Sel ation Review in Psychiatry

Eighth 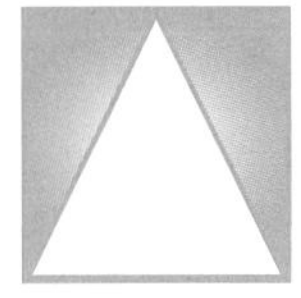 Edition

Contributing Editors

Matt Biel, M.D.

Instructor in Psychiatry and Fellow in Child Psychiatry, New York University School of Medicine, New York, New York

Nikole Benders, M.D.

Instructor in Psychiatry, New York University School of Medicine, New York, New York

KAPLAN & SADOCK'S

Study Guide and Self-Examination Review in Psychiatry

EIGHTH 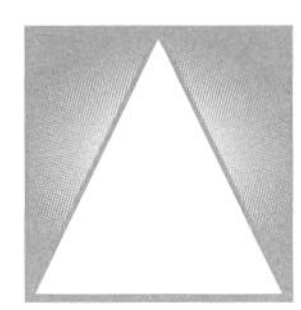 EDITION

Benjamin James Sadock, M.D.

Menas S. Gregory Professor of Psychiatry and Vice Chairman,
Department of Psychiatry, New York University School of Medicine;
Attending Psychiatrist, Tisch Hospital;
Attending Psychiatrist, Bellevue Hospital Center;
Consulting Psychiatrist, Lenox Hill Hospital,
New York, New York

Virginia Alcott Sadock, M.D.

Professor of Psychiatry, Department of Psychiatry,
New York University School of Medicine;
Attending Psychiatrist, Tisch Hospital;
Attending Psychiatrist, Bellevue Hospital Center,
New York, New York

Ze'ev Levin, M.D.

Clinical Associate Professor of Psychiatry,
Department of Psychiatry,
New York University School of Medicine,
New York, New York

Wolters Kluwer | Lippincott Williams & Wilkins
Health

Philadelphia • Baltimore • New York • London
Buenos Aires • Hong Kong • Sydney • Tokyo

Acquisitions Editor: Charles W. Mitchell
Managing Editor: Joyce A. Murphy
Developmental Editor: Katey Millet
Associate Director of Marketing: Adam Glazer
Production Editor: Bridgett Dougherty
Senior Manufacturing Manager: Benjamin Rivera
Design Coordinator: Stephen Druding
Compositor: Aptara, Inc
Printer: Quebecor World-Taunton

530 Walnut Street
Philadelphia, PA 19106 USA
LWW.com

Printed in the USA

Library of Congress Cataloging-in-Publication Data

Sadock, Benjamin J., 1933–
Kaplan & Sadock's study guide and self-examination review in psychiatry / Benjamin James Sadock, Virginia Alcott Sadock. —8th ed.
p. cm.
Includes bibliographical references and index.
ISBN 978-0-7817-8043-8 (alk. paper)
1. Psychiatry—Examinations—Study guides. 2. Psychiatry—Examinations, questions, etc. I. Sadock, Virginia A. II. Title. III. Title: Kaplan and Sadock's study guide and self-examination review in psychiatry. IV. Title: Study guide and self-examination review in psychiatry.
RC454.K36 2007
616.890076—dc22

2007010764

Care has been taken to confirm the accuracy of the information presented and to describe generally accepted practices. However, the authors, editors, and publisher are not responsible for errors or omissions or for any consequences from application of the information in this book and make no warranty, expressed or implied, with respect to the currency, completeness, or accuracy of the contents of the publication. Application of this information in a particular situation remains the professional responsibility of the practitioner.

The authors, editors, and publisher have exerted every effort to ensure that drug selection and dosage set forth in this text are in accordance with current recommendations and practice at the time of publication. However, in view of ongoing research, changes in government regulations, and the constant flow of information relating to drug therapy and drug reactions, the reader is urged to check the package insert for each drug for any change in indications and dosage and for added warnings and precautions. This is particularly important when the recommended agent is a new or infrequently employed drug.

Some drugs and medical devices presented in this publication have Food and Drug Administration (FDA) clearance for limited use in restricted research settings. It is the responsibility of the health care provider to ascertain the FDA status of each drug or device planned for use in their clinical practice.

To purchase additional copies of this book, call our customer service department at (800) 638-3030 or fax orders to (301) 223-2320. International customers should call (301)223-2300.

Visit Lippincott Williams & Wilkins on the Internet: at LWW.com. Lippincott Williams & Wilkins customer service representatives are available from 8:30 am to 6 pm, EST.

10 9 8 7 6 5 4 3 2 1

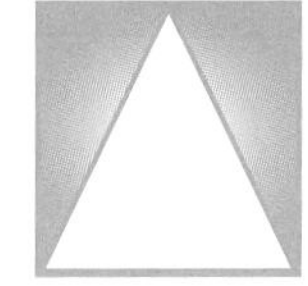

Preface

This new and improved eighth edition of *Study Guide and Self-Examination Review in Psychiatry* is designed to stand alone as a separate textbook to serve as a guide to the mastery of a tremendous amount of material relating to psychiatry and the behavioral sciences. The student will find questions of varying complexity that cover the etiology, diagnosis, and treatment of every known psychiatric disorder. This is coupled with a comprehensive discussion that covers not only correct answers but wrong answers as well. By carefully studying both questions and answers, the reader will gain a thorough understanding of material useful to prepare for examinations of all types. This book was written to meet the needs of medical students, psychiatric physicians, and mental health professionals from all fields. It is designed especially to help those preparing for the United States Medical Licensing Examination (USMLE) and the American Board of Psychiatry and Neurology (ABPN); it will also prove of value to all who want to test their knowledge in psychiatry as part of their continuing medical education.

The authors have added new and different questions to each edition of *Study Guide* and modified and updated material from earlier editions. This *Study Guide* contains more than 1,500 questions, more than any other book of its kind, and the format of each question is standardized to follow that used by the USMLE and ABPN. In addition, the allocation of topics is carefully weighted with attention to both clinical and theoretical issues.

The authors of the last edition of *Study Guide* are particularly pleased that Ze'ev Levin, M.D., a close personal and professional associate and outstanding academician, has joined them as third author. Dr. Levin is Associate Director of Residency Training in Psychiatry at NYU Medical Center and his participation has immeasurably facilitated and enhanced the preparation of this work. In addition, we wish to thank our two Contributing Editors: Matt Biel M.D. served as Contributing Editor in Child Psychiatry, and Nikole Benders, M.D. served as Contributing Editor in Adult Psychiatry.

COMPREHENSIVE TEACHING SYSTEM

Study Guide forms one part of a comprehensive system developed by the authors to facilitate the teaching of psychiatry and the behavioral sciences. At the head of the system is *Comprehensive Textbook of Psychiatry*, which is global in depth and scope; it is designed for and used by psychiatrists, behavioral scientists, and all other workers in the mental health field. *Kaplan & Sadock's Synopsis of Psychiatry* is a relatively brief, highly modified, original, and current version useful for medical students, psychiatric residents, practicing psychiatrists, and other mental health professionals. A special edition of *Synopsis, Concise Textbook of Clinical Psychiatry*, covers just the diagnosis and treatment of all psychiatric disorders. Other parts of the system are the pocket handbooks: *Pocket Handbook of Clinical Psychiatry, Pocket Handbook of Psychiatric Drug Treatment, Pocket Handbook of Emergency Psychiatric Medicine*, and *Pocket Handbook of Primary Care Psychiatry*. These books cover the diagnosis and the treatment of mental disorders, psychopharmacology, psychiatric emergencies, and primary care psychiatry, respectively, and are compactly designed and concisely written to be carried in the pocket by clinical clerks and practicing physicians, whatever their specialty, to provide a quick reference. Finally, *Comprehensive Glossary of Psychiatry and Psychology* provides simply written definitions for psychiatrists and other physicians, psychologists, students, and other mental health professionals. Together, these books create a multiple approach to teaching, studying, and learning of psychiatry.

HOW TO USE THIS BOOK

Each chapter begins with an introduction that emphasizes areas of special significance about which the student should be aware. The authors have also prepared lists of helpful hints—now expanded and in alphabetical order—that present key terms and concepts essential to a basic knowledge of psychiatry. Students should be able to define and discuss each of the terms in depth as preparation for examinations.

The section *Objective Examinations in Psychiatry* provides the student with helpful hints on how to take the examinations. If the student understands how questions are constructed, his or her chances of answering correctly are greatly improved. This book defines distractors (wrong answers) as well as correct answers in each discussion.

To use this book most effectively, the student should attempt to answer all the questions in a particular chapter. By allowing about 1 minute for each answer, the student can approximate the time constraints of an actual written examination. The answers should be verified by referring to the corresponding answer section in each chapter. Pay particular attention to the discussion of the wrong answers, a feature unique to this book. If further information is needed, the reader is referred to the current editions of either the *Synopsis of Psychiatry* or the *Comprehensive Textbook of Psychiatry*.

ACKNOWLEDGEMENTS

In addition to the contributing editors mentioned above, we wish to thank Regina Furner who served as Project Editor and whose knowledge of the complex organization and format of the text was invaluable. Nitza Jones, Project Editor of *Synopsis* and *Comprehensive Textbook of Psychiatry*, also assisted in the preparation of the book. Others we wish to thank are Mryl Manley, M.D., Caroly S. Pataki, M.D., Norman Sussman, M.D., Michael Stanger, M.D., and Kathleen Rey.

We especially acknowledge James Sadock, M.D., and Victoria Gregg, M.D., for their help in their areas of expertise, emergency adult and emergency pediatric medicine, respectively.

At Lippincott Williams & Wilkins, we thank Joyce Murphy, Katey Millet, and Charley Mitchell. At Aptara we thank Judi Rohrbaugh.

We want to express our deep thanks to Robert Cancro, M.D., who retired after 28 years serving as Chairman of Psychiatry at New York University School of Medicine and who gave us his full support. He was succeeded as Chair in 2006 by Dolores Malaspina, M.D., to whom we extend a warm welcome as she leads the Department of Psychiatry into the 21st century.

Finally, we want to acknowledge and thank Alan and Marilyn Zublatt for their generous support of this and other *Kaplan & Sadock* textbooks. Over the years they have been unselfish benefactors to many educational, clinical and research projects at the NYU Medical Center. We are deeply grateful for their help. We thank them not only for ourselves but also on behalf of all those at NYU—students, clinicians, and researchers—who have benefited from their extraordinary humanitarian vision.

B.J.S.
V.A.S.
New York University School of Medicine
New York, New York

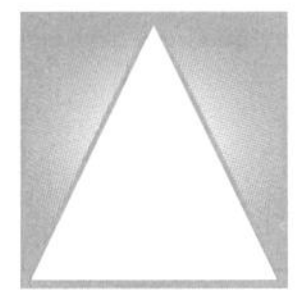

Contents

1 The Patient–Doctor Relationship

The patient–doctor relationship is at the core of the practice of medicine. It is of utmost concern to all physicians and should be evaluated in all cases. It is essential that all clinicians consider the nature of this relationship, the factors in themselves and their patients that influence the relationship, and the ways in which good rapport can be achieved.

Rapport is the spontaneous, conscious feeling of harmonious responsiveness that promotes the development of a constructive therapeutic relationship. It implies an understanding and trust between the doctor and patient. Medicine is an intensely human and personal endeavor, and the patient–doctor relationship itself becomes part of the therapeutic process.

The bio-psycho-social model of disease stresses an integrated approach to human behavior and disease. Each system in this model, the biological, psychological and social, affects and is affected by the others. It does not consider illness as a direct result of a person's psychological or sociocultural makeup, but rather promotes a more comprehensive understanding of disease and treatment. This model provides a conceptual framework for dealing with disparate information and serves as a reminder that there may be important issues to consider beyond the biological.

The interactions between a doctor and patient can take different shapes, and it is helpful to be aware of the models that have been formulated to describe these interactions. The paternalistic model, the informative model, the interpretive model, and the deliberative model are guides for thinking about the patient–doctor relationship. A talented, sensitive physician uses different approaches with different patients and may have different approaches with the same patient as time and medical circumstances vary.

Doctors and patients may have divergent, distorted, and unrealistic views about each other. Transference and countertransference, terms originating in psychoanalytic theory, are hypothetical constructs that are extremely useful as organizing principles for explaining certain developments of the patient–doctor relationship that can be upsetting and that can interfere with good medical care. Students must be aware of and familiar with these concepts in order to fully understand the complexities of the patient–doctor interaction. The patient–doctor relationship is one of the most important factors in issues of treatment compliance, or adherence. Compliance decreases when communication problems arise. Doctors should be familiar with the factors that increase and decrease treatment adherence, and the clinician must explore the reasons for noncompliance rather than dismiss the patient as uncooperative.

In addition to the vast amount of knowledge and the skills required for the practice of medicine, an effective physician must also develop the capacity for balancing compassionate concern with discompassionate objectivity, the wish to relieve pain with the ability to make painful decisions, and the desire to cure and control with an acceptance of one's human limitations. William Osler, M. D. discussed the characteristics and qualities of the physician in his book *Aequanimitas*. Although rarely reached, all students of medicine should be familiar with them, and strive to reach them.

Students should test their knowledge by addressing the following questions and answers.

HELPFUL HINTS

The key terms listed below should be understood by the student.

- active versus passive patients
- aggression and counteraggression
- authority figures
- belligerent patients
- biopsychosocial
- biopsychosocial model
- burnout
- closed-ended questions
- compliance
- compliance versus noncompliance
- confrontation
- content versus process
- countertransference
- cultural attitudes
- defensive attitudes
- distortion
- patient–doctor models
- early social pressures
- emotional reactions
- emotionally charged statements
- empathy
- George Engel
- "good patients"
- humor
- identification
- illness behavior
- individual experience
- insight
- interpretation
- listening
- misperception
- misrepresentation

- mutual participation
- need–fear dilemma
- open-ended questions
- overcompensatory anger
- personality
- psychodynamics
- rapport
- reflection
- self-monitoring
- sick role
- socioeconomic background
- sublimation
- therapeutic limitations
- transference
- unconscious guilt
- unresolved conflicts

QUESTIONS

Directions

Each of the questions or incomplete statements below is followed by five suggested responses or completions. Select the *one* that is *best* in each case.

1.1 Transference feelings

A. are based on doctors projecting their feelings to the patient
B. is a main reason for lawsuits filed by mistreated patients
C. do no occur with a highly experienced physician
D. are based on a patient projecting feelings from past relationships to the doctor
E. none of the above

1.2 Rapport is

A. based on doctors projecting their feelings to the patient
B. based on a patient projecting feelings from past relationships to the doctor
C. a feeling of harmony that promotes a therapeutic relationship
D. of little significance in obtaining the history
E. none of the above

1.3 What percent of patients comply with treatment in the medical setting at any given time?

A. 90 percent
B. 75 percent
C. 50 percent
D. 30 percent
E. 10 percent

1.4 Illness behavior refers to

A. the role society ascribes to the sick person
B. being excused from responsibilities
C. the influence of culture on illness
D. the way the condition presents itself
E. all of the above

1.5 Which of the following models guides us in thinking about the patient–doctor relationship?

A. The paternalistic model
B. The deliberative model
C. The informative model
D. The interpretive model
E. All of the above

1.6 Which of the following statements about transference is *true*?

A. Transference reactions may be strongest with psychiatrists.
B. Transference is a conscious process.
C. Transference occurs only in patient interactions with psychiatrists, not with clinicians from other disciplines.
D. Transference toward physicians is exclusively positive because patients know doctors are trying to help them.
E. Transference implies that the way a clinician interacts with their patient has no direct bearing on the emotional reactions of the patient.

1.7 Which of the following patient factors is associated with treatment compliance?

A. Socioeconomic status
B. Educational level
C. Subjective feelings of distress
D. Intelligence
E. All of the above

1.8 Which of the following doctor factors is associated with treatment compliance?

A. Positive physician attitude
B. Short waiting room time
C. Older doctors with experience
D. Increased frequency of visits
E. All of the above

1.9 Which of the following is considered important in establishing rapport with a patient?

A. Putting the patient at ease
B. Expressing compassion
C. Evaluating a patient's insight
D. Showing expertise
E. All of the above

1.10 Which of the following is true about the techniques used when interviewing a patient?

A. Confrontation is used to test a patient's ability to remain calm.
B. Reflection allows the doctor an opportunity to share with the patient his or her personal feelings.
C. Silence is used as a way of withholding empathy.
D. Interpretations should be made early and as often as possible.
E. Clarification is a way for the doctor to get further details about what has already been revealed.

1.11 All of the following statements about illness behavior are correct *except*

A. It is affected by a person's cultural beliefs about disease.
B. It always involves the experience of illness as a loss.
C. It involves the sick role that society ascribes to people when they are ill.
D. It is affected by prior illness episodes of standard severity.
E. It can be affected by psychological factors such as personality.

1.12 In which instance is an autocratic patient–doctor relationship most appropriate?

A. A patient who has a life-threatening illness with various treatment options.
B. A woman who is a carrier of the gene for cystic fibrosis consults her doctor about whether she and her husband should conceive.
C. A 54-year-old woman with hypertension wishes to monitor her own blood pressure at home.
D. A 22-year-old man is brought into the emergency room with a gunshot wound to the chest.
E. A young woman confides in her doctor about wanting to have an abortion.

1.13 Compared to nonpsychiatric medical patients, psychiatric patients

A. do not have to deal with the stigma attached to being a patient
B. are more likely to tolerate a traditional interview format
C. are twice as likely to visit a primary care physician
D. exhibit a higher degree of compliant behavior
E. never need family members or friends to provide medical histories

1.14 Which of the following is *not* considered a necessary part of a psychiatric patient–doctor relationship?

A. Discussion of payment
B. The understanding that confidentiality may be broken in some situations
C. Awareness of the consequences for missed appointments
D. The patient's familiarity with the doctor's personal life
E. Clarification of the doctor's availability between scheduled appointments

Directions

Each set of lettered headings below is followed by a list of numbered words or statements. For each numbered word or statement, select the *one* lettered heading most closely associated with it. Each lettered heading may be selected once, more than once, or not at all.

Questions 1.15–1.18

A. Open-ended questions
B. Closed-ended questions

1.15 Intent of question is vague
1.16 May invite yes or no answers
1.17 Low time efficiency
1.18 Patient selects topic

Questions 1.19–1.23

A. Active–passive model
B. Teacher–student model
C. Mutual participation model
D. "Friendship" model

1.19 A patient is admitted to the hospital with a sudden onset of altered mental status when found thrashing about in bed. After a workup, a physician restrains him to perform a lumbar puncture.
1.20 A 64-year-old woman with diabetes mellitus visits her physician after repeatedly drawing high blood glucose levels during home monitoring.
1.21 After a patient's complete recovery from illness, her physician continues to phone and visit her—and declares his love for her.
1.22 Three days after abdominal surgery, a 32-year-old man has mild basal rales by auscultation. His surgeon tells him to ambulate.
1.23 The doctor of a 16-year-old girl with persistent abdominal problems tells her that she must go for a lower gastrointestinal (GI) series.

Questions 1.24–1.28

A. Composure
B. Equanimity
C. Imperturbability
D. Idealism
E. Bravery

1.24 The ability to maintain calm and steadiness
1.25 The ability to handle stressful situations with an even temper
1.26 Forming standards, and living under their influence
1.27 Calmness of mind, bearing, and appearance
1.28 The capacity to face or endure events with courage

Questions 1.29–1.32

A. Transference
B. Countertransference
C. Both transference and countertransference

1.29 Can be upsetting and interfere with good medical care
1.30 A patient sees her doctor as overly critical because her mother had always criticized her life choices
1.31 May be encouraged as integral to some intensive psychiatric treatment
1.32 A doctor is hostile to a patient who he assumes will be "difficult" and noncompliant because she reminds him of his ex-wife

ANSWERS

1.1 The answer is D

Transference describes the process of *patients unconsciously projecting feelings from their past relationships to the doctor.* A patient may come to see the doctor as cold, harsh, critical, threatening, seductive, caring, or nurturing, not because of anything the physician says or does, but because that has been the patient's experience in the past. The residue of the experience leads the patient unwittingly to "transfer" the feeling from past relationships to the doctor. The transference can be positive or negative, and it can swing back and forth—sometimes abruptly—between the two. Many a physician has become unsettled when a pleasant, cooperative, and admiring patient suddenly and for no discernible reason becomes enraged and breaks off the relationship or threatens a lawsuit. Physicians are not immune to distorted perceptions of the patient–doctor relationship. When *doctors unconsciously project their feelings to the patient*, the process is called countertransference, not transference.

While physicians can be sued for anything, like any other person, transference feelings are not one of the *main reasons for lawsuits filed by mistreated patients.*

A doctor's level of expertise does not have any effect on whether transference feelings will occur or not.

1.2 The answer is C

Rapport is the spontaneous, conscious *feeling of harmonious responsiveness that promotes the development of a constructive relationship.* It implies an understanding and trust between the doctor and patient. With rapport, patients feel accepted with both their assets and liabilities. Frequently, the doctor is the only person to whom they can talk about things that they cannot tell anyone else. Most patients trust their doctors to keep secrets, and this confidence must not be disobeyed.

Transference describes the process of *patients unconsciously projecting feelings from their past relationships to the doctor.* When *doctors unconsciously project their feelings to the patient*, the process is called countertransference; these feelings are not directly related to rapport.

1.3 The answer is C

An overall figure derived from a number of studies indicates that *54 percent of patients comply with treatment at any given time.* One study found that up to 50 percent of patients with hypertension do not comply at all with treatment and that 50 percent of those who do leave treatment within 1 year.

1.4 The answer is E (all)

The term *illness behavior* describes patients' reactions to the experience of being sick. Aspects of illness behavior have sometimes been termed the *sick role, the role that society ascribes to people when they are ill.* The sick role *can include being excused from responsibilities* and the expectation of wanting to obtain help to get well. *Illness behavior and the sick role* are *affected by people's previous experiences with illness and by their cultural beliefs about disease.* The influence of culture on reporting and manifestation of symptoms must be evaluated. For some disorders this varies little among cultures, whereas for others *the way a person deals with the disorder may strongly shape the way the condition presents itself.* The relation of illness to family processes, class status, and ethnic identity is also important. The attitudes of peoples and cultures about dependency and helplessness greatly influence whether and how a person asks for help, as do such psychological factors as personality type and the personal meaning the person attributes to being ill.

1.5 The answer is E (all)

In thinking about the patient–doctor relationship, it is helpful to formulate models of interaction. In a *paternalistic model* between doctor and patient, it is assumed that the doctor knows best. The doctor prescribes the treatment, and the patient is expected to comply. In this model, the doctor asks most of the questions and generally dominates the interaction. This approach may be of value in an emergency situation, when the doctor needs to take control and make potentially life-saving decisions without long deliberation. In the *deliberative model*, the physician acts as a counselor to the patient, actively advocating a particular course of action. It is used commonly to modify injurious behaviors like trying to get patients to stop smoking or to lose weight. In the *informative model*, the doctor dispenses information. All available data are freely given, but the choice is left wholly up to the patient. This model may be appropriate for certain one-time consultations where the patient will be returning to the regular care of a known physician. The *interpretive model* is used by doctors who have come to know their patients better and understand something of the circumstances of their lives, their families, their values and their hopes and aspirations, and are better able to make recommendations that take into account the unique characteristics of an individual patient.

1.6 The answer is A

Transference describes *the process of patients unconsciously attributing to their doctors aspects of important past relationships*, especially those with their parents. Transference is ubiquitous, and *plays a role in the interaction of all patients with all clinicians.* The *transference can be positive or negative*, and it can swing back and forth between the two. *Transference reactions may be strongest with psychiatrists*, especially when the therapeutic modality used requires the psychiatrist to be more neutral. The more neutral the psychiatrist is, the more transferential fantasies and concerns are mobilized in the patient and transferred onto the doctor. The words and deeds of doctors have powerful effects on their patients because of the unique authority the doctor has, and the patients' dependence on them. How a particular physician behaves and interacts has a direct bearing on the emotional, and even the physical, reactions of the patient.

1.7 The answer is C

A highly significant factor associated with treatment compliance is the patients' *subjective feelings of distress* or illness, as opposed to doctors' often objective medical estimates of the disease and required therapy. Patients who believe they are ill tend toward compliance. Asymptomatic patients, such as those with hypertension, are at greater risk for noncompliance than are patients with symptoms. There is no clear association between compliance and a patient's sex, marital status, race, religion, *socioeconomic status, intelligence*, or *educational level.*

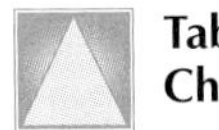

Table 1.1
Checklist for Clinicians

The following checklist allows clinicians to rate their skills in establishing and maintaining rapport. It helps them detect and eliminate weaknesses in interviews that failed in some significant way. Each item is rated "yes," "no." or "not applicable."

	Yes	No	N/A
1. I put the patient at ease.	______	______	______
2. I recognized the patient's state of mind.	______	______	______
3. I addressed the patient's distress.	______	______	______
4. I helped the patient warm up.	______	______	______
5. I helped the patient overcome suspiciousness.	______	______	______
6. I curbed the patient's intrusiveness.	______	______	______
7. I stimulated the patient's verbal production.	______	______	______
8. I curbed the patient's rambling.	______	______	______
9. I understood the patient's suffering.	______	______	______
10. I expressed empathy for the patient's suffering.	______	______	______

1.8 The answer is E (all)

Compliance increases when physicians have a *positive attitude* and are enthusiastic and nonpunitive. *Older doctors with experience*, the amount of time spent talking to patients, *a short waiting room time*, and *increased frequency of visits* are also associated with high compliance rates. The patient–doctor relationship, or match, is one of the most important factors in compliance issues. When a doctor and patient have different priorities and beliefs and different styles of communication (including a different understanding of medical advice and different medical expectations), compliance decreases.

1.9 The answer is E (all)

Establishing rapport is the first step of a psychiatric interview. It encompasses six strategies, as defined by Ekkhard and Sieglinde Othmer: *putting patients at ease*, finding patient's pain and *expressing compassion*, evaluating patient's pain and expressing compassion, *evaluating patient's insight* and becoming an ally, *showing expertise*, establishing authority and balancing the roles of empathic listener, expert, and authority. As part of a strategy for increasing rapport, Othmer and Othmer developed a checklist that enables interviewers to recognize problems and refine their skills in establishing rapport. The first ten questions in the checklist are shown in Table 1.1.

1.10 The answer is E

In *clarification*, doctors attempt to get details from patients about what they have already said. *Confrontation* is meant to point out to a patient something that the doctor thinks the patient is not paying attention to, is missing, or is in some way denying. Confrontation must be done skillfully so that patients are not forced to become hostile and defensive. The confrontation is meant to help patients face whatever needs to be faced in a direct but respectful way. In the technique of *reflection*, a doctor repeats to the patient, in a supportive manner, something that the patient has said. The goal of reflection is twofold: to assure the doctor that he or she has correctly understood what the patient is trying to say and to let the patient know that the doctor perceives what is being said. It is an empathic response meant to let the patient know that the doctor is both listening to the patient's concerns and understanding them. *Silence* may be used to allow patients to contemplate, cry, or just sit in an accepting, supportive environment in which the doctor makes it clear that not every moment must be filled with talk. *Interpretation* is most often used when a doctor states something about a patient's behavior or thinking that the patient may not be aware of. The technique is a sophisticated one and should generally be used only after the doctor has established some rapport with the patient and has a reasonably good idea of what some inter-relationships are.

1.11 The answer is B

The term *illness behavior* describes patients' reactions to the experience of being sick. Aspects of illness behavior have sometimes been termed the *sick role, the role that society ascribes to people when they are ill*. The sick role can include being excused from responsibilities and the expectation of wanting to obtain help to get well. Illness behavior and the sick role are *affected by people's previous experiences with illness* and *by their cultural beliefs about disease*. The influence of culture on reporting and manifestation of symptoms must be evaluated. For some disorders this varies little among cultures, whereas for others the way a person deals with the disorder may strongly shape the way a condition presents itself. The relation of illness to family processes, class status, and ethnic identity is also important. The attitudes of peoples and cultures about dependency and helplessness greatly influence whether and how a person asks for help, as do such *psychological factors as personality type* and the personal meaning the person attributes to being ill. People react to illness in different ways, which depend on their habitual modes of thinking, feeling, and behaving. *Some people experience illness as an overwhelming loss; others see in the same illness a challenge they must overcome or a punishment they deserve*. Mack Lipkin, Jr. created a list of essential areas to be addressed in the assessment of illness behavior, which included questions about *prior illness episodes, especially illnesses of standard severity* (childbirth, renal stones, surgery); cultural degree of stoicism; cultural beliefs concerning the specific problem; personal meaning of or beliefs about the specific problem; and several questions to ask to elicit the patient's explanatory model.

1.12 The answer is D

In a paternalistic, or *autocratic*, patient–doctor relationship, it is assumed that the doctor knows best. He or she will prescribe treatment, and the patient is expected to comply without questioning. Moreover, the doctor may decide to withhold information when it is believed to be in the patient's best interests. In this model, the physician asks most of the questions and generally dominates the interview.

There are circumstances in which an autocratic approach is desirable. In *emergency situations* the doctor needs to take control and make potentially life-saving decisions without long deliberation. In addition, some patients feel overwhelmed by their illness and are comforted by a doctor who can take charge. In general, however, the paternalistic autocratic approach risks a clash of values, especially in situations with many alternatives and potentially life-changing decisions in which the patient must play a role, such as a *life-threatening illness* like cancer, or issues concerning *high-risk conception* or *abortion*. In most instances, illnesses which can be monitored and controlled by the combined efforts of the doctor and patient, such as *hypertension*, should also not be treated autocratically.

1.13 The answer is C

Psychiatric patients must often contend with stresses and pressures that *differ from* those suffered by *patients who do not have a psychiatric disorder*. These stresses include *stigma attached to being a psychiatric patient* (it is more acceptable to have a medical or surgical problem than a mental problem); communication difficulty because of disorders of thinking, and oddities of behavior and impairments of insight and judgment that *might make compliance with treatment difficult*. Because psychiatric patients often find it difficult to describe fully what is going on, physicians must be prepared to obtain information from other sources. *Family members, friends, and spouses can provide critical data* such as past psychiatric history, responses to medication, and precipitating stresses that patients may not be able to describe themselves.

Studies show that 60 percent of all patients with mental disorders visit a nonpsychiatric physician during any 6-month period and that *patients with mental disorders are twice as likely to visit a primary care physician as are other patients*. Nonpsychiatric physicians should be knowledgeable about the special problems of psychiatric patients and the specific techniques used to treat them. One such problem is *compliance* with treatment. In general, *psychiatric patients exhibit a higher degree of noncompliant behavior than do medical patients*. Compliance increases when physicians have such characteristics as enthusiasm and a nonpunitive attitude, and when physicians explain to patients the value of a particular treatment outcome and emphasize that following the recommendation will produce this outcome.

1.14 The answer is D

Before psychiatric clinicians can establish an ongoing relationship with patients, it is *necessary to address certain issues*. For example, they must *openly discuss payment of fees*. Discussing these issues and any other questions about fees from the beginning of the relationship can minimize misunderstanding later. Psychiatrists should also discuss the extent and limitations of *confidentiality* with patients, so that patients are clear about what can and cannot remain confidential. As much as physicians must legally and ethically respect patients' confidentiality, it may be wholly or partially *broken in some specific situations*. For example, if a patient makes clear that he or she intends to harm someone, the doctor has a responsibility to notify the intended victim.

Patients need to be informed about a doctor's *policies for missed appointments*. Some doctors ask patients to give 24 hours' notice to avoid being billed for a missed session. Others bill for missed sessions regardless of advance notification. Still others decide on a case-by-case basis or perhaps state a 24-hour rule but make exceptions when warranted. Some doctors state that if they receive advance notice and can fill the appointment time, they won't charge for missed sessions; others do not charge for missed appointments at all. The choice is up to the individual physician, but patients must know in advance to make an informed decision about whether to accept the doctor's policy or to choose another doctor. Though a clinician may choose to reveal aspects of his or her personal life when appropriate, it is not necessary to the patient–doctor relationship that the patient be *familiar with the doctor's personal life*. Limited, discreet self-disclosure, or self-revelation, by physicians may be useful in certain situations, and physicians should feel at ease and should communicate a sense of self-comfort. Conveying this sense may involve answering a patient's questions about whether a physician is married and where he or she comes from. A doctor who practices self-revelation excessively, however, is using a patient to gratify unfulfilled needs in his or her own life and is abusing the role of the physician. If a doctor feels that a piece of information will help a patient be more comfortable, the doctor can decide in each case whether to be self-revealing. The decision depends on whether the information will further a patient's care or if it will provide nothing useful.

Answers 1.15–1.18

1.15 The answer is A

1.16 The answer is B

1.17 The answer is A

1.18 The answer is A

Interviewing any patient involves a fine balance between allowing the patient's story to unfold at will and obtaining the necessary data for diagnosis and treatment. Most experts on interviewing agree that the ideal interview is one in which an interviewer begins with broad, open-ended questioning, continues by becoming more specific, and closes with detailed direct questioning.

The early part of the interview is generally the most open ended, in that physicians allow patients to speak as much as possible in their own words. A closed-ended, or directive, question is one that asks for specific information and that allows a patient few options in answering. Too many closed-ended questions, especially in the early part of an interview, can lead to a restriction of the patient's responses. Sometimes, directive questions are necessary to obtain important data, but when used too often, a patient may think that information is to be given only in response to direct questioning by the doctor. An example of an open-ended question is, "Can you tell me more about that?" Closed-ended questions, however, can be effective in generating quick responses about a clearly delineated topic. Closed-ended questions have been shown to be useful in eliciting information about the absence of certain symptoms (for example, auditory hallucinations and suicidal ideation). Closed-ended questions have also

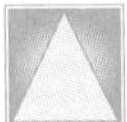

Table 1.2
Pros and Cons of Open-Ended and Closed-Ended Questions

Aspect	Broad, Open-Ended Questions	Narrow, Closed-Ended Questions
Genuineness	High They produce spontaneous formulations.	Low They lead the patient.
Reliability	Low They may lead to nonreproducible answers.	High Narrow focus, but they may suggest answers.
Precision	Low Intent of question is vague.	High Intent of question is clear.
Time efficiency	Low Circumstantial elaborations.	High May invite yes or no answers.
Completeness of diagnostic coverage	Low Patient selects topic.	High Interviewer selects topic.
Acceptance by patient	Varies Most patients prefer expressing themselves freely; others feel guarded and insecure.	Varies Some patients enjoy clear-cut checks; others hate to be pressed into a yes or no format.

Reprinted with permission from Othmer E., Othmer SC. *The Clinical Interview Using DSM-IV.* Washington, DC: American Psychiatric Press; 1994.

been found to be effective in assessing such factors as frequency, severity, and duration of symptoms. With open-ended questions, *the intent is purposefully vague*, the patient is allowed to *select the topic*, and they tend by their nature to be of *lower time efficiency* than closed-ended questions. Table 1.2 summarizes some of the pros and cons of open-ended and closed-ended questions.

Answers 1.19–1.23

1.19 The answer is A

1.20 The answer is C

1.21 The answer is D

1.22 The answer is B

1.23 The answer is B

The patient–doctor relationship has a number of potential models. Often, neither the physician nor the patient is fully conscious of choosing one or another model. The models derive most often from the personalities, expectations, and needs of both the physician and the patient. The fact that their personalities, expectations, and needs are largely unspoken and may differ can lead to miscommunication and disappointment for both participants, physician and patient, in the relationship. The physician must be consciously aware of which model is operating with which patient and should be able to shift models, depending on the particular needs of specific patients and on the treatment requirements of varying clinical situations. Models of the patient–doctor relationship include the active–passive model, the teacher–student (or parent–child or guidance–cooperation) model, the mutual participation model, and the "friendship" (or socially intimate) model.

The *active–passive model* implies passivity on the part of the patient and the taking over by the physician that necessarily results. In this model, patients assume no responsibility for their own care and play no active role in treatment. The model is appropriate when a patient is unconscious, immobilized, or delirious. The sudden onset of the patient's altered mental status can be a potentially life-threatening situation. Possible causes of the profoundly changed mental status are trauma, vascular disorders, brain tumors, meningitis, encephalitis, and toxicological, metabolic, endocrine, and psychiatric disorders. For some patients with an altered mental status, *a lumbar puncture* is necessary and should be performed, as long as increased intracranial pressure, which can cause brainstem herniation, is not suspected. A computed tomographic (CT) scan or an eye examination that checks for papilledema may aid in the assessment before a lumbar puncture is performed.

In the *teacher–student model* the physician's dominance is assumed and emphasized. The physician is paternalistic; the patient is essentially dependent and accepting. The model is often observed *after surgery* and before such diagnostic tests as a *GI series*.

The *mutual participant model* implies equality between the physician and the patient: both participants in the relationship require and depend on each other's input. The need for a patient–doctor relationship based on a model of mutual, active participation is most obvious in the treatment of such chronic illnesses as renal failure and *diabetes*, in which a patient's knowledge and acceptance of treatment is critical to success. The model may also be effective in more subtle situations—for example, in pneumonia.

The *"friendship" model* of the patient–doctor relationship is generally considered dysfunctional, and can lead to unethical behavior. It is most often prompted by an underlying psychological problem in the physician, who may have an emotional need to turn the care of the patient into a relationship of mutual sharing of personal information and *love*. The model often involves a blurring of boundaries between professionalism and intimacy and an indeterminate perpetuation of the relationship, rather than an appropriate ending and termination of treatment.

Answers 1.24–1.28

1.24 The answer is C

1.25 The answer is B

1.26 The answer is D

1.27 The answer is A

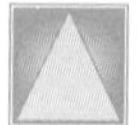

Table 1.3
Character and Qualities of the Physician As Described by William S. Osler, M.D., in *Aequanimitas*

Imperturbability	The ability to maintain extreme calm and steadiness
Presence of mind	Self-control in an emergency or embarrassing situation so that one can say or do the right thing
Clear judgment	The ability to make an informed opinion that is intelligible and free of ambiguity
Ability to endure frustration	The capacity to remain firm and deal with insecurity and dissatisfaction
Infinite patience	The unlimited ability to bear pain or trial calmly
Charity toward others	To be generous and helpful, especially toward the needy and suffering
The search for absolute truth	To investigate facts and pursue reality
Composure	Calmness of mind, bearing, and appearance
Bravery	The capacity to face or endure events with courage
Tenacity	To be persistent in attaining a goal or adhering to something valued
Idealism	Forming standards and ideals and living under their influence
Equanimity	The ability to handle stressful situations with an undisturbed, even temper

1.28 The answer is E

See Table 1.3.

Answers 1.29–1.32

1.29 The answer is C

1.30 The answer is A

1.31 The answer is A

1.32 The answer is B

Doctors and patients may have divergent, distorted, and unrealistic views about each other, about what happens during a clinical encounter, and about what the patient has a right to expect. *Transference* and *countertransference* are terms originating in psychoanalytic theory. They are purely hypothetical constructs, but they have proved extremely useful as organizing principles for explaining certain developments of the patient–doctor relationship that *can be upsetting* and that *can interfere with good medical care.*

Transference describes the process of patients unconsciously attributing to their doctors aspects of important past relationships, *especially those with their parents.* A patient may come to see the doctor as cold, harsh, *critical*, threatening, seductive, caring, or nurturing, not because of anything the physician says or does, but because that has been the patient's experience in the past. The residue of the experience leads the patient to unwittingly "transfer" the feeling from past relationships to the doctor. The transference can be positive or negative, and it can swing back and forth—sometimes abruptly—between the two.

Transference reactions may be strongest with psychiatrists, for a number of reasons. For example, as part of *intensive*, insight-oriented psychotherapy, the *encouragement of transference feelings is an integral part of treatment.* In some types of therapy, a psychiatrist is more or less neutral. The more neutral or less information the patient has about the psychiatrist, the more transferential fantasies and concerns are mobilized and projected onto the doctor. Once the fantasies are stimulated and projected, the psychiatrist can help patients gain insight into how these fantasies and concerns affect all the important relationships in their lives.

Physicians themselves are not immune to distorted perceptions of the patient–doctor relationship. When doctors unconsciously ascribe motives or attributes to patients that come from the *doctor's past relationships*, the process is called *countertransference*. Countertransference may take the form of negative, disruptive feelings, but it may also encompass disproportionately positive, idealizing, or even eroticized reactions. Just as patients have expectations for physicians—for example, competence, objectivity, comfort, and relief—physicians often have unconscious or unspoken expectations of patients. Most commonly patients are thought of as "good" patients if their expressed severity of symptoms correlates with an overtly diagnosable biological disorder, if they are compliant and generally nonchallenging with treatment, if they are emotionally controlled, and if they are grateful. If these expectations are not met, even if this is a result of the unconscious unrealistic needs on the part of the physician, the patient may be blamed and considered unlikable, untreatable, or "difficult."

2

Interviewing Techniques with Special Patient Populations

Different types of patients fall under the rubric of special patient populations. They include patients with urgent issues, the severely mentally ill, patients from different cultural backgrounds, and patients with particular personality problems that make them difficult to engage.

Psychotic patients have poor reality testing and need a focused and structured interview. There are essential techniques to be aware of in the handling of delusions, hallucinations, thought disorders, and suspiciousness. Similarly, potentially suicidal patients need to be assessed in a clear, open way, with a thorough assessment of their suicidal potential.

Somatic patients are often frustrating in light of their resistance to considering a psychological exploration of their symptoms. Seductive patients often require direct responses by the clinician, to maintain boundaries. Dependent patients need firm limit setting, and demanding patients should be treated respectfully, but firmly, with a clear understanding of what will and won't be tolerated in the clinical setting.

Narcissistic patients may initially idealize the doctor and, very soon after, be contemptuous of them. Potentially violent patients need to be assessed in a way that is safe for the patient and the doctor.

Familiarity with these different types of patients and issues will help the treating clinician establish a safe space in which the patient and doctor can work together to treat the problem at hand.

Students should test their knowledge by addressing the following questions and answers.

HELPFUL HINTS

The key terms listed below should be understood by the student.

- agitative patients
- belligerent patients
- boundary violation
- coercion
- close-ended questions
- cross cultural issues
- cultural attitudes
- defensive attitudes
- demanding patients
- dependant patients
- derailments
- emotional reactions
- emotionally charged statements
- "good patients"
- grid iron abdomen
- grievance collector
- help rejecting complainers
- isolated patients
- limit setting
- listening
- malingering
- methods of suicide
- narcissistic patients
- nationality
- noneuphemistic question
- obsessive patients
- open-ended questions
- passive suicidal patients
- personality
- psychological advantage
- psychomotor agitation
- race
- reflection
- religion
- reunion fantasy
- ruminative patients
- secondary gain
- seductive patients
- self-monitoring
- slippery slope
- somatizing patients
- thought disorder
- uncooperative patients
- world of fantasy

QUESTIONS

Directions

Each of the questions or incomplete statements below is followed by five suggested responses or completions. Select the *one* that is *best* in each case.

2.1 The psychiatric interview serves all of the following functions *except*

A. to assess the nature of the problem
B. to demonstrate to the patient their expertise
C. to establish a therapeutic relationship
D. to implement a treatment plan
E. None of the above

2.2 When steering a patient in an interview, which of the following is *not* used?

A. redirection
B. coercion
C. continuation

D. echoing
E. All of the above

2.3 Which of the following is *not* a specific technique used in a psychiatric interview?

A. Privilege
B. Silence
C. Confrontation
D. Transition
E. All of the above

2.4 When ending a psychiatric interview, the doctor should

A. end the interview on time
B. leave unfinished business for the next appointment
C. give the patient the opportunity to ask questions
D. all of the above
E. None of the above

2.5 Confronting a patient with the topic of suicide in a psychiatric interview

A. increases the chances of depressed patients attempting or committing suicide
B. is necessary with all depressed patients
C. hinders the doctor's rapport
D. should not be done in a straightforward manner
E. None of the above

2.6 Choose the answer that best fits the example given in the below case study:
A 45-year-old man was convinced he had acquired immune deficiency syndrome (AIDS), despite having no risk factors. He repeatedly sought out human immunodeficiency virus (HIV) testing and blood cell counts. When tests reported that he was not HIV positive, he felt considerable, but short-lived, relief. He soon began to doubt the accuracy of the tests and reporting. "Can you tell me with certainty, that there is 100 percent no chance of error?" he asked his medical doctor. Over several months, his anxiety and depression increased, and he accepted referral to a psychiatrist.

A. A somatizing patient
B. A depressed patient
C. A noncooperative patient
D. A lying patient
E. None of the above

2.7 Which type of patient would say the following: "I have a friend who is in the business and is great friends with some very famous celebrities. I could introduce you to them . . ."

A. A somatizing patient
B. A seductive patient
C. A noncooperative patient
D. A lying patient
E. None of the above

2.8 With paranoid patients a physician

A. should be as relaxed and friendly as possible
B. should be prepared to explain in detail every decision
C. should not take seriously a patient's hostile or conspiratorial misperception of a neutral event
D. must react defensively to a patient's suspicions
E. should not allow a patient to remain evasive

2.9 Antisocial patients

A. rarely malinger
B. must be approached with a heightened sense of vigilance
C. rarely present as socially adept or intelligent
D. should never be confronted directly about inappropriate behavior
E. seldom cause physicians to feel threatened

2.10 At the beginning of an appointment, a patient wants to discuss her perception of why she felt ill, but the physician wants to know the chronology of her symptoms. The physician should

A. allow the patient to complete her thoughts
B. politely interrupt the patient and continue with closed-ended questions
C. inform her that time is of the essence
D. inform her that an extra charge will be made if more time is needed for the appointment
E. immediately discuss how compliance will be affected by her perceptions and responses

2.11 In the interview of the psychotic patient, which of the following is *true*?

A. Less structure works best.
B. Open-ended questions are most useful.
C. Delusions should be addressed with clear disbelief.
D. Short questions are the easiest for the patient to follow.
E. None of the above.

2.12 Mr. M, a 60-year-old man, 10 months after the death of his wife of 40 years, reluctantly told his daughter that he wished he were dead, but would never act on these wishes. Alarmed, she took him to a psychiatrist for an evaluation. Which of the following is *true*?

A. Asking this man about suicide may increase his risk.
B. Euphemistic inquiries about his suicide risk would foster rapport.
C. Feeling this way is a normal grief reaction, so no action is required.
D. Detailed questions about his suicidality are essential for prevention.
E. His daughter has overreacted in light of the absence of described intent.

2.13 Somatizing patients

A. experience emotional distress in terms of physical symptoms
B. may resist self-reflection
C. often fear that their symptoms are not being taken seriously

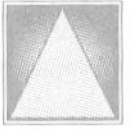

Table 2.1
Three Functions of the Medical Interview

Functions	Objectives	Skills
I. Determining the nature of the problem	1. To enable the clinician to establish a diagnosis or recommend further diagnostic procedures, suggest a course of treatment, and predict the nature of the illness	1. Knowledge base of diseases, disorders, problems, and clinical hypotheses from multiple conceptual domains: biomedical, sociocultural, psychodynamic, and behavioral 2. Ability to elicit data for the above conceptual domains (encouraging the patient to tell his or her story; organizing the flow of the interview, the form of questions, the characterization of symptoms, the mental status examination).
II. Developing and maintaining a therapeutic relationship	1. The patient's willingness to provide diagnostic information 2. Relief of physical and psychological distress 3. Willingness to accept a treatment plan or a process of negotiation	1. Defining the nature of the relationship 2. Allowing the patient to tell his or her story 3. Hearing, bearing, and tolerating the patient's expression of painful feelings 4. Appropriate and genuine interest, empathy, support, and cognitive understanding
III. Communicating information and implementing a treatment plan	1. Patient's understanding of the illness 2. Patient's understanding of the suggested diagnostic procedures 3. Patient's understanding of the treatment possibilities	1. Determining the nature of the problem (function I) 2. Developing a therapeutic relationship (function II) 3. Establishing the differences in perspective between physician and patient

Adapted from Lazare A, Bird J, Lipkin M Jr, Putnam S. Three functions of the medical interview: An integrative conceptual framework. In: Lipkin Jr M, Putnam S, Lazare A, eds. *The Medical Interview*. New York: Springer; 1989:103.

D. are often harmed by aggressive and unwarranted medical interventions
E. all of the above

2.14 Which of the following minimizes agitation and the risk of harm by potentially violent patients?

A. Evaluating the patient in a nonstimulating environment
B. Asking the patient if he is carrying a weapon
C. Heeding one's subjective sense of fear
D. Terminating the interview if necessary
E. All of the above

ANSWERS

2.1 The answer is B

Three functions of medical interviews are: to *assess the nature of the problem, to develop and maintain a therapeutic relationship*, and *to communicate information* and implement a treatment plan. See Table 2.1. While showing expertise may be a good way to establish rapport, it is *not* a function of psychiatric interview.

2.2 The answer is B

During the interview, the doctor may steer the flow of information. *Continuation*, *echoing*, and *redirection* are three ways to steer in an interview.

With *continuation*, the interviewer tends to the patient's talk by raising eyebrows or uttering *hmms* to signal the patient nonverbally to continue. He or she may use short tracking phrases, such as "And?" "Then what?" or "How is that?", if his or her nonverbal signals get ignored. The interviewer may also use phrases, such as "That's interesting" or "Really?", to encourage the patient to continue.

With *echoing*, the interviewer may echo a part of what the patient has said. He or she may intent to prod the patient to continue or shift the emphasis.

Redirection may be used to steer a patient if the patient introduces a new productive topic. The interviewer follows the new lead and may delay the transition: "What you are saying is very important. We will come back to this topic. But before we do, let's finish up on . . . (old topic)."

Coercion is defined as the act of forcing a person to act or think in a certain way by use of pressure, threats, or intimidation. This is *not* one of the ways in which to steer a patient.

2.3 The answer is A

There are several specific techniques that are used in a psychiatric interview, they include: *silence, confrontation and transition*.

The technique of *silence* can be used in many ways in normal conversations, even to indicate disapproval or disinterest. In the patient–doctor relationship, however, silence may be constructive and in certain situations may allow patients to contemplate, to cry, or just to sit in an accepting, supportive environment in which the doctor makes it clear that not every moment must be filled with talk.

The technique of *confrontation* is used to point out to a patient something that the doctor thinks the patient is not paying attention to, is missing, or is in some way denying. Confrontation must be done skillfully so that patients are not forced to become hostile and defensive. The confrontation is meant to help patients face whatever needs to be faced in a direct but respectful way. For example, a patient who has just made a suicidal gesture but is telling the doctor that it was not serious may be confronted with the statement, "What you have done may not have killed you, but it's telling me that you are in serious trouble right now and that you need help so that you don't try suicide again."

The technique of *transition* allows doctors to convey the idea that enough information has been obtained on one subject; the doctor's words encourage patients to continue on to another subject. For example, a doctor may say, "You've given me a good sense of that particular time in your life. Perhaps now you could tell me a bit more about an even earlier time in your life."

Privilege is not an interviewing technique. Privilege is the right to maintain secrecy or confidentiality in the face of a subpoena. Privileged communications are statements made by certain persons within a relationship—such as husband–wife, priest–penitent, or patient–doctor—that the law protects from forced disclosure on the witness stand. The right of privilege belongs to the patient, not to the physician, and so the patient can waive the right.

2.4 The answer is C

Physicians want patients to leave an interview feeling understood and respected and believing that all the pertinent and important information has been conveyed to an informed, empathic listener. To this end, *doctors should give patients a chance to ask questions* and should let patients know as much as possible about future plans. Doctors should thank patients for sharing the necessary information and let patients know that the information conveyed has been helpful in clarifying the next steps. Any prescription of medication should be spelled out clearly and simply, and doctors should ascertain whether patients understand the prescription and how to take it. *It is not as imperative to end a session on time,* as it is to ascertain the patient understands prescriptions and future plans. If a doctor has *unfinished business* such as explaining medications and its effects to the patient, this *should not be left until the next session.* Doctors should make another appointment or give a referral and some indication about how patients can reach help quickly if it is necessary before the next appointment.

2.5 The answer is B

All patients must be asked about suicidal thoughts; however, depressed patients may need to be questioned more fully. A thorough assessment of suicide potential addresses intent, plans, means, and perceived consequences, as well as history of attempts and family history of suicide. Many patients mention their thoughts of suicide spontaneously. If not, the examiner can begin with a somewhat general question, such as "Do you ever have thoughts of hurting yourself?" or "Does it ever seem that life isn't worth living?" These questions can then be followed up with more specific questions. The examiner must feel comfortable enough to ask simple *straightforward,* noneuphemistic questions. *Asking about suicide does not increase the risk.* The psychiatrist is not raising a topic that the patient has not already contemplated. Specific, detailed questions are essential for prevention. Confronting a patient with the topic of suicide *does not hinder the psychiatrist's rapport.*

2.6 The answer is A

Some patients experience and describe emotional distress in terms of physical symptoms. *This is certainly true for the group of somatoform disorders.* Many somatizing patients live with the fear that their symptoms are not taken seriously and the parallel fear that something medically serious may be overlooked. Psychiatrists' main task in dealing with these patients is to acknowledge the suffering conveyed by the symptoms without necessarily accepting that patient's explanation for the symptoms. It is essential that somatizing patients feel that their physical complaints are not being dismissed. An important goal of treatment is to minimize the harm caused by aggressive and unwarranted medical interventions. These patients often do better with frequent, short medical consultations that are scheduled in advance, rather than urgent visits prompted by new symptoms.

2.7 The answer is B

Sex is not the only enticement with which psychiatrists can be seduced. Patients may offer insider information for profitable trading in the stock market, *may promise an introduction to a movie star friend,* or may suggest that they will dedicate their next novel to the psychiatrist. Although it is easy to understand that some offers by patients, such as the possibility of a sexual involvement, cannot be accepted without considerable harm to the patient, others may seem more innocuous. However, because they nearly always introduce a different agenda into the therapy than that originally contracted for, and because they create additional, more ambiguous levels of obligation between therapist and patient, any psychiatric work is inevitably contaminated, and the ability to help the patient is compromised. Consequently, gaining any material or social benefit from the patient other than the agreed-on fee is unethical.

2.8 The answer is B

Paranoid patients fear that people want to hurt them and intend to do them harm. Doctors *should be able to explain in detail every decision* and planned procedure to paranoid patients and should react nondefensively to patients' suspicions. Patients may misperceive cues in their environment to the degree that they see *conspiracies in neutral events.* They are critical, *evasive,* and suspicious. They are often called grievance seekers because they tend to blame others for everything bad that happens in their lives. They are extremely mistrustful and may question everything that doctors advise doing. Physicians must remain somewhat formal, albeit always respectful and courteous, with these patients, as they often view expressions of warmth and empathy with suspicion ("What does he want from me?").

2.9 The answer is B

Doctors must treat antisocial patients with respect but also *with a heightened sense of vigilance.* These patients can inspire fear in others, often legitimately so, as many have violent histories. Doctors who *feel threatened by patients* should unashamedly seek assistance and not feel compelled to see the patients alone. Firm limits must be set on behavior (for example, no drugs in the hospital and no sexual activity with other patients), and the consequences of transgressing must be stated firmly and adhered to (for example, discharge from the hospital if the patient is medically stable, isolation if not). If inappropriate behavior is discovered, patients *must be confronted directly* and nonangrily, and they must be held responsible for their actions. On the surface these patients may appear charming, socially adept, and intelligent, because over many years they have perfected the behaviors they know to be appropriate, and they perform almost as actors. *Antisocial patients often malinger*, the term for willfully feigning illness for a clear secondary gain (for example, to obtain drugs, get a bed for the night, or hide from people pursuing them). They obviously get sick, as nonantisocial people do, and when they are sick they need to be cared for in the same ways as others.

2.10 The answer is A

The early part of the interview is generally the most open ended, in that the physician allows patients to speak as much as possible in their own words by asking open-ended questions and also permits them to *finish*. An example of an open-ended question is, "Can you tell me more about that?" That type of questioning is important to establish rapport, which is the first step in an interview. In one survey of 700 patients, the patients substantially agreed that physicians do not have the time or the inclination to listen and to consider the patient's feelings, that physicians do not have enough knowledge of the emotional problems and socioeconomic background of the patient's family, and that physicians increase the patient's fear by giving explanations in technical language. Psychosocial and economic factors exert a profound influence on human relationships, so the physician should have as much understanding as possible of the patient's environment and subculture.

As for *time* and *charges*, physicians should inform patients about their fee policies but should not interrupt patients to do so. Instead, those areas of business should be dealt with before the initial visit, so that an ongoing relationship with a patient can be established. The matter of fees must be discussed openly from the outset: the physician's charges, whether the physician is willing to accept insurance payments directly (known as assignments), the policy concerning payment for missed appointments, and whether the physician is part of a managed care plan. Discussing those questions and any other questions about fees at the beginning of the relationship can minimize misunderstandings later.

A discussion of compliance with a medical plan is important, but premature early in the interview. Furthermore, *compliance*, which is the degree to which the patient carries out clinical recommendations by the treating physician, is a two-way street. Studies have shown that noncompliance is associated with physicians perceived as rejecting and unfriendly. Noncompliance is also associated with asking a patient for information without giving any feedback and with failing to explain a diagnosis or the cause of the presenting symptoms. A physician who is aware of the patient's belief system, feelings, and habits and who enlists the patient in establishing a treatment regimen increases compliant behavior.

2.11 The answer is D

Psychotic patients have poor or absent reality testing. Therefore, the evaluation of a patient with psychotic symptoms *needs to be more focused and structured* than that of other patients. *Open-ended questions* and long periods of silence may be disorganizing. *Short questions are easier to follow than long ones.* Delusional patients often come to psychiatric evaluation having had their beliefs dismissed or belittled by friends and family. They are on guard for similar reactions from the examiner. In asking questions about delusions, the doctor *should not reveal their disbelief*; this only hurts the treatment alliance and hampers any rapport being formed with the patient.

2.12 The answer is D

A thorough assessment of suicide potential addresses intent, plans, means, and perceived consequences, as well as a history of attempts and family history of suicide. The examiner must ask clear, straightforward, *noneuphemistic questions. Asking about suicide does not increase risk*; the psychiatrist is not raising a topic that the patient has not already contemplated. Some patients may report a wish that they were dead, but would never intentionally do anything to take their own lives. Others express greater degrees of determination. Either way, any expression of a wish to die should be considered and evaluated seriously. It should *never be considered lightly or as a part of a "normal" grief reaction*. There are some patients who tell no one of their suicide plans and proceed in a deliberate, systematic manner. The *daughter did not overreact* since her father suffered a loss and suicidal statements need to be taken seriously.

2.13 The answer is E (all)

Somatizers *experience and describe emotional distress in terms of physical symptoms*. They pose a number of difficulties for the psychiatrist because they may be *reluctant to engage in self-reflection* and psychological exploration. They live with the fear that their *symptoms are not being taken seriously* and the parallel fear that something medically serious may be overlooked. An important goal of treatment is to minimize *the harm caused by aggressive and unwarranted medical interventions*.

2.14 The answer is E (all)

Most unpremeditated violence is preceded by a prodrome of accelerating psychomotor agitation. Several steps can be taken to minimize the agitation and potential risk. The interview should be conducted in a *quiet, nonstimulating environment*. The psychiatrist should avoid any behavior that could be misconstrued as menacing, like standing over the patient, staring, or touching. The psychiatrist should *ask whether the patient is carrying any weapons* and may ask the patient to leave the weapon with a guard or in a holding area. If the agitation continues to increase, *the psychiatrist may need to terminate the interview*. The physician should *always heed his or her own sense of comfort or fear*.

3 Normality

Normality and mental health are central issues in psychiatric theory and practice but are difficult to define. For example, normality has been defined as patterns of behavior or personality traits that are typical or that conform to some standard of proper and acceptable ways of behaving and being. The use of terms such as typical or acceptable, however, has been criticized because they are ambiguous, involve value judgments, and vary from one culture to another. To overcome this objection psychiatrist and historian George Mora devised a system to describe behavioral manifestations that are normal in one context but not in another, depending on how the person is viewed by the society. This paradigm, however, may give too much weight to peer group observations and judgments. The World Health Organization (WHO) defines normality as a state of complete physical, mental, and social well-being; but again, this definition is limited, because it defines physical and mental health simply as the absence of physical or mental disease.

The text revision of the fourth edition of *Diagnostic and Statistical Manual of Mental Disorders* (DSM-IV-TR) offers no definition of normality or mental health, although a definition of mental disorder is presented. According to DSM-IV-TR, a mental disorder is conceptualized as a behavioral or psychological syndrome or pattern that is associated with distress (e.g., a painful symptom) or disability (i.e., impairment in one or more important areas of functioning). In addition, the syndrome or pattern must not be merely an expected and culturally sanctioned response to a particular event, such as the death of a loved one. DSM-IV-TR emphasizes that neither deviant behavior (e.g., political, religious, or sexual) nor conflicts that are primarily between the individual and society are mental disorders.

Students should test their knowledge by addressing the following questions and answers.

HELPFUL HINTS

The student should know the following theories, theorists and terms.

- autonomy versus shame and doubt
- conflict-free ego functions
- ego identity versus role confusion
- ego integrity versus despair
- ego mechanisms
- Erik Erikson
- Karl Jaspers
- Carl Gustav Jung
- Theodore Lidz
- life cycle theory
- generativity versus stagnation
- George Mora
- industry versus inferiority
- initiative versus guilt
- intimacy versus isolation
- mature defenses
- normality as utopia
- normality as average
- normality as process
- normality as health
- Jean Piaget
- *Three Essays on the Theory of Sexuality*
- trust versus mistrust

QUESTIONS

Directions

Each of the questions or incomplete statements below is followed by five suggested responses or completions. Select the *one* that is *best* in each case.

3.1 According to Dr. George Mora, a heteronormal person is

A. seen as abnormal by his or her own society
B. seen as unusual by members of another society
C. seen as normal by members of another society
D. seen as normal by his or her own society
E. None of the above

3.2 Which of the following is not a healthy defense mechanism?

A. Humor
B. Suppression
C. Sublimation
D. Altruism
E. Denial

3.3 Autonomous functions of the ego include

A. perception
B. intuition
C. comprehension

D. language
E. all of the above

3.4 According to Karl Jaspers, the personal world is abnormal when

A. it separates the person from others emotionally
B. the person cannot live without fear, guilt, or anxiety
C. the person cannot adjust to the external world with contentment
D. the person does not have the ability to achieve insight into one's self
E. all of the above

3.5 According to Theodore Lidz, which of the following is *true*?

A. The acquisition of many abilities must wait for the physical maturation of the organism.
B. Cognitive development plays a significant role in creating phasic shifts.
C. Society establishes roles and sets expectation for persons of different ages and statuses.
D. Children attain many attributes and capacities for directing the self and controlling impulses.
E. All of the above

Directions

Each set of lettered headings below is followed by a list of numbered words or statements. For each numbered word or statement, select the *one* lettered heading most closely associated with it. Each lettered heading may be selected once, more than once, or not at all.

Questions 3.6–3.9

A. Normality as process
B. Normality as health
C. Normality as average
D. Normality as utopia

3.6 Traditional approach
3.7 Harmonious and optimal functioning
3.8 Based on bell-shaped curve
3.9 The end result of interacting systems

Questions 3.10–3.14

A. Sigmund Freud
B. Kurt Eissler
C. Melanie Klein
D. Erik Erikson
E. Laurence Kubie

3.10 Absolute normality cannot be obtained because the normal person must be totally aware of his or her thoughts and feelings.
3.11 Normality is the ability to master the periods of life: trust vs. mistrust; autonomy vs. shame and doubt; initiative vs. guilt; industry vs. inferiority; identity vs. role confusion; intimacy vs. isolation; generativity vs. stagnation; and ego integrity vs. despair.
3.12 Normality is an idealized fiction.
3.13 Normality is characterized by strength of character, the capacity to deal with conflicting emotions, the ability to experience pleasure without conflict and the ability to love.
3.14 Normality is the ability to learn by experience, to be flexible, and to adapt to a changing environment.

ANSWERS

3.1 The answer is D

Normality and mental health are central issues in psychiatric theory and practice but are difficult to define. For example, *normality* has been defined as patterns of behavior or personality traits that are typical or that conform to some standard of proper and acceptable ways of behaving and being. The use of terms such as *typical* or *acceptable*, however, has been criticized because they are ambiguous, involve value judgments, and vary from one culture to another. To overcome this objection psychiatrists and historians devised a system to describe *behavioral manifestations that are normal in one context but not in another, depending on how the person is viewed by the society* (Table 3.1).

3.2 The answer is E

Denial is not a healthy defense mechanism because it prevents the person from becoming aware of either internal or external reality.

Humor, sublimation, suppression and altruism are all healthy defense mechanisms.

Humor is a defense mechanism that allows the overt expression of feelings and thoughts without personal discomfort or immobilization and does not produce an unpleasant effect on others. Humor allows the individual to tolerate and yet focus on what is too terrible to be borne. It differs from wit, a form of displacement that involves distraction from the affective issue.

Sublimation is an unconscious defense mechanism in which the energy associated with unacceptable impulses or drives is diverted into personally and socially acceptable channels. Unlike other defense mechanisms, sublimation offers some minimal gratification of the instinctual drive or impulse.

Suppression is the conscious act of controlling and inhibiting an unacceptable impulse, emotion or idea. Suppression is

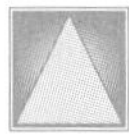

Table 3.1
Normality in Context

Term	Concept
Autonormal	Person seen as normal by his or her own society
Autopathological	Person seen as abnormal by his or her own society
Heteronormal	Person seen as normal by members of another society observing him or her
Heteropathological	Person seen as unusual or pathological by members of another society observing him or her

Data from George Mora, M.D.

differentiated from repression in that repression is an unconscious process.

Altruism involves getting pleasure from giving to others what an individual himself or herself would have liked to receive. It is closely linked with ethics and morals; Freud recognized altruism as the only basis for the development of community interest.

3.3 The answer is E (all)

The psychoanalyst Heinz Hartmann conceptualized normality by describing the "autonomous functions of the ego." These psychological capacities present at birth are conflict free, that is, uninfluenced by the internal psychic world. They include *perception, intuition, comprehension, thinking, language*, certain aspects of motor development, learning, and intelligence. The concept of autonomous and conflict-free functions of the ego helps explain the mechanisms whereby some persons lead relatively normal lives in the presence of extraordinary external experiential traumas—the so-called invulnerable child, that is, a child who is invulnerable to the "slings and arrows of outrageous fortune" by virtue of autonomous ego strengths.

3.4 The answer is A

Karl Jaspers (1883–1969), the German psychiatric and philosopher, described a "personal world"—the way a person thinks or feels—that could be normal or abnormal. According to Jaspers, the personal world is abnormal when it (1) springs from a condition that is recognized universally as abnormal, such as schizophrenia, (2) *when it separates the person from others emotionally*, and (3) when it does not provide the person with a sense of "spiritual and material" security.

According to Otto Rank, normality is the capacity *to live without fear, guilt, or anxiety* and to take responsibility for one's own actions.

According to Karl Menninger, normality is the ability to *adjust to the external world with contentment* and to master the task of acculturation.

According to R.E. Money-Kryle, normality is the *ability to achieve insight into one's self*, an ability that is never fully accomplished.

3.5 The answer is E (all)

Theodore Lidz, a major exponent of life cycle theory describes several factors that account for the phasic nature of the life cycle.

1. *The acquisition of many abilities must wait for the physical maturation of the organism.* For example, the infant cannot become a toddler until the pyramidal nerve tracts that permit voluntary discrete movements of the lower limbs become functional. Then, after such maturation occurs, it takes considerable practice to gain the skills needed to master a function, but the function becomes amenable to training and education. Adequate mastery of simple skills must precede their incorporation into more complex activities. In a somewhat different way, shifts in the physiological equilibrium can initiate a new phase in the life cycle, as when the new inner forces that come with puberty require changes in personality functioning, whatever the preparation in prior phases of childhood.

2. *Cognitive development plays a significant role in creating phasic shifts.* The ability to communicate needs and desires verbally and to understand what parents say is a major factor in ending the period of infancy, and children's ability to attend school depends to a great extent on their gaining the ability to form concrete categories at the age of 5 or 6. Cognitive development does not progress at an even pace, because qualitatively different capacities emerge in rather discrete stages.

3. *Society establishes roles and sets of expectation for persons of different age and statuses.* At age 5 or 6, a child becomes a schoolchild with new demands and opportunities. As adults, interpersonal relationships such as marriage require that the person attend to the needs of the other.

4. *Children attain many attributes and capacities for directing the self and controlling impulses* by internalizing parental characteristics to gradually overcome the need for surrogate egos to direct their lives and provide security. Such internalizations take place in stages in relation to the child's physical, intellectual, and emotional development.

5. Finally, time itself is a determinant of phasic changes not only because of the need to move into age-appropriate roles but because changes in physical make-up at puberty and old age require changes in self-concepts and attitudes. Awareness of the passage of time also fosters entry into new stages of life, as when personas realize that more time lies behind than ahead of them as they enter late middle age.

Answers 3.6–3.9

3.6 The answer is B

3.7 The answer is D

3.8 The answer is C

3.9 The answer is A

The normality as health perspective is the traditional medical psychiatric approach to health and illness. Most physicians equate normality with health and view health as an almost universal phenomenon. As a result, behavior is assumed to be within normal limits when no manifest psychopathology is present. If all behavior were to be put on a scale, normality would encompass the major portion of the continuum, and abnormality would be the small remainder.

The normality as utopia perspective conceives of normality as that harmonious and optimal blending of the diverse elements of the mental apparatus that culminates in optimal functioning. Such a definition emerges when psychiatrists or psychoanalysts talk about the ideal person, when they grapple with a complex problem, or when they discuss their criteria for a successful treatment. This approach can be traced back to Sigmund Freud, who when discussing normality stated, "A normal ego is like normality in general, an ideal fiction."

The normality as average perspective is commonly used in normative studies of behavior and is based on a mathematical principle of the bell-shaped curve. This approach considers the middle range normal and both extremes deviant. The normative approach based on this statistical principal describes each individual in terms of general assessment and total score. Variability

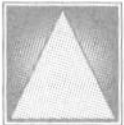

Table 3.2
Psychoanalytic Concepts of Normality

Theorist	Concept
Sigmund Freud	Normality is an idealized fiction
Kurt Eissler	Absolute normality cannot be obtained because the normal person must be totally aware of his or her thoughts and feelings
Melanie Klein	Normality is characterized by strength of character, the capacity to deal with conflicting emotions, the ability to experience pleasure without conflict, and the ability to love
Erik Erikson	Normality is the ability to master the periods of life: trust vs. mistrust; autonomy vs. shame and doubt; initiative vs. guilt; industry vs. inferiority; identity vs. role confusion; intimacy vs. isolation; generativity vs. stagnation; and ego integrity vs. despair
Laurence Kubie	Normality is the ability to learn by experience to be flexible, and to adapt to a changing environment

is described only within the context of groups, not within the context of the individual.

The normality as process perspective stresses that normal behavior is the end result of interacting systems. Based on this definition, temporal changes are essential to a complete definition of normality. In other words, the normality-as-process perspective stresses changes or processes rather than a cross-sectional definition of normality.

Answers 3.10–3.14

3.10 The answer is B

3.11 The answer is D

3.12 The answer is A

3.13 The answer is C

3.14 The answer is E
See Table 3.2.

4 Human Development

The life cycle represents the stages through which all humans pass from birth to death. The fundamental assumption of all life cycle theories is that development occurs in successive, clearly defined stages. This sequence is invariant; that is, it occurs in a particular order in every person's life, whether or not all stages are completed. A second assumption of life cycle theory is the epigenetic principle, which maintains that each stage is characterized by events or crises that must be resolved satisfactorily for development to proceed smoothly. According to the epigenetic model, if resolution is not achieved within a given life period, all subsequent stages reflect that failure in the form of physical, cognitive, social, or emotional maladjustment. A third assumption is that each phase of the life cycle contains a dominant feature, complex of features, or a crisis point that distinguishes it from phases that either preceded or will follow it.

Charting of the life cycle lies within the study of developmental psychology and involves such diverse elements as biological maturity, psychological capacity, adaptive techniques, defense mechanisms, symptom complexes, role demands, social behavior, cognition, perception, language development, and interpersonal relationships. Various models of the life cycle describe the major developmental phases but emphasize different elements. Taken together however, they demonstrate that there is an order to human life, despite the fact that each person is unique.

Jean Piaget studied the cognitive and intellectual development of children, from birth to adolescence. Not all contemporary theorists agree with his findings or observations, but his work is evocative and seminal, and offers a striking theory of cognitive development through different ages. Sigmund Freud's observations and theories about psychosexual development are provocative and challenging. No one can argue with the profound and lasting effect his thinking had on 20th-century culture nor on the increased understanding of psychodynamic forces that shape behavior. A new psychology is evolving for the current century that will rely on many of Freud's observations but which will differ in concepts still to be defined.

Erik Erikson formulated age-specific crises that he observed to occur in correlation with specific psychosocial phases. Margaret Mahler viewed development through a perspective of attachment, and defined what she felt was the challenge of the first 3 years of life, in terms of separation-individuation. More recent theorists, such as Daniel Levinson and Carol Gilligan, have continued to expand and clarify different aspects of development and life stresses.

The student should study the questions and answers below for a useful review of all of these topics.

HELPFUL HINTS

Readers should be aware of the following theories, theorists, and developmental stages as they relate to human development throughout the life cycle.

- adolescent homosexuality
- adoption
- adultery
- affectional bond
- age-30 transition
- age-related cell changes
- ageism
- Mary Ainsworth
- alimony
- anal personality
- attachment
- autonomous ego functions
- John Bowlby's stages of bereavement
- castration anxiety
- characteristics of thought:
  - concrete operations
  - formal operations
  - preoperational phase
  - sensorimotor phase (object permanence)
- climacterium
- cognitive decline
- concepts of normality
- core identity
- crushes
- cults
- death and children
- death criteria
- delayed, inhibited, and denied grief
- dependence
- developmental landmarks
- developmental tasks
- divorce
- dreams in children
- dual-career families
- effects of divorce
- egocentrism
- Electra complex
- empty-nest syndrome
- epigenetic principle
- Erik Erikson:
  - eight psychosocial stages
- failure to thrive
- family planning
- family size
- fathers and attachment
- feeding and infant care
- fetal development
- formal operations and morality
- foster parents
- Anna Freud
- gender expectations

- gender identity
- generativity
- genetic counseling
- geriatric period
- Arnold Gesell
- goodness of fit
- grief
- Roy Grinker
- Heinz Hartmann
- hormones
- integrity
- intimacy
- Carl Jung
- Melanie Klein
- Elisabeth Kübler-Ross
- language development
- learning problems
- Daniel Levinson
- linkage objects
- Madonna complex
- Margaret Mahler:
  - infant-developmental stages
- marriage
- Masters and Johnson
- masturbation
- maternal behavior
- maternal neglect
- menarche
- midlife crisis
- mourning
- "Mourning and Melancholia"
- mutuality
- negativism
- neural organization of infancy
- normal autistic and normal symbiotic phases
- play and pretend
- postpartum mood disorders and psychosis
- pregnancy:
  - marriage and alternative lifestyle
  - sexuality and prenatal diagnosis
  - teenage
- pregnancy and childbirth
- primary and secondary sex characteristics
- pseudodementia
- psychosexual moratorium
- puberty
- racism, prejudice
- reactions to authority
- reflexes (i.e., rooting, grasp, Babinski, Moro)
- religious behavior
- remarriage
- retirement
- Dame Cicely Saunders
- school adjustment, behavior, refusal
- self-blame
- senility
- separation
- separation-individuation process:
  - differentiation
  - practicing
  - rapprochement
  - consolidation
- sex in the aged
- sibling and parental death
- sibling rivalry
- single-parent home
- smiling
- social deprivation syndromes (anaclitic depression-hospitalism)
- somnambulism
- spacing of children
- René Spitz
- spouse and child abuse
- stepparents and siblings
- stranger and separation anxiety
- stress reaction
- suicide in the aged
- Harry Stack Sullivan
- superego
- surrogate mother
- survivor guilt
- Thomas Szasz
- temperament
- thanatology
- toilet training
- uncomplicated bereavement

QUESTIONS

Directions

Each of the questions or incomplete statements below is followed by five suggested responses or completions. Select the *one* that is *best* in each case.

4.1 Pruning refers to

A. excitotoxicity
B. the addition of cells to the nervous system during development
C. the process of eliminating the branching of dendrites of the brain
D. the programmed elimination of neurons, synapses and axons
E. all of the above

4.2 Which percentage of women uses alcohol during pregnancy?

A. 10 percent
B. 20 percent
C. 35 percent
D. 45 percent
E. 60 percent

4.3 Which of the following is *not* a characteristic of fetal alcohol syndrome?

A. Microphthalmia
B. CNS manifestations
C. Hyperactivity
D. Attention deficits
E. Withdrawal-like symptoms

4.4 In which period is the "band-aid phase" present?

A. Toddler period
B. Preschool period
C. Infancy period
D. Middle years period
E. None of the above

4.5 Which percentage of teenagers ages 15 to 19 use at least one method of birth control?

A. 25 percent
B. 50 percent
C. 65 percent
D. 75 percent
E. 95 percent

4.6 Children born to teenage mothers have a greater chance of

A. becoming teenage parents
B. joining a gang
C. dying before the age of five
D. becoming addicted to a narcotic
E. all of the above

4.7 The psychological separation from parents in adolescence is called

A. first individuation
B. second individuation
C. third individuation
D. fourth individuation
E. none of the above

4.8 The transition from adolescence to young adulthood is characterized by

A. the establishment of an adult work identity
B. the need for an intimate relationship
C. separation from family
D. achievement of mental maturity
E. none of the above

4.9 Which of the following is *true* about Piaget's approach to cognitive development?

A. Cognitive growth occurs in invariant stages.
B. The sensorimotor stage is from ages 2 years to 7 years.
C. Object constancy is the ability to remember an object once it is out of sight.
D. Preoperational thought is nonsymbolic.
E. Concrete operational thought is illogical.

4.10 Which of the following is a factor to be considered in adolescent misuse or rejection of contraceptives?

A. The belief that it interferes with pleasure
B. Lack of education from schools
C. Self-consciousness about use
D. Access to and/or cost of contraceptives
E. All of the above

4.11 Which of the following medical interventions requires parental consent for adolescents under the age of 16?

A. Alcohol counseling
B. Treatment for a sexually transmitted disease
C. Inpatient mental health treatment
D. Birth control pills or other contraception
E. Treatment for an AIDS-related illness

4.12 Compared to nonadopted children, adopted children are more likely to have:

A. problems with drug abuse
B. aggressive behavior
C. learning disturbances
D. conduct disorders
E. all of the above

4.13 According to Robert Butler, the themes of stock taking; reassessing commitments to family, work, and marriage; and dealing with parental illness and death are most common in which stage of life?

A. Adolescence
B. Young adulthood
C. Old age
D. Middle adulthood
E. All of the above

4.14 Which of the following is *not* one of the basic personality traits found to remain relatively stable throughout life?

A. Openness to experience
B. Confidence
C. Conscientiousness
D. Neuroticism
E. Extraversion

4.15 Positive physiological effects of exercise and nutrition in old age include:

A. increased heart volume and weight
B. increased muscle mass and body density
C. decreased heart rate at rest
D. decreased systolic blood pressure
E. all of the above

4.16 In an infant, social smiling is elicited preferentially by the mother at

A. under 4 weeks of age
B. 4 to 8 weeks
C. 8 to 12 weeks
D. 3 to 4 months
E. more than 4 months

4.17 A child will refer to him or herself by name at which age?

A. 18 months
B. 2 years
C. 3 years
D. 4 years
E. 6 years

Directions

Each set of lettered headings below is followed by a list of numbered words or statements. For each numbered word or statement, select the *one* lettered heading most closely associated with it. Each lettered heading may be selected once, more than once, or not at all.

Questions 4.18–4.21

A. Testosterone
B. Estrogen
C. Both
D. Neither

4.18 Low levels may be associated with depressed mood
4.19 Influence CNS functioning
4.20 Responsible for masculinization of males
4.21 Levels correlate with libido and are manifested by sex drive

Questions 4.22–4.26

A. 2 months
B. 6 months
C. 1.5 to 2.5 years
D. 3 to 5 years
E. 5 years

4.22 End of baby talk
4.23 Cooing
4.24 Subtleties of tone and inflection
4.25 Babbling
4.26 First sentence

Questions 4.27–4.29

A. Pre-conventional morality
B. Conventional role-conformity
C. Self-accepted principles

4.27 Children try to conform to gain approval
4.28 Punishment and obedience to the parent are determining factors
4.29 Children comply with rules on the basis of a concept of ethical principles

Questions 4.30–4.33

A. Marriage counseling
B. Marital therapy
C. Both marriage counseling and marital therapy

4.30 Only discusses a particular conflict related to the immediate concerns of the family
4.31 Emphasizes helping partners cope with their problems effectively
4.32 Places emphasis on restructuring the interaction between the couple
4.33 Encourages personality growth and development

Questions 4.34–4.38

A. Sigmund Freud
B. Erik Erikson
C. Heinz Kohut
D. Bernice Neugarten
E. Daniel Levinson

4.34 Old age is a time of reconciliation with others and resolution of grief over the death of others and the approaching death of self.
4.35 The maintenance of self-esteem is a major task of old age.
4.36 People who are narcissistic and too heavily invested in body appearance are liable to become preoccupied with death.
4.37 Increased control of the ego and id with aging results in increased autonomy.
4.38 The major conflict of old age relates to giving up the position of authority and evaluating achievements and former competence.

Questions 4.39–4.43

A. Grief/bereavement
B. Depression
C. Both grief and depression

4.39 Loss of appetite
4.40 Clinically significant distress or impairment
4.41 Dysphoria triggered by reminders of the deceased
4.42 Rarely includes suicidal ideation
4.43 Diminished interest in the world

ANSWERS

4.1 The answer is D

Pruning refers to *the programmed elimination during development of neurons, synapses, axons* and other brain structures from the original number, present at birth, to a lesser number. Thus, the developing brain contains structures and cellular elements that are absent in the older brain. The fetal brain generates more neurons than it will need for adult life. For example, in the visual cortex neurons increase from birth to 3 years of age at which point they diminish in number. Another example is that the adult brain contains a lesser number of neural connections than were present during the early and middle years of childhood. Approximately twice as many synapses are present in certain parts of the cerebral cortex during early postnatal life than during adulthood. Pruning occurs to rid the nervous system of cells that have served their function in the development of the brain. Some neurons, for example, exist to produce neurotrophic or growth factors and are then programmed to die—a process called apoptosis—when that function is fulfilled.

The developing white matter of the human brain prior to 32 weeks gestation is especially sensitive to damage from hypoxic and ischemic injury and metabolic insults. Neurotransmitter receptors located on synaptic terminals are subject to injury from excessive stimulation by excitatory amino acids (e.g., glutamate, aspartate), a process referred to as *excitotoxicty*.

The addition of cells to the nervous system during development is not known as pruning. The human brain weighs about 350 g at birth and 1,450 g at full adult development, a fourfold increase, mainly in the neocortex. This increase is almost entirely due to growth in the number and *branching of dendrites establishing new connections*. Pruning *does not refer to the elimination of these branching dendrites*.

4.2 The answer is B

Alcohol use in pregnancy is a major cause of serious physical and mental birth defects in children. Each year, up to 40,000 babies are born with some degree of alcohol-related damage. The National Institute on Drug Abuse (NIDA) reports that *19 percent of pregnant women used alcohol during their pregnancy*, the highest rate being among white women.

4.3 The answer is E

Fetal alcohol syndrome is characterized by growth retardation of prenatal origin (height, weight); minor anomalies, including *microphthalmia (small eyeballs)*, short palpebral fissures, midface hypoplasia (underdevelopment), a smooth or short philtrum, and a thin upper lip; and *CNS manifestations*, including microcephaly (head circumference below the third percentile), a history of delayed development, *hyperactivity*, *attention deficits*, learning disabilities, intellectual deficits, and seizures. *Withdrawal-like symptoms is not a characteristic of fetal alcohol syndrome*; however, infants born to mothers dependent on narcotics go through a withdrawal syndrome at birth.

4.4 The answer is B

Children between the ages of 3 and 6 years are aware of their bodies, of the genitalia, and of differences between the sexes. In their play, doctor–nurse games allow children to act out their sexual fantasies. Their awareness of their bodies extends beyond the genitalia; they show a preoccupation with illness or injury, so much that *the preschool period has been called "the Band-Aid phase."* Every injury must be examined and taken care of by a parent.

The *toddler period* is marked by accelerated motor and intellectual development. The ability to walk gives toddlers some control over their own actions; this mobility enables children to determine when to approach and when to withdraw. The acquisition of speech profoundly extends their horizons. Typically, children learn to say "no" before they learn to say "yes." Toddlers' negativism is vital to the development of independence, but if it persists, oppositional behavior connotes a problem.

The *infancy period* begins with the delivery of the fetus. Reflexes are present at birth. They include the rooting reflex (puckering of the lips in response to perioral stimulation), the grasp reflex, the plantar (Babinski) reflex, the knee reflex, the abdominal reflex, the startle (Moro) reflex, and the tonic neck reflex. In normal children, the grasp reflex, the startle reflex and the tonic neck reflex disappear by the fourth month. The Babinksi reflex usually disappears by the twelfth month.

4.5 The answer is E

Currently, *98 percent of teenagers ages 15 to 19 years are using at least one method of birth control.* The two most common methods are condoms and birth control pills. Sexually transmitted diseases (STDs) are still high among teenagers. Approximately one in four sexually active teens contracts an STD every year and half of all new HIV infections occur in people under the age of 25.

4.6 The answer is C

Teenage pregnancy creates a plethora of health risks for both mother and child. Children born to teenage mothers have a greater chance of *dying before the age of five*. Those who survive are more likely to perform poorly in school and are at greater risk of abuse and neglect. Teenage mothers are less likely to gain adequate weight during pregnancy, increasing the risk of premature births and low birth weight. Low-birth weight babies are more likely to have organs that are not fully developed resulting in bleeding in the brain, respiratory distress syndrome and intestinal problems.

4.7 The answer is B

The psychological separation from parents in adolescence has been called the second individuation. The continuous process of elaboration of self and differentiation from others that occurs in the developmental phases of young (20 to 40 years of age) and middle (40 to 60 years of age) adulthood is influenced by all important adult relationships. At its core are ties to children, spouse and parents (i.e., the family), the same psychological constellation that shaped the first and second individuations. The continued elaboration of these themes in young adulthood has been called the *third individuation*.

The *first individuation* is a rather exclusive affair among infant, mother, and father. As children grow, young parents reengage memories of their own childhoods and fuse their experiences as parents with memories of their own progenitors from a generation ago. The separation-individuation process in infancy is responsible for establishing a stable sense of self and the capacity to relate to others.

The *fourth individuation* refers to the elaboration of separation-individuation processes in middle adulthood (40 to 60 years of age). One of the most powerful influences on these processes in midlife is the ironic awareness that one will die and will be deprived of involvement with loved ones at the very time that a mature understanding of the importance of others for one's health, happiness, and security is at its peak.

4.8 The answer is C

The transition from adolescence to young adulthood is characterized by *real and intrapsychic separation from the family of origin* and the engagement of new, phase-specific tasks. This process is the shedding of family dependencies to become a member of society at large, the shift from preadolescent idealized parental images to postadolescent idealized ethics and values, and the gradual shift from the family of origin to the family of procreation.

4.9 The answer is A

Piaget explains cognitive maturation by using a biological model that focuses on schemes, organized ways for children's developing brains to make sense of their experiences. To structure such schemes, children use complementary processes, assimilation and accommodation. According to Piaget, *cognitive growth occurs in stages that are always in a fixed order, invariant*. Overall, cognitive maturity is defined by a child's increasingly more refined ability to both internally and externally conceptualize space. In the *sensorimotor phase, from birth to 2 years*, infants use body senses and activity to explore the environment. Cognitive growth results in forming new skills, such as object permanence, which is the ability to remember an object once it is out of sight. *Object* constancy is a concept that arises from theories of attachment, and Margaret Mahler's psychoanalytic theory that proposes a complex sequence whereby an infant arrives at a basic sense of self. During the second phase, the *preoperational phase,* between the ages of 2 and 7, children become intuitive, anticipating experiences with consequences. Children in this phase *think symbolically* but illogically and with egocentricity and a direct inability to perceive self from others in their environment. Between the ages of 7 and 11, children enter a *concrete operational phase,* which involves the ability to think logically and in an organized fashion. At the end of this stage, age 11, children develop the capacity to think abstractly.

4.10 The answer is E (all)

The number of teenagers who engage in sexual intercourse is increasing. Each year about 1 million teenage girls under the age of 19 become pregnant. Only one third of sexually active teenagers use contraceptives; most are uneducated about contraceptive use or are unwilling or unable to obtain contraceptives. There are several factors that may affect *adolescents' misuse or rejection of contraceptives*. These include: (1) Denial, or the belief that pregnancy cannot occur; (2) Opportunism, or taking advantage of the opportunity (possibly unexpected) for coitus without regard for the consequences; (3) Love, whereby coitus is driven by passionate enthusiasm with the expectation of marriage if pregnancy occurs; (4) Embarrassment, or *self-consciousness about using a condom or inserting a diaphragm in front of the partner*; (5) Entrapment, which involves the desire to impregnate or to become pregnant to force the partner to become attached emotionally; (6) Eroticism, or the belief that contraceptive use decreases or *interferes with erotic pleasure*; (7) Nihilism, or the belief that contraceptives are ineffective or useless; (8) Fear and anxiety, in which coitus is associated with high levels of anxiety, or fear of performance ability interferes with contraceptive use; (9) Abortion, or the belief that if one gets pregnant, an abortion can be obtained so a contraceptive is not needed; (10) Education, or when there is a *lack of education about effective contraceptive use from parents and school*; and (11) Availability, in which *access to, or cost of, contraception prohibits its use*.

4.11 The answer is C

The law defines a minor as a person under the age of 18; at 18, for legal matters, a person is considered an adult. In many situations, however, adolescents can make their own health care decisions. For example, a minor can *consent to care for sexually transmitted diseases* without parental consent, including *treatment for illnesses related to AIDS*. Similarly, *birth control pills, like all other forms of contraception,* must be made available to minors without parental consent. Parental consent is also not necessary for a minor to *receive alcohol counseling* (although in some states counselors may tell parents). *However, a minor must be 16 or over to consent to inpatient mental health treatment.*

4.12 The answer is E (all)

Adoption is defined as the process by which a child is taken into a family by one or more adults who are not the biological parents but are recognized by law as the child's parents. Emotional and behavior disorders such as *aggressive behavior*, stealing, and *learning disturbances* have been reported to be higher among adopted than nonadopted children. The later the age of adoption, the higher the incidence and the more severe the behavioral problems. Adopted children are also more likely to develop *conduct disorders, problems with drug abuse*, and antisocial personality traits. It is unclear whether these problems result from the process of adoption or whether parents who give up children for adoption are more likely to pass along a genetic predisposition for these behaviors.

4.13 The answer is D

Robert Butler described several underlying themes in *middle adulthood* that appear to be present regardless of marital and family status, gender, or economic level. The themes include aging (as changes in bodily functions are noticed in middle adulthood); taking stock of accomplishments and setting goals for the future; reassessing commitments to family, work, and marriage; dealing with parental illness and death; and attending to all the developmental tasks without losing the capacity to experience pleasure or to engage in playful activity.

4.14 The answer is B

Some developmental theorists have focused on defining core personality traits within the individual and determining their course over the life span. Several well-designed longitudinal studies that have followed individuals over periods ranging from 10 to 50 years have found strong evidence for *stability in five basic personality traits*: *extraversion, neuroticism, agreeableness, openness to experience*, and *conscientiousness*. Some studies found slight decreases in extraversion and slight increases in agreeableness as individuals move into the oldest-old category (those over 85), which contrasts with early theories that proposed that personality rigidifies as individuals age.

4.15 The answer is E (all)

Diet and exercise play a role in preventing or ameliorating chronic diseases of older persons, such as arteriosclerosis and hypertension. Hypertensive geriatric patients can often correct their condition by moderate exercise and decreased salt intake (less than 3 g a day) without the addition of drugs. A regimen of daily moderate exercise (walking for 30 minutes a day) has been associated with a reduction in cardiovascular disease, decreased incidence of osteoporosis, improved respiratory function, the maintenance of ideal weight, and a general sense of well-being. Exercise has been shown to improve strength and function even among the very old. In many cases a disease process has been reversed and even cured by diet and exercise, without additional medical or surgical intervention. Positive and healthy physiological effects of exercise and nutrition include *increases* in strength of bones, ligaments, and muscles; *muscle mass and body density*; articular cartilage thickness; *heart volume and weight*; and cardiac stroke volume; and *decreases* in *heart rate at rest*; pulmonary ventilation during submaximal work; body fatness; and *systolic blood pressure*.

4.16 The answer is B

Arnold Gesell, a developmental psychologist and physician, described developmental schedules that outline the qualitative sequence of motor, adaptive, language, and personal-social behavior of the child from the age of 4 weeks to 6 years. Gesell's approach is normative; he viewed development as the unfolding of a genetically determined sequence. According to his schedules, at birth all infants have a repertoire of reflex behaviors—breathing, crying, and swallowing. By 1 to 2 weeks of age, the infant smiles. The response is endogenously determined, as evidenced by smiling in blind infants. By 2 to 4 weeks of age, visual fixation and following are evident. *By 4 to 8 weeks, social smiling is elicited preferentially by the face or the voice of the caretaker.*

4.17 The answer is B

To understand normal development, one must take a comprehensive approach and have an internal map of the age-expected norms for various aspects of human development. The areas of neuromotor, cognitive, and language milestones have many empirical normative data. The normal child is able to accomplish specific tasks at certain ages. For example, by *18 months,* children can walk up the stairs with one hand held; at *2 years,* they can *refer to themselves by name;* and at 3 years, they can *put on their shoes.* A cross can be copied at *4 years,* a square can be copied at 5 years, and a triangle can be copied at *6 years.* Some children may be able to perform a task at an earlier or later age and still fall within the normal range.

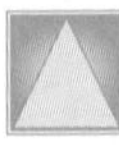

Table 4.1
Landmarks of Normal Behavioral Development

Age	Motor and Sensory Behavior	Adaptive Behavior	Personal and Social Behavior
Under 4 weeks	Makes alternating crawling movements Moves head laterally when placed in prone position	Responds to sound of rattle and bell Regards moving objects momentarily	Quiets when picked up Impassive face
16 weeks	Symmetrical postures predominate Holds head balanced Head lifted 90 degrees when prone on forearm Visual accommodation	Follows a slowly moving object well Arms activate on sight of dangling object	Spontaneous social smile (exogenous) Aware of strange situations
28 weeks	Sits steadily, leaning forward on hands Bounces actively when placed in standing position	One-hand approach and grasp of toy Bangs and shakes rattle Transfers toys	Takes feet to mouth Pats mirror image Starts to imitate mother's sounds and actions
40 weeks	Sits alone with good coordination Creeps Pulls self to standing position Points with index finger	Matches two objects at midline Attempts to imitate scribble	Separation anxiety manifest when taken away from mother Responds to social play, such as pat-a-cake and peekaboo Feeds self cracker and holds own bottle
52 weeks	Walks with one hand held Stands alone briefly	Seeks novelty	Cooperates in dressing

Adapted from Stella Chess, M.D.

Other landmarks of normal behavioral development are listed in Table 4.1.

Answers 4.18–4.21

4.18 The answer is B

4.19 The answer is C

4.20 The answer is A

4.21 The answer is A
Sex hormone levels increase slowly throughout adolescence and correspond to bodily changes. From ages 16 and 17, a large increase seems to occur in average testosterone levels, which then decrease and stabilize at the adult level. *Testosterone* is the hormone *responsible for masculinization of boys*, and estradiol (an estrogen) is the hormone responsible for feminization of girls. *Both testosterone and estrogen also influence CNS functioning*, including mood and behavior. *Low estrogen levels may be associated with depressed mood* (as happens in some women's premenstrual periods). High testosterone levels have been correlated with aggression and impulsivity in some men. *Testosterone levels correlate with libido and are manifested by sex drive* and masturbation in both sexes. In boys, androgens are produced by the testes and the adrenal gland; in girls, by the adrenal gland only. Levels are usually much higher in boys than in girls, and the effect of hormone changes on sexual behavior is usually more pronounced in boys than in girls.

Answers 4.22–4.26

4.22 The answer is E

4.23 The answer is A

4.24 The answer is D

4.25 The answer is B

4.26 The answer is C
See Table 4.2.

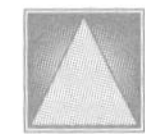

Table 4.2
Language Achievements

Average Age	Achievements
Gestational	
Infancy	
Birth-3 mos	Understands phonemes; responds to sound; can distinguish speech sounds; Noam Chomsky's language acquisition device
2 mos	Cooing; turn-taking with caregivers
16–28 wks	
28–40 wks	Knows friendly from unfriendly voices Native language discrimination
6 mos	Babbling; self-expressions for needs
40 wks–1 yr	Words connected to meaning; first words
$1^1/_2$–$2^1/_2$ yrs	First sentence—2 words; 50-word vocabulary
Early childhood	
2–3 yrs	Three-word sentences; uses small words, morphemes, to alter meaning; marked rise in vocabulary; girls greater vocabulary
3–5 yrs	Subtleties of tone and inflection; vocabulary increases to 14,000 words
5 yrs	End of baby talk: end of second language ease Child can make self fully understood
Middle childhood	
6–11 yrs	Metalinguistics understood; child improves inflection, pronouncement
Adolescence	
11 yrs and older	

Answers 4.27–4.29

4.27 The answer is B

4.28 The answer is A

4.29 The answer is C

For most persons, developing a well-defined sense of morality is a major accomplishment of late adolescence and adulthood. *Morality* is defined as conformity to shared standards, rights, and duties. Jean Piaget described morality as developing gradually, in conjunction with the stages of cognitive development. Lawrence Kohlberg integrated Piaget's concepts of morality and described three major levels of morality seen in adolescence. The first level is *pre-conventional morality*, in which *punishment and obedience to the parent are the determining factors*. The second level is morality of *conventional role-conformity*, in which *children try to conform to gain approval* and to maintain good relationships with others. The third and highest level is morality of *self-accepted principles*, in which children voluntarily *comply with rules on the basis of a concept of ethical principles* and make exceptions to rules in certain circumstances.

Answers 4.30–4.33

4.30 The answer is A

4.31 The answer is C

4.32 The answer is B

4.33 The answer is B

Marital therapy is a form of psychotherapy for married persons in conflict with each other. A trained person establishes a professional contract with the patient-couple and, through definite types of communication, attempts to alleviate the disturbance, to reverse or change maladaptive patterns of behavior, and to *encourage personality growth and development*. In *marriage counseling, only a particular conflict related to the immediate concerns of the family is discussed*; marriage counseling is conducted much more superficially by persons with less psychotherapeutic training than is marital therapy. Marriage therapy places greater *emphasis on restructuring the interaction between the couple*—including, at times, exploration of the psychodynamics of each partner. *Both therapy and counseling emphasize helping marital partners cope effectively with their problems*.

Answers 4.34–4.38

4.34 The answer is B

4.35 The answer is C

4.36 The answer is E

4.37 The answer is A

4.38 The answer is D

Early personality theorists proposed that development was completed by the end of childhood or adolescence. *Erik Erikson* was one of the first development theorists to propose that personality continues to develop and grow over the life span, and others have since also defined development into old age. Erikson believed that development proceeded through a series of psychological stages, each with its own conflict that is resolved by the individual with greater or lesser success. According to Erikson, the central conflict in old age is between integrity, *the sense of satisfaction people feel reflecting on a life lived productively, and despair, the sense that life has little purpose or meaning*. Contentment in old age comes only with getting beyond narcissism and into intimacy and generativity.

Sigmund Freud believed that *increasing control of the ego and id with aging results in increased autonomy*, but regression may permit primitive modes of functioning to reappear.

The theorist *Heinz Kohut* proposed that old people must continually cope with narcissistic injury as they attempt to adapt to the biological, psychological, and social losses associated with the aging processes. *The maintenance of self-esteem is a major task of old age*.

According to *Bernice Neugarten, the major conflict of old age relates to giving up the position of authority and evaluating achievements and former competence*. It is a *time of reconciliation with others and resolution of grief over the death of others and the approaching death of self*.

Finally, *Daniel Levinson* believed that ages 60 to 65 is a transition period ("the late adult transition") and that *people who are narcissistic and too heavily invested in body appearance are liable to become preoccupied with death*. Creative mental activity is a normal and healthy substitute for reduced physical activity.

Answers 4.39–4.43

4.39 The answer is C

4.40 The answer is B

4.41 The answer is A

4.42 The answer is A

4.43 The answer is C

Grief and depression share many features: sadness, tearfulness, *loss of appetite*, poor sleep, and *diminished interest in the world*. There are, however, enough differences that psychiatrists regard them as separate syndromes. Symptoms of bereavement may meet syndromal criteria for major depressive episode, but grieving persons *rarely have* morbid feelings of guilt and worthlessness, *suicidal ideation*, or psychomotor retardation. The mood disturbance in depression is typically pervasive and unremitting; fluctuations in grief are common. Persons often describe grief coming in waves, washing over them, and then subsiding. Even in intense grief, moments of lightheartedness and happy reminiscence are possible. Furthermore, functional impairment in bereavement is transient and mild, while a hallmark of depression is *clinically significant distress or impairment*. In grief, *dysphoria is often triggered by thoughts or reminders of the deceased*, whereas dysphoria in depression is often independent of the deceased. The realization that grief is time limited is very important. Whereas depression can occur at any time and often becomes chronic, intermittent, or episodic, grief occurs within the first 2 months of bereavement and has depressive symptoms that last less than 2 months. Many persons suffering from major depression lack hope; they cannot imagine ever feeling better. Persons who have experienced previous depression are at risk for becoming depressed at times of major loss and a bereaved person's clinical history may be helpful in judging a current reaction. Depressed persons threaten suicide more often than grieving persons, who, except in unusual instances—for example, physically dependent and older persons—do not seriously wish to die, even if they claim that life is unbearable. Physicians must determine when grief has become pathological and has evolved into major depressive disorder. Grief is a normal, albeit intensely painful state that responds to support, empathy, and the passage of time. Major depressive disorder is potentially a medical emergency that requires immediate intervention to forestall a complication such as suicide.

5 The Brain and Behavior

Simply defined, neuropsychiatry is the study of brain-behavior relationships. Neuropsychiatry seeks to understand how the brain, through structural and neural networks, produces and controls behavior and mental processes, including emotions, personality, thinking, learning and memory, problem solving, and consciousness. The field is concerned with how behavior may influence the brain and related physiological processes. The explosion of data derived from psychopharmacology, functional neuroimaging, and human neurogenetics makes this one of the most exciting fields of medicine. The psychiatrist must be able to critically review new data and research and apply this knowledge to evaluating new drugs, treatments, and diagnostic techniques.

A basic understanding of behavioral neuroanatomy provides knowledge of classical syndromes, such as those of lobar dysfunction. The basal ganglia, limbic structures, hypothalamus, and lobes of the cerebral cortex are of special relevance. It is also crucial to understand the ultrastructure of individual brain cells, the details of synaptic connectivity, the functional organization of the brain, and the behavioral consequences of pathological processes in the central nervous system. Students should be knowledgeable about the vast functional diversity of brain cells and their organization. Students must also have a thorough grasp of the structure and function of neurotransmission. The role of genetics in psychiatric disorders includes knowledge about gene expression, DNA replication, messenger RNA synthesis and translation into protein, and the consequences of mutations at each of these stages.

Of central importance to clinical psychopharmacology is a thorough knowledge of the neurotransmitters, including the brainstem location of the biogenic amine neurotransmitter nuclei and the widespread distribution of their axonal projections. Excitatory neurotransmitters (e.g., glutamate), inhibitory neurotransmitters (e.g., γ-aminobutyric acid [GABA]), the monoamine neurotransmitters (e.g., serotonin, dopamine, norepinephrine, epinephrine, histamine, and acetylcholine), and the peptide neurotransmitters (e.g., endorphins and enkephalins) are crucial to an understanding of current psychotherapeutic medications.

Finally, a knowledge of the major neuroimaging techniques, including clinical and research indications, and the limitations of each technique, is essential. These methods include magnetic resonance imaging (MRI), computed tomography (CT), magnetic resonance spectroscopy (MRS), single photon emission computed tomography (SPECT), proton emission tomography (PET), electroencephalography (EEG), and magnetoencephalography (MEG), among others.

Students should test their knowledge by addressing the following questions and answers.

HELPFUL HINTS

- aphasia: Broca's, Wernicke's, conduction, global, transcortical motor, transcortical sensory, anomic, mixed transcortical
- apraxias: limb-kinetic, ideomotor, ideational
- autonomic sensory and motor systems
- basal ganglia and cerebellum and clinical syndromes
- behavioral neuroanatomy: arousal and attention, memory, language, emotions
- biological rhythms
- cerebral cortex
- chronobiology
- cytoarchitectonics and cortical columns
- development of cortical networks; plasticity
- dopamine and serotonin hypothesis of schizophrenia
- electrophysiology: membranes and charge; ion channels, action potentials, chemical neurotransmission
- epilepsy: complex partial seizures, temporal lobe epilepsy, TLE personality, *déjà vu*
- five primary senses (somatosensory, visual, auditory, olfaction, taste)
- frontal, parietal, temporal and occipital lobes and clinical syndromes
- GABA and serotonin hypothesis of anxiety disorders
- glutamate, GABA, glycine, dopamine, norepinephrine, epinephrine, serotonin, acetylcholine, histamine, opioids, substance P, neurotensin, cholecystokinin, somatostatin, vasopressin, oxytocin, neuropeptide Y
- gray matter and white matter
- inheritance patterns: autosomal dominant, autosomal recessive, sex-linked

- ligand-gated ion channel; G protein-coupled receptor; second messenger
- limbic system: amygdala, hippocampus, Papez circuit
- molecular genetics: pedigree, positional cloning, candidate gene, mutations
- neuroimaging: CT, MRI, MRS, fMRI, SPECT, PET, EEG, MEG, TMS, EP, ERP
- neurons and glial cells
- neurotransmitters: biogenic amines, amino acids, peptides, nucleotides, gases, eicosanoids, anandamides
- norepinephrine and serotonin hypothesis of mood disorders
- organization of sensory and motor systems; hemispheric lateralization
- prefrontal lobe syndromes
- psychoneuroendocrinology: hormones and hormone receptors, adrenal axis, thyroid axis, growth hormone, estrogens
- psychoneuroimmunology: placebo effect, cancer, infection, AIDS
- synapses: presynaptic membrane, synaptic compartment, postsynaptic membrane

QUESTIONS

Directions

Each of the questions or incomplete statements below is followed by five suggested responses or completions. Select the *one* that is *best* in each case.

5.1 Which of the following statements concerning astrocytes is *false*

A. They are the most numerous class of glial cells.
B. They help form the blood-brain barrier.
C. They remove neurotransmitters from the synaptic cleft.
D. They may have a nutritive function.
E. They buffer the intracellular sodium concentrations.

5.2 The site of origin of an action potential is at the

A. synaptic cleft
B. axon hillock
C. Nodes of Ranvier
D. gap junction
E. voltage-gated sodium channel

5.3 All of the following statements about neuronal connections are true *except*?

A. Many connections between brain regions are reciprocal.
B. The locus ceruleus is an example of a convergent neuronal system.
C. Visual input is conveyed in a serial or hierarchical fashion.
D. Regions of the brain are specialized for different functions.
E. The role of any specific brain region in the production of specific behaviors must be viewed in the context of neural connections with other brain regions.

5.4 Circadian influences arise from all of the following *except*

A. pontine reticular formation
B. suprachiasmatic nucleus
C. hypothalamus
D. supraoptic nucleus
E. external cues

5.5 The basal ganglia include

A. the lentiform nucleus
B. the substantia nigra
C. the subthalamic nucleus
D. the caudate nucleus
E. all of the above

5.6 In schizophrenia

A. no abnormalities in neural migration have been hypothesized.
B. reductions of 50 to 60 percent are reported in overall temporal lobe size.
C. there is decreased prefrontal cerebral blood flow on PET scans during certain tasks (when compared to healthy controls).
D. there is a proliferation of glial cells.
E. there is an associated increase in the size of the amygdala.

5.7 All of the following are medical causes of amnesia *except*

A. Vitamin deficiencies
B. Infection
C. Alcoholism
D. Migraine
E. Cocaine intoxication

5.8 The following CT image in Figure 5.1 shows enlargement of the ventricles due to atrophy of the head of the caudate nucleus. The disease displayed in this image is

A. Alzheimer's disease
B. Pick's disease
C. Huntington's disease
D. Parkinson's disease
E. Lewy Body disease

5.9 The one advantage of CT over MRI in psychiatric clinical practice is

A. CT has superior resolution.
B. CT can distinguish between white matter and gray matter.
C. CT has the ability to take thinner slices through the brain than does MRI.

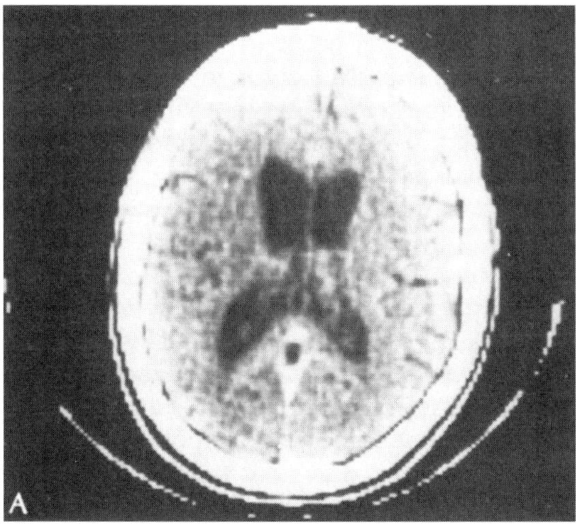

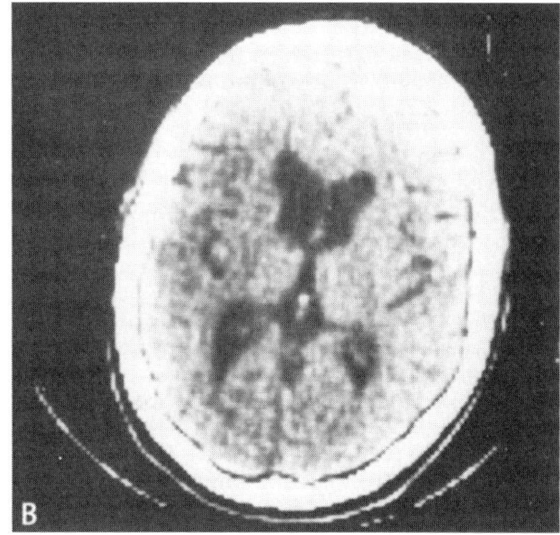

FIGURE 5.1
A and **B**, CT scans at two axial levels show ventricular enlargement with atrophy of the caudate nucleus, particularly the head of the caudate. (Reprinted with permission from Rowland LP, ed. *Merritt's Textbook of Neurology.* 9th ed. Baltimore: Lippincott Williams & Wilkins; 1995:698.)

D. CT is superior in detecting calcified brain lesions.
E. CT avoids exposing patients to radiation.

5.10 The following image in Figure 5.2 shows small petechial hemorrhages in the mammillary bodies of this brain. This image most closely represents which of the following?

A. Vascular stroke
B. Wernicke's disease
C. Pyridoxine deficiency
D. Lewy Body disease
E. Cluster headache

5.11 True statements about the relationship of GABA to seizure activity include all of the following *except*

A. Blockage of GABA inhibition can result in seizures.
B. Benzodiazepines and barbiturates act at GABA receptors.

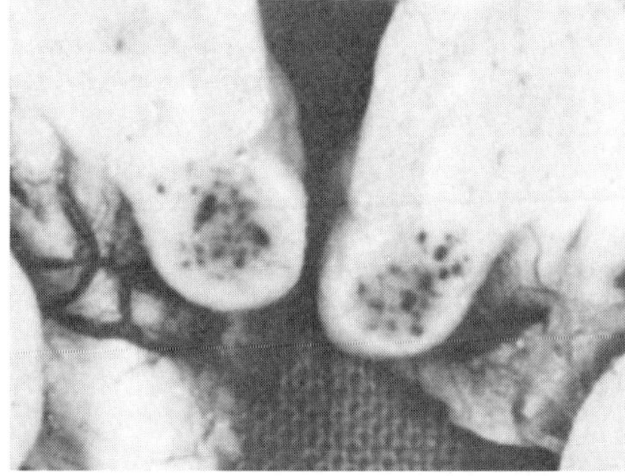

FIGURE 5.2
Petechial hemorrhages in the mamillary bodies. (Reprinted with permission from Lewis AJ. *Mechanisms of Neurological Disease.* Boston: Little, Brown and Company; 1976:414.)

C. Manipulation of GABA-receptor function has little effect on seizure activity.
D. Enhancement of GABA-receptor function raises the seizure threshold.
E. Reduction of GABA clearance by inhibition of GABA uptake is clinically effective in reducing seizures.

5.12 Which of the following statements about melatonin is *false?*

A. It is released by the pineal body.
B. It is secreted when the eye perceives light.
C. It is synthesized from serotonin.
D. It is involved in the regulation of circadian rhythms.
E. It is implicated in the pathophysiology of depression.

5.13 PET and SPECT scans

A. entail the injection of radioactively labeled drugs.
B. provide exquisitely detailed images of brain structure.
C. produce two-dimensional information.
D. are similar to MRI in creating fine visual detail.
E. are commonly used in clinical practice.

5.14 Which of the following personality disorders is most commonly associated with HIV infection?

A. Borderline
B. Narcissistic
C. Antisocial
D. Dependent
E. Histrionic

5.15 Serotonin is

A. primarily located in the CNS.
B. able to cross the blood-brain barrier.

C. not dependent on tryptophan concentration for its synthesis.
D. directly affected by carbohydrate intake in its synthesis.
E. synthesized from the amino acid tryptophan.

5.16 All of the following associations between aspects of the basal ganglia and their respective disorders are correct *except*

A. subthalamic nucleus—hemiballismus
B. caudate nucleus—obsessive-compulsive disorder
C. caudate nucleus—Huntington's disease
D. globus pallidus—Wilson's disease
E. substantia nigra—Alzheimer's disease

5.17 Which of the following is commonly associated with epilepsy?

A. Schizophreniform psychosis
B. Depression
C. Personality changes
D. Hyposexuality
E. None of the above

5.18 MRI studies

A. prove that there are specific, structural brain changes in a significant number of schizophrenic patients.
B. provide some evidence that there may be structural brain changes in major depressive disorder.
C. prove that caudate enlargement occurs early in the course of schizophrenia.
D. are inferior to CT with regard to visualizing gray versus white matter in the brain.
E. suggest no brain changes secondary to alcohol dependence.

5.19 Techniques that reflect regional brain activity by measuring neuronal activity rather than blood flow include

A. xenon-133 (^{133} Xe) single proton emission computed tomography (SPECT)
B. fluorine-18 [^{18}F]-fluorodeoxyglucose (FDG) positron emission tomography (PET)
C. technetium-99 (^{99}Tc) hexamethylpropyleneamine oxime (HMPAO) SPECT
D. nitrogen-13 (^{13}N) PET
E. functional magnetic resonance imaging (fMRI)

5.20 True statements regarding arousal include

A. The ascending reticular activating system (ARAS) sets the level of consciousness.
B. Both the thalamus and the cortex fire rhythmic bursts of neuronal activity.
C. During wakefulness, the ARAS stimulates the thalamic interlaminar nuclei.
D. Small discrete lesions of the ARAS may produce a stuporous state.
E. All of the above

5.21 A patient is brought to your office for cognitive testing. The patient is given the task of scanning a long list of random letters and is told to identify only the letter "A." She is unable to continue this task for more than a minute. What is the most likely location of her lesion?

A. thalamus
B. lateral corticospinal tract
C. basal ganglia
D. frontal lobe
E. substantia nigra

5.22 A patient with intractable epilepsy undergoes surgical removal of both hippocampi and amygdalae. Which of the following is the most likely side effect of this procedure?

A. impaired learning ability
B. impaired skill-related memory
C. impaired factual memory
D. ataxia
E. loss of vision

5.23 A patient suffers a stroke of the left hemisphere. Which of the following is the most likely sequela?

A. denial of illness
B. inability to move the left hand
C. loss of narrative aspects of dreams
D. failure to respond to humor
E. depression

5.24 A patient is diagnosed with temporal lobe epilepsy (TLE) but does not experience the classic grand mal seizures. Which of the following behaviors is the patient likely to exhibit?

A. hyposexuality
B. hypersexuality
C. placidity
D. hypermetamorphosis
E. lack of emotion to visual stimuli

5.25 Korsakoff's syndrome is a classic example of which type of amnesia?

A. Hippocampal amnesia
B. Diencephalic amnesia
C. Lateralized amnesia
D. Traumatic injury-induced amnesia
E. Transient global amnesia

Directions

Each group of questions below consists of lettered headings followed by a list of numbered words or statements. For each numbered word or statement, select the *one* lettered heading that is most closely associated with it. Each lettered heading may be selected once, more than once, or not at all.

Questions 5.26–5.30

A. Vascular dementia
B. Pick's disease
C. HIV dementia

D. Huntington's disease
E. Creutzfeldt-Jakob disease

5.26 John is a highly successful merger-acquisition attorney. Immediately after his 50th birthday, John announces he plans to give up his partnership in his law firm and investigate the Lincoln assassination, which he believes is a communist conspiracy. He spends all the family savings and is irritable with those who doubt him. He is found on the street one evening psychotic, delusional, very fidgety, and unable to sit still. His father died in a psychiatric hospital with similar symptoms.

5.27 A patient presents with loss of short-term memory, loss of sense of time, and a progressive decline in other cognitive abilities as well. This loss is variable, however, and some days are better than others. At times, she seems to suffer from episodes of acute confusion. She is quite aware of this new disability and is very bothered. Her personality remains intact, although she does experience "mood swings" regularly.

5.28 A 25-year-old homosexual man cohabitates with his partner. He has yearly serological tests and has a normal CD4 lymphocyte count. Despite feeling systemically well, he begins reporting "memory problems" with difficulty thinking and concentrating, along with an overwhelming sense of apathy. Also, he reports insomnia, morning fatigue, and poor appetite. His mini mental status exam score is 29 of 30. The neurological exam shows normal gait, strength, coordination, sensation, and cranial nerves.

5.29 A patient is suffering from rapidly progressing dementia over the last 6 months. She has become withdrawn and forgetful, and often cannot find the right words to express herself in conversation. She also has become unsteady on her feet, and frequently has spasms in her arms and legs.

5.30 A 40-year-old woman presents to your office after her family has noted her to be more aggressive and irritable. In your office, she laughs inappropriately and makes rude comments to your nurse. Loss of memory, difficulty planning, and lack of motivation are also among her complaints. Her mother and uncle developed similar signs of dementia while in their 50s.

Questions 5.31–5.33

A. Dorsolateral prefrontal cortex lesion
B. Medial prefrontal cortex lesion
C. Orbitofrontal prefrontal cortex lesion

5.31 A normally kind and quiet woman suddenly becomes loud, boisterous, and rude to her husband and friends. Her husband reports she shows no remorse or concern about these actions, quite a change from her usual self. She also acts strangely and inappropriately, having an affair with a 15-year-old high school sophomore.

5.32 A bank executive often referred to as a "workaholic" suddenly loses all motivation to excel on the job. Although previously in the middle of planning numerous projects, he now is unable to plan or direct the simplest of tasks. Remaining focused at work for a full 8 hours becomes nearly impossible for him, despite a previously consistent 12-hour work schedule.

5.33 A business professional is suddenly found to be mute. On further observation, she appears to be relatively akinetic as well, with hardly any initiation of movements. She understands when spoken to, but appears apathetic concerning her condition.

Questions 5.34–5.38

A. Serotonin
B. Glycine
C. Norepinephrine
D. Acetylcholine
E. Dopamine

5.34 Median and dorsal raphe nuclei
5.35 Locus ceruleus
5.36 Nucleus basalis of Meynert
5.37 Substantia nigra
5.38 Spinal cord

Questions 5.39–5.43

A. Prosencephalon
B. Mesencephalon
C. Rhombencephalon

5.39 Telencephalon
5.40 Diencephalon
5.41 Pons
5.42 Midbrain
5.43 Cerebral cortex

Questions 5.44–5.47

A. Left brain localization
B. Right brain localization

5.44 Recognition of faces
5.45 Language functions
5.46 Prosody
5.47 Maintenance of attention

Questions 5.48–5.52

A. Dopamine
B. Serotonin
C. Melatonin
D. Anticholinergic drugs
E. Growth hormone

5.48 Cause(s) dry mouth, constipation, blurred vision, urinary retention
5.49 Synthesized by serotonin, released by pineal body
5.50 Amphetamines cause release, cocaine blocks uptake
5.51 Dietary variations in tryptophan can affect brain levels
5.52 Released in pulses

Questions 5.53–5.55

A. Ideational apraxia
B. Ideomotor apraxia
C. Limb-kinetic apraxia

5.53 Inability to perform an isolated motor act upon command
5.54 Inability to perform components of a sequence as a whole
5.55 Inability to use the contralateral hand in the presence of preserved strength

ANSWERS

5.1 The answer is E

In addition to neurons, the brain also contains several types of glial cells, which are at least ten times more numerous than neurons. *Astrocytes, the most numerous class of glial cells*, appear to serve a number of functions, *including participation in the formation of the blood-brain barrier, removal of certain neurotransmitters from the synaptic cleft*, buffering of the *extracellular potassium (not sodium) concentration*, and, given their close contact with both neurons and blood vessels, possibly a nutritive function as well.

Oligodendrocytes and Schwann cells, found in the CNS and peripheral nervous system, respectively, are relatively small cells that wrap their membranous processes around axons in a tight spiral. The resulting myelin sheath facilitates the conduction of action potentials along the axon. The third class of glial cells, the *microglia*, is actually derived from macrophages and functions as scavengers, eliminating the debris resulting from neuronal death and injury. Recent studies have discovered additional roles for glial cells in brain function and produced data suggesting that alterations in glia may contribute to the pathophysiology of schizophrenia and depression.

5.2 The answer is B

The propagation of an action potential along an axon is described as an all-or-none phenomenon; that is, once an action potential has been triggered, it is propagated at full strength for the entire length of the axon. Determination of whether an action potential is generated is by the summation of excitatory and inhibitory chemical influences that act on the *axon hillock*, which originates the action potential. The action potential causes the release of neurotransmitter molecules into the *synaptic cleft*, the small space between the presynaptic neuron and the postsynaptic neuron. *Nodes of Ranvier* are segments of bare axonal membrane not covered by myelin. *Gap junctions*, also called electrical synapses, allow direct transfer of ions between two neurons as a form of interneuronal neurochemical communication. Once the threshold potential is reached at the axon hillock, the action potential is propagated by the opening of *voltage-gated sodium channels*.

5.3 The answer is B

Many neuronal connections are either divergent or convergent in nature. A divergent system involves the conduction of information from one neuron or a discrete group of neurons to a much larger number of neurons that may be located in diverse portions of the brain. *The locus ceruleus*, a small group of norepinephrine-containing neurons in the brainstem that sends axonal projections to the entire cerebral cortex and other brain regions, *is an example of a divergent neuronal system, not a convergent system*. In contrast, the output of multiple brain regions may be directed toward a single area, forming a convergent system.

Many, but not all, connections between brain regions are reciprocal; that is, each region tends to receive input from those regions to which it sends axonal projections. In some cases, the axons arising from one region may directly innervate the reciprocating projection neurons in another region; in other cases, local circuit interneurons are interposed between the incoming axons and the projection neurons that furnish the reciprocal connections. For some projections, the reciprocating connection is indirect, passing through one or more additional brain regions and synapses before innervating the initial brain region.

The connections among regions may be organized in a hierarchical or parallel fashion, or both. For example, *visual input is conveyed in a serial or hierarchical fashion* through several populations of neurons in the retina to the lateral geniculate nucleus, to the primary visual cortex, and then progressively to the multiple visual association areas of the cerebral cortex. Within the hierarchical scheme, different types of visual information (e.g., motion, form) may be processed in a parallel fashion through different portions of the visual system.

Regions of the brain are specialized for different functions. For example, lesions of the left inferior frontal gyrus (Broca's area) produce a characteristic impairment in speech production. However, speech is a complex faculty that depends not only on the integrity of Broca's area but also on the processing of information across a number of brain regions through divergent and convergent, serial and parallel interconnections. Thus, the role of any specific brain region in the production of specific behaviors cannot be viewed in isolation but *must be viewed within the context of the neural circuits connecting those neurons with other brain regions*.

5.4 The answer is D

Sleep is one of several biological rhythms within the body. Circadian biological rhythms are set by internal and external forces, generally called zeitgebers (time givers, time clues, synchronizers), which constitute a widely distributed set of nuclei. The principal circadian influences emanate from the *pontine reticular formation* as well as the *suprachiasmatic nucleus of the hypothalamus*. Recent evidence has shown that the suprachiasmatic nucleus can entrain circadian rhythms even in the absence of physical synaptic connections with the remainder of the hypothalamus, suggesting that this zeitgeber may act through elaboration of diffusible substances. *External cues* such as sunlight and temperature also influence circadian rhythms. The *supraoptic nucleus* controls the synthesis and secretion of vasopressin and is not involved in controlling circadian rhythms.

5.5 The answer is E (all)

The basal ganglia are a collection of nuclei that have been grouped together on the basis of their interconnections. These nuclei play an important role in regulating movement and in certain disorders of movement (dyskinesias), which include jerky movements (chorea), writhing movements (athetosis), and rhythmic movements (tremors). In addition, recent studies have shown that certain components of the basal ganglia play an important role in many cognitive functions.

The basal ganglia are generally considered to include the *caudate nucleus*, the putamen, the globus pallidus (referred to as the paleostriatum or pallidum), the *subthalamic nucleus*, and the *substantia nigra*. The term *striatum* refers to the *caudate nucleus* and the *putamen* together; the term corpus striatum refers to the caudate nucleus, the putamen, and the globus pallidus; and the term *lentiform nucleus* refers to the putamen and the globus pallidus together.

5.6 The answer is C

Neuroimaging with SPECT and PET can investigate the functioning of brain regions in vivo. By imaging subjects during tasks, cerebral activity patterns reflect the functioning of neural networks necessary to perform the tasks. In numerous studies, individuals with schizophrenia show dysfunction within frontal-parietal-temporal networks, even during different tasks that utilize these cerebral areas. In these patients *there is decreased prefrontal cerebral blood flow on PET blood flow scans during certain tasks (when compared to healthy controls).* An example is the Wisconsin Card Sorting Test, an abstract problem-solving test requiring attention and working memory. Monozygotic twins discordant for schizophrenia underwent PET blood flow scans while performing this test. In all but one pair the ill twin had relatively decreased prefrontal cerebral blood flow; the area of temporal lobe limbic region in the ill twin was invariably hyperactive. In vivo studies do not speak to when or how the functional abnormality arose. However, finding functional consequences as the result of cerebral areas defined as abnormal in neuropathological investigations is essential in correlating neurodevelopmental abnormalities with the clinical symptoms of schizophrenia.

Imaging the brain with MRI allows for volumetric measurements of brain structure. In schizophrenia, *reductions of 10 to 15 percent, not 50 to 60 percent, are reported in overall temporal lobe size,* in temporal lobe gray matter, and in specific temporal lobe structures. Recent MRI studies suggest subtle volumetric reductions in widespread cortical areas, including the frontal and parietal secondary association areas, and in the thalamus.

Schizophrenia is associated with enlarged ventricles and a *decrease (not increase) in the size of the amygdala,* hippocampus, and parahippocampal gyrus. There is a *lack, not a proliferation, of glial cells in schizophrenia.* A proliferation of glial cells is seen in degenerative brain conditions and encephalopathies that arise after birth. This does not occur in schizophrenia and suggests that whatever causes the brain abnormalities in schizophrenia does so before the third trimester of gestation because glial cells become responsive to injury only after the third trimester.

Of considerable interest in understanding the developmental neurobiology of schizophrenia are studies exploring cortical cytoarchitecture, particularly in the networks showing in vivo dysfunction. In the cortex of individuals with schizophrenia, heterotopic groups of neurons belonging to layer II are found displaced into layer III. *This may indicate abnormal neuronal migration* that results in heterotopic neuronal islands and abnormal cytoarchitecture. Layer II of the prefrontal cortex of persons with schizophrenia shows reduced numbers of small neurons, with higher densities of pyramidal neurons in layer V.

5.7 The answer is E

Medical causes of amnesia include *alcoholism*, seizures, *migraine*, drugs, *vitamin deficiencies*, trauma, strokes, tumors, *infections*, and degenerative diseases. Herpes simplex encephalitis is the paradigmatic infectious etiology for an amnestic disorder. Herpetic infection of the central nervous system (CNS) preferentially involves the temporal lobes and produces a hemorrhagic necrosis that can be fatal. Survivors often display a profound amnestic disorder due to destruction of medial temporal lobe structures, whereas other cognitive functions are largely intact.

A hallmark of the classic alcoholic "blackout" is the lack of memory for the actual blackout and for events leading up to it. This represents acute anterograde amnesia with inability to encode new memories during the period of intoxication and inability to retrieve memories encoded proximate to the blackout. Chronic alcoholism, persistent vomiting, malabsorption syndromes, and severe malnutrition can lead to vitamin deficiencies that may lead to an amnestic syndrome. Deficiency of thiamine or vitamin B_1 has been identified as the cause of Wernicke's encephalopathy and Korsakoff's syndrome.

Migraines have also been implicated as a cause of transient global amnesia in some cases. *Intoxication with common drugs of abuse, such as cocaine and heroin, is not associated with amnesia per se.* Chronic use, however, can produce cognitive dysfunction.

5.8 The answer is C

Huntington's disease (formerly Huntington's chorea) is an autosomal dominant neurodegenerative disorder characterized by midlife onset, a relentlessly progressive course, and a combination of motor, psychiatric, and cognitive symptoms. The disease is caused by a CAG repeat expansion mutation in the huntington gene on chromosome 4. Gross pathology of Huntington's disease often shows enlarged lateral ventricles, atrophy of the caudate and putamen, and atrophy of the cerebral cortex due to neuronal loss in these areas. Huntington's disease remains an important example of subcortical dementia and the prominence of the psychiatric consequences of neurodegenerative disorders.

In *Alzheimer's disease*, there is cerebral atrophy, mainly in the frontal, temporal, and parietal regions. As a consequence, there is ex vacuo ventricular dilation. The cerebral atrophy with *Pick's disease* is lobar and typically involves the frontal and temporal lobes. This atrophy is so striking that it is "knife-like" in appearance. This atrophy may be asymmetrical. Microscopically, there is marked loss of cortical neurons with gliosis. Pick bodies, cytoplasmic inclusions that are highlighted by silver stain, are seen in the cortex. In *Parkinson's disease*, Lewy bodies are found in the substantia nigra of the midbrain, coupled with the loss of pigmented neurons. In persons with the dementia of diffuse *Lewy body disease*, there are Lewy bodies in the neocortex. Some persons have the Lewy bodies in both locations. The basal ganglia and diencephalon may also be involved in some cases.

5.9 The answer is D

One reason to order a CT scan in preference to an MRI scan is that *CT is superior in detecting calcified brain lesions.* Whether to order a CT or a more expensive MRI is one of the common clinical questions in psychiatric practice. The resolution of both techniques is under 1 mm, but *MRI has the capability of taking thinner slices through the brain, does have superior resolution,* and *can better distinguish between white matter and gray matter.* CT is based on X-ray technology; MRI utilizes magnetic fields. Therefore, *MRI, not CT, avoids exposing patients to radiation.*

5.10 The answer is B

The small petechial hemorrhages in the mammillary bodies seen here are characteristic of *Wernicke's disease*, a complication of chronic alcoholism with thiamine deficiency. *Neither vascular stroke, pyridoxine deficiency, Lewy body disease, nor cluster headaches present with hemorrhages in the mammillary bodies.*

5.11 The answer is C

GABA and GABA-receptor subtypes play a central role in the expression of seizures. GABA, as the major inhibitory neurotransmitter in the CNS, can be found in up to 30 percent of CNS synapses. In general, for the mature brain, loss or *blockade of GABA inhibition can result in increased hyperexcitability that results in seizures.* Several GABAergic drugs are widely used in the treatment of epilepsy. *Benzodiazepines and barbiturates act at GABA receptors* to enhance inhibition. Both have been shown to be effective in the control of partial, complex partial, and generalized tonic–clonic seizures. Benzodiazepines are also effective in the short-term treatment of generalized absence seizures, but a functional tolerance tends to develop, thereby reducing their efficacy. Barbiturates may exacerbate generalized absence seizures. Benzodiazepines are also effective in the treatment of atypical absence and myoclonic seizures. Anticonvulsant benzodiazepines and barbiturates are highly sedating, which limits their use.

Other evidence that the GABAergic system is important in the expression of seizures is that *manipulation of GABA has major effects on seizures.* It *can cause, exacerbate, or reduce seizure activity.* The mushroom poison picrotoxin antagonizes GABA receptors and can elicit seizures. Penicillin given at high doses (especially in renal failure patients or intrathecally) can also result in partial or generalized seizures. Penicillin reduces GABA-induced chloride current flow by blocking the ion channel pore.

In the mature or adult brain, *enhancement of GABA-receptor function raises the seizure threshold.* Certain naturally occurring and synthetic steroids are potent modulators of GABA that may be associated with menstrually related epilepsy. *Reduction of GABA clearance, or raising the GABA level, is clinically effective* in reducing seizures. Several of the pharmacological effects of ethanol are mediated through effects on GABA in chronic alcoholism, thus accounting for seizure activity.

5.12 The answer is B

Melatonin is released by the pineal body, which also contains many other peptides and hormones. Melatonin is secreted when the eye perceives *darkness (not light)*; its release is inhibited when the eye perceives light. *Melatonin is synthesized from serotonin* by the action of two enzymes: serotonin-N-acetylase and 5-hydroxyindole-O-methyltransferase. *Melatonin is involved in the regulation of circadian rhythms and has been implicated in the pathophysiology of depression.*

5.13 The answer is A

The two radiotracer methods of neuroimaging, PET and SPECT, *entail the injection of radioactively labeled drugs.* The imaging and measurement over time of the distribution of these radiotracers is used to assess the neurochemistry, blood flow, or metabolism of the brain. The three methods based on nuclear magnetic resonance are MRI, functional MRI (fMRI), and MRS. In general terms, MRI provides *exquisitely detailed images of brain structure*; fMRI provides images of local neuronal activity with high spatial and temporal resolution; and MRS provides measurements of the concentrations of numerous chemicals in the brain without the radiation exposure of PET and SPECT but with much lower sensitivity.

In PET and SPECT, a biological process of interest is studied by synthetically incorporating a radionuclide into a molecule of known physiological relevance. The so-called radiopharmaceutical is then administered to a patient either by inhalation, ingestion, or most commonly by intravenous injection. As radioactivity distributes within the subject, the radiotracer's uptake into the brain is measured over time and is used to obtain information about the physiological process of interest. *PET and SPECT rely on sophisticated principles to produce three-, not two-, dimensional information* (as in a chest X-ray). In order to understand this process, a basic understanding of the physics of photon emission is required.

Although some of the methods, such as structural MRI, have been a standard component of the clinical assessment of patients with neurological disorders for more than a decade, similar *clinical applications have not yet been found for patients with psychiatric disorders.* These methods are largely restricted to research studies. Neuroimaging is also attractive to the field of psychiatry because it provides direct measurements of the brain and therefore passes the limitations of peripheral measures (e.g., concentrations of plasma hormones or urinary catecholamine metabolites), which generate only indirect assessments of central nervous system function.

5.14 The answer is C

Personality disorders represent extremes of normal personality characteristics and are disabling conditions. Prevalence rates of personality disorders among HIV-infected (19 to 36 percent) and HIV at-risk (15 to 20 percent) individuals are high and significantly exceed rates found in the general population (10 percent). *Antisocial personality disorder is the most common and is a risk factor for HIV infection.* Individuals with personality disorder, particularly antisocial personality disorder, have high rates of substance abuse and are more likely to inject drugs and share needles, compared with those without an Axis II diagnosis. Approximately one-half of drug abusers meet criteria for a diagnosis of antisocial personality disorder. Antisocial personality disorder individuals are also more likely to have higher numbers of lifetime sexual partners, engage in unprotected anal sex, and contract STDs compared with individuals without antisocial personality disorder.

5.15 The answer is E

Peripheral serotonin is located in platelets, mast cells, and enterochromaffin cells of the gastrointestinal system. The *CNS contains less than 2 percent of the serotonin in the body;* despite the abundance of peripheral serotonin, it is *unable to cross the blood-brain barrier,* necessitating the synthesis of serotonin within the brain. *Serotonin is synthesized from the amino acid tryptophan,* which is derived from the diet. The rate-limiting step in serotonin synthesis is the hydroxylation of tryptophan by the enzyme tryptophan hydroxylase to form 5-hydroxytryptophan (5HTP). Under normal circumstances this enzyme is not saturated by substrate, *so tryptophan concentration can affect the rate of serotonin synthesis.* Because tryptophan competes with other large neutral amino acids for transport, brain uptake of this amino acid is determined both by the amount of circulating tryptophan and by the ratio of tryptophan to other large neutral amino acids. This ratio *may be elevated by carbohydrate intake,* which induces insulin release and the uptake of many large-chain amino acids into peripheral tissues. Conversely, high-protein foods tend to be relatively low in tryptophan, thus lowering this ratio. The administration of specialized low-tryptophan diets has been found to produce significant declines in brain serotonin levels. Following tryptophan hydroxylation, 5-HTP is rapidly decarboxylated by aromatic amino acid decarboxylase to form serotonin.

5.16 The answer is E

The basal ganglia, a subcortical group of gray matter nuclei, appear to mediate postural tone. There are four functionally distinct ganglia: the striatum, the pallidum, the substantia nigra, and the subthalamic nucleus. The caudate nucleus plays an important role in the modulation of motor acts. When functioning properly, it acts as a gatekeeper to allow the motor system to perform only those acts that are goal directed. *Anatomic and functional neuroimaging studies have correlated decreased activation of the caudate with obsessive-compulsive behavior. The caudate also shrinks dramatically in Huntington's disease.* This disorder is characterized by rigidity, on which is gradually superimposed choreiform or "dancing" movements. Psychosis may be a prominent feature of Huntington's disease, and suicide is not uncommon.

The globus pallidus contains two parts. The internal and external parts of the globus pallidus are nested within the concavity of the putamen. The globus pallidus receives input from the corpus striatum and projects fibers to the thalamus. *This structure may be severely damaged in Wilson's disease* and in carbon monoxide poisoning, which are characterized by dystonic posturing and flapping movements of the arms and legs.

The substantia nigra is named the black substance because the presence of melanin pigment causes it to appear black to the naked eye. It *degenerates in Parkinson's disease (not Alzheimer's disease). Parkinsonism* is characterized by rigidity and tremor and is associated with depression in over 30 percent of the cases.

Lesions in the subthalamic nucleus yield ballistic movements, which are sudden limb jerks of such velocity that they are compared to projectile movement (hemiballismus).

5.17 The answer is E (none)

Epilepsy is associated with a range of psychiatric disorders; however, *most patients with epilepsy have no other comorbid psychiatric conditions.* Studies from communities, epilepsy clinics, and psychiatric hospitals demonstrate an increased prevalence of psychiatric problems among epileptic patients as compared to nonepileptic patients. Among epileptic patients, much of the psychopathology results from electrophysiological, structural, or chemical changes in the temporal limbic system, and, possibly, the frontal lobes. Although most patients with epilepsy are healthy, one-fourth or more have *schizophreniform psychoses, depression, personality changes,* or *hyposexuality.* These behavioral changes may be chronic and present between seizure episodes. Other behaviors are episodic and directly related to the seizure discharges. Epileptic patients may have auras with psychic content, nonconvulsive status epilepticus, prodromal symptoms, postictal confusion, or a periictal psychosis that is distinct from the schizophreniform psychosis of epilepsy.

5.18 The answer is B

MRI studies *have provided some evidence that there may be structural brain changes in major depressive disorder.* Although there have been fewer studies of mood disorders than of schizophrenia, some consistent findings have emerged. In major depressive disorder, smaller volumes of the frontal lobe, the cerebellum, the caudate, and the putamen have been reported. On the basis of these observations, neuroanatomic models of mood regulation involving specific frontosubcortical circuits have been proposed.

In patients with bipolar I disorder, the most commonly reported finding is the presence of an enlarged third ventricle. As the third ventricle lies adjacent to the hypothalamus, some researchers have suggested that hypothalamic dysfunction may play a role in the pathogenesis of bipolar I disorder. Less commonly, decreased volumes of the cerebellum and temporal lobes have also been noted.

In terms of pathological findings, several groups have reported an increased incidence of white matter hyperintensities in individuals with bipolar I disorder; unfortunately, neither the cause nor the clinical significance of these hyperintensities has been clearly established.

Even with the increased resolution provided by MRI scanning, it remains *as yet unproved (not proved) whether there are relatively specific structural brain changes in patients with schizophrenia or if cerebral mass reduction is nonspecific.* Several studies have provided convincing data regarding reduced volume in specific cortical regions, including prefrontal cortex and temporal cortical regions. Such changes have even been found in patients early in the course of illness, suggesting that the structural changes observed in the cortex are present at the onset of the illness and do not stem from progression of the illness or from iatrogenic factors. *Enlargement of caudate volume* has also been reported early in the course of the illness, but multiple studies suggest that caudate enlargement may be secondary to treatment with typical dopamine-receptor antagonist agents. More recently it has been suggested that this enlargement recedes with clozapine (Clozaril) treatment.

Of the substance abuse disorders, alcohol dependence has been the most thoroughly studied using MRI. *Current evidence suggests that alcohol dependence leads to generalized reductions in brain mass* as reflected by decreases in cortical gray and white matter and increased cerebrospinal fluid volume of the cerebral ventricles, particularly the lateral ventricles. Many of the changes may be at least partially reversed during sustained periods of abstinence. *MRI is superior (not inferior) to CT in visualizing gray versus white matter.*

5.19 The answer is B

Fluorine-18 [^{18}F]-fluorodeoxyglucose (FDG) is an analogue that the brain cannot metabolize. Glucose is by far the predominant energy source available to brain cells, and its utilization is therefore a highly sensitive indicator of the rate of brain metabolism. Thus, the brain regions with the highest metabolic rate and the highest blood flow take up the most FDG but are unable to metabolize and excrete the usual metabolic products. The concentration of ^{18}F builds up in these neurons and is detected by the PET camera. FDG PET, therefore, measures glucose metabolism.

Each of the other choices measures blood flow rather than metabolism. Blood flow generally is proportional to brain metabolism and may be measured by a wider variety of clinical techniques. *Xenon-133* is a noble gas that is inhaled directly and is detected by SPECT scanners. The xenon quickly enters the blood and is distributed to areas of the brain as a function of regional blood flow. It may therefore be referred to as the regional cerebral blood flow (rCBF) technique. Because of technical factors, xenon SPECT can measure blood flow only on the surface of the brain. This limitation is important because many mental tasks require communication between the cortex and subcortical structures, and the latter activity is missed by xenon SPECT. Assessment of blood flow over the whole brain with SPECT requires the injectable tracers, *technetium-99* (^{99}Tc) *d,l-hexamethylpropyleneamine oxime* (*HMPAO*) SPECT.

These radiotracers are highly lipophilic, cross the blood-brain barrier rapidly, and enter cells. Once inside a cell, the ligands are enzymatically converted to charged ions, which remain trapped in the cell. Thus, over time, the tracers are concentrated in areas of relatively higher blood flow. Although blood flow is usually assumed to be the major variable tested in HMPAO SPECT, local variations in the permeability of the blood-brain barrier and in the enzymatic conversion of the ligands in cells also contribute to regional differences in signal levels. In *nitrogen-13* (^{13}N) PET, the radioactive nitrogen isotope (^{13}N) is usually linked to another molecule that is distributed into cells as a function of blood flow.

5.20 The answer is E (all)

Arousal, or the establishment and maintenance of an awake state, appears to require at least three brain regions. Within the brainstem, *the ascending reticular activating system (ARAS), a diffuse set of neurons, appears to set the level of consciousness.* The ARAS projects to the intralaminar nuclei of the thalamus, and these nuclei in turn project widely throughout the cortex. Electrophysiological studies show that *both the thalamus and the cortex fire rhythmic bursts of neuronal activity* at the rates of 20 to 40 cycles per second. During sleep, these bursts are not synchronized. *During wakefulness, the ARAS stimulates the thalamic intralaminar* nuclei, which in turn coordinate the oscillations of different cortical regions. The greater the synchronization, the higher the level of wakefulness. The absence of arousal produces stupor and coma. In general, *small discrete lesions of the ARAS may produce a stuporous state*, whereas at the hemispheric level, large bilateral lesions are required to cause the same depression in alertness. One particularly unfortunate but instructive condition involving extensive, permanent bilateral cortical dysfunction is the persistent vegetative state. Sleep–wake cycles may be preserved, and the eyes may appear to gaze, but there is no registering of the external world and no evidence of conscious thought.

5.21 The answer is D

The maintenance of attention appears to require an intact right *frontal lobe.* For example, a widely used test of persistence requires scanning and identifying only the letter "A" from a long list of random letters. *Normal individuals can usually maintain performance of such a task for several minutes, but in patients with right frontal lobe dysfunction, this capacity is curtailed severely.* Lesions of similar size in other regions of the cortex usually do not affect persistence tasks. In contrast, the more generally adaptive skill of maintaining a coherent line of thought is distributed diffusely throughout the cortex. Major causes of confusion are listed in Table 5.1.

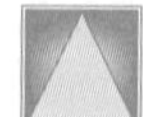

Table 5.1
Major Causes of Acute Confusion

Toxic
Prescription drugs
Nonprescription drugs
Drug withdrawal
Metabolic
Hypoxia
Hypoglycemia
Uremia
Hepatic disease
Thiamine deficiency
Electrolyte disturbances
Endocrinopathies
Infectious and inflammatory
Meningitis
Encephalitis
Vasculitis
Abscess
Epileptic
Postictal state
Complex partial status epilepticus
Absence status epilepticus
Vascular
Stroke
Subarachnoid hemorrhage
Traumatic
Concussion
Severe traumatic brain injury
Neoplastic
Deep midline tumors
Increased intracranial pressure
Postsurgical
Preoperative atropine
Hypoxia
Analgesics
Electrolyte imbalance
Fever

Reprinted with permission from Filley CM. *Neurobehavioral Anatomy.* Niwot, CO: University Press of Colorado; 1995:52.

5.22 The answer is C

The most famous human subject in the study of memory is H. M., a man with intractable epilepsy, whose entire hippocampus and amygdala were surgically removed. The epilepsy was thus controlled, but he was left with *a complete inability to form and recall memories of facts.* The finding that H. M.'s *learning and memory skills were relatively preserved* has led to the suggestion that factual memory may be separate within the brain from skill-related memory. A complementary deficit in skill-related memory with preservation of factual memory may be seen in individuals with Parkinson's disease, in whom dopaminergic neurons of the nigrostriatal tract degenerate. Because this deficit in skill-related memory can be ameliorated with levodopa, which is thought to potentiate dopaminergic neurotransmission in the nigrostriatal pathway, a role has been postulated for dopamine in skill-related memory. Additional case reports have implicated the amygdala and the afferent and efferent fiber tracts of the hippocampus as being essential to the formation of memories. Lesional studies have also suggested a mild lateralization of hippocampal function in which the left hippocampus is more efficient at forming verbal memories and the right hippocampus tends to form nonverbal memories. After unilateral lesions in humans, however, the remaining hippocampus may compensate to a large extent. Medical causes of amnesia include alcoholism, seizures, migraine, drugs, vitamin deficiencies, trauma, strokes, tumors, infections, and degenerative diseases. *Ataxia and loss of vision are unrelated to the hippocampus and amygdalae.*

5.23 The answer is C

Several studies have suggested a hemispheric dichotomy within the cortex of emotional representation. The left hemisphere houses the analytical mind but may have a limited emotional repertoire. Lesions to the right hemisphere, which cause profound functional deficits, may be noted with indifference by the intact left hemisphere. *The denial of illness (called anosognosia) and inability to move the left hand are associated with injury to the right hemisphere.*

In contrast, *left hemisphere lesions*, which cause profound aphasia, *may trigger a catastrophic depression*, as the intact right hemisphere struggles with the realization of the loss. The right hemisphere appears dominant for affect, socialization, and body image.

Damage to the left hemisphere produces intellectual disorder and a loss of the narrative aspect of dreams. Damage to the right hemisphere produces affective disorders, loss of the visual aspects of dreams, *and a failure to respond to humor*, shadings of metaphor, and connotations.

5.24 The answer is A

Within the hemispheres, the temporal and frontal lobes play a prominent role in emotion. The temporal lobe exhibits a high frequency of epileptic foci. TLE is of particular interest in psychiatry because temporal lobe seizures may often manifest bizarre behavior without the classic grand mal shaking movements caused by seizures in the motor cortex. *A proposed TLE personality is characterized by hyposexuality, emotional intensity, and a perseverative approach to interactions, termed viscosity.* Patients with left TLE may generate references to personal destiny and philosophical themes and may display a humorless approach to life. In contrast, patients with right TLE may display excessive emotionality, ranging from elation to sadness. Although TLE patients may display excessive aggression between seizures, the seizure itself may evoke fear.

The inverse of a TLE personality appears in people with bilateral injury to the temporal lobes after head trauma, cardiac arrest, herpes simplex encephalitis, or in Pick's disease. This lesion resembles the one described in the Kluver-Bucy syndrome, an experimental model of temporal lobe ablation in monkeys. *Behavior in this syndrome is characterized by hypersexuality, placidity, a tendency to explore the environment with the mouth, inability to recognize the emotional significance of visual stimuli, and constantly shifting attention, called hypermetamorphosis.*

5.25 The answer is B

The diencephalic structures involved in memory include the mammillary bodies, the medial dorsal thalamic nuclei, the internal medullary lamina, and the mamillothalamic tracts. Degeneration of the mammillary bodies is the neuropathological hallmark of a Korsakoff's psychosis. The mammillary bodies might functionally be of importance as repositories of neurotransmitters vital to memory. *Korsakoff's syndrome is the classic example of diencephalic amnesia.*

The hippocampi have primary roles in new learning and anterograde memory but not in retrograde memory. Hippocampi are involved in explicit or declarative memory but not in implicit memory, such as the nonconscious, automatic performance of previously learned skills (e.g., putting a golf ball or driving a car). The frequency of motor vehicle accidents makes *traumatic brain injury* (TBI) the fastest growing etiology for amnestic disorders. The temporal lobes are at particular risk for high-speed impact-related trauma, as they abut the bony prominences of the temporal bone. Head trauma, particularly closed head injury (also known as concussion), produces a well-circumscribed amnestic disorder.

Laterality refers to the hemispheric specialization of certain types of memory; it is not a form of amnesia. Unilateral damage to either hippocampus produces deficits in memory related to its function. However, profound amnestic syndromes are not seen unless there is bilateral damage. *Transient global amnesia* causes sudden and severe attacks of forgetful confusion for time, places and other people. The prognosis for transient global amnesia is good with the confusion quickly clearing up and a total recovery, unlike Korsakoff's syndrome where the prognosis is variable.

Answers 5.26–5.30

5.26 The answer is D

5.27 The answer is A

5.28 The answer is C

5.29 The answer is E

5.30 The answer is B

Huntington's disease is an autosomal dominant genetic condition, and therefore there is usually a family history of the disease. Usually diagnosed in the late 30s or early 40s, Huntington's disease affects men and women equally. Emotional symptoms often appear early and include irritability, depression, or psychosis. Later, cognitive disturbance appears; this is marked by psychomotor slowing, loss of spontaneity, and memory defect. Motor abnormalities, due to reduction in levels of GABA and acetylcholine, include the development of choreoathetotic movements, which eventually yield to profound bradykinesia.

Vascular dementia, like other dementias, includes loss of short-term memory, loss of sense of time, and a progressive decline in other abilities. However, in vascular dementia, the memory loss is typically much more variable than in Alzheimer's disease and patients can be much better on some days than others. There may be long periods with no change in the memory loss, and then an episode of acute confusion (often associated with a new mini stroke) followed by a step down in the person's memory. Other characteristic features of vascular dementia are that people usually have a greater degree of awareness of their disability than is the case in Alzheimer's disease. There may be a relative preservation of personality and an increased likelihood of problems with unpredictable behavior or changeable emotions.

One-third of asymptomatic individuals with HIV and one-half of individuals with acquired immunodeficiency syndrome (AIDS) show evidence of cognitive impairment. Those individuals with *HIV-associated dementia complex* appear apathetic and slowed. Apathy is a common early symptom, often causing a noticeable withdrawal by the patient from social activity. In some cases, the dementia is not due to the effects of HIV on the CNS but rather to the effects of accompanying opportunistic lesions of the brain (e.g., toxoplasmosis and lymphoma), in which case dementia should be attributed to those lesions. Overall, HIV-associated dementia is rapidly progressive, usually ending in death within 2 years.

Due to a transmissible prion, *Creutzfeldt-Jakob disease* is characterized by dementia, periodic bursts of EEG activity, involuntary movements (often myoclonic or choreoathetotic in nature), and ataxia. Patients with CJD may become rather withdrawn and forgetful, and soon develop problems in finding the right words and having a conversation. Brain imaging may show nonspecific atrophy. Usually, the disease develops after 40 years of age and progresses rapidly over the course of several months.

Pick's disease usually appears in a patient's 40s or 50s, an earlier age than other types of dementia such as Alzheimer's disease. The disorder affects the frontal and temporal lobes of the brain, making this one of several forms of frontotemporal dementia. Pick's disease is characterized by personality change, including disinhibited behavior and language abnormalities, later followed by deterioration in memory. Structural brain imaging often reveals frontal atrophy. At autopsy, intraneuronal Pick inclusion bodies are identified.

Answers 5.31–5.33

5.31 The answer is C

5.32 The answer is A

5.33 The answer is B

The frontal lobes, the region that determines how the brain acts on its knowledge, constitute a category unto themselves. In comparative neuroanatomical studies, the massive size of the frontal lobes is the main feature that distinguishes the human brain from that of other primates and that lends it uniquely human qualities. Within the prefrontal cortex, there are three regions, lesions of which produce distinct syndromes: the orbitofrontal, the dorsolateral, and the medial.

Dysfunction of the *orbitofrontal area* causes disinhibition and lack of remorse. Insight and judgment are impaired. The *dorsolateral area* appears to be the executive headquarters of the brain. Lesions in this region lead to deficiencies of planning and motivation. Patients may be unable to use foresight and feedback to maintain goal directedness, focus, and sustained effort. Dorsolateral frontal lobe injury may also produce mood disorders. The *medial area* appears to initiate a wide range of activities. Ablation of this region may produce profound apathy characterized by limited spontaneous movement, gesture, and speech. In the extreme, there may be a state of akinetic mutism, without any initiation of activity at all.

Answers 5.34–5.38

5.34 The answer is A

5.35 The answer is C

5.36 The answer is D

5.37 The answer is E

5.38 The answer is B

The major site of *serotonergic cell bodies* is in the upper pons and the midbrain—specifically, the *median and dorsal raphe nuclei*. These neurons project to the basal ganglia, the limbic system, and the cerebral cortex.

The major concentration of *norepinephrine* in the cell bodies that project upward in the brain is in the *locus ceruleus* in the pons. The axons of these neurons project through the medial forebrain bundle to the cerebral cortex, the limbic system, the thalamus, and the hypothalamus.

A group of *acetylcholine* producing neurons in the *nucleus basalis of Meynert* project to the cerebral cortex, the limbic system, the hypothalamus, and the thalamus. Some patients with dementia of the Alzheimer's type or Down's syndrome appear to have degeneration of the neurons in the nucleus basalis of Meynert.

The three most important *dopaminergic* producing tracts for psychiatry are the nigrostriatal tract, the mesolimbic-mesocortical tract, and the tuberoinfundibular tract. The nigrostriatal tract projects from its cell bodies in the *substantia nigra* to the corpus striatum. When the dopamine (D_2) receptors at the end of this tract are blocked by classic antipsychotic drugs, parkinsonian side effects emerge. In Parkinson's disease the nigrostriatal tract degenerates and results in the motor symptoms of the disease. Because of the significant association between Parkinson's disease and depression, the nigrostriatal tract may also be involved with the control of mood, in addition to its classic role in motor control.

The receptor for the inhibitory amino acid neurotransmitter *glycine is present in highest quantities in the spinal cord*. Mutations in the glycine receptor cause a rare neurological condition called hyperekplexia, which is characterized by an exaggerated startle response.

Answers 5.39–5.43

5.39 The answer is A

5.40 The answer is A

5.41 The answer is C

5.42 The answer is B

5.43 The answer is A

In the early stages of human brain development, three primary vesicles can be identified in the neural tube: the *prosencephalon*, the *mesencephalon*, and the *rhombencephalon*. Subsequently, *the prosencephalon divides to become the telencephalon and the diencephalon*. The telencephalon gives rise to the cerebral cortex, the hippocampal formation, the amygdala, and some components of the basal ganglia. The diencephalon becomes the thalamus, the hypothalamus, and several other related structures. *The mesencephalon gives rise to the midbrain structures of the adult brain. The rhombencephalon divides into the metencephalon and the myelencephalon*. The metencephalon gives rise to the *pons and the cerebellum*; the medulla is the derivative of the myelencephalon. See Table 5.2.

Answers 5.44–5.47

5.44 The answer is A

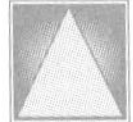

Table 5.2
Derivatives of the Neural Tube

Primary Vesicles	Secondary Vesicles	Brain Components
Prosencephalon	Telencephalon	Cerebral cortex Hippocampus Amygdala Striatum
	Diencephalon	Thalamus Hypothalamus Epithalamus
Mesencephalon	Mesencephalon	Midbrain
Rhombencephalon	Mesencephalon	Pons Cerebellum
	Myelencephalon	Medulla

5.45 The answer is A

5.46 The answer is B

5.47 The answer is B

Hemispheric lateralization of function is a key feature of higher cortical processing. The primary sensory cortices for touch, vision, hearing, smell, and taste are represented bilaterally. However, *recognition of faces* appears localized to the left brain. The clearest known example of hemispheric lateralization is the localization *of language functions* to the left hemisphere. *Prosody*, the emotional components of language, appears to be localized in the right brain.

The maintenance of attention appears to require an intact right frontal lobe. One widely diagnosed disorder of attention is attention-deficit/hyperactivity disorder (ADHD). No pathological findings have been associated consistently with this disorder. Functional neuroimaging studies have variously documented either frontal lobe or right hemisphere hypometabolism in ADHD patients.

Answers 5.48–5.52

5.48 The answer is D

5.49 The answer is C

5.50 The answer is A

5.51 The answer is B

5.52 The answer is E

Blockade of *anticholinergic and cholinergic* receptors is a common pharmacodynamic effect of many psychotropic drugs. *Blockage of these receptors leads to the commonly seen side effects of blurred vision, dry mouth, constipation, and difficulty in initiating urination.* Excessive blockage of cholinergic receptors causes confusion and delirium.

Melatonin is secreted from the pineal body when the eye perceives darkness, and its release is inhibited when the eye perceives light. *Melatonin is synthesized from serotonin* by the action of two enzymes: serotonin-*N*-acetylase anal 5-hydroxyindole-*O*-methyltransferase. Melatonin is involved in the regulation of circadian rhythms and has been implicated in the pathophysiology of depression.

Substances that affect the dopamine system include amphetamine and cocaine. *Amphetamines cause the release of dopamine and cocaine blocks the uptake of dopamine.* Thus, both substances increase the amount of dopamine present in the synapse. Cocaine and methamphetamine (Desoxyn) are among the most addicting substances. Their use may permanently deplete the brain's stores of dopamine. The dopaminergic systems may be particularly involved in the brain's so-called reward system, and this involvement may explain the high addiction potential of cocaine. Mutant "knockout mice," in which the dopamine transport gene has been experimentally deleted, do not respond biochemically or behaviorally to cocaine. This suggests that the dopamine transporter is necessary for the pharmacological effects of cocaine.

The precursor amino acid to *serotonin* is tryptophan. *Dietary variations in tryptophan can measurably affect serotonin levels in the brain.* Tryptophan depletion causes irritability and hunger, whereas tryptophan supplementation may induce sleep, relieve anxiety, and increase a sense of well-being. Once synthesized, serotonin is packaged into vesicles for release upon the arrival of an action potential. The synaptic action of serotonin concludes by reuptake into the presynaptic terminal.

The components of the *growth hormone* axis are growth hormone–releasing hormone (GHRH) and growth hormone–release-inhibiting factor (GHRIF), also known as somatostatin, from the hypothalamus, and growth hormone itself from the anterior pituitary. *Growth hormone is released in pulses throughout the day.* The pulses are closer together during the first hours of sleep than at other times. Growth hormone regulation has been studied particularly in schizophrenia and mood disorders, in which some data suggest a disordered regulation of the growth hormone axis.

Answers 5.53–5.55

5.53 The answer is B

5.54 The answer is A

5.55 The answer is C

The skillful use of the hands is called praxis, and deficits in skilled movements are termed apraxias. The three levels of apraxia are limb-kinetic, ideomotor, and ideational. *Limb-kinetic apraxia is the inability to use the contralateral hand in the presence of preserved strength*; it results from isolated lesions in the supplementary motor area, which contains neurons that stimulate functional sequences of neurons in the motor strip. *Ideomotor apraxia is the inability to perform an isolated motor act upon command*, despite preserved comprehension, strength, and spontaneous performance of the same act. Ideomotor apraxia simultaneously affects both limbs and involves functions so specialized that they are localized to only one hemisphere. *Ideational apraxia occurs when the individual components of a sequence cannot be organized and executed as a whole.* For example, the sequence of opening an envelope, removing the letter, unfolding it, and placing it on the table cannot be performed in order, even though the individual acts can be performed in isolation.

6

Contributions of the Psychosocial Sciences to Human Behavior

The psychosocial sciences include psychology, anthropology, sociology, ethology, and epidemiology, among others. Our understanding of human behavior has been enriched by the work of professionals in each of these fields.

Students should be able to define these disciplines, and a brief description of each follows: *Psychology* is concerned with behavior and its related mental and physiological processes. There are several types, ranging from *clinical psychology* that specializes in applying psychological theory to persons with emotional or behavioral disorders to *educational psychology,* which is the application of psychological principles to problems of teaching and learning. *Anthropology* is the branch of science concerned with the origin and development of humans in all their physical, social, and cultural relationships. *Sociology* is the study of the collective behaviors of human beings, including the developmental structure and interactions of their social institutions. *Ethology* is the study of animal behaviors and *epidemiology* is the study of the various factors that determine the frequency and distribution of diseases.

Jean Piaget (1896–1980) focused on the ways that children think and develop cognitive abilities, describing four major stages leading to more adult organizations of thought. John Bowlby (1907–1990) focused on the development of attachment and the belief that normal attachment in infancy is essential to ongoing healthy development. René Spitz (1887–1974) described anaclitic depression, or hospitalism, in which normal children who were separated for long periods from adequate caregiving in institutions failed to thrive and, therefore, became depressed and nonresponsive. Ethologists, such as Konrad Lorenz (1903–1989) and Harry Harlow (1905–1981), studied bonding and attachment behaviors in animals, and showed how studying animal behavior could help to illuminate human behavior.

Learning theory was developed by such behavioral researchers as Ivan Pavlov (1849–1936), John B. Watson (1878–1958), and B. F. Skinner (1904–1990). Tenets of learning theory, including operant and classical conditioning, underlie behavioral treatments of various mental disorders.

The questions and answers below will help students test their knowledge of the subjects highlighted.

HELPFUL HINTS

The student should know the following terms, theoreticians, and concepts.

- abstract thinking
- accommodation
- acculturation
- adaptation
- aggression
- Mary Ainsworth
- anaclitic depression
- animistic thinking
- anxiety hierarchy
- *Aplysia*
- assimilation
- attachment
- attachment phases
- attribution theory
- aversive stimuli
- basic study design
- behavior disorders
- Ruth Benedict
- bias
- biostatistics
- bonding
- John Bowlby
- catharsis
- chronic stress
- cognitive dissonance
- cognitive organization
- cognitive strategies
- cognitive triad
- concrete operations
- contact comfort
- cross-cultural studies and syndromes: amok, *latah, windigo, piblokto, curandero, esperitismo*, voodoo
- culture-bound syndromes
- deductive reasoning
- deviation, significance
- double-blind method
- drift hypothesis
- egocentric
- epidemiology
- epigenesis
- escape and avoidance conditioning
- ethology
- experimental neurosis
- extinction
- family types, studies
- Faris and Dunham
- fixed and variable ratios
- formal operations
- frequency
- frustration-aggression hypothesis
- genetic epistemology
- Harry Harlow
- Hollingshead and Redlich
- Holmes and Rahe
- hospitalism
- Clark L. Hull
- illness behavior
- imprinting
- incidence
- indirect surveys
- inductive reasoning
- information processing
- inhibition

- Eric Kandel
- learned helplessness
- learning theory
- Alexander Leighton
- H. S. Liddell
- lifetime expectancy
- Konrad Lorenz
- Margaret Mead
- Midtown Manhattan study
- monotropic
- Monroe County study
- motivation
- New Haven study
- normative
- object permanence
- operant and classical conditioning
- operant behavior
- organization
- Ivan Petrovich Pavlov
- phenomenalistic causality
- Jean Piaget
- positive and negative reinforcement
- preattachment stage
- preoperational stage
- prevalence
- protest-despair-detachment
- punishment
- randomization
- reciprocal determinism
- reciprocal inhibition
- reliability
- respondent behavior
- risk factors
- schema
- segregation hypothesis
- Hans Selye
- semiotic function
- sensorimotor stage
- sensory deprivation
- separation anxiety
- signal indicators
- B. F. Skinner
- social causation and selection theory
- social class and mental disorders
- social isolation and separation
- social learning
- sociobiology
- René Spitz
- stimulus generalization
- Stirling County study
- strange situation
- stranger anxiety
- surrogate mother
- syllogistic reasoning
- symbolization
- systematic desensitization
- tension-reduction theory
- therapist monkeys
- Nikolaas Tinbergen
- type I and type II errors
- use of controls
- validity
- variation, average
- vulnerability theory
- John B. Watson
- Joseph Wolpe

QUESTIONS

Directions

Each question or incomplete statement below is followed by five suggested responses or completions. Select the *one* that is *best* in each case.

6.1 In which of the following age groups is the stage of preoperational thought present?

A. Birth to 2 years
B. 2 to 7 years
C. 7 to 11 years
D. 11 through the end of adolescence
E. None of the above

6.2 Premack's principle states that

A. high frequency behaviors can be used to reinforce low-frequency behavior
B. a person can learn by imitating the behavior of another person
C. persons will attribute others' behavior to stable their own personality traits
D. the more people feel capable of controlling a threatening event, the less anxious they will be
E. persons will attribute their own behavior to situational causes

6.3 Learning can be reflected in neural changes in which of the following ways?

A. The growth of new neurons
B. The expansion of existing neurons
C. Changes in connectivity between existing neurons
D. All of the above
E. None of the above

6.4 Cross-cultural studies

A. are free from experimental bias
B. show that depression is not a universally expressed symptom
C. show that incest is not a universal taboo
D. show that schizophrenic persons are universally stigmatized as social outcasts
E. show that the nuclear family of mother, father, and children is a universal unit

6.5 True statements about violence and aggression include all of the following *except*

A. In the United States, homicide is the second leading cause of death among people 15 to 25 years of age.
B. A young black man is 8 times more likely to be murdered than is a white man of the same age.
C. Less than 50 percent of people who commit homicides or assaultive behavior have imbibed significant amounts of alcohol immediately beforehand.
D. The best predictor of violent acts is a previous violent act.
E. More than 70 percent of homicides are committed with handguns.

6.6 Which of the following statements regarding punishment is *not* true?

A. Punishment is often more useful than reinforcement.
B. Punishment produces aggressive behavior.
C. Punishment is less useful than extinction.
D. Use of punishment should be carefully supervised.
E. Self-injurious behaviors are the main instances where punishment should be used.

6.7 Which of the following chromosomal abnormalities has been implicated as having an influence on aggressive behavior?

A. 45-XO
B. 47-XYY
C. 47-XXY

D. 48-XXXY
E. 47-XXX

6.8 Learned helplessness studies

A. used Rhesus monkeys as experimental animals
B. are used as paradigms for clinical depression in humans
C. demonstrated that outcomes were contingent on behavior
D. suggest that cortisol may be specifically decreased in helpless animals
E. involved peer separations

6.9 Which of the following is *not* characteristic of a primate totally deprived of social contact?

A. Abnormally fearful of peers
B. Unable to nurture their young
C. No recovery if greater than 12 months isolation
D. Rapid reattachment if mother returns
E. Self-orality is common

6.10 Prevalence is the

A. proportion of a population that has a condition at one moment in time
B. ratio of persons who acquire a disorder during a year's time
C. risk of acquiring a condition at some time
D. standard deviation
E. rate of first admissions to a hospital for a disorder

6.11 Asian patients seem to achieve a clinical response comparable to those of non-Asian patients, even though they require a significantly lower dose of

A. lithium
B. antipsychotics
C. tricyclics
D. benzodiazepines
E. all of the above

6.12 The "choo-choo" phenomenon is associated with which of the following types of social deprivation in monkeys?

A. Total isolation-reared monkeys
B. Mother-only-reared monkeys
C. Peer-only-reared monkeys
D. Partial isolation-reared monkeys
E. Separation-reared monkeys

6.13 The increased frequency of aggressive behavior in certain children defined as abnormal has been correlated with all of the following *except*

A. brain injury
B. faulty identification models
C. cultural environment
D. violence in movies
E. curiosity

6.14 Which of the following statistical procedures is used to evaluate the frequency of events in a population?

A. Analysis of Variance (ANOVA)
B. Chi-squared test
C. T-test
D. Discriminant analysis
E. Z-score

6.15 Attachment theory states that

A. Infants are generally polytropic in their attachments.
B. Attachment occurs instantaneously between the mother and the child.
C. Attachment is synonymous with bonding.
D. Attachment disorders may lead to a failure to thrive.
E. Separation anxiety is most common when an infant is 5 months old.

6.16 Which of the following statements regarding crossover studies is *true?*

A. Eliminate selection bias.
B. Is a variation of the double-blind study.
C. Contain a treatment group and a control group.
D. Are a type of prospective study.
E. All of the above

Directions

Each set of lettered headings below is followed by a list of numbered phrases. For each numbered phrase, select

A. if the item is associated with A only
B. if the item is associated with B only
C. if the item is associated with both A and B
D. if the item is associated with neither A nor B

Questions 6.17–6.21

A. Behavioral Model of learning
B. Psychoanalytic Model of learning

6.17 Theory is based on experimentation
6.18 Subjective methods of interpretation
6.19 Childhood experiences are the focus of the analysis
6.20 Testable hypotheses that can be evaluated through experimentation
6.21 Theory is predominantly based on case histories

Questions 6.22–6.27

A. Classical conditioning
B. Operant conditioning

6.22 Instrumental conditioning
6.23 Learning takes place as a result of the contiguity of environmental events
6.24 Learning occurs as the consequence of action
6.25 Repeated pairing of a neutral stimulus with one that evokes a response
6.26 Ivan Petrovich Pavlov
6.27 B. F. Skinner

Directions

Each set of lettered headings below is followed by a list of numbered statements. For each numbered statement, select the *best* lettered heading. Each heading may be used once, more than once, or not at all.

Questions 6.28–6.29

A. Type I error
B. Type II error

6.28 When the null hypothesis is retained where it should have been rejected
6.29 When the null hypothesis is rejected where it should have been retained

Questions 6.30–6.34

A. Fixed-ratio schedule
B. Variable-ratio schedule
C. Fixed-interval schedule
D. Variable-interval schedule

6.30 Leads to the most rapid rate of response
6.31 Seen with the use of slot machines
6.32 Associated with scalloping
6.33 Generates an oscillating rate of response
6.34 Seen with the three-strike rule of baseball

Questions 6.35–6.38

A. Ivan Petrovich Pavlov
B. Eric Kandel
C. Konrad Lorenz
D. Harry Harlow

6.35 Imprinting
6.36 Surrogate mother
6.37 Experimental neurosis
6.38 *Aplysia*

Questions 6.39–6.42

A. John Bowlby
B. Harry Harlow
C. Mary Ainsworth
D. René Spitz

6.39 "Secure base" effect
6.40 Protest, despair, detachment
6.41 First described anaclitic depression
6.42 Primarily associated with ethological studies

Questions 6.43–6.47

A. Positive reinforcement
B. Negative reinforcement
C. Punishment
D. Classical conditioning

6.43 Anorexic woman begins eating and gaining weight in order to get out of the hospital
6.44 Child has his favorite toy taken away every time he wets his bed
6.45 A woman gives her dog a treat every time he sits when told
6.46 A man begins leaving home earlier in the morning to avoid rush hour traffic
6.47 Dog begins salivating to the sound of a bell after learning food is coming soon after

ANSWERS

6.1 The answer is B

The state of preoperational thought is present in children 2 to 7 years old. During this stage, children use symbols and language more extensively than in the sensorimotor stage. Thinking and reasoning are intuitive; children learn without the use of reasoning. Preoperational thought is midway between socialized adult thought and the completely autistic Freudian unconscious.

Piaget used the term sensorimotor to describe the first stage, present from birth to 2 years of age. Infants begin to learn through sensory observation, and they gain control of their motor functions through activity, exploration, and manipulation of the environment. *The stage of concrete operations is present in children from 7 to 11 years of age.* The stage of concrete operations is so named because in this period, children operate and act on the concrete, real, and perceivable world of objects and events. Egocentric thought is replaced by operational thought, which involves dealing with a wide array of information outside the child. Therefore, children can now see things from someone else's perspective.

The stage of formal operations is present from 11 years of age through the end of adolescence. This stage is named so because young persons' thought operates in a formal, highly logical, systematic, and symbolic manner. This stage is characterized by the ability to think abstractly, to reason deductively, and to define concepts. It is also characterized by the emergence of skills for dealing with permutations and combinations; young persons can grasp the concept of probabilities.

6.2 The answer is A

A concept developed by David Premack states that a behavior engaged in with high frequency can be used to reinforce a low-frequency behavior. In one experiment, Premack observed that children spent more time playing with a pinball machine than eating candy when both were freely available. When he made playing with the pinball machine contingent on eating a certain amount of candy, the children increased the amount of candy they ate. In a therapeutic application of this principle, patients with schizophrenia were observed to spend more time in a rehabilitation center sitting down doing nothing than they did working at a simple task. When being able to sit down for 5 minutes was made contingent on a certain amount of work, the work output was considerably increased, as was the skill acquisition. This principle is also known as Grandma's rule ("If you eat your spinach, you can have dessert").

The social learning theory relies on role modeling, identification, and human interactions. This theory states that *a person can learn by imitating the behavior of another person*, but personal factors are involved.

The attribution theory is a cognitive approach concerned with how a person perceives the causes of behavior. *According to the attribution theory, persons are likely to attribute their own behavior to situational causes but are likely to attribute others' behavior to stable internal dispositions (personality traits).*

The self-efficacy theory predicts that the more people feel capable of predicting and controlling threatening events, the less vulnerable they are to anxiety and stress disorders in response to traumatic experiences.

6.3 The answer is D (all)

The growth and selective connectivity of neurons is the basic mechanism of all learning and adaptation. Learning can be reflected in neural changes in a number of ways, including *(1) the growth of new neurons, (2) the expansion of existing neurons, and (3) the changes in the connectivity between existing neurons.* All of these changes are expressions of plasticity or the ability of the nervous system to change. The birth of new neurons, or neurogenesis, is a controversial field of study. Some recent research suggests that new neurons are generated in different areas of primate and human brains, especially in regions involved with new learning, such as the hippocampus, the amygdala, and the frontal and temporal lobes.

6.4 The answer is E

Cross-cultural studies examine and compare various cultures along a number of parameters: attitudes, beliefs, expectations, memories, opinions, roles, stereotypes, prejudices, and values. Usually, the cultures studied have differing languages and political organizations.

The nuclear family of mother, father, and children is a universal unit in all cultures. The extended family—in which grandparents, parents, children, and other relatives all live under the same roof—is no longer as common in the United States, but it is still prevalent in less industrialized cultures. In the United States, more than 85 percent of the men and women between the ages of 35 and 45 are husbands or wives in a nuclear family.

Cross-cultural studies *are not free from experimental bias;* in fact, they are subject to extreme bias because of problems in translation and other areas of information gathering. Questions have to be asked in ways that are clearly understood by the group under study. One of the best-known cross-cultural studies, *Psychiatric Disorder among the Yoruba* by Alexander Leighton, was his attempt to replicate in Nigeria the Stirling County study he had conducted in Canada. The study was criticized because not only did it fail to distinguish psychophysiological symptoms from those associated with infections, parasites, and nutritional diseases, but also it assumed that the indicators of sociocultural disintegration in Stirling County could be used among the Yoruba. All cultures are relative; that is, each must be examined within the context of its own language, customs, and beliefs.

6.5 The answer is C

People may have violent thoughts or fantasies but unless they lose control, thoughts do not become acts. Any set of conditions that produces increased aggressive impulses in the context of diminished control may produce violent acts. Situations with combinations of factors include toxic and organic states, developmental disabilities, florid psychosis, conduct disorder, and overwhelming psychological and environmental stress.

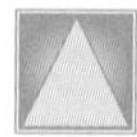

Table 6.1
Commonly Cited Predictors of Dangerousness to Others

High degree of intent to harm
Presence of a victim
Frequent and open threats
Concrete plan
Access to instruments of violence
History of loss of control
Chronic anger, hostility, or resentment
Enjoyment in watching or inflicting harm
Lack of compassion
Self-view as victim
Resentful of authority
Childhood brutality or deprivation
Decreased warmth and affection in home
Early loss of parent
Fire setting, bed-wetting, and cruelty to animals
Prior violent acts
Reckless driving

Table 6.1 summarizes some of the best-known concepts of violence predictors. *One of the best predictors of violent acts is a previous violent act.* Any predictor, however, is merely a guideline for the possibility of an increased risk for violence, and many potentially violent people do not fit any particular profile.

Violent acts are most often committed by persons who know or knew each other. Homicides are most prevalent among strangers (55 percent); *more than 70 percent of homicides are committed with handguns.* In the United States, *homicide is the second leading cause of death among people 15 to 25 years of age. Furthermore, a young black man is eight times more likely to be murdered than is a white man of the same age.*

Generally, the probability of aggressive behavior increases when people become psychologically decompensated, perhaps also when the onset of a mental disorder is rapid. Otherwise, little is known about the relationship between the course of illness and aggression. Episodic decompensation may occur in those who ingest large quantities of alcohol; *more than 50 percent (not less than 50 percent)* of *people who commit criminal homicides or assaultive behavior are reported to have imbibed significant amounts of alcohol immediately beforehand.*

6.6 The answer is A

Punishment is *less useful as a therapeutic procedure than reinforcement or extinction*, because it may produce unwanted effects, such as *aggressive behavior*, and the possibility of inflicting physical damage is always present. For the most part, punishment is *used only in situations in which the behavior to be changed is injurious to the patient.* A clinical example of such a condition is rumination disorder in which infants regurgitate their food mouthful by mouthful, which leads to malnutrition and dehydration and is frequently life threatening. One treatment is to use the principle of punishment, making an unpleasant event contingent on each episode of regurgitation.

The use of punishment in a clinical situation should be carefully supervised and should follow certain rules. The behavior to be addressed should have been resistant to appropriate behavior-change procedures involving the use of positive reinforcement. Behaviors incompatible with the problem behavior can often be reinforced, and the problem thus can be eliminated. In addition, the behavior to be changed should be severely incapacitating and should threaten physical integrity (e.g., the self-injurious behavior of some children with autistic disorders). Punishment procedures that cause tissue damage should not be used. The behavior to be changed should be observed, measured, and recorded, so that the effects of punishment and the amount of punishment used can be seen. If effectively used, punishment rapidly brings a behavior under control, and behaviors can then be built up with the use of positive reinforcement.

6.7 The answer is B

Behavior research involving the influence of chromosomes on aggressive behavior has concentrated primarily on abnormalities in X and Y chromosomes, particularly the *47-XYY syndrome.* Early studies indicated that persons with the syndrome could be characterized as tall, of below-average intelligence, and likely to be apprehended and in prison for engaging in criminal behavior. Subsequent studies indicated however, that, at most, the XYY syndrome contributes to aggressive behavior in only a small percentage of cases. Studies of the androgen and gonadotropin characteristics of persons with XYY syndrome have been inconclusive. However, *none of the other listed chromosomal abnormalities have been associated with increases in aggressive behavior.*

6.8 The answer is B

The animal model of learned helplessness relates closely to some important aspects of *clinical depression,* particularly cognitive aspects. Those cognitive aspects are reflected in feelings of helplessness and hopelessness. Etiological theories, as well as therapeutic approaches, have developed from that cognitive view of depression.

In the original experimental study with animals, *dogs (not monkeys) were observed in one of three situations.* In the first situation, they were put in harnesses and subjected to electric shock that they could terminate by touching a panel; not surprisingly, they learned to escape the shock rather quickly. In the second situation, the dogs were prepared as in the preceding situation, but when the shock was given, they were unable to terminate it. Finally, to control for the effect of the shock itself, dogs were put in harnesses but were not subjected to shock at all. In Phase 2 of the study, dogs were given electric shock while unharnessed in a shuttle box. Normally, dogs have no difficulty learning to avoid the shock by going to the other side of the box, which proved to be true for the dogs that had been exposed to escapable shock while in the harness. However, the dogs that had been exposed to inescapable shock failed to learn that they could escape from the electric shock in Phase 2 by jumping over a barrier that separated the two sides of the shuttle box. They were described as being initially agitated in reaction to the shock, but instead of running around frantically until they discovered that they could escape the shock by crossing the barrier, they would sit or lie down, whining quietly—that is, they acted as if they were helpless and incapable of escaping. The interpretation was that the inescapable shock they had experienced earlier made them unable to cope with the present situation. One explanation was that they had learned during their initial experience *that outcomes were not contingent on their behavior.* No matter what they did, it did no good; they learned to be helpless.

Studies suggest that *cortisol may be specifically elevated (not decreased) in helpless animals.* Norepinephrine depletions in the locus ceruleus also have been found. Peer separation studies have been used with *Rhesus monkeys.* In general, the behavioral reaction to *peer separation is* quite similar to that following maternal separation in terms of the classic protest-despair response. Furthermore, when peer groups are formed and separations are repeated, the response is seen with each separation.

6.9 The answer is D

It is the monkeys who are separated from their caretakers after a bond has developed, *not those who are totally isolated,* who show rapid reattachment when returned to their mother.

The name most associated with isolation and separation studies is Harry Harlow. His work showed that the long-term effects of 6 months of total social isolation produce adolescent monkeys that are both *abnormally aggressive and abnormally fearful.* The isolates *exhibit aggression against agemates who are more physically adept than they.*

Infant monkeys that survive a 3-month, rather than a 6-month, total social isolation can *make remarkable social adjustment through the development of play.*

Monkeys totally isolated for a 12-month period, however, *are totally unresponsive to the new physical and social world with which they are presented and do not recover.* Totally deprived monkeys also show an *inability to nurture their young,* as well as displaying *self-orality* and self-clasping.

6.10 The answer is A

Prevalence is the *proportion of a population that has a condition at one moment in time.* The *ratio of persons who acquire a disorder during a year's time* (new cases) is called the annual incidence. In a stable situation, the prevalence is approximately equal to the annual incidence times the average duration, measured in years, of the condition. The *risk of acquiring a condition at some time* in the future is the accumulation of age-specific annual incidence rates over a period of time.

Standard deviation (SD) is a statistical measure of variability within a set of values so defined that, for a normal distribution, about 68 percent of the values fall within one SD of the mean, and about 95 percent lie within two SDs of the mean. It is sometimes presented by Σ, the Greek letter sigma.

The rate of first admissions to a hospital for a disorder is the ratio of all first admissions to an average general hospital during a particular time.

6.11 The answer is E (all)

Asian patients require lower dosages of dopamine receptor antagonist (typical antipsychotic) medications than comparable non-Asian patients to achieve a desirable clinical outcome. Also, when treated on a fixed-dosage schedule, Asians seem to develop significantly greater extrapyramidal adverse effects. One study found a 52 percent higher plasma concentration of haloperidol (Haldol) in Chinese schizophrenic patients living in China than in non-Asian schizophrenic patients residing in the United States when both groups received treatment on a fixed-dosage schedule.

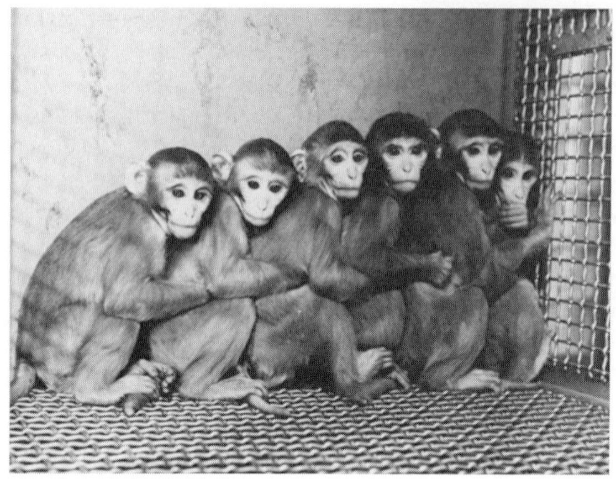

FIGURE 6.1
Choo-choo phenomenon in peer-only–reared infant rhesus monkeys.

Another study demonstrated that Chinese schizophrenic patients residing in Taiwan and Taipei achieved haloperidol plasma concentrations comparable to those of white, African-American, and Hispanic patients hospitalized in San Antonio while using significantly lower daily dosages of haloperidol.

As is the case with neuroleptics, studies with *tricyclic drugs have shown that average dosages prescribed for Asians are significantly lower* (up to 50 percent lower) than dosages prescribed in the United States for non-Asians. The reasons for this responsiveness have not been clearly established, although preliminary evidence suggests differential responsiveness of relevant receptors, differences in resulting plasma concentrations, or both.

Studies of prescription patterns as well as those comparing the pharmacokinetics and pharmacodynamics of benzodiazepines across ethnic groups have established the *enhanced sensitivity of Asians to the effects of benzodiazepines.* Typically prescribed doses are one-half to two-thirds those of similar nonminority populations. The ethnic differences in benzodiazepine metabolism are most often linked to polymorphisms in the (S)-mephenytoin phenotype, yielding a higher percentage of poor metabolizers in the Chinese ethnic group. Additional mechanisms, both genetic and environmental, have been invoked by other investigators.

As with tricyclic drugs, antipsychotics, and benzodiazepines, *Asians seem to achieve clinical responses comparable to those of non-Asian patients using significantly lower dosages and with serum concentrations of lithium 0.5 to 0.7 mEq/L versus the 0.8 to 1.2 mEq/L generally required by white populations.*

6.12 The answer is C

An area of animal research that has relevance to human behavior and psychopathology is the longitudinal study of nonhuman primates. Monkeys have been observed from birth to maturity, not only in their natural habitats and laboratory facsimiles but also in laboratory settings that involve various degrees of social deprivation early in life. Socially isolated monkeys are raised in varying degrees of isolation and are not permitted to develop normal attachment bonds. Social isolation techniques illustrate the effects of an infant's early social environment on subsequent development and separation techniques, which illustrate the effects of loss of a significant attachment figure. The *choo-choo phenomenon is observed in peer-only-reared infant rhesus monkeys* and is the actual physical alignment these monkeys have been observed to form, in addition to behavior such as becoming easily frightened, clinging to each other, being reluctant to explore, and engaging in minimal play. (Figure 6.1).

6.13 The answer is E

Curiosity and aggression show no correlation. In the normal child, aggression can be effectively understood in terms of the motives (for example, defense and mastery) for which aggressiveness is a suitable mediator. Its increased frequency in abnormal children can be correlated with defects in the organism, as in the case of *brain injury,* or with distortions in the child's environment, as in the case of *faulty identification models.* Moreover, the frequency of the display of aggressive behavior is a function of the child's *cultural environment.* Aggressive fantasy materials (*violence in movies,* crime comics, and television) rather than affording catharsis for instinctual aggressiveness generate the very tensions they profess to release.

A central issue is the meaning to be ascribed to the term "aggression." If a boy is observed taking apart a watch, that behavior may be aggressive if, for example, the watch belongs to the child's father, and the father has just punished him. However, if the watch is an old one in his stock of toys, the boy's motive may be curiosity about its mechanism, especially if he takes delight in reassembling it. If he strikes another child, that act may be motivated by aggression if the victim is the baby sister his parents have just embraced. Or the blow may be defensive if the victim has made a threatening gesture or has tried to seize the boy's favorite toy. Anecdotes make the point, but documented experimental examples of aggressive children are also available: children emulating adult models, children systematically subjected to frustration, and children watching films or television of aggressive behavior, all of whom show predictable increases in aggressiveness.

6.14 The answer is B

The *chi-square test* is used to evaluate the relative frequency or proportion of events in a population that fall into well-defined categories. Research on whether parents who were abused as children are more likely to abuse their children could be tested using the chi-square test of association. A *t-test* is a statistical procedure designed to compare two sets of observations. *Analysis of variance, or ANOVA,* is a set of statistical procedures designed to compare two or more groups of observations. *Discriminate analysis* is a multivariate method for finding the relation between a single discrete outcome and a linear combination of two or more predictors. The *z-score* is the deviation of a score from its group mean expressed in standard deviations.

6.15 The answer is D

Attachment disorders are characterized by biopsychosocial pathology that results from maternal deprivation, a lack of care by and interaction with the infant's mother or caretaker. Psychosocial dwarfism, separation anxiety disorder, avoidant personality disorder, depressive disorders, delinquency, learning disorders, borderline intelligence, and *failure to thrive have been traced to negative attachment experiences.* Failure to thrive results in the infant's being unable to maintain viability outside a hospital setting. When maternal care is deficient because the mother is mentally ill, because the child is institutionalized for a long time, or because the primary object of attachment dies, the child suffers emotional damage.

John Bowlby formulated a theory that states normal attachment is crucial to healthy development. According to Bowlby, attachment occurs when the infant has a warm, intimate, and continuous relationship with its mother, and both mother and infant find satisfaction and enjoyment. *Infants are generally monotropic, not polytropic, in their attachments,* but multiple attachments may also occur; attachment may be directed toward the father or a surrogate. *Attachment does not occur instantaneously between the mother and the child;* it is a gradually developing phenomenon. Attachment results in one person's wanting to be with a preferred person who is perceived as stronger, wiser, and able to reduce anxiety or distress. Attachment produces a feeling of security in the infant. It is a process that is facilitated by interaction between the mother and the infant. The amount of time together is less important than the quality of activity between the two.

Attachment is not synonymous with bonding; they are different phenomena. Bonding concerns the mother's feelings for her infant. It differs from attachment in that a mother does not normally rely on her infant as a source of security, a requirement of attachment behavior. A great deal of research on the bonding of a mother to her infant reveals that it occurs when they have skin-to-skin contact or other types of contact, such as voice and eye contact.

Separation from the attachment person may or may not produce intense anxiety, depending on the child's developmental level and the current phase of attachment. Separation anxiety is expressed as tearfulness or irritability, in a child who is isolated or separated from its mother or caretaker. *Separation anxiety is most common when an infant is 10 to 18 months of age (not 5 months),* and it disappears generally by the end of the third year. Table 6.2 delineates aspects of normal attachment at different ages.

6.16 The answer is E (all)

A crossover study is a variation of the double-blind study. The treatment group and the control or placebo group change places at some point, so that the placebo group gets the treatment and the treatment group now receives the placebo. *That procedure eliminates selection bias because,* if the treatment group improves in both instances and the placebo group does not, one can conclude that the makeup of the two groups was truly random. Each group serves as the control for the other.

Answers 6.17–6.21

6.17 The answer is A

6.18 The answer is B

6.19 The answer is B

6.20 The answer is A

6.21 The answer is B

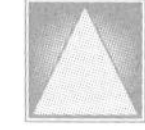

Table 6.2
Normal Attachment

Birth to 30 days
- Reflexes at birth
  - Rooting
  - Head turning
  - Sucking
  - Swallowing
  - Hand-mouth
  - Grasp
  - Digital extension
  - Crying—signal for particular kind of distress
  - Responsiveness and orientation to mother's face, eyes, and voice
- 4 days—anticipatory approach behavior at feeding
- 3 to 4 weeks—infant smiles preferentially to mother's voice

Age 30 days through 3 months
- Vocalization and gaze reciprocity further elaborated from 1 to 3 months; babbling at 2 months, more with the mother than with a stranger
- Social smile
- In strange situations increased clinging response to mother

Age 4 through 6 months
- Briefly soothed and comforted by sound of mother's voice
- Spontaneous, voluntary reaching for mother
- Anticipatory posturing to be picked up
- Differential preference for mother intensifies
- Subtle integration of responses to mother

Age 7 through 9 months
- Attachment behaviors further differentiated and focused specifically on mother
- Separation distress, stranger distress, strange-place distress

Age 10 through 15 months
- Crawls or walks toward mother
- Subtle facial expressions (coyness, attentiveness)
- Responsive dialogue with mother clearly established
- Early imitation of mother (vocal inflections, facial expression)
- More fully developed separation distress and mother preference
- Pointing gesture
- Walking to and from mother
- Affectively positive reunion responses to mother after separation or, paradoxically, short-lived, active avoidance or delayed protest

Age 16 months through 2 years
- Involvement in imitative jargon with mother (12 to 14 months)
- Head-shaking "no" (15 to 16 months)
- Transitional object used during the absence of mother
- Separation anxiety diminishes
- Mastery of strange situations and persons when mother is near
- Evidence of delayed imitation
- Object permanence
- Microcosmic symbolic play

Age 25 months through 3 years
- Able to tolerate separations from mother without distress when familiar with surroundings and given reassurances about mother's return
- Two- and three-word speech
- Stranger anxiety much reduced
- Object consistency achieved—maintains composure and psychosocial functioning without regression in absence of mother
- Microcosmic play and social play; cooperation with others begins

Based on material by Justin Call, M.D.

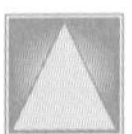

Table 6.3
Behavioral and Psychoanalytic Models

Behavioral Model	Psychoanalytic Model
Behavior is determined by current contingencies, reinforcement history, and genetic endowment	Behavior is determined by intrapsychic processes
Problem behavior is the focus of study and treatment	Behavior is but a symbol of intrapsychic processes and a symptom of unconscious conflict; the underlying conflict is the focus of treatment
Contemporary variables, such as contingencies of reinforcement, are the focus of the analysis	Historical variables, such as childhood experiences, are the focus of the analysis
Treatment entails the application of the principles of operant or classical conditioning	Treatment consists of bringing unconscious conflicts into consciousness
Objective observation, measurement, and experimentation are the methods used; the focus is on observable behavior and environmental events (antecedents and consequences)	Subjective methods of interpretation of behavior and inference regarding unobservable events (e.g., intrapsychic processes) are used
Theory is based on experimentation	Theory is predominantly based on case histories
Tenets can be formulated into testable hypotheses and evaluated through experimentation	Many tenets cannot be formulated into testable hypotheses to be evaluated through experimentation

Reprinted with permission from Dorsett PC. Behavioral and social learning psychology. In: Stoudemire A, ed. *Human Behavior: An Introduction for Medical Students*. Philadelphia: JB Lippincott; 1990:105.

Attempts have been made to reconcile behavioral theory and freudian psychodynamics by stressing the commonalities between the two. In tension reduction theory of behavior, behavior is motivated by an organism's attempt to reduce tension produced by unsatisfied or unconscious drives. Similarly, Sigmund Freud's pleasure principle is a tension-reducing force and, consequently, a strong motivator. When a drive is repressed, anxiety occurs and acts as an acquired drive; a person's behavior may be motivated by an attempt to reduce that anxiety. Adults may avoid situations that are likely to stimulate anxiety, but they may be completely unaware of their avoidance patterns. Therapy, in part, is an unlearning process. The patient learns that certain behaviors can reduce anxiety, and avoidance patterns are replaced by approach patterns. Table 6.3 gives a comparison of the behavioral and psychoanalytic models.

Answers 6.22–6.27

6.22 The answer is B

6.23 The answer is A

6.24 The answer is B

6.25 The answer is A

6.26 The answer is A

6.27 The answer is B

Among the building blocks of learning theory are classical and operant conditioning. In *classical conditioning*, learning is thought to take place as a result of the *contiguity of environmental events*: When events occur closely together in time, people will probably come to associate the two. In the case of *operant conditioning*, learning is thought to occur as a result of the *consequences of a person's actions* and the resultant effect on the environment. As *B. F. Skinner* (1904–1990) stated, "A person does not act upon the world, the world acts upon him."

Classical or respondent conditioning results from the repeated pairing of a neutral (conditioned) stimulus with one that evokes a response (unconditioned stimulus), such that the neutral stimulus eventually comes to evoke the response. The time relation between the presentation of the conditioned and unconditioned stimuli is important and varies for optimal learning from a fraction of a second to several seconds.

The Russian physiologist and Nobel prize winner, *Ivan Petrovich Pavlov* (1849–1936), observed in his work on gastric secretion that a dog salivated not only when food was placed in its mouth but also at the sound of the footsteps of the person coming to feed the dog, even though the dog could not see or smell the food. Pavlov analyzed these events and called the saliva flow that occurred with the sound of footsteps a *conditioned response* (CR)—a response elicited under certain conditions by a particular stimulus.

In a typical Pavlovian experiment, a *stimulus* (S) that had no capacity to evoke a particular response before training did so after consistent association with another stimulus. For example, under normal circumstances, a dog does not salivate at the sound of a bell, but when the bell sound is always followed by the presentation of food, the dog ultimately pairs the bell and the food. Eventually, the bell sound alone elicits salivation (CR).

Skinner's theory of learning and behavior is known as operant or *instrumental conditioning*. Whereas in classical conditioning an animal is passive or restrained and behavior is reinforced by the experimenter, in operant conditioning the animal is active and behaves in a way that produces a reward; thus *learning occurs as a consequence of action*. For example, a rat receives a reinforcing stimulus (food) only when it responds correctly by pressing a lever. Food, approval, praise, good grades, or any other response that satisfies a need in an animal or a person can serve as a reward.

Operant conditioning is related to trial-and-error learning, as described by the American psychologist Edward L. Thorndike

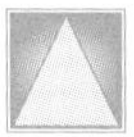

Table 6.4
Reinforcement Schedules in Operant Conditioning

Reinforcement Schedule	Example	Behavioral Effect
Fixed-ratio (FR) schedule	Reinforcement occurs after every 10 responses (10:1 ratio); 10 bar presses release a food pellet; workers are paid for every 10 items they make.	Rapid rate of response to obtain the greatest number of rewards. Animal knows that the next reinforcement depends on a certain number of responses being made.
Variable-ratio (VR) schedule	Variable reinforcement occurs (e.g., after the third, sixth, then second response, and so on).	Generates a fairly constant rate of response because the probability of reinforcement at any given time remains relatively stable.
Fixed-interval (FI) schedule	Reinforcement occurs at regular intervals (e.g., every 10 minutes or every third hour).	Animal keeps track of time. Rate of responding drops to near 0 after reinforcement and then increases at about the expected time of reward.
Variable-interval (VI) schedule	Reinforcement occurs after variable intervals (e.g., every 3, 6, and then 2 hours), similar to VR schedule.	Response rate does not change between reinforcements. Animal responds at a steady rate to get the reward when it is available; common in trout fishing, use of slot machines, checking mailbox.

(1874–1949). In trial-and-error learning, a person or an animal attempts to solve a problem by trying different actions until one proves successful: A freely moving organism behaves in a way that is instrumental in producing a reward. For example, a cat in a Thorndike puzzle box must learn to lift a latch to escape from the box. For this reason, operant conditioning is sometimes called *instrumental conditioning*. Thorndike's law of effect states that certain responses are reinforced by reward and the organism learns from these experiences.

Four kinds of instrumental or operant conditioning are described in Table 6.4.

Answers 6.28–6.29

6.28 The answer is B

6.29 The answer is A

The null hypothesis states that observed differences or variation in scores can be attributed to random sources. When the null hypothesis is rejected, observed differences between groups are deemed to be improbable by chance alone. For example, if drug A is compared to a placebo for its effects on depression and the null hypothesis is rejected, the investigator concludes that the observed differences most likely are not explainable simply by sampling error. When offering this conclusion, the investigator has the odds on his or her side. However, what are the chances of the statement being incorrect?

In statistical inference there is no way to say with certainty that rejection or retention of the null hypothesis was correct. There are two types of potential errors.

Type I errors occur when the null hypothesis is rejected but should have been retained, such as when a researcher decides that two means are different. He or she might conclude that the treatment works or that groups are not sampled from the same population, whereas in reality the observed differences are attributable only to a sampling error. In a conservative scientific setting, type I errors should be made rarely. There is a great disadvantage to advocating treatments that really do not work. The probability of a type I error is denoted with the Greek letter alpha (α). Because of the desire to avoid type I errors, statistical models have been created so that the investigator has control over the probability of a type I error. At the 0.05 significance or alpha level, a type I error is expected to occur in 5 percent of all cases. At the 0.01 level, it may occur in 1 percent of all cases. Thus, at the 0.05 α level, one type I error is expected to be made in each of 20 independent tests. At the 0.01 α level, one type I error is expected to be made in each 100 independent tests.

In a type II error the null hypothesis is retained when it really was wrong and should have been rejected. For example, an investigator may reach the conclusion that a treatment does not work when in fact it is efficacious. The probability of a type II error is symbolized by the Greek letter beta (β).

Answers 6.30–6.34

6.30 The answer is A

6.31 The answer is D

6.32 The answer is C

6.33 The answer is C

6.34 The answer is A

Often given in the form of attention and praise contingent on certain behaviors, reinforcement is a basic ingredient of most therapists' repertoire. Much is known about various schedules of reinforcement, defined as the pattern or frequency with which a reward is delivered as a consequence of behavior. The most frequently used schedules are listed in Table 6.4. The fixed-ratio schedule leads to the *most rapid rate of response* and is seen in *baseball rules when a player is called out after three strikes*. The use of *slot machines* demonstrates a variable-interval schedule of reinforcement. The fixed-interval schedule has an *oscillating rate of response* that increases near the expected time of reward, a concept known as *scalloping*.

Answers 6.35–6.38

6.35 The answer is C

6.36 The answer is D

6.37 The answer is A

6.38 The answer is B

Imprinting has been described as the process by which certain stimuli become capable of eliciting certain innate behavior patterns during a critical period of an animal's behavioral development. The phenomenon is associated with *Konrad Lorenz,* who in 1935 demonstrated that the first moving object (in that case, Lorenz himself) a duckling sees during a critical period shortly after hatching is regarded and reacted to thereafter as the mother duck.

Harry Harlow is associated with the concept of the *surrogate mother* from his experiments in the 1950s with Rhesus monkeys. Harlow designed a series of experiments in which infant monkeys were separated from their mothers during the earliest weeks of life. He found that the infant monkeys, if given the choice between a wire surrogate mother and a cloth-covered surrogate mother, chose the cloth-covered surrogates even if the wire surrogates provided food.

Ivan Petrovich Pavlov coined the terms *"experimental neurosis"* to describe disorganized behavior that appears in the experimental subject (in Pavlov's case, dogs) in response to an inability to master the experimental situation. Pavlov described extremely agitated behavior in his dogs when they were unable to discriminate between sounds of similar pitch or test objects of similar shapes.

Eric Kandel contributed to the knowledge of the neurophysiology of learning. He demonstrated in the study of the snail *Aplysia* that synaptic connections are altered as a result of learning. His work earned him the Nobel Prize in Medicine in 2001.

Answers 6.39–6.42

6.39 The answer is C

6.40 The answer is A

6.41 The answer is D

6.42 The answer is B

Attachment can be defined as the emotional tone between children and their caregivers and is evidenced by an infant's seeking and clinging to the caregiving person, usually the mother. By their first month, infants usually have begun to show such behavior, which is designed to promote proximity to the desired person.

John Bowlby, a British psychoanalyst (1907–1990), formulated the theory that normal attachment in infancy is crucial to healthy development. Bowlby described a predictable set and sequence of behavior patterns in children who are separated from their mothers for long periods (more than 3 months): *protest,* in which the child protests against the separations by crying, calling out, and searching for the lost person; *despair,* in which the child appears to lose hope that the mother will return; and *detachment,* in which the child emotionally separates himself or herself from the mother. Bowlby believed that this sequence involves ambivalent feelings toward the mother; the child both wants her and is angry at her for her desertion.

Mary Ainsworth built on Bowlby's observations and found that the interaction between the mother and her baby during the attachment period influences the baby's current and future behavior significantly. Many observers believe that patterns of infant attachment affect future adult emotional relationships. Patterns of attachment vary among babies; for example, some babies signal or cry less than others. Sensitive responsiveness to infant signals, such as cuddling the baby when it cries, causes infants to cry less in later months. Close bodily contact with the mother when the baby signals for her is also associated with the growth of self-reliance, rather than with a clinging dependence, as the baby grows older. Unresponsive mothers produce anxious babies; these mothers often have lower intelligence quotients (IQs) and are emotionally more immature and younger than responsive mothers.

Ainsworth also confirmed that attachment serves the purpose of reducing anxiety. What she called the *secure base effect* enables a child to move away from the attachment figures and to explore the environment. Inanimate objects, such as a teddy bear or a blanket (called the transitional object by Donald Winnicott), also serve as a secure base, one that often accompanies children as they navigate the world.

Harry Harlow's *ethological studies* with monkeys are relevant to attachment theory. Harlow demonstrated the emotional and behavioral effects of isolating monkeys from birth and keeping them from forming attachments. The isolates were withdrawn, unable to relate to peers, unable to mate, and incapable of caring for their offspring.

Anaclitic depression, also known as hospitalism, was first described by René Spitz in infants who had made normal attachments but were then separated suddenly from their mothers for varying times and placed in institutions or hospitals. The children became depressed, withdrawn, nonresponsive, and vulnerable to physical illness but recovered when their mothers returned or when surrogate mothering was available.

Answers 6.43–6.47

6.43 The answer is B

6.44 The answer is C

6.45 The answer is A

6.46 The answer is B

6.47 The answer is D

In operant conditioning, learning is thought to occur as a result of the consequences of one's actions and the resultant effect on the environment. In *classical conditioning*, in contrast, learning is thought to take place as the result of the contiguity of environmental events; when events occur closely together in time, persons will probably come to associate the two. An example is Pavlov's salivating dogs experiment.

In operant conditioning, *positive reinforcement* is the process by which certain consequences of a response increase the probability that the response will occur again. Food, water, praise, and money, as well as substances such as opium, cocaine, and nicotine, all may serve as positive reinforcers.

Negative reinforcement is the process by which a response that leads to the removal of an aversive event increases that response. Any behavior that enables one to avoid or escape a punishing consequence is strengthened; therefore, a patient with anorexia nervosa eating and gaining weight in order to get out of the hospital (presuming she prefers going home to a prolonged hospitalization), as well as getting up early to avoid traffic are examples of negative reinforcement.

Negative reinforcement is not punishment. *Punishment* is an aversive stimulus (for example, a slap, or the removal of a desired object) that is presented explicitly to weaken or suppress an undesired response. Punishment reduces the probability that a response will occur.

7 Clinical Neuropsychological Testing

Clinical neuropsychological tests of intelligence and personality are useful to measure specific aspects of a person's intelligence, thinking, or personality in particular clinical situations.

Intelligence testing is necessary to establish the degree of mental retardation. Neuropsychological tests help quantify and localize brain damage. The clinical neuropsychologist integrates the medical and psychosocial history with the reported complaints and the patterns of performance on neuropsychological procedures to determine whether results are consistent with a particular area of brain damage or a particular diagnosis.

The aim of neuropsychological tests is to achieve quantifiable and reproducible results that can be compared with the test scores of normal people of comparable age and demographic background. They are indicated to identify cognitive defects, to differentiate incipient depression from dementia, to determine the course of an illness, to assess neurotoxic effects, to evaluate the effects of treatment, and to evaluate learning disorders.

Projective tests present stimuli to whose meanings are not immediately obvious; the ambiguity forces the patient to project his or her own needs into the test situation. Those being tested impute meanings to the stimulus, apparently based on psychological and emotional factors.

Most commonly used assessment instruments are standardized against normal control subjects. This ensures that test administration and scoring are invariant across time and examiners. The data show whether the test is valid and reliable.

The student should be familiar with the types of neuropsychological assessment tests that are available, how they are administered, and their indications for use.

HELPFUL HINTS

- abstract reasoning
- accurate profile
- attention
- attention-deficit/ hyperactivity disorder
- average IQ
- battery tests
- behavioral flexibility
- bell-shaped curve
- Bender Visual Motor Gestalt test
- Alfred Binet
- catastrophic reaction
- clang association
- classification of intelligence
- coping phase
- dementia
- dressing apraxia
- dysgraphia
- dyslexia
- EEG abnormalities
- Eysenck personality inventory
- fluency
- full-scale IQ
- Gestalt psychology
- Halstead-Reitan
- House-Tree-Person test
- individual and group tests
- intelligence quotient (IQ)
- learning disability
- left versus right hemisphere disease
- Luria-Nebraska Neuropsychological Battery (LNNB)
- manual dexterity
- maturational levels
- memory: immediate, recent, recent past, remote
- mental age
- mental status cognitive tasks
- MMPI
- motivational aspects of behavior
- neuropsychiatric tests
- objective tests
- organic dysfunction
- orientation
- performance subtests
- perseveration
- personality functioning
- personality testing
- primary assets and weaknesses
- prognosis
- projective tests
- prosody
- psychodynamic formulations
- Raven's Progressive Matrices
- reaction times
- recall phase
- reliability
- response sets
- Rorschach test
- scatter pattern
- Shipley Abstraction test
- standardization
- Stanford-Binet
- stimulus words
- TAT
- temporal orientation
- test behavior
- validity
- verbal subtests
- visual-object agnosia
- WAIS
- WISC
- word-association technique

QUESTIONS

7.1 Which of the following about the Rorschach Test is *true*?

A. A standard set of fifteen inkblots serves as the stimulus for the test.
B. All the blots are black and white.
C. It has an inquiry phase to determine aspects of the responses that are crucial to the scoring.
D. There is no order to the ways in which the cards are shown.
E. It is named after a German psychiatrist.

7.2 The Minnesota Multiphasic Personality Inventory (MMPI) is most correctly described as

A. composed of 200 questions
B. generally used as a good diagnostic tool
C. the most widely used personality assessment instrument
D. a good indication of a subject's disorder when the person scores high on one particular clinical scale
E. in the form of ten clinical scales, each of which was derived empirically from heterogeneous groups

7.3 Neuropsychological referrals are made for

A. establishing a baseline of performance for assessing future change
B. diagnostic purposes
C. ascertaining if brain impairment is present
D. planning for rehabilitation
E. all of the above

7.4 Neuropsychological testing is used to assess

A. normal aging
B. early dementia
C. competence
D. a diagnosis of pseudodementia
E. all of the above

7.5 Neuropsychological deficits associated with left hemisphere damage include all of the following *except*

A. aphasia
B. right-left disorientation
C. finger agnosia
D. visuospatial deficits
E. limb apraxia

7.6 True statements about projective personality tests include

A. They tend to be more direct and structural than objective personality instruments.
B. The variety of responses is limited.
C. Instructions are usually specific.
D. They often focus on latent or unconscious aspects of personality.
E. None of the above

7.7 An intelligence quotient (IQ) of 100 corresponds to intellectual ability for the general population in the

A. 20th percentile
B. 25th percentile
C. 40th percentile
D. 50th percentile
E. 65th percentile

7.8 After taking the Wechsler Adult Intelligence Scale (WAIS), a patient showed that poor concentration and attention had adversely influenced the answers on one of the subtests. Select the WAIS subtest that most likely screened the patient for these symptoms.

A. arithmetic
B. block design
C. digit symbol
D. comprehension
E. picture completion

7.9 The Bender Visual Motor Gestalt test is administered to test

A. maturation levels in children
B. organic dysfunction
C. loss of function
D. visual and motor coordination
E. all of the above

7.10 Which is *not* true of the Wisconsin Card Sorting Test?

A. It assesses abstract reasoning
B. The patient is told during testing whether their responses are correct or incorrect
C. The examiner changes the principle of sorting when the task is mastered
D. The examiner records the number of trials required to achieve ten consecutive correct responses
E. It assesses parietal lobe dysfunction

7.11 In the Wechsler Adult Intelligence Scale (WAIS)

A. digit span is a subtest of the verbal component of the test
B. the average range of IQ is 100 to 120
C. mental retardation corresponds to the lowest 1% of the population
D. the verbal scale is more sensitive to normal aging
E. its latest revision is designed for persons aged 16 to 60

Directions

Each group of questions below consists of lettered headings followed by a list of numbered words or statements. For each numbered word or statement, select the *one* lettered heading most closely associated with it. Each lettered heading may be selected once, more than once, or not at all.

Questions 7.12–7.16

A. Frontal lobes
B. Dominant temporal lobe
C. Nondominant parietal lobe
D. Dominant parietal lobe
E. Occipital lobe

7.12 The loss of gestalt, loss of symmetry, and distortion of figures
7.13 Patient not able to name a camouflaged object but able to name it when it is not camouflaged
7.14 Two or more errors or two or more 7-second delays in carrying out tasks of right-left orientation
7.15 Any improper letter sequence in spelling "earth" backward
7.16 Patient not able to name common objects

Questions 7.17–7.21

A. Rorschach test
B. Luria-Nebraska Neuropsychological Battery
C. Halstead-Reitan Battery of Neuropsychological Tests
D. Stanford-Binet Intelligence Scale
E. None of the above

7.17 Consists of ten tests, including the trail-making test and the critical flicker frequency test
7.18 Is extremely sensitive in identifying discrete forms of brain damage, such as dyslexia
7.19 Consists of 120 items, plus several alternative tests, applicable to the ages between 2 years and adulthood
7.20 Furnishes a description of the dynamic forces of personality through an analysis of the person's responses
7.21 A test of diffuse cerebral dysfunction to which normal children by the age of 7 years respond negatively

Questions 7.22–7.24

A. Short-term memory loss
B. Signs of organic dysfunction
C. Korsakoff's syndrome
D. Posterior right hemisphere lesion
E. Damage to frontal lobes or caudate

7.22 Wechsler Memory Scale
7.23 Wisconsin Card Sorting Test
7.24 Benton Visual Retention Test

Questions 7.25–7.29

A. Wechsler Adult Intelligence Scale (WAIS)
B. Thematic Apperception Test (TAT)
C. Shipley Abstraction Test
D. Sentence Completion Test
E. Raven's Progressive Matrices

7.25 A broad set of complex verbal and visuospatial tasks that are normatively summarized by three scales
7.26 Impaired performance is associated with posterior lesions of either cerebral hemisphere
7.27 Series of 20 black-and-white pictures depicting individuals of different ages and sexes involved in a variety of settings
7.28 More direct than most projective tests in soliciting responses from the patient
7.29 Requires the patient to complete logical sequences

Questions 7.30–7.34

A. Executive functions
B. Attention and concentration
C. Visuospatial–constructional
D. Motor
E. None of the above

7.30 Clock drawing and facial recognition
7.31 Finger tapping
7.32 Trail-making test
7.33 Digit span
7.34 Wisconsin Card Sorting Test

Questions 7.35–7.37

A. Stanford-Binet Intelligence Scale
B. Wechsler Preschool and Primary Scale of Intelligence (WPPSI)
C. Wechsler Intelligence Scale for Children (WISC)—Third Edition
D. All of the above
E. None of the above

7.35 Appropriate for children at least 6 years of age to 16 years
7.36 Appropriate for children beginning at $2^1/_2$ years of age
7.37 Yields a composite IQ score, and scores for verbal reasoning, abstract visual reasoning, quantitative reasoning, and short-term memory

Questions 7.38–7.42

A. Immediate memory
B. Episodic memory
C. Semantic memory
D. Recent past memory
E. Implicit memory

7.38 Memory for automatic skills, like speaking grammatically or driving a car
7.39 Recall of perceived material within thirty seconds of presentation
7.40 Memory for specific events, like a phone message
7.41 Retention of information over the past few months, like current events
7.42 Memory for knowledge and facts, like the first president of the United States

Directions

Each set of lettered headings below is followed by a list of numbered phrases. For each numbered phrase, select

A. if the item is associated with A only
B. if the item is associated with B only
C. if the item is associated with both A and B
D. if the item is associated with neither A nor B

Questions 7.43–7.44

A. Brief Psychiatric Rating Scale (BPRS)
B. Schedule for Affective Disorders and Schizophrenia (SADS)

7.43 Ratings are made on the basis of mental status interview and do not require that the examiner ask any specific questions

7.44 Highly structured interview

ANSWERS

7.1 The answer is C

The Rorschach Test was devised by Hermann Rorschach, *a Swiss psychiatrist*. It involves *an inquiry phase to determine important aspects of each response that are crucial to its scoring*. It comprises *a standard set of 10 inkblots*, which serve as a stimulus for associations. *Five of the blots are black and white; the other five include colors. The cards are shown to a patient in a particular order*, and the psychologist keeps a record of the patient's verbatim responses, along with initial reaction times and total time spent on each card. See Figure 7.1.

7.2 The answer is C

The *MMPI* is composed of over 500 *statements, not* 200 *questions*. It is the *most widely used* personality assessment instrument. Although the test was initially thought to be a *diagnostic tool*, workers now use the inventory to interpret the patterning of the entire profile obtained from the clinical scales. Researchers have identified personality correlates of various configurations produced on the inventory, which can serve as diagnostic aids. Therefore, a *good indication of a subject's disorder is not a single high score on one scale;* the complete results are examined for an interpretation, and at least two of the highest scores are used to arrive at a diagnosis. The inventory is in the form of clinical scales, but these scales *were derived from homogeneous groups of psychiatric patients, not from heterogenous groups of people*.

7.3 The answer is E (all)

Most neuropsychological referrals are made for diagnostic purposes, to ascertain if brain impairment is present, or to differentiate among neurological or psychiatric disorders. Other important uses of testing include establishing a baseline of performance for assessing future change and planning for rehabilitation or management of behaviors affected by brain impairment. The specific methods of neuropsychological assessment reflect the individual's unique presentation of symptoms and complaints, history and development, the perspective of the neuropsychologist, and the referral question.

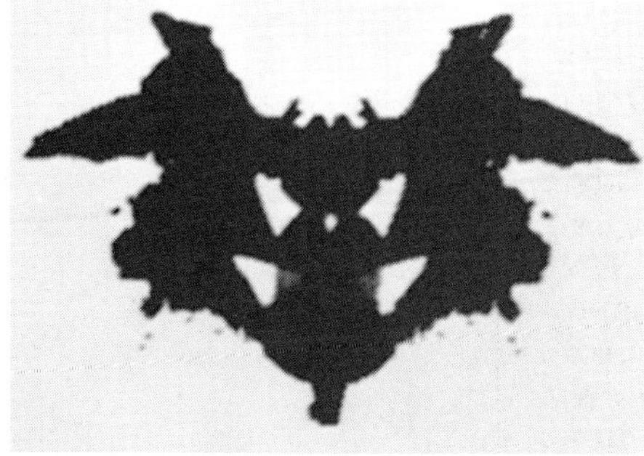

FIGURE 7.1
Plate 1 of the Rorschach test. (Reprinted with permission from Huber Medical Publisher, Bern.)

A common referral issue involves documentation of level of functioning for a variety of purposes, including assessment of change or competence, especially in the presence of diagnoses such as dementia, stroke, and head injury.

7.4 The answer is E (all)

Neuropsychological testing provides a detailed, objective picture of different aspects of memory and attention, which can be helpful in reassuring healthy persons about their abilities. It also provides an opportunity for assessing undetected mood or anxiety disorders that may be reflected in cognitive concerns and offers suggestions about mnemonic strategies that can sharpen everyday function.

When concerns about a person's memory functioning are expressed by relatives instead of the patient, there is a higher probability of a neurological basis for the functional problems. Neuropsychological testing combined with a good clinical history and other medical screening tests is *highly effective in distinguishing early dementia* from the milder forms of *declining memory that can be seen with normal aging*. Neuropsychological evaluation is particularly helpful in documenting cognitive deterioration and differentiating among forms of dementia, such as Alzheimer's disease and frontal lobe dementia.

Neuropsychologists are often asked to consult in *determining individuals' competence* to make decisions or to manage personal affairs. Neuropsychological testing can be useful in these cases by documenting areas of clear and significant impairment and identifying areas of strength and well-preserved skill. However, opinions about competence should not be based on test findings alone but must include other, more indirect observations (e.g., in-home assessment, collateral interviews) of everyday functioning.

A substantial minority of patients with severe depression exhibit serious generalized impairment of cognitive functioning. In addition to problems with attention and slowing of thought and action, there may be significant forgetfulness and difficulties with reasoning. By examining the pattern of cognitive impairments, neuropsychological testing can help to identify *pseudodementia*, a dementia-like condition seen in elderly patients with depressive disorders. Perhaps more common is a mixed presentation, in which depression coexists with various forms of cognitive decline, increasing the severity of cognitive dysfunction beyond what would be expected from the neurological impairment alone. Neuropsychological testing can provide a baseline for measuring the effectiveness of antidepressant therapy in alleviating cognitive and mood symptoms.

7.5 The answer is D

Many functions are mediated by both the right and left cerebral hemispheres. However, important qualitative differences between the two hemispheres can be demonstrated in the presence of lateralized brain injury. Various cognitive skills that have been linked to the left or right hemisphere in right-handed people are listed in Table 7.1. Although *language* is the most obvious area that is largely controlled by the left hemisphere (with injuries leading to aphasias), the left hemisphere is also generally considered to be dominant for *limb praxis* (i.e., performing complex movements, such as brushing teeth, commanding, or imitation) and has been associated with a cluster of deficits identified as Gerstmann syndrome (i.e., *finger agnosia*, dyscalculia,

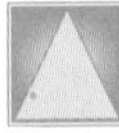

Table 7.1
Selected Neuropsychological Deficits Associated with Left or Right Hemisphere Damage

Left Hemisphere	Right Hemisphere
Aphasia	Visuospatial deficits
Right-left disorientation	Impaired visual perception
Finger agnosia	Neglect
Dysgraphia (aphasic)	Dysgraphia (spatial, neglect)
Dyscalculia (number alexia)	Dyscalculia (spatial)
Constructional apraxia (details)	Constructional apraxia (Gestalt)
Limb apraxia	Dressing apraxia
	Anosognosia

dysgraphia, and *right-left disorientation*). In contrast, the right hemisphere is thought to play a more important role in controlling *visuospatial abilities and hemispatial attention*, which are associated with the clinical presentations of constructional apraxia and neglect, respectively.

Although lateralized deficits such as these are typically characterized in terms of damage to the right or left hemisphere, it is important to keep in mind that the patient's performance can also be characterized in terms of preserved brain functions. In other words, it is the remaining intact brain tissue that drives many behavioral responses following injury to the brain and not only the absence of critical brain tissue.

7.6 The answer is D

Projective personality tests, in contrast to objective personality instruments, are more indirect and unstructured. Unlike objective tests, in which the patient may simply mark "true" or "false" to given questions, the variety of responses to projective personality tests is almost unlimited. Instructions are usually general, allowing the patient's fantasies to be expressed. Patients generally do not know how their responses will be scored or analyzed, making it difficult to obtain a desired result. Projective tests typically do not measure one particular personality characteristic such as type A personality (i.e., narrow-band measurement) but instead are designed to assess a personality as a whole (i.e., broad-band measurement).

Projective tests often focus on latent or unconscious aspects of personality. Obviously, psychologists and others differ in the degree to which they rely on unconscious information. In many projective techniques, patients are simply shown a picture of something and asked to tell what the picture reminds them of. Projective techniques assume that when presented with an ambiguous stimulus such as an inkblot, for which there are an almost unlimited number of responses, the patients' responses will reflect fundamental aspects of their personalities. The ambiguous stimulus is a sort of screen on which individuals project their own needs, thoughts, or conflicts. Different persons have different thoughts, needs, and conflicts and hence will have different responses. In particular, a schizophrenic patient's responses will often reflect a rather bizarre, idiosyncratic view of the world.

Hundreds of different projective techniques have been developed—most of which are not used widely today.

7.7 The answer is D

An intelligence quotient (IQ) of 100 corresponds to the *50th percentile* in intellectual ability for the general population. Modern psychological testing began in the first decade of the 20th century when Alfred Binet (1857–1911), a French psychologist, developed the first intelligence scale to separate the mentally defective youngsters (who were to be given special education) from the rest of the children (whose school progress was to be accelerated).

7.8 The answer is A

The *arithmetic* subtest showed that the patient's ability to do simple arithmetic was influenced adversely by poor attention and concentration. The *block design* subtest requires a subject to arrange a series of pictures to tell a story. This process tests performance and cognitive styles. The *digit symbol* subtest requires a subject to match digits and symbols in as little time as possible, as a test of performance. The *comprehension* subtest reveals a subject's ability to adhere to social consequences and to understand social judgments when the subject answers questions about how people should behave. On the *picture completion* subtest a subject must complete a picture with a missing part. Visuospatial defects appear when errors are made on this procedure.

7.9 The answer is E (all)

The Bender Visual Motor Gestalt test, devised by the American neuropsychiatrist Lauretta Bender in 1938, is a technique that consists of nine figures that are copied by the subject (Fig. 7.2). It is administered as a means of evaluating *maturation levels in children* and *organic dysfunction.* Its chief applications are to determine retardation, *loss of function,* and organic brain defects in children and adults. The designs are presented one at a time to

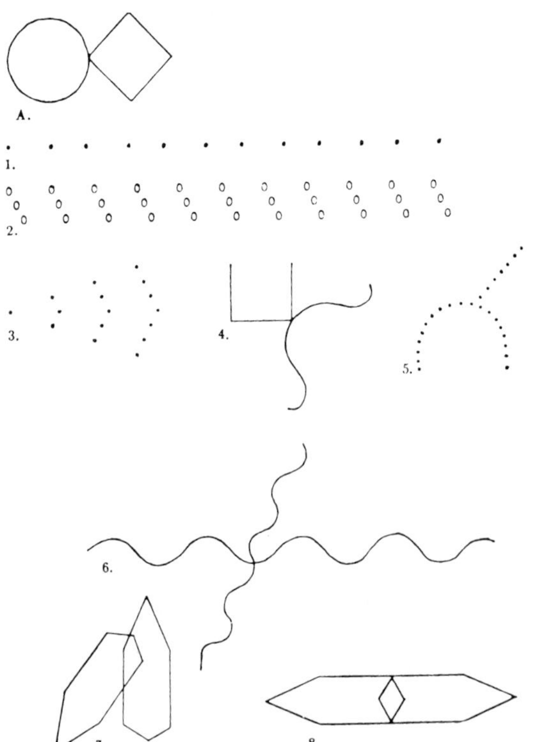

FIGURE 7.2

Test figures from the Bender Visual Motor Gestalt test, adapted from Max Wertheimer. (Reprinted with permission from Bender L. *A Visual Motor Gestalt Test and Its Clinical Use.* New York: American Orthopsychiatric Association; 1938:33.)

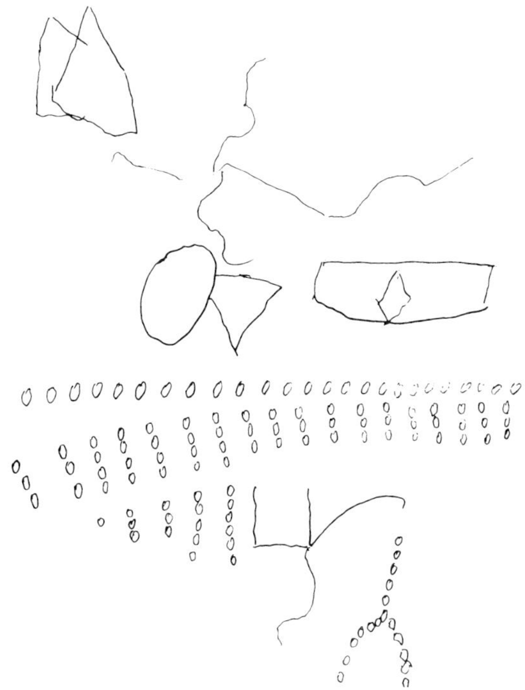

FIGURE 7.3
Bender Visual Motor Gesalt test drawings of a 57-year-old brain-damaged woman.

the subject, who is asked to copy them onto a sheet of paper. The subject then is asked to copy the designs from memory (Figs. 7.3 and 7.4); thus, the Bender designs can be used as a test of both *visual and motor coordination* and immediate visual memory.

7.10 The answer is E

Persons with damage to the frontal lobes or to the caudate nucleus, and some patients with schizophrenia give abnormal responses to the Wisconsin Card Sorting Test (WCST). *It does not address parietal lobe damage.* This *test assesses abstract reasoning* and flexibility in problem solving. Stimulus cards are presented to patients to sort into groups according to a principle established by the examiner but unknown to the patient. As the patient sorts the cards, *he or she is told whether the responses are correct or incorrect. The number of trials required to achieve ten consecutive responses is recorded.* When or if the patient has mastered the task, *the examiner changes the principle of sorting*, and the number of trials required to achieve correct sorting is recorded.

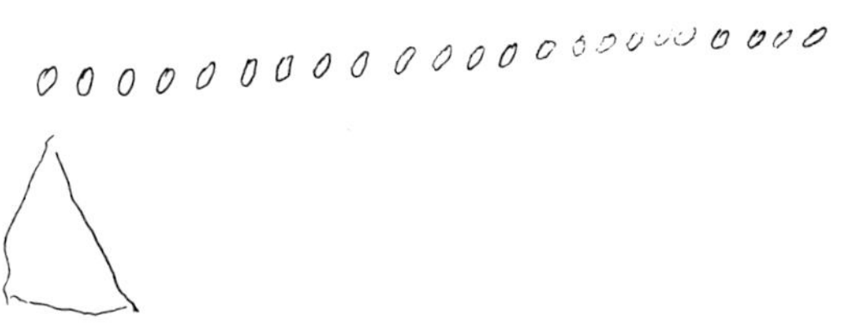

FIGURE 7.4
Bender Visual Motor Gesalt test recall by the 57-year-old brain-damaged patient who drew Figure 7.3.

7.11 The answer is A

The Wechsler Adult Intelligence Scale (WAIS) comprises 11 subtests made up of six verbal (information, comprehension, arithmetic, similarities, *digit span*, vocabulary), and five performance (picture completion, block design, picture arrangement, object assembly, digit symbol) subtests, which yield a verbal IQ, a performance IQ, and a combined full-scale IQ. *The latest edition, the WAIS-III, is designed for persons 16 to 89 years of age.* There are scales for children ages 4 to 6.5 and 5 through 15. *The average or normal range of IQ is 90 to 110*; IQ scores of at least 120 are considered superior. *Mental retardation, defined as IQ below 70, corresponds to the lowest 2.2 percent of the population*; 2 of every 100 people have IQ scores consistent with mental deficiency. *The performance scale is more sensitive to normal aging than the verbal scale*, which is more sensitive to education.

Answers 7.12–7.16

7.12 The answer is C

7.13 The answer is E

7.14 The answer is D

7.15 The answer is A

7.16 The answer is B

Numerous mental status cognitive tasks are available to test and localize various brain dysfunctions. Construction apraxia—*the loss of gestalt, loss of symmetry, and distortion of figures*—seen in the task of copying the outline of simple objects, is localized to the *nondominant parietal lobe*. Dysfunction of the *occipital lobes* is suggested when a *patient cannot name a camouflaged object but can name it when it is not camouflaged. Two or more errors or two or more 7-second delays in carrying out tasks of right-left orientation* (for example, place left hand to right ear, right elbow to right knee) are localized to dysfunction of the *dominant parietal lobe*. A dysfunction in concentration is thought to be localized to the *frontal lobes* and can be tested by eliciting *any improper letter sequence in spelling "earth" backward*. In anomia the *patient cannot name common objects* (for example, watch, key); the impairment is localized to the *dominant temporal lobe*.

Answers 7.17–7.21

7.17 The answer is C

7.18 The answer is B

7.19 The answer is D

7.20 The answer is A

7.21 The answer is E

Various neuropsychiatric tests, including the Halstead-Reitan and the Luria-Nebraska batteries, are sometimes useful in bringing to light subtle organic dysfunctions that are undetected in standard psychiatric, psychological, and even neurological assessments. The *Halstead-Reitan Battery of Neuropsychological Tests consists of ten tests, including the trail-making test and the critical flicker frequency test.* It was developed in an attempt to improve the reliability of the criteria used to diagnose brain damage. Assessment data were gathered on a group of patients with left hemisphere injury, right hemisphere injury, and global involvement. The trail-making test is a test of visuomotor perception and motor speed, and the critical flicker frequency test (noting when a flicker light becomes steady) tests visual perception.

The *Luria-Nebraska Neuropsychological Battery (LNNB) is extremely sensitive in identifying discrete forms of brain damage, such as dyslexia* (an impairment in the ability to read) and dyscalculia (an inability to perform arithmetical operations), rather than more global forms.

The *Stanford-Binet Intelligence Scale* is one of the tests most frequently used in the individual examination of children. It *consists of 120 items, plus several alternative tests, applicable to the ages between 2 years and adulthood.* The tests have a variety of graded difficulties, both verbal and performance, designed to assess such functions as memory, free association, orientation, language comprehension, knowledge of common objects, abstract thinking, and the use of judgment and reasoning.

The *Rorschach test* is a psychological test consisting of ten inkblots that the person is asked to look at and interpret. It *furnishes a description of the dynamic forces of personality through an analysis of the person's responses.*

The face-hand test, devised by Lauretta Bender, is *a test of diffuse cerebral dysfunction to which normal children by the age of 7 years respond negatively.* The person, whose eyes are closed, is touched simultaneously on the cheek and the hand; retesting is done with the person's eyes open. The results are considered positive if the person fails consistently to identify both stimuli within ten trials.

Answers 7.22–7.24

7.22 The answer is C

7.23 The answer is E

7.24 The answer is A

The *Wechsler Memory Scale* screens for verbal and visual memory and yields a memory quotient. The results can reveal whether a subject has *amnestic Korsakoff's syndrome. The Wisconsin Card Sorting Test* assesses a person's abstract reasoning ability and flexibility in problem solving. The results can reveal whether a person has *damage to the frontal lobes or to the caudate.*

The *Benton Visual Retention Test* screens for *short-term memory loss.*

Signs of organic dysfunction may be screened for by the Bender Visual Motor Gestalt test. *Posterior right-hemisphere lesions* can be revealed through a Facial Recognition Test.

Answers 7.25–7.29

7.25 The answer is A

7.26 The answer is E

7.27 The answer is B

7.28 The answer is D

7.29 The answer is C

Assessment of intellectual functioning serves as the cornerstone of the neuropsychological examination. The Wechsler intelligence scales, based on carefully developed normative standards, have represented the traditional gold standard in intellectual assessment for many years. The scope and variety of subtests on which the summary intelligence quotient (IQ) values are based also provide useful benchmarks against which to compare performances on other tests of specific abilities. The latest revision of this instrument is the Wechsler Memory Scale III. In general, *the Wechsler intelligence scales use a broad set of complex verbal and visuospatial tasks that are normatively summarized as a Verbal IQ, a Performance IQ, and Full Scale IQ.* In the context of a neuropsychological examination, the patient's performance across the procedures provides useful information regarding longstanding abilities as well as current functioning. Most neuropsychologists recognize that the summary IQ values provide only a ball-park range for characterizing an individual's general level of functioning. Therefore, it is usually more appropriate and meaningful to characterize an individual's intellectual functioning in terms of the range of functioning (e.g., borderline, low average, average, high average, superior) represented by the IQ value rather than the specific value.

Raven's Progressive Matrices require the patient to complete a design by selecting from a multiple-choice pictorial display the stimulus that completes a design in which a part is omitted.The difficulty of the discrimination increases over trials in the lengthy test. A briefer, less difficult version (Color Matrices) is especially useful for patients who are unable to complete the standard test, which can require 30 to 45 minutes. *Impaired performance is associated with poor visuoconstructive ability and with posterior lesions of either cerebral hemisphere,* but receptive language deficit may contribute to poor performance in patients with dominant hemisphere damage.

Although the Rorschach test is clearly the most frequently used projective personality test, the *Thematic Apperception Test* (TAT) is probably in second place. Many clinicians include both the TAT and the Rorschach test in a battery of tests for personality assessment. *The TAT consists of a series of 20 black-and-white pictures that depict individuals of both sexes and of different age groups involved in a variety of different settings.* For example, on Card 1, a young boy is shown sitting at a table, looking at a violin. Card 2 depicts a farm scene in which a young woman in the foreground is carrying books in her hands; a man is working in the fields nearby, and an older woman is seen in the background. Typically, a patient is shown ten TAT cards and asked to make up stories about them. The patient is asked to tell what is going on in the picture, what was going on before the picture was taken, what the individuals in the picture are thinking and feeling, and what is likely to happen in the future. An example of a TAT card is presented in Figure 7.5.

Henry Murray developed the TAT at the Harvard Psychological Clinic in 1943. The stories the patient make up concerning the pictures, according to the projective hypothesis, reflect the patient's own needs, thoughts, feelings, stresses, wishes, desires, and view of the future.

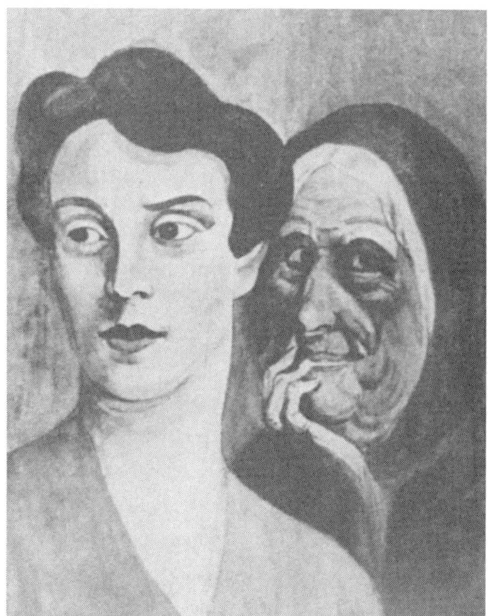

FIGURE 7.5
Card 12F of the Thermatic Apperception Test. (Reprinted with permission from Murray HA. *Thematic Apperception Test,* Cambridge, MA: Harvard University Press, Copyright ©1943 President and Fellows of Harvard College, © 1971 Henry A. Murray.)

Although a projective instrument, the Sentence Completion Test is much more direct in soliciting responses from the patient. The patient is simply presented with a series of incomplete sentences and asked to complete each sentence stem with the first response that comes to mind. Examples of possible incomplete sentences are as follows:

My father seldom . . .
Most people don't know that I'm afraid of . . .
When I was a child, I . . .
When encountering frustration, I usually . . .

The purpose of the test is to elicit, somewhat indirectly, information about the patient that cannot be elicited by other measures. Since the patient responds in writing, the examiner's time is limited. The length of time it takes to complete this test varies greatly, depending on the number of incomplete sentences. Tests can range from fewer than ten sentences to more than 75.

There are many variations of sentence completion tests. Some clinicians have developed their own. One form developed by Julian Rotter has some established validity and reliability, but most sentence completion tests do not. Special-purpose sentence completion tests have been developed to measure different problem areas. For example, one sentence completion test is used with patients who have chronic pain, and another to assess issues concerning transsexual patients. The sentence completion test is seldom, if ever, used alone but is combined with other appropriate instruments.

Advantages of the sentence completion are short administration time, ease of administration, variety of instruments, and ease of construction. Disadvantages are lack of reliability and validity studies and ease of fabrication and deception.

The *Shipley Abstraction Test requires the patient to complete logical sequences;* it assesses the patient's capacity to think abstractly. Because performance on a test of this type is related to educational background, an accompanying vocabulary test is also given to the patient, and a comparison is made between the patient's performances on the two tests. A low abstraction score in relation to vocabulary level is interpreted as reflecting an impairment in conceptual thinking.

Answers 7.30–7.34

7.30 The answer is C

7.31 The answer is D

7.32 The answer is A

7.33 The answer is B

7.34 The answer is A

Digit Span is the auditory-verbal measure of simple span of attention (*Digits Forward*) and cognitive manipulation of increasingly longer strings of digits (*Digits Backward*). *Facial Recognition* assesses matching and discrimination of unfamiliar faces. *Clock Drawing* is a useful screening technique sensitive to organization and planning as well as constructional ability. *Finger Tapping* is the standard measure of simple motor speed; particularly useful for documenting lateralized motor impairment. The *Wisconsin Card Sorting Test* is the measure of problem-solving efficiency and is particularly sensitive to executive deficits of perseveration and impaired ability to generate alternative strategies flexibly in response to feedback. The *Trail-Making Test* requires rapid and efficient integration of attention, visual scanning, and cognitive sequencing.

Answers 7.35–7.37

7.35 The answer is C

7.36 The answer is A

7.37 The answer is A

The most frequently used general intelligence batteries for children are the WISC, the Stanford-Binet Test, and the Wechsler Preschool and Primary Scale of Intelligence (WPPSI). A relatively low level of general intelligence is probably the most constant behavioral result of brain damage in children.

Generally, a comprehensive evaluation screens each relevant domain to establish integrity of function. The decision to administer more detailed testing within a domain is based on the referral question, the response to screening measures, and behaviors observed during the test session. A growing number of tests is available for inclusion in an individually designed session. The choice depends on examiner experience and preference.

Intelligence and academic achievement tests vary and the choice of instrument is based in part on the age of the child. For example, *the Stanford-Binet Intelligence Scale is appropriate for children beginning at $2^1/_2$ years of age. It yields a composite IQ score and scores for four scales: verbal reasoning, abstract visual reasoning, quantitative reasoning, and short-term memory.*

Intelligence and achievement tests are not validated with respect to brain function, but they provide valuable data for a neuropsychological evaluation. *The Wechsler Intelligence Scale for Children—Third Edition is the most commonly administered general intelligence test for children at least 6 years of age.* It is a battery comprising 13 subtests (ten core tests and 32 alternates). Three summary IQs are obtained: (1) the Verbal IQ, based on five verbal subtests; (2) the Performance IQ, based on five performance subtests; and (3) the averaged index of general intellectual functioning, the Full Scale IQ. Language expression, comprehension, and application of verbal skills in problem solving are assessed within the verbal scale. Nonverbal visuoperceptual analysis, synthesis, expression, psychomotor speech, and visuomotor efficiency are assessed within the Performance Scale. Neither scale assesses several important factors that influence successful performance, such as motivation, creativity, organizational skills, or study habits. Four additional index scores can be obtained. The Verbal Comprehension Index is based on performances on the information, similarities, vocabulary, and comprehension subtests. The perceptual Organizational Index is based on performances on the picture completion, picture arrangement, block design, and object assembly subtests. The Freedom from Distractibility Index is based on arithmetic and digit-span performances. The Processing Speed Index is based on coding and symbol search performances. The *Wechsler Preschool and Primary Scale of Intelligence (WPPSI)* is a scale for children ages 4 to 6 years, extending the range of assessment downward in age.

Answers 7.38–7.42

7.38 The answer is E

7.39 The answer is A

7.40 The answer is B

7.41 The answer is D

7.42 The answer is C

Immediate (or short-term) memory may be defined as the reproduction, recognition, or recall of perceived material within a period up to 30 seconds after presentation. It is most often assessed by digit repetition and reversal (auditory) and memory-for-designs (visual) tests. Both an auditory-verbal task, such as digit span or memory for words or sentences, and a nonverbal visual task, such as memory for designs or for objects or faces, should be given to assess a patient's immediate memory. Patients can also be asked to listen to a standardized story and then repeat it as accurately as possible. Patients with lesions of the right hemisphere are likely to show more severe defects on visual nonverbal tasks than on auditory verbal tasks. Conversely, patients with left hemisphere disease, including those who are not aphasic, are likely to show severe deficits on the auditory verbal tests, with variable performance on the visual nonverbal tasks.

Recent past memory concerns the retention of information over the past few months. Patients can be asked questions about current events.

Remote memory is the ability to remember events in the distant past. It is commonly believed that remote memory is well preserved in patients who show pronounced defects in recent memory, but the remote memory of senile and amnesic patients is usually significantly inferior to that of normal persons of comparable age and education. Even patients who appear to be able to recount their past fairly accurately show gaps and inconsistencies in their recitals on close examination.

Memory theorists have described three other types of memories: *episodic*, for specific events (e.g., a telephone message); *semantic*, for knowledge and facts (e.g., the first president of the United States); and *implicit*, for automatic skills (e.g., speaking grammatically or driving a car). Semantic and implicit memory do not decline with age, and persons continue to accumulate information over a lifetime. A minimal decline in episodic memory with aging may relate to impaired frontal lobe functioning.

Answers 7.43–7.44

7.43 The answer is A

7.44 The answer is B

One of the more commonly used interview rating scales is the Brief Psychiatric Rating Scale (BPRS). To use the BPRS, the psychologist or psychiatrist completes a mental status interview with the patient and then rates that patient on a series of 18 psychiatric symptoms such as motor retardation, blunted affect, conceptual disorganization, anxiety, and guilt. Expanded definitions of each of these terms are provided to the examiner. The interviewer rates each domain on a seven-point scale from "not present," the lowest rating, to "extremely severe," the highest rating. An experienced interviewer can complete the ratings in 2 or 3 minutes. The BPRS has been used extensively in drug outcome and other studies. The advantages of the BPRS are the reasonably high interrater reliability, the ease and speed of rating, and the well-defined symptom description. *The BPRS ratings are made on the basis of a mental status interview and do not require that the examiner ask any specific questions of the patient.* This approach allows flexibility but results in considerable variation due to interview style. A flexible interview results in different information being gathered by different interviewers.

The SADS *is a highly structured interview instrument.* The interviewer is required to ask each patient a series of prescribed questions to ensure that all relevant areas are addressed. For example, a patient is asked a question similar to the following: "Have you ever heard voices or other things that weren't there or that other people couldn't hear or see?" Based on the patient's response, the examiner asks other detailed, prescribed follow-up questions concerning hallucinations, or if the response was negative, the interviewer moves on to the next question in a different area. This approach ensures that all areas are covered in a comprehensive fashion. The SADS is especially helpful for establishing a reliable diagnosis. The SADS can also be used as an index of behavioral severity. Behavioral changes can be determined by repeated administration. The SADS is quite time-consuming, mainly because it is comprehensive. After an initial evaluation using the complete SADS, a condensed SADS (SADS/C) can be used for follow-up.

The advantage of the test is that it is comprehensive and has reasonably good reliability. One disadvantage is its length; another is that in the structured interview the interviewer must read questions from a lengthy booklet, which makes it difficult to establish eye contact and rapport with the patient. The SADS has been used for both research and clinical purposes, probably more frequently for the former.

8 Theories of Personality and Psychopathology

All psychiatrists should be familiar with the essential aspects of certain theoretical frameworks of personality and psychopathology. Psychoanalysis is the bedrock of psychodynamic understanding and forms the fundamental point of reference for a variety of types of therapeutic intervention. It embraces not only psychoanalysis itself, but also various forms of psychoanalytically oriented psychotherapies, and related therapies involving psychodynamic concepts.

All major psychological theories of personality involve the basic premise that a person's early psychosocial development shapes what comes later: that the impact of childhood events, beliefs, experiences, and fantasies continue, consciously or unconsciously, throughout life and account for adult behavior.

The most important personality theorist of the modern era was Sigmund Freud (1856–1939). His revolutionary contributions to the understanding of the human mind and psyche continue to stimulate, provoke, and challenge students of personality and psychopathology today. His basic tenets of the unconscious mind, psychosexual development, and psychodynamics remain the bedrock of psychoanalytic theory, even though many have disagreed with, modified, or expanded on his ideas. No matter how a particular theorist may feel about Freud's ideas, each must begin with a thorough knowledge of his contributions.

There have been many psychoanalytic personality theorists with widely varying views on development. These include Alfred Adler (1870–1937), Erik Erikson (1902–1994), Karen Horney (1885–1952), Carl Gustav Jung (1875–1961), Melanie Klein (1882–1960), Harry Stack Sullivan (1892–1949), and Heinz Kohut (1913–1981). Schools of thought, encompassing a variety of different theories, include ego psychology, object relations, self psychology, and interpersonal psychology, among others. Each approach has its own perspective on personality development and the development of psychopathology.

Students should study the questions and answers below to test their knowledge in this area.

HELPFUL HINTS

The student should know the various theorists, their schools of thought, and their theories.

- Karl Abraham
- abreaction
- acting out
- Alfred Adler
- Franz Alexander
- Gordon Allport
- analytical process
- attention cathexis
- Michael Balint
- behaviorism
- Eric Berne
- Wilfred Bion
- birth trauma
- Joseph Breuer
- cathexis
- Raymond Cattell
- character traits
- condensation
- conflict
- conscious
- day's residue
- defense mechanisms
- displacement
- dream work
- ego functions
- ego psychology
- Erik Erikson
- Eros and Thanatos
- Ronald Fairbairn
- Sandor Ferenczi
- Anna Freud
- free association
- Erich Fromm
- fundamental rule
- Kurt Goldstein
- Heinz Hartmann
- Karen Horney
- hypnosis
- hysterical phenomena
- infantile sexuality
- instinctual drives
- interpretation
- Carl Gustav Jung
- Søren Kierkegaard
- Melanie Klein
- Heinz Kohut
- latent dream
- Kurt Lewin
- libido
- libido and instinct theories
- manifest dream
- Abraham Maslow
- Adolph Meyer
- multiple self-organizations
- Gardner Murphy
- Henry Murray
- narcissism
- narcissistic, immature, neurotic, and mature defenses
- nocturnal sensory stimuli
- object constancy
- object relations
- parapraxes
- Frederick S. Perls
- preconscious
- preconscious system
- pregenital
- primary and secondary gains
- primary autonomous functions

- primary process
- psychic determinism
- psychoanalytic theory
- psychodynamic thinking
- psychoneurosis
- psychosexual development
- Sandor Rado
- Otto Rank
- reality principle
- reality testing
- regression
- Wilhelm Reich
- repetition compulsion
- repression
- resistance
- secondary process
- secondary revision
- signal anxiety
- structural model
- *Studies on Hysteria*
- Harry Stack Sullivan
- symbolic representation
- symbolism
- synthetic functions of the ego
- talking cure
- *The Ego and the Id*
- *The Interpretation of Dreams*
- topographic theory
- transference
- unconscious motivation
- Donald Winnicott
- wish fulfillment

QUESTIONS

Directions

Each of the questions or incomplete statements below is followed by five suggested responses or completions. Select the *one* that is *best* in each case.

8.1 According to Wilhelm Reich, which of the following attributes can be recognized in a person with a compulsive character?

A. Stiffly walking
B. A cold appearance
C. Excessive complaining
D. Sexually suggestive body movement
E. All of the above

8.2 Which of the following theorists is considered the founder of the attachment theory?

A. Heinz Kohut
B. Adolf Meyer
C. John Bowlby
D. Melanie Klein
E. Otto Kernberg

8.3 According to Erich Fromm, which of the following character types are typical of modern capitalist society?

A. Receptive
B. Exploitative
C. Hoarders
D. Marketers
E. All of the above

8.4 The Oedipus complex as described by Freud involves all of the following *except*

A. intense love relationships
B. rivalries
C. adult sexuality
D. both mother and father
E. anal phase

8.5 The Oedipus complex is resolved according to Freud through

A. the castration complex
B. the acting out of symbolic rivalries
C. moving on to the genital stage of development
D. the realization of one's gender identity
E. the identification with the opposite sex parent

8.6 According to Otto Rank, *death fear* is

A. the fear of dying "before one's time"
B. the fear of losing all ties in the process of becoming separate
C. the fear of losing one's identity by fusing with another person
D. the fear of dying usually associated with a phobia
E. none of the above

8.7 A young woman presents to you complaining of lack of energy, trouble sleeping, depression, and hopelessness that has been present for the last year. You diagnose her with major depressive disorder. Which of the following would have been Freud's explanation of this disorder?

A. She feels despair that her self-object needs will not be met by others.
B. Her internal good objects have been destroyed by aggression and greed.
C. She never mastered the trust versus mistrust stage of ego development.
D. Her depression is actually internally directed anger.
E. She is being persecuted by a tormenting internal object.

8.8 Erik Erikson's epigenetic principle states

A. each sequential stage must be satisfactorily resolved for development to proceed smoothly.
B. the genetic component of personality must be explored to fully understand the ego.
C. each developmental stage must be completed, but in no particular order.
D. development spans the entire life cycle, from infancy through old age and senescence.
E. none of the above

8.9 Separation and individuation

A. involve a "practicing" sub-phase
B. begins at approximately 8 or 9 months of age
C. involve attaining a sense of object permanence
D. is based on the work of Dan Stern, M.D.
E. has no associated anxiety

8.10 Freud declared the road to understanding the unconscious lies in which of the following?

A. Mastering the phases of ego development
B. Understanding infant sexuality
C. Interpretation of dreams
D. Instinct control
E. Repression of preconscious desires

8.11 A patient of yours reports having recurrent dreams of snakes shedding their skins. According to Carl Gustav Jung, this image is an example of which of the following?

A. Manifest content
B. Archetypes
C. Primary process
D. Illusions
E. Phallic symbol

8.12 You have a 72-year-old patient who has been very concerned with her appearance ever since you met her. She has had three facelifts, never leaves the house without makeup, and refuses to allow her grandchildren to call her "grandmother." Which of the following of Erikson's stages is this woman having difficulty mastering?

A. Integrity versus despair
B. Narcissistic
C. Generativity versus stagnation
D. Egocentric
E. Identity versus role confusion

8.13 Attachment theory

A. studies the "stranger situation"
B. is associated with Mary Main
C. relates patterns of adult interactions with significant objects to early infant attachment
D. defines four categories of infant behavior
E. all of the above

8.14 Erikson differs from Freud by his placing greater emphasis on

A. psychosexual development
B. object relations
C. interpersonal relationships
D. cultural factors in development
E. instinctual drives

8.15 Which of the following is *not* considered a mature defense?

A. Anticipation
B. Suppression
C. Somatization
D. Altruism
E. Asceticism

8.16 The work of Anna Freud, daughter of Sigmund Freud, included all of the following *except*

A. Contradictions to her father's claims about psychosexual development
B. Expansion on individual defense mechanisms
C. Development of modern ego psychology
D. Contributions to child psychoanalysis
E. Studies on the function of the ego in personality development

8.17 According to Carl Gustav Jung, archetypes are

A. instinctual patterns
B. expressed in representational images
C. expressed in mythological images
D. organizational units of the personality
E. all of the above

8.18 Which of the following statements regarding Freud's view of hypnosis is *not* true?

A. Freud eventually abandoned the use of hypnosis for the use of free association.
B. Freud believed hypnosis concealed aspects of transference.
C. Freud believed no patient was completely refractory to hypnosis.
D. Freud felt hypnosis encouraged the patient to please the hypnotist.
E. None of the above

8.19 Lacanian theory

A. places heavy emphasis on linguistics
B. has no place for biology or drives
C. postulates that an individual is embedded in political and societal structure
D. views the analytical process as an effort to recognize alienation from one's true self
E. all of the above

8.20 All of the following statements concerning the concept of the preconscious are true *except*

A. It is those mental events brought to consciousness by focusing attention.
B. It interfaces with both the unconscious and the conscious.
C. It acts as a censor to unacceptable wishes and desires.
D. It is part of the topographical model of the mind formulated by Freud.
E. It is characterized by primary process thinking.

8.21 Which of the following about Melanie Klein is *false*?

A. She stressed the role of intrapsychic fantasy.
B. She coined the term "persecutory anxiety."
C. She described the "depressive position."
D. She denounced Freud's "death instinct."
E. She was a child analyst.

Directions

Each set of lettered headings below is followed by a list of numbered words or statements. For each numbered word or statement, select the *one* lettered heading most closely associated with it. Each lettered heading may be selected once, more than once, or not at all.

Questions 8.22–8.25

A. Urethral Stage
B. Genital Stage
C. Latency Stage
D. Anal Stage
E. Phallic Stage

8.22 The ultimate separation from dependence on and attachment to the parents.
8.23 Lying the foundation for gender identity
8.24 Further integration of oedipal identifications
8.25 Striving for separation from dependence and control by parents.

Questions 8.26–8.30

A. Basic trust versus basic mistrust
B. Integrity versus despair
C. Initiative versus guilt
D. Intimacy versus isolation
E. Identity versus role diffusion

8.26 Infancy
8.27 Early childhood
8.28 Puberty and adolescence
8.29 Early adulthood
8.30 Late adulthood

Questions 8.31–8.35

A. Anna Freud
B. Erik Erikson
C. Sigmund Freud
D. Melanie Klein
E. Harry Stack Sullivan

8.31 Civilization and its Discontents
8.32 Envy and Gratitude
8.33 Schizophrenia as a Human Process
8.34 The Ego and the Mechanisms of Defense
8.35 Childhood and Society

Questions 8.36–8.40

A. Franz Alexander
B. Donald Winnicott
C. Karen Horney
D. Melanie Klein
E. Heinz Kohut

8.36 Introduced the concept of the transitional object
8.37 Believed that oedipal strivings are experienced during the first year of life, wherein gratifying experiences with the good breast reinforce basic trust
8.38 Emphasized cultural factors and disturbances in interpersonal and intrapsychic development
8.39 Introduced the concept of the corrective emotional experience
8.40 Expanded Freud's concept of narcissism; his/her theories are known as self psychology

Questions 8.41–8.45

A. Initiative versus guilt
B. Intimacy versus isolation
C. Trust versus mistrust
D. Industry versus inferiority
E. Generativity versus stagnation

8.41 Care
8.42 Hope
8.43 Love
8.44 Purpose
8.45 Competence

Questions 8.46–8.49

A. Projection
B. Displacement
C. Sublimation
D. Repression
E. Reaction formation

8.46 A young woman gets into an argument with her boyfriend. Although very upset, she remains silent as he tells her she is worthless. Once she gets home, the young woman picks a fight with her younger sister over nothing and begins yelling at her.
8.47 A young man is very envious of his best friend. Although it is difficult to admit, he believes his friend is more successful, better looking, and is always the life of the party. To the contrary, this young man tells his family that his best friend is envious of him, despite there being no evidence that this is so.
8.48 An 18-year-old male lives alone with his mother and despises her. He is embarrassed that he has these feelings, and compensates by hovering over her, attending to her every need.
8.49 A middle-aged man has had an unconscious desire to control others for as long as he can remember. To fulfill this need, he became a prison guard.

Questions 8.50–8.53

A. Manifest dream content
B. Latent dream content
C. Dream work
D. Secondary revision

8.50 Unconscious thoughts and wishes
8.51 What is recalled by the dreamer
8.52 Mental operation of making the unconscious known
8.53 Work of organizing aspects of a dream into less bizarre form

Questions 8.54–8.58

A. Narcissistic defense
B. Immature defense
C. Neurotic defense
D. Mature defense

8.54 Humor
8.55 Displacement
8.56 Regression
8.57 Denial
8.58 Sublimation

Questions 8.59–8.61

A. Prototaxic mode
B. Parataxic mode
C. Syntaxic mode

8.59 Events are causally related because of temporal or serial connections
8.60 Most logical, rational, and mature type of cognitive functioning
8.61 Undifferentiated thought that cannot separate the whole into parts

ANSWERS

8.1 The answer is A

According to Wilhelm Reich (1897–1957), individuals with compulsive character are tense and restrained, *walk stiffly*, and sit rigidly. They are overconcerned about orderliness, tend to ruminate, and are indecisive and distrusting. They experience a blockage between their thoughts and feelings. Because they have little access to their feelings, they have little ability to prioritize their actions, to make decisions, or to sense others' reactions to them. The compulsive character avoids expression of repressed impulses by rigid overcontrol. Because of this, these individuals are very threatened by trivial changes in routine.

The hysterical character has the least body armoring, hence the most lability of function. Body movements tend to be soft, rolling, and *sexually suggestive*. Phallic-narcissistic people *appear cold*, reserved, and prickly. Masochistic individuals suffer, *complain*, and damage and deprecate themselves in ways that provoke and torture others.

8.2 The answer is C

John Bowlby is generally considered the founder of attachment theory. He formed his ideas about attachment in the 1950s while he was consulting with the World Health Organization on the problems of homelessness in children. He stressed that the essence of attachment is proximity (i.e., the tendency of a child to stay close to the mother or caregiver). A basic sense of security and safety is derived from a continuous and close relationship with the caregiver, according to Bowlby. He felt that without this early proximity to the mother or caregiver, the child does not develop a secure base, which he considered a launching pad for independence. In the absence of a secure base, the child feels frightened or threatened, and development is severely compromised.

Heinz Kohut is best known for his writings on narcissism and the development of self psychology. *Adolf Meyer* introduced the concept of common sense psychiatry, which focused on the ways in which a patient's current life situation could be realistically improved. *Melanie Klein* evolved a theory of internal object relations that was intimately likened to drives. *Otto Kernberg* works as one of the most influential object relations theorists in the United States.

8.3 The answer is E (all)

As a social philosopher and critic, Fromm did not really develop a systematic theory of psychopathology. He identified three major mechanisms of retreat from individuation. Some individuals, he said, may seek an authoritarian solution, trying to live through someone or something external to themselves, relying on that for their sense of adequacy. Others may become destructive, attacking anything that confronts them with their separateness and aloneness. Most individuals develop a conformist attitude, warding off the anxiety of experiencing their own intentionality by accepting socially offered thoughts, roles, and attitudes.

These mechanisms result in four different unproductive orientations or characters typical of modern capitalist society: receptive, exploitative, hoarding, and marketing. The *receptive character* often appears to be cooperative and open; however, the primary agenda is to establish a passive relationship with a leader who solves problems magically. *Exploitative characters* are likewise interested in filling themselves up from the outside; however, they aggressively manipulate and usurp whatever reduces their terror. *Hoarders* collect, store, and close in on themselves, often being cold and aloof in their efforts to feel secure. *Marketers* treat themselves as a plastic commodity to be manipulated as needed to achieve externally validated success.

8.4 The answer is E

The *phallic period*, during which the Oedipus complex emerges, is a critical phase of development for the budding formation of the child's own sense of gender identity—as decisively male or female—based on the child's discovery and realization of the significance of anatomical sexual differences. *Adult sexual adjustment* is said to rely on the *attachment to one parent and the identification with the other*. The events associated with the phallic phase also set the stage for the developmental predisposition to later psychoneuroses. Freud used the term Oedipus complex to refer to the *intense love relationships*, together with their associated *rivalries*, hostilities, and emerging identifications, formed during this period between the child and parents.

8.5 The answer is A

There is some differentiation between the sexes in the pattern of development. Freud explained the nature of this discrepancy in terms of genital differences. Under normal circumstances, he believed that, for boys, the *oedipal situation was resolved by the castration complex*. Specifically, the boy had to give up his strivings for his mother because of the threat of castration—castration anxiety. In contrast, the Oedipus complex in girls was also evoked by reason of the castration complex, but unlike the boy, the little girl was already castrated, and as a result, she turned to her father as bearer of the penis out of a sense of disappointment over her own lack of a penis. The little girl was thus more threatened by a loss of love than by actual castration fears.

8.6 The answer is C

Death fear is *the fear of losing one's identity by fusing with another person*. The weaker one's personal identity, the stronger the death fear.

Life fear, by contrast, is *fear of losing all ties in the process of becoming separate*. Every person experiences the cycle of movement from union to separation and back again as part of the life process. This movement takes place at various levels: family, societal, artistic, and spiritual. At each level, there is one or more movement toward union and rebirth. Each person, for example, usually yields to a love experience in which personal differences are set aside to experience unity with another, to experience self-worth, and to be relieved of the sense of difference. The yielding to another ends when the will asserts its separateness, and a new affirmation of individuality occurs.

Fear of dying *associated with a phobia* or "*before one's time*" are not ideas associated with Otto Rank.

8.7 The answer is D

Freud originally understood *depression as internally directed anger*. In his view the self-reproaches and the loss of self-esteem commonly experienced by depressed patients are directed not at the self, but rather, at an ambivalently experienced introject. He noted that in some cases the only way the ego can give up an object is to introject it, so the anger directed at the ambivalently held object takes on the clinical manifestation of the depression.

From the self-psychological point of view associated with Heinz Kohut, *depression is related to a sense of despair about ever getting one's self object needs met by people in the environment*. Melanie Klein suggested that depression is linked to a reactivation of the depressive position; depressed patients are convinced that they have *destroyed their internal good objects because of their own aggression and greed*. As a result, they feel persecuted by internal bad objects while longing for the lost love objects.

Erikson hypothesized that the depressed patient's experience of being empty and of being no good is an outgrowth of a *developmental derailment* that causes oral pessimism to predominate. Depression therefore results from failing to develop a basic sense of trust or the virtue of hope. From an object relations perspective, many depressed patients unconsciously experience themselves to be at the mercy of a *tormenting internal object* that is unrelenting in its persecution of them. In cases of psychosis, that primitive forerunner of the superego may actually be hallucinated as a voice that is unrelentingly critical.

8.8 The answer is A

Erikson's formulations were based on the concept of epigenesis, a term borrowed from embryology. His *epigenetic principle holds that development occurs in sequential, clearly defined stages, and that each stage must be satisfactorily resolved* for *development to proceed smoothly*. According to the epigenetic model, if successful resolution of a particular stage does not occur, all subsequent stages reflect the failure in the form of physical, cognitive, social, or emotional maladjustment.

8.9 The answer is A

Margaret Mahler has conceptualized the process of development in terms of phases of separation and individuation. The *"practicing" sub-phase* of this process follows upon the first or "hatching" sub-phase, which arises at approximately *4 or 5 months of age*. The third sub-phase, "rapproachement" *involves separation anxiety*. The child's wishes to be separate from the mother are tempered by an increasing awareness of the need for and dependence on the mother. The fourth, and final phase, the sub-phase of "object constancy," involves consolidation of individuality and mature psychological involvement with others. *Object permanence*, the knowledge that objects in the external world have an existence independent of the child's actions on them or interactions with them is a major accomplishment of Piaget's sensorimotor period of intellectual development. *Dan Stern*, a psychiatrist and psychoanalyst, who focused his work on infant observation, brought into clearer focus the intense affective and interactional matrix between mother and child and directed attention more specifically to the emergence of a sense of self.

8.10 The answer is C

Freud became aware of the significance of dreams when he noted that patients frequently reported their dreams in the process of free association. Through their further associations to dream content, he learned that dreams were definitely meaningful, even though meanings were often hidden or disguised. Most of all, Freud was struck by the intimate connection between dream content and unconscious memories or fantasies that were long repressed. This observation led Freud to declare that *the interpretation of dreams was the royal road to understanding the unconscious*.

8.11 The answer is B

Carl Gustav Jung believed *archetypes* to be instinctual patterns. All psychic energy is transmitted in forms of experience, behavior, and emotion, which are expressed in representational or mythological images. Thus, the archetypes represent the basic motivations and drives that become organizational units of the personality. Snakes shedding their skins are usually interpreted as a symbol for change and renewal. *Primary processes, manifest content of dreams, and phallic representations are concepts of Freud*.

8.12 The answer is A

Erikson's theory of psychosocial development centers around eight stages of ego development throughout the life cycle. *Integrity versus despair* is the last of the stages and takes place between age 65 and death. If this stage is successfully mastered, the individual arrives at a peaceful acceptance of his/her own mortality without losing interest in life. This patient in this case, however, is clearly having difficulties with this stage as she attempts to deny the passage of time and refuses to prepare for this endpoint of the life cycle. A person in a stage of despair is unconsciously fearful of death, and lives in basic self-contempt.

Generativity versus stagnation is another of Erikson's stages that takes place from ages 40 to 65, and is focused on raising children with nurturance and love and not living in isolation. The stage of *identity versus role confusion* occurs between age 11 and the end of adolescence, where the adolescent must begin to establish a future role in adult society.

8.13 The answer is E (all)

Attachment theory takes its origin in the work of John Bowlby. *It relates patterns of early infant attachment to patterns of adult interaction with significant objects*. It emphasizes the significance of the mother's empathic responsivity to infant needs for self-development and relatedness, the importance of the mother-child involvement for personality development, and the role of the mother as catalyst for age-appropriate development. Using the Adult Attachment Interview (AAI), developed by *Mary Main*, these theorists document the nature if internal working models of early attachment relations. Study of infant responses in the *stranger situation*, an arrangement for observing the quality of parent-child interaction and the effects of separation, has led to *the definition of four categories of infant behavior: secure, avoidant, resistant and disorganized-disoriented.*

8.14 The answer is D

Erikson's work concentrated on the effects of social, cultural, and psychological factors in development. Although Erikson acknowledged the important role of sexuality, it was less central to his theory. *The concepts of instinctual drives and psychosexual development are essential parts of Freud's theories, not Erikson's. Object relations*, which refer not to interpersonal relationships but to the interactions of internalized constructs of external relationships, is the central idea in object relation psychology.

8.15 The answer is C

Somatization is an immature defense. In it, psychic derivatives are converted into bodily symptoms, and patients react with somatic manifestations rather than psychic manifestations. All the others are mature defenses. *Anticipation* is goal directed and involves realistic anticipation or planning for future inner discomfort. *Suppression* involves the conscious postponement of attention to a conscious impulse or conflict. *Altruism* uses constructive and instinctually satisfying service to others to undergo a vicarious experience. *Asceticism* involves the assignment of value to specific pleasure and is directed against all base pleasures.

8.16 The answer is A

Anna Freud, the daughter of Sigmund Freud, ultimately made her own set of unique contributions to psychoanalysis. Whereas her father focused primarily on repression as the central defense mechanism, Anna Freud greatly *elaborated on individual defense mechanisms*, including reaction formation, undoing, introjection, identification, projection, turning against the self, reversal, and sublimation. She was also a key figure in the *development of modern ego psychology* in that she emphasized that there was "depth in the surface." In other words, the defenses marshaled by the ego to avoid unacceptable wishes from the id were in and of themselves complex and worthy of attention. Up to that point the primary focus had been on uncovering unconscious sexual and aggressive wishes. She also made seminal contributions to *the field of child psychoanalysis* and studied the *function of the ego in personality development*. She founded the Hampstead child therapy course and clinic in London in 1947 and served as its director. *Anna Freud was not known to have contradicted her father's claims on psychosexual development.*

8.17 The answer is E (all)

Carl Gustav Jung believed archetypes to be *instinctual patterns*. All psychic energy is transmitted in forms of experience, behavior, and emotion, which are *expressed in representational* or *mythological images*. Thus, the archetypes represent the basic motivations and drives that become *organizational units of the personality*.

8.18 The answer is C

Freud's concept of transference was to become a cornerstone of psychoanalytic theory and technique, a discovery that eventually contributed to his abandonment of hypnosis as a tool. Freud first observed that *many patients were simply refractory to hypnosis*. When a patient could be hypnotized, he noted following the discovery of transference that *hypnosis concealed aspects of the transference*, so that these aspects could not be investigated as part of the process. He also felt that *hypnosis encouraged the patient to please the hypnotist*, instead of learning about the origins and the meanings of symptoms. By the late 1890s, Freud abandoned hypnosis. Instead, he had the patient lie on the couch and say whatever came to mind without censorship, which is the method of *free association* that remains a central part of psychoanalytic technique today.

8.19 The answer is E (all)

The French psychoanalyst Jacques Lacan (1901–1981) made a lasting impression on French psychoanalysis as well as on literary and film criticism in academic departments throughout the world. *Lacan's reading of Freud relies heavily on linguistics.* The notion that the human being is constituted by language is one of three basic principles endorsed by Lacan. *The unconscious is structured like a language that consists only of signifiers—biology and drives have no place in his theory.* Second, the ego does not exist as an autonomous structure. *A third principle is that an individual is inevitably embedded in political and societal structure that cannot be transcended.*

Lacan preferred to speak of "orders" rather than stages of development, and he identified three orders relevant to understanding the human condition. From 6 to 18 months there is an imaginary order involving a mirror stage, during which infants delight in identifying with their reflection. This preverbal and presymbolic order gives way to a symbolic order involving the acquisition of language and a split between the inner and the outer world. The inner world is connected with a misrecognition in the mirror stage where the "I" or the self is identified, with the father's laws and the cultural standards associated with those laws: The final order is that of the "real," which is stark factual reality and exists somewhere outside of language; this is viewed as unreachable and indefinable by Lacan.

Lacan thrived on being unorthodox. He denied the significance of diagnoses, rules, or established schools of thought. *He saw the analytical process as an effort to recognize the alienation from one's true self.* Analysis was also designed to bring out underlying structures and contexts in the unconscious. Historical reconstruction is downplayed whereas desire for the "Other" is examined in all its many forms.

Lacanian analysis has had little influence on the clinical practice of psychoanalysis in North America, although literary critics within American universities have made many applications of Lacan in their analyses of texts. Its anti-empirical basis, its denial of the importance of preverbal human experience, and the impenetrability of much of the prose written by Lacan and Lacanian disciples have made it less popular among American clinicians than those in Europe and South America.

8.20 The answer is E

The publication of *The Interpretation of Dreams* in 1900 heralded the arrival of Freud's topographical model of the mind, in which he divided the mind into three regions: the conscious system, the preconscious system, and the unconscious system. The preconscious system comprises those mental events, processes, and contents that can be *brought to conscious awareness by the act of focusing attention*. Although most persons are not consciously aware of the appearance of their first-grade teacher, they ordinarily can bring this image to mind by deliberately focusing attention on the memory. Conceptually, *the preconscious interfaces with both the unconscious and conscious* regions of the mind. To reach conscious awareness, contents of the unconscious must become linked with words and thus become preconscious. The preconscious also serves to maintain the repressive barrier and to *censor unacceptable wishes and desires. It is the unconscious system (not the preconscious) that is characterized by primary process thinking.*

8.21 The answer is D

Melanie Klein thought that *Freud's concept of the death instinct was central* to understanding aggression, hatred, sadism, and other forms of badness, which she viewed as derivatives of the death instinct. Her perspective grew largely from her *psychoanalytic work with children.* She became impressed with *the role of unconscious intrapsychic fantasy*, and proposed that infants project derivatives of the death instinct into the mother, and then fear attack from the "bad mother," a phenomenon referred to as *persecutory anxiety*. This anxiety is associated with Klein's paranoid-schizoid position. Through the integration of good and bad internal object relations, infants develop concern for the mother toward whom they have developed harmful fantasies. This concern results in reparation, and the entering of the *depressive position.*

Answers 8.22–8.25

8.22 The answer is B

8.23 The answer is E

8.24 The answer is C

8.25 The answer is D

The awareness of the external world of objects develops gradually in infants. Soon after birth, they are primarily aware of physical sensations, such as hunger, cold, and pain, which give rise to tension, and caregivers are regarded primarily as persons who relieve their tension or remove painful stimuli. Recent infant research, however, suggests that awareness of others begins much sooner than Freud originally thought. Table 8.1 provides a summary of the objectives for the stages of psychosexual development and the object relationships associated with each stage.

Answers 8.26–8.30

8.26 The answer is A

8.27 The answer is C

8.28 The answer is E

8.29 The answer is D

8.30 The answer is B

The first of Erik Erikson's developmental stages, *infancy* (birth to 1 year), is characterized by the first psychosocial crisis the infant must face, that of *basic trust versus basic mistrust.* The crisis takes place in the context of the intimate relationship between the infant and its mother. The infant's primary orientation to reality is erotic and centers on the mouth. The successful resolution of the stage includes a disposition to trust others, a basic trust in oneself, a capacity to entrust oneself, and a sense of self-confidence.

During *early childhood* (ages 3 to 5 years), the crisis addressed by the child is *initiative versus guilt.* As the child struggles to resolve the oedipal struggle, guilt may grow because of aggressive thoughts or wishes. Initiative arises as the child begins to desire to mimic the adult world and as the child finds enjoyment in productive activity.

The stage of *puberty and adolescence* (age 11 years through the end of adolescence) is characterized by *identity versus role diffusion,* during which the adolescent must begin to establish a future role in adult society. During this psychosocial crisis, the adolescent is peculiarly vulnerable to social and cultural influences.

Early adulthood (21 to 40 years) is characterized by *intimacy versus isolation.* The crisis is characterized by the need to establish the capacity to relate intimately and meaningfully with

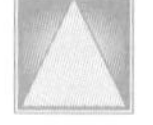

Table 8.1
Stages of Psychosexual Development and their objectives

Stage	Objective
Oral	To establish a trusting dependence on nursing and sustaining objects, to establish comfortable expressing and gratification of oral libidinal needs without excessive conflict or ambivalence from oral sadistic wishes.
Anal	The anal period is essentially a period of striving for independence and separation from the dependence on and control by the parent. The objectives of sphincter control without overcontrol (fecal retention) or loss of control (messing) are matched by the child's attempts to achieve autonomy and independence without excessive shame or self-doubt from loss of control.
Urethral	Issues of control and urethral performance and loss of control. It is not clear whether or to what extent the objectives of urethral functioning differ from those of the anal period.
Phallic	The objective of this phase is to focus erotic interest in the genital area and genital functions. This focusing lays the foundation for gender identity and serves to integrate the residues of previous stages of psychosexual development into a predominantly genital-sexual orientation. The establishing of oedipal situation is essential for the furtherance of subsequent identifications that will serve as the basis for important and enduring dimensions of character organization.
Latency	The primary objective in this period is the further integration of oedipal identifications and a consolidation of sex-role identity and sex roles. The relative quiescence and control of instinctual impulses allow for the development of ego apparatuses and mastery skills. Further identificatory components may be added to the oedipal ones on the basis of broadening contacts with other significant figures outside the family, such as teachers, coaches, and other adults.
Genital	The primary objectives of this period are on the ultimate separation from dependence on and attachment to the parents and the establishment of mature, nonincestuous object relations. Related to this are the achievement of a mature sense of personal identity and acceptance and the integration of a set of adult roles and functions that permit new adaptive integrations with social expectations and cultural values.

others in mutually satisfying and productive interactions. The failure to achieve a successful resolution of that crisis results in a sense of personal isolation. *Late adulthood* (65 and older) is characterized by *integrity versus despair.* The crisis implies and depends on the successful resolution of all the preceding crises of psychosocial growth. It entails the acceptance of oneself and of all the aspects of life and the integration of their elements into a stable pattern of living. The failure to achieve ego integration often results in a kind of despair and an unconscious fear of death. The person who fails this crisis lives in basic self-contempt.

Answers 8.31–8.35

8.31 The answer is C

8.32 The answer is D

8.33 The answer is E

8.34 The answer is A

8.35 The answer is B

Anna Freud is probably best known for her book "*The Ego and the Mechanisms of Defense*." In it she gives a particularly clear description of how the defenses work, including some special attention to adolescents' use of defenses. *Melanie Klein's "Envy and Gratitude"* contains papers from 1946 until her death in 1960, and two papers published posthumously. In it, she introduces her theory of primary envy. In *"Civilization and Its Discontents," Sigmund Freud* proposes that the conflict between sexual needs and societal mores is the source of mankind's propensity for dissatisfaction, aggression, hostility and ultimately violence. *Erik Erikson, in "Childhood and Society,"* writes about the influence of society on culture and child development. He correlated personality growth with parental and societal values. *Harry Stack Sullivan, in "Schizophrenia as a Human Process,"* expounded the idea that schizophrenia developed as a result of the cultural forces that bore on the individual.

Answers 8.36–8.40

8.36 The answer is B

8.37 The answer is D

8.38 The answer is C

8.39 The answer is A

8.40 The answer is E

Donald Winnicott (1897–1971) was an influential contributor to object relations theory. He focused on the conditions that make it possible for a child to develop awareness as a separate person. One of the conditions is the provision of an environment termed "good-enough mothering." Good-enough mothering enables the child to be nurtured in a nonimpinging environment that permits the emergence of the true self. Winnicott *introduced the concept of the transitional object,* something that helps the child gradually shift from subjectivity to external reality. Such a material possession, usually blankets or a soft toy, exists in an intermediate realm as a substitute for the mother and as one of the first objects a child begins to recognize as separate from the self.

Melanie Klein (1882–1960) modified psychoanalytic theory, particularly in its application to infants and very young children. In contrast to orthodox psychoanalytic theory, which postulates the development of the superego during the fourth year of life, Klein's theory maintains that a primitive superego is formed during the first and second years. Klein further believed that aggressive, rather than sexual, drives are preeminent during the earliest stages of development. She deviated most sharply from classic psychoanalytic theory in her formulations concerning the Oedipus complex. She *believed that oedipal strivings are experienced during the first year of life,* as opposed to the classic formulation of its occurring between the ages of 3 and 5. She also believed that, *during the first year, gratifying experiences with the good breast reinforce basic trust* and that frustrating experiences can lead to a depressive position.

Karen Horney (1885–1952) was an American psychiatrist who ascribed great importance to the influence of sociocultural factors on individual development. She raised questions about the existence of immutable instinctual drives and developmental phases or sexual conflict as the root of neurosis while recognizing the importance of sexual drives. Rather than focusing on such concepts as the Oedipus complex, Horney *emphasized cultural factors and disturbances in interpersonal and intrapsychic development* as the cause of neuroses in general.

Franz Alexander (1891–1964) founded the Chicago Institute for Psychoanalysis. He *introduced the concept of the corrective emotional experience.* The therapist, who is supportive, enables the patient to master past traumas and to modify the effects of those traumas. Alexander was also a major influence in the field of psychosomatic medicine.

Heinz Kohut (1913–1981) *expanded Sigmund Freud's concept of narcissism.* In *The Analysis of the Self,* published in 1971, Kohut wrote about a large group of patients suffering from narcissistic personality disorder whom he believed to be analyzable but who did not develop typical transference neuroses in the classic sense. The conflict involves the relation between the self and archaic narcissistic objects. Those objects are the grandiose self and the idealized parent image, the reactivations of which constitute a threat to the patient's sense of integrity. Kohut's *theories are known as self psychology.*

Answers 8.41–8.45

8.41 The answer is E

8.42 The answer is C

8.43 The answer is B

8.44 The answer is A

8.45 The answer is D

See Table 8.2.

Answers 8.46–8.49

8.46 The answer is B

8.47 The answer is A

8.48 The answer is E

8.49 The answer is C

In freudian psychoanalytic theory, defense mechanisms represent the ego's attempts to mediate between the pressure of the

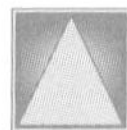

Table 8.2
Erikson's Psychosocial Stages

Psychosocial Stage	Associated Virtue
Trust vs. mistrust (birth—)	Hope
Autonomy vs. shame and doubt (~18 months—)	Will
Initiative vs. guilt (~3 years—)	Purpose
Industry vs. inferiority (~5 years—)	Competence
Identity vs. role confusion (~13 years—)	Fidelity
Intimacy vs. isolation (~20s—)	Love
Generativity vs. stagnation (~40s—)	Care
Integrity vs. despair (~60s—)	Wisdom

Adapted from Erikson E. *Insight and Responsibility*. New York: WW Norton; 1964; Erikson E. *Identity: Youth and Crisis*. New York: WW Norton: 1968.

instinctual drives emerging from the id, and the restrictions imposed by the societal rules from the superego.

Displacement is the shifting of unacceptable emotions or impulses to a more appropriate object. Although the woman is angry at her boyfriend, she waits until she gets home and displaces this anger on her younger sibling, a less dangerous outlet. *Projection* is a defense mechanism in which the patient reacts to an inner unacceptable impulse as if it were outside the self. In this case, the man projects his envy as coming from his friend, when it is actually an inner unacceptable impulse. In *reaction formation*, an unacceptable unconscious impulse is transformed into its opposite. The teenage boy, rather than accepting his feelings of hatred towards his mother, treats her with love and constant attention. *Sublimation* is satisfaction of an objectionable impulse obtained by using socially acceptable means. The man in this case is therefore channeling his urges to control others, rather than preventing them. *Repression* is the unconscious act of preventing a thought or feeling from entering consciousness.

Answers 8.50–8.53

8.50 The answer is B

8.51 The answer is A

8.52 The answer is C

8.53 The answer is D

Freud distinguished between two layers of dream content. The *manifest content* refers to what is recalled by the dreamer; the *latent content* involved the unconscious thoughts and wishes that threaten to awaken the dreamer. Freud described the unconscious mental operations by which latent dream content is transformed into manifest dream as the *dream work*. Repressed wishes and impulses must attach themselves to innocent or neutral images to pass the scrutiny of the dream censor. This process involves selection of apparently meaningless or trivial images from the dreamer's current experience, images that are dynamically associated with the latent images that they resemble in some respect. *Secondary revision* is the process by which primitive aspects of dreams are made into more coherent and less bizarre form.

Answers 8.54–8.58

8.54 The answer is D

8.55 The answer is C

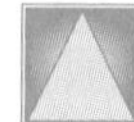

Table 8.3
Defense Mechanisms

Denial. A mechanism in which the existence of unpleasant realities is disavowed. The mechanism keeps out of conscious awareness any aspects of external reality that, if acknowledged, would produce anxiety. A narcissistic defense.

Displacement. A mechanism by which the emotional component of an unacceptable idea or object is transferred to a more acceptable one. A neurotic defense.

Humor. The overt expression of feelings without personal discomfort or immobilization and without unpleasant effects on others. Humor allows one to bear, yet focus on, what is too terrible to be borne, in contrast to wit, which always involves distraction or displacement away from the affective issues. A mature defense.

Regression. A mechanism in which a person undergoes a partial or total return to early patterns of adaptation. Regression is observed in many psychiatric conditions, particularly schizophrenia. An immature defense.

Sublimation. A mechanism in which the energy associated with unacceptable impulses or drives is diverted into personally and socially acceptable channels. Unlike other defense mechanisms, sublimation offers some minimal gratification of the instinctual drive or impulse. A mature defense.

8.56 The answer is B

8.57 The answer is A

8.58 The answer is D

George Valliant classified four types of defense mechanisms: mature, immature, neurotic, and narcissistic. *Humor and sublimation are considered mature defenses*. Mature defense mechanisms are healthy and adaptive, and they are seen in normal adults. *Displacement is considered a neurotic defense*. Neurotic defenses are seen in obsessive-compulsive patients, hysterical patients, and adults under stress. *Regression is considered an immature defense*. Immature defenses are seen in adolescents and are also seen in psychopathological states such as depression. They are the most primitive defense mechanisms. *Denial is considered a narcissistic defense*, which is characteristic of young children and psychotic adults. At times, some of the defensive categories overlap; for instance, neurotic defenses may be seen in normally healthy, mature adults. These defense mechanisms are defined in Table 8.3.

Answers 8.59–8.61

8.59 The answer is B

8.60 The answer is C

8.61 The answer is A

Harry Stack Sullivan described three modes of experiencing and thinking about the world. The *prototaxic mode* is undifferentiated thought that cannot separate the whole into parts or use symbols. It occurs normally in infancy and also appears in patients with schizophrenia. In the *parataxic mode*, events are causally related because of temporal or serial connections. Logical relationships, however, are not perceived. The *syntaxic mode* is the logical, rational, and most mature type of cognitive functioning of which a person is capable. These three types of thinking and experiencing occur side by side in all persons; it is the rare person who functions exclusively in the syntaxic mode.

9

Clinical Examination of the Psychiatric Patient

The psychiatric evaluation comprises two sections. The first is a series of histories: psychiatric, medical, and family. The second is the mental status examination, which reviews the patient's emotional and cognitive functioning at the time of the interview. Because diagnosis in psychiatry is not etiologically based, and because it does not have any external validating criteria, a psychiatric diagnosis is as good as the knowledge and skill of the clinician making it. The *Diagnostic and Statistical Manual of Mental Disorders* (DSM) diagnostic system, with which all American psychiatrists are intimately familiar, is based on descriptive phenomenology rather than inferred date, and has greatly increased the reliability of psychiatric diagnoses.

A structured history and mental status examination is a guide for organizing the patient's history. While it is not intended as a rigid plan for interviewing a patient, attending to all its sections does allow for greater completeness of assessment. It ensures that the clinician attends to issues other than only symptoms, like a developmental history, sexual history, and attention to the patient biologically, psychologically, and socially.

In this day and age of increased monitoring of medical care by third parties, the astute clinician must be aware of good documentation of care, and attend to the medical record. Reviews of cases are often conducted by persons with little or no background in psychiatry who do not recognize the complexities of psychiatric diagnosis and treatment. "Inadequate information" in a chart is unacceptable.

Similarly, psychiatrists must have a knowledge and understanding of physical signs and symptoms. They must often decide whether a patient needs a medical examination, and what that should include. There are numerous medical conditions that can manifest psychiatric symptoms. Each of these diagnoses argues for a different set of laboratory or diagnostic tests. Advances in neuropsychiatry and biological psychiatry have made laboratory tests more and more useful. Laboratory tests are also used to monitor dosing, treatment adherence, and toxic effects of various psychotropic medications.

The student should address the following questions and study the answers to gain knowledge of the clinical examination of the psychiatric patient.

HELPFUL HINTS

Students should familiarize themselves with these terms, especially the acronyms and names of laboratory tests.

- adulthood
- anamnesis
- antipsychotics
- appearance, behavior, attitude, and speech
- appropriateness
- carbamazepine
- catecholamines
- chief complaint
- clang associations
- concentration, memory, and intelligence
- confabulation
- consciousness and orientation
- countertransference
- CSF
- CT
- current social situation
- cyclic antidepressants
- data
- do's and don'ts of treating violent patients
- dreams, fantasies, and value systems
- DSM-IV-TR and Axes I–V
- early, middle, and late childhood history
- EEG
- eliciting delusional beliefs
- family history
- history of present illness; previous illnesses
- initial interview and greeting
- interviewing variations
- judgment and insight
- lithium
- marital history
- medical history
- mental status examination
- military history
- mood, feelings, and affect
- neologisms
- occupational and educational history
- paraphasia
- patient questions
- perception
- PET
- polysomnography
- prenatal history
- prognosis
- psychiatric history
- psychiatric report
- psychodynamic formulation
- psychosexual history
- punning
- rapport
- reliability
- religious background
- resistance
- sensorium and cognition
- sexuality
- social activity
- stress interview
- style
- subsequent interviews
- therapeutic alliance
- thought process
- time management
- transference
- treatment plan
- TRH
- TSH
- uncovering feelings
- VDRL
- word salad

QUESTIONS

Directions

Each of the questions or incomplete statements below is followed by five suggested responses or completions. Select the *one* that is *best* in each case.

9.1 The psychiatric history

A. focuses exclusively on information obtained from the patient
B. has no formal structure
C. focuses primarily on symptoms
D. does not address medical issues
E. attends to the patient's anamnesis

9.2 The medical record

A. cannot be used by regulatory agencies
B. is absolutely confidential
C. cannot be used in malpractice litigation
D. is accessible to patients
E. is used only by the treating team

9.3 Formal thought disorders include

A. circumstantiality
B. clang associations
C. neologisms
D. flight of ideas
E. all of the above

9.4 True statements about diagnostic tests in psychiatric disorders include

A. serum amylase may be increased in bulimia nervosa
B. serum bicarbonate may be decreased in panic disorder
C. decreased serum calcium has been associated with depression
D. serum bicarbonate may be elevated in bulimia nervosa
E. all of the above

9.5 Which of the following is *not* part of the sensorium category of the mental status examination?

A. Fund of knowledge
B. Abstract thinking
C. Alertness
D. Judgment
E. Concentration

9.6 Tests of concentration include all of the following *except*

A. calculations
B. repeating a series of random numbers
C. proverb interpretation
D. spelling "world" backward
E. repeating three or four unrelated objects after 5 to 10 minutes

9.7 Which of the following is included in the medical record of a patient admitted to an inpatient psychiatric unit?

A. The treatment plan
B. Summaries of case conferences
C. Reports of diagnostic evaluations
D. Legal admission documents
E. All of the above

9.8 Hypothyroidism in the elderly may commonly present with all of the following *except*

A. lassitude
B. fatigue
C. cognitive impairment
D. anorexia
E. constipation

9.9 True statements about the lengths of time drugs of abuse can be detected in urine include

A. morphine for 8 days
B. benzodiazepine for 2 to 3 weeks
C. alcohol for 7 to 12 hours
D. marijuana for 24 to 48 hours
E. cocaine for 1 to 2 weeks

9.10 A good test for recent memory is to ask patients

A. their date of birth
B. what they had to eat for their last meal
C. how many siblings they have
D. to subtract 7 from 100
E. who is the president of the United States

9.11 Common pretreatment lithium tests include

A. ECG
B. pregnancy test
C. serum electrolytes
D. serum BUN
E. all of the above

9.12 Polysomnography (sleep EEG) abnormalities include

A. a decrease in the amount of REM sleep in major depressive disorder
B. a lengthened REM latency in major depressive disorder
C. an increase in REM sleep in dementia
D. an increased sleep latency in schizophrenia
E. none of the above

9.13 The first sign of beginning cerebral disease is impairment of

A. immediate memory
B. recent memory
C. long-term memory
D. remote memory
E. none of the above

9.14 In a psychiatric interview

A. the psychiatrist may have to medicate a violent patient before taking a history
B. a violent patient should be interviewed alone to establish a patient–doctor relationship
C. delusions should be challenged directly

D. the psychiatrist must not ask depressed patients if they have suicidal thoughts
E. the psychiatrist should have a seat higher than the patient's seat

9.15 Which of the following substances has been implicated in mood disorders with a seasonal pattern?

A. luteotropic hormone (LTH)
B. gonadotropin-releasing hormone (GnRH)
C. testosterone
D. estrogen
E. melatonin

9.16 Each of the following statements is true *except*

A. Sodium lactate provokes panic attacks in a majority of patients with panic disorder.
B. Sodium lactate can trigger flashbacks in patients with posttraumatic stress disorder.
C. Hyperventilation is as sensitive as lactate provocation in inducing panic attacks.
D. Panic attacks triggered by sodium lactate are not inhibited by propranolol.
E. Panic attacks triggered by sodium lactate are inhibited by alprazolam.

9.17 If a patient receiving clozapine shows a white blood count (WBC) of 2,000 per cc, the clinician should

A. increase the dosage of clozapine at once
B. terminate any antibiotic therapy
C. stop the administration of clozapine at once
D. monitor the patient's WBC every 10 days
E. institute weekly complete blood count (CBC) tests with differential

9.18 Which of the following liability issues about the medical record are *true*?

A. Failure to keep medical records violates state statutes.
B. Failure to keep medical records violates licensing provisions.
C. Psychiatrists in private practice are obligated to maintain medical records of their patients.
D. Records need to be kept for the time determined by state laws.
E. All of the above.

Directions

Each set of lettered headings below is followed by a list of numbered words or statements. For each numbered word or statement, select the *one* lettered heading most closely associated with it. Each lettered heading may be selected once, more than once, or not at all.

Questions 9.19–9.23

A. Epstein-Barr virus (EBV)
B. Mean corpuscular volume (MCV)
C. Creutzfeldt-Jakob disease
D. Bulimia nervosa
E. Bromide intoxication

9.19 Elevated in alcoholism and vitamin B_{12} and folate deficiency
9.20 Causative agent for infectious mononucleosis; associated with depression, fatigue, and personality change
9.21 Decreased serum chloride
9.22 Psychosis, hallucinations, delirium
9.23 Biphasic or triphasic slow bursts on EEG

Questions 9.24–9.28

A. Hyperthyroidism
B. Hypothyroidism
C. Porphyria
D. Hepatolenticular degeneration
E. Pancreatic carcinoma

9.24 Jaundice, sense of imminent doom
9.25 Dry skin, myxedema madness
9.26 Kayser-Fleischer rings, brain damage
9.27 Abdominal crises, mood swings
9.28 Tremor, anxiety, hyperactivity

Questions: 9.29–9.33

A. Elevated level of 5-HIAA
B. Decreased level of 5-HIAA

9.29 Carcinoid tumors
9.30 Phenothiazine medications
9.31 Aggressive behavior
9.32 High banana intake
9.33 Suicidal patients

Questions 9.34–9.38

A. Circumstantiality
B. Derailment
C. Preservation
D. Flight of ideas
E. Thought blocking

9.34 Multiple associations so that thoughts move abruptly from idea to idea
9.35 A sudden break in the flow of ideas
9.36 Overinclusion of trivial details that impedes getting to the point
9.37 A breakdown in the logical connection between ideas and overall goal-directedness
9.38 Repetition of words, phrases, or ideas that are out of context

ANSWERS

9.1 The answer is E

The patient's personal and developmental history or, *anamnesis, is an essential focus of the psychiatric history* (Table 9.1). The history, which includes psychiatric, *medical* and family information, comes from the patient, but is often supplemented by collateral *information from family members, social referral agencies, previous treating physicians, and old hospital records.*

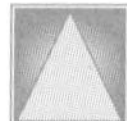

Table 9.1
Outline of Psychiatric History

I. Identifying data
II. Chief complaint
III. History of present illness
  A. Onset
  B. Precipitating factors
IV. Past illnesses
  A. Psychiatric
  B. Medical
  C. Alcohol and other substance history
V. Family history
VI. Personal history (anamnesis)
  A. Prenatal and perinatal
  B. Early childhood (through age 3)
  C. Middle childhood (ages 3–11)
  D. Late childhood (puberty through adolescence)
  E. Adulthood
    1. Occupational history
    2. Marital and relationship history
    3. Military history
    4. Educational history
    5. Religion
    6. Social activity
    7. Current living situation
    8. Legal history
  F. Sexual history
  G. Fantasies and dreams
  H. Values

It allows the psychiatrist to understand where the patient is, where the patient has come from, and where the patient is likely to go in the future, *focusing on much more than a symptom check-list. It has a structure*, which is not a rigid plan for interviewing a patient, but is a guide for organizing the psychiatrist's thoughts and questions.

9.2 The answer is D

Patients have a legal right to access their medical records. This right derives from the belief that medical care is a collaborative process between doctor and patient. The medical record is a narrative that documents all events that occur during the course of treatment. *It is used not only by the treating team, but also by regulatory agencies, and managed care companies.* It is also crucial in *malpractice litigation*. Although in theory it is accessible to authorized persons only and is safeguarded for confidentiality, *absolute confidentiality cannot be guaranteed.*

9.3 The answer is E (all)

The form of thought refers to the way in which ideas are linked, not the ideas themselves. Thoughts may be logically associated and goal directed. If they are not, a disorder of thought (also called formal thought disorder or sometimes, thought disorder) may exist. No thought disorder is pathognomonic for a particular disorder. However, a specific disorder of thought form is sometimes more characteristic of one diagnosis than another and may thereby convey diagnostic significance. For example, *clang associations* and *flight of ideas* are most closely associated with manic states. *Neologisms* and *circumstantiality* are associated with schizophrenia. There may be overlap, however.

9.4 The answer is E (all)

The patient's history and physical examination typically dictate which tests are ordered. Laboratory abnormalities are typically useful when they optimize outcomes; that is, if the test results will contribute to the detection of a previously unrecognized medical condition or otherwise influence treatment. Diagnostic testing can also serve a therapeutic function by reassuring the patient or family that other serious medical problems do not appear to be present.

Serum amylase may be increased in bulimia nervosa. Serum bicarbonate may be decreased in panic disorder and may be *elevated in patients with bulimia nervosa. Serum calcium may be decreased in depression* in addition to hyperparathyroidism and bone metastases.

9.5 The answer is D

Many aspects of a patient's judgment are assessed during the course of taking a psychiatric history; however, *judgment* is its own category in the mental status examination. It is more formally tested by asking questions directed at assessing if the patient understands the outcome of his/her behavior, and whether or not he/she is influenced by this understanding. The sensorium part of the mental status examination assesses brain function. It focuses on *alertness*, orientation, *concentration* and calculation, memory, *fund of knowledge, and abstract thinking*.

9.6 The answer is C

Concentration describes the ability to sustain attention over time. Patients who forget the examiner's question, are distracted by extraneous stimuli, or lose track of what they are saying have impaired concentration. Concentration may be tested in several ways.

Memory, which involves concentration, must be evaluated across the spectrum of immediate to remote. One test of immediate recall is to *say* (without inflection or verbal spacing) *a series of random numbers and have the patient repeat the series.* A progressively longer sequence of numbers is presented, and both forward and backward recall are tested. Most adults can easily recall five or six numbers forward and three or four in reverse. Recent memory is for events several minutes to hours old and may be evaluated by *giving patients* the *names of three or four unrelated objects and asking them to repeat them after 5 to 10 minutes.* Remote memory describes events 2 or more years old. It is usually revealed in the course of obtaining patients' histories, although it may be necessary to confirm facts through collateral sources.

Calculations describe the ability to manipulate numbers mentally. Simple addition, subtraction, or multiplication questions may be used. Problems of money and change are often helpful with patients with limited educational background. For example, if a magazine costs $3.50 and you pay with a ten dollar bill, how much change should you be given? Other tests of concentration include counting backward by 3s, reciting the alphabet backward, *spelling "world" backward*, and naming the months of the year backward.

Abstract reasoning describes the ability to mentally shift back and forth between general concepts and specific examples. A frequently used way to test abstract reasoning is asking *proverb interpretation.* For example, a clinician might ask the patient, "What does it mean when someone says, 'People who live in glass houses shouldn't throw stones'?" A conventional response, one that is able to generalize from the specifics of the proverb to the generalization, might be, "Don't criticize others of what you are guilty yourself." A nonabstract response would address the

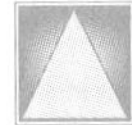

Table 9.2
Medical Record

There shall be an individual record for each person admitted to the psychiatric inpatient unit. Patient records shall be safeguarded for confidentiality and be accessible only to authorized persons. Each case record shall include

1. Legal admission documents
2. Identifying information on the individual and family
3. Source of referral, date of commencing service, and name of staff member carrying overall responsibility for treatment and care
4. Initial, intercurrent, and final diagnoses, including psychiatric or mental retardation diagnoses in official terminology
5. Reports of all diagnostic examinations and evaluations, including findings and conclusions
6. Reports of all special studies performed, including X-rays, clinical laboratory tests, clinical psychological testing, electroenchephalograms, psychometric tests
7. The individual written plan of care, treatment, and rehabilitation
8. Progress notes written and signed by all staff members having significant participation in the program of treatment and care
9. Summaries of case conferences and special consultations
10. Dated and signed prescriptions or orders for all medications, with notation of termination dates
11. A closing summary of the course of treatment and care
12. Documentation of any referrals to another agency

Adapted from the 1995 guidelines of the New York State Office of Mental Health.

concrete particulars without grasping the larger meaning; for example, "You would break the glass." (Some answers will be idiosyncratic and difficult to classify as either abstract or concrete: "The police would see you and would come to arrest you.")

9.7 The answer is E (all)

The New York State Office of Mental Health has written guidelines for what material needs to be incorporated into the medical record of a patient on an inpatient unit (Table 9.2). It requires an individual record for each person admitted to a psychiatric inpatient unit that is safeguarded for confidentiality and accessible only to authorized personnel. In it are *the legal admission documents*, the patient's identifying information, the referral source, date of admission and the name of the staff member bearing overall responsibility for the patient's treatment and care. Diagnoses, initial and final *reports of all examinations and evaluations*, reports of all tests and studies, and *treatment plans* must all be included in this document. Progress notes, *summaries of case conferences* and special consultations, and dated and signed prescriptions must also be included. The medical record must also include a closing summary of the course of treatment, and documentation of any referrals to another agency.

9.8 The answer is D

Thyroid disease in the elderly is common and can present with an atypical picture. Nonspecific symptoms such as *lassitude, constipation*, cold intolerance, *fatigue*, and *cognitive impairment may occur.* These symptoms may be attributed to depression or degenerative dementia. Severe hypothyroidism (myxedema) is a medical emergency that occurs primarily in patients over age 50. *Anorexia is more common in older patients with hyperthyroidism.* They present with typical symptoms of heat intolerance, weight loss, tremor, palpitations, and atrial fibrillation.

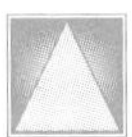

Table 9.3
Drugs of Abuse That Can Be Tested in Urine

Drug	Length of Time Detected in Urine
Alcohol	7–12 hours
Amphetamine	48 hours
Barbiturate	24 hours (short-acting) 3 weeks (long-acting)
Benzodiazepine	3 days
Cocaine	6–8 hours (metabolites 2–4 days)
Codeine	48 hours
Heroin	36–72 hours
Marijuana	3 days to 4 weeks (depending on use)
Methadone	3 days
Methaqualone	7 days
Morphine	48–72 hours
Phencyclidine (PCP)	8 days
Propoxyphene	6–48 hours

9.9 The answer is C

The laboratory is useful for detecting substances of abuse and for evaluating the impact the substance use is having on the patient's body. Often the laboratory detection of abused substances and certain diagnostic test abnormalities related to the substance abuse (e.g., abnormal liver function tests in alcohol-abusing patients) are used therapeutically to confront the denial of a patient with a substance abuse disorder and to help engage the patient in treatment.

The most commonly used specimen for the detection of drugs of abuse is urine, although toxicological analyses can also be performed on blood specimens. The period of time that the clinician can detect drugs in blood specimens is typically shorter than the length of time drugs can be detected in urine specimens because drugs and their metabolites are excreted and detectable in the urine for longer periods of time than they are detectable in blood. However, the length of time that a particular drug of abuse can be detected in the urine is somewhat variable, depending on the specific drug, the duration and amounts of the substance used, and concomitant medical problems (e.g., liver or kidney disease). *Table 9.3 provides a list of some common drugs of abuse that can be detected in urine specimens, along with a typical length of time* after recent use that the substance can be detected. Other specimens that have been studied to detect substance abuse include saliva and hair samples.

9.10 The answer is B

Recent memory is the ability to remember what has been experienced within the past few hours, days, or weeks. It is assessed by asking patients to describe how they spent the last 24 hours, such as *what they had to eat for their last meal.*

Remote memory or long-term memory is the ability to remember events in the distant past. Memory for the remote past can be evaluated by inquiring about important dates in patients' lives, such as *their date of birth, or how many siblings they have.* The answers must be verifiable. *Subtracting 7 from 100* is more a test of concentration. Asking *who the president of the United States is* tests the general fund of information.

9.11 The answer is E (all)

The therapeutic and toxic blood levels of lithium are very close to one another, and in certain individuals even seem to overlap. Additionally, lithium has effects on a number of organ systems of which the clinician should be aware. Lithium therapy is associated with a benign elevation of the white blood cell count (WBC), which may reach 15,000 cells per mm^3. This WBC elevation can sometimes be mistaken for signs of infection or wrongly attributed to lithium in the context of other signs of infection (e.g., fever, cough, discomfort on urination, malaise). Furthermore, lithium can have adverse effects on electrolyte balance (especially in patients on thiazide diuretics), thyroid function, the kidney, and the heart. The common lithium pretreatment tests include *serum electrolytes, BUN,* serum creatinine, urinalysis, thyroid function tests (TFTs) (e.g., TSH, T_4, T_3RU), and an *ECG.* In patients with a history suggestive of possible kidney problems, a 24-hour urine test for creatinine and protein clearance is recommended. Some clinicians routinely order this test in patients about to begin lithium therapy. It has been argued that antithyroid antibody testing is helpful in assessing the potential of lithium-induced hypothyroidism. Because of the potential cardiac teratogenicity of lithium, *a pregnancy test* in potentially child-bearing women should be ordered. Periodic follow-up of serum electrolytes, BUN, creatinine, TFTs, ECG, and 24-hour urine for creatinine and protein clearance are recommended. The frequency and exact makeup of the follow-up testing battery should be dictated by the patient's medical condition.

9.12 The answer is D

EEG obtained during sleep is a potentially powerful biological marker of psychiatric illness. Sleep EEG abnormalities described in major depressive disorder include *an increase in the overall amount of rapid-eye movement (REM) sleep,* not a decrease, and a *shortened (not lengthened) REM latency.* Medical conditions giving rise to pseudodepressions are typically associated with decreased REM sleep. *Patients with dementia usually have increased amounts of non-REM sleep. In schizophrenia, an increased sleep latency* has been reported, especially during relapse.

9.13 The answer is B

Memory impairment, most notably in *recent* or short-term *memory, is usually the first sign of beginning cerebral disease.* Memory is a process by which anything that is experienced or learned is established as a record in the central nervous system, where it persists with a variable degree of permanence and can be recollected or retrieved from storage at will. *Immediate memory* is the reproduction, recognition, or recall of perceived material after a period of 10 seconds or less has elapsed after the initial presentation. *Recent memory* covers a time period from a few hours to a few weeks after the initial presentation. *Long-term memory or remote memory* is the reproduction, recognition, or recall of experiences or information from the distant past. That function is usually not disturbed early in cerebral disease.

9.14 The answer is A

Psychiatrists often encounter violent patients in a hospital setting. Frequently, the police bring a patient into the emergency room in some type of physical restraint (for example, handcuffs). The psychiatrist must establish whether effective verbal contact can be made with the patient or whether the patient's sense of reality is so impaired that productive interviewing is impossible. If impaired reality testing is an issue, *the psychiatrist may have to medicate a violent patient before taking a history.*

With or without restraints, *a violent patient should not be interviewed alone* to establish a patient–doctor relationship. At least one other person should always be present; in some situations that other person should be a security guard or a police officer. Other precautions include leaving the interview room's door open and sitting between the patient and the door, so that the interviewer has unrestricted access to an exit should it become necessary. The psychiatrist must make it clear, in a firm but nonangry manner, that the patient may say or feel anything but is not free to act in a violent way.

Delusions should never be directly challenged. Delusions are fixed false ideas that may be thought of as a patient's defensive and self-protective, albeit maladaptive, strategy against overwhelming anxiety, low self-esteem, and confusion. Challenging a delusion by insisting that it is not true or possible only increases the patient's anxiety and often leads the patient to defend the belief desperately. However, clinicians should not pretend that they believe the patient's delusion. Often, the best approach is for clinicians to indicate that they understand that the patient believes the delusion to be true but that they do not hold the same belief.

Being mindful of the possibility of suicide is imperative when interviewing any depressed patient, even if a suicidal risk is not apparent. *The psychiatrist must ask depressed patients if they have suicidal thoughts.* Doing so does not make patients feel worse. Instead, many patients are relieved to talk about their suicidal ideas. The psychiatrist should ask specifically, "Are you suicidal now?" or "Do you have plans to take your own life?" A suicide note, a family history of suicide, or previous suicidal behavior by the patient increases the risk for suicide. Evidence of impulsivity or of pervasive pessimism about the future also places patients at risk. If the psychiatrist decides that the patient is in imminent risk for suicidal behavior, the patient must be hospitalized or otherwise protected.

The way chairs are arranged in the psychiatrist's office affects the interview. *The psychiatrist should not have a seat higher than the patient's seat.* Both chairs should be about the same height, so that neither person looks down on the other.

9.15 The answer is E

Melatonin is the substance that has been implicated in mood disorders with seasonal pattern. Melatonin's exact mechanism of action is unknown, but its production is stimulated in the dark, and it may affect the sleep–wake cycle. Melatonin is synthesized from serotonin, an active neurotransmitter. Decreased nocturnal secretion of melatonin has been associated with depression. A number of other substances also affect behavior, and some known endocrine diseases (for example, Cushing's disease) have associated psychiatric signs. Symptoms of anxiety or depression may be explained in some patients by changes in endocrine function or homeostasis.

Luteotropic hormone (LTH) is an anterior pituitary hormone whose action maintains the function of the corpus luteum.

Gonadotropin-releasing hormone (GnRH), produced by the hypothalamus, increases the pituitary secretion of LTH and the follicle-stimulating hormone (FSH). GnRH is secreted in a pulsatile manner that is critical for the control of LTH and FSH from the pituitary. GnRH also acts as a neurotransmitter whose exact function is unknown.

Testosterone is the hormone responsible for the secondary sex characteristics in men. A decreased testosterone level has been associated with erectile dysfunction and depression. Testosterone is formed in greatest quantities by the interstitial cells of the testes, but it is also formed in small amounts by the ovaries and the adrenal cortex.

Estrogen is produced by the granulosa cells in the ovaries and it is responsible for pubertal changes in girls. Exogenous estrogen replacement therapy has been associated with depression.

9.16 The answer is C

Even though hyperventilation can trigger panic attacks in predisposed persons, *hyperventilation is not as sensitive as lactate provocation in inducing panic attacks. Sodium lactate provokes panic attacks* in a majority (up to 72 percent) of patients with panic disorder. Therefore, lactate provocation is used to confirm a diagnosis of panic disorder. *Sodium lactate can also trigger flashbacks in patients with posttraumatic stress disorder.* Carbon dioxide (CO_2) inhalation also precipitates panic attacks in those so predisposed. *Panic attacks triggered by sodium lactate are not inhibited by* peripherally acting β-blockers, such as *propranolol* (Inderal), but are *inhibited by alprazolam* (Xanax) and tricyclic drugs.

9.17 The answer is C

A patient who shows a white blood count of 2,000 while taking clozapine (Clozaril) is at high risk for agranulocytosis. If agranulocytosis develops (that is, if the WBC is less than 1,000) and there is evidence of severe infection (for example, skin ulcerations), the patient should be placed in *protective isolation on a medical unit.* The clinician should *stop the administration of clozapine at once,* not increase the dosage of clozapine. The patient may or may not have clinical symptoms, such as fever and sore throat. *If the patient does have such symptoms, antibiotic therapy* may be necessary. Depending on the severity of the condition, the physician should *monitor the patient's WBC every 2 days, not 10 days,* or institute *daily, not weekly, CBC tests* with differential.

9.18 The answer is E (all)

Properly kept medical records can be the psychiatrist's best ally in malpractice litigation. The *failure to keep records may violate state statutes or licensing provisions.* Out-patient records are also subject to scrutiny by third parties, and *psychiatrists in private practices* are under the same obligation to maintain a record of the patient in treatment as hospital psychiatrists. Records need not be kept indefinitely; the *length of time varies according to state laws.*

Answers 9.19–9.23

9.19 The answer is B

9.20 The answer is A

9.21 The answer is D

9.22 The answer is E

9.23 The answer is C

There are major psychological changes that occur in psychiatric disorders, which have led many doctors to believe that all mental illness is accompanied by such changes, even though current laboratory tests do not allow all of them to be demonstrated. In some cases, as listed in Table 9.4, those

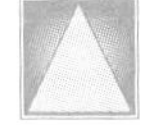

Table 9.4
Some Laboratory Findings in Mental Disorder

Test	Major Psychiatric Indication	Comments
Mean corpuscular volume (average volume of a red blood cell)	Alcohol abuse	Elevated in alcoholism and vitamin B_{12} and folate deficiency
Epstein-Barr Virus (EBV); cytomegalovirus (CMV)	Cognitive/medical workup	Part of herpes virus group EBV is causative agent for infectious mononucleosis, which can present with depression, fatigue, and personality change
	Anxiety	CMV can produce anxiety, confusion, mood disorders
	Mood disorders	EBV may be associated with chronic mononucleosis-like syndrome associated with chronic depression and fatigue
Chloride (Cl), serum	Eating disorders	Decreased in patients with bulimia and psychogenic vomiting
	Panic disorder	Mild elevation in hyperventilation syndrome, panic disorder
Bromide (Br), serum	Dementia	Bromide intoxication can cause psychosis, hallucinations, delirium
	Psychosis	Part of dementia workup, especially when serum chloride is elevated
Electroencephalogram (EEG)	Cognitive/medical workup	Seizures, brain death, lesions; shortened REM latency in depression High-voltage activity in stupor; low-voltage fast activity in excitement, functional nonorganic cases (e.g., dissociative states), alpha activity present in the background, which responds to auditory and visual stimuli Biphasic or triphasic slow bursts seen in dementia of Creutzfeldt-Jakob disease

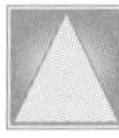

Table 9.5
Medical Problems That May Present as Psychiatric Symptoms

Medical Problem	Sex and Age Prevalence	Common Medical Symptoms	Psychiatric Symptoms and Complaints	Impaired Performance and Behavior	Diagnostic Problems
Hyperthyroidism (thyrotoxicosis)	Females 3:1, 30 to 50	*Tremor*, sweating, loss of weight and strength	*Anxiety* if rapid onset; depression if slow onset	Occasional *hyperactivity* or grandiose behavior	Long lead time; a rapid onset resembles anxiety attack
Hypothyroidism (myxedema)	Females 5:1, 30 to 50	Puffy face, *dry skin*, cold intolerance	Anxiety with irritability, thought disorder, somatic delusions, hallucinations	*Myxedema madness*; delusional, paranoid belligerent behavior	Madness may mimic schizophrenia; mental status is clear, even during most disturbed behavior
Porphyria—acute intermittent type	Females, 20 to 40	*Abdominal crises*, paresthesias, weakness	Anxiety—sudden onset, severe *mood swings*	Extremes of excitement or withdrawal; emotional or angry outbursts	Patients often have truly abnormal lifestyles; crises resemble conversion disorder or anxiety attacks
Hepatolenticular degeneration (Wilson's disease)	Males 2:1; adolescence	Liver and extrapyramidal symptoms, *Kayser-Fleischer rings*	Mood swings—sudden and changeable; anger—explosive	Eventual *brain damage* with memory and IQ loss; combativeness	In late teens, disorder may resemble adolescent storm, incorrigibility, or schizophrenia
Pancreatic carcinoma	Males 3:1, 50 to 70	Weight loss, abdominal pain, weakness, *jaundice*	Depression, *sense of imminent doom* but without severe guilt	Loss of drive and motivation	Long lead time; exact age and symptoms of involutional depression

changes are very much in evidence and are useful in confirming diagnoses.

Answers 9.24–9.28

9.24 The answer is E

9.25 The answer is B

9.26 The answer is D

9.27 The answer is C

9.28 The answer is A

The clinician should be aware of the many medical problems that may present as psychiatric symptoms. For example, *tremor, anxiety,* and *hyperactivity* are often associated with *hyperthyroidism; dry skin* and *myxedema madness* (which may mimic schizophrenia) are associated with *hypothyroidism; abdominal crises* and *mood swings* are associated with *porphyria; Kayser-Fleischer rings* and *brain damage* are associated with *hepatolenticular*

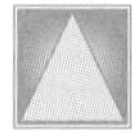

Table 9.6
Formal Thought Disorders

Circumstantiality. Overinclusion of trivial or irrelevant details that impede the sense of getting to the point.
Clang associations. Thoughts are associated by the sound of words rather than by their meaning, e.g., through rhyming or assonance.
Derailment. (Synonymous with loose associations) A breakdown in both the logical connection between ideas and the overall sense of goal-directedness. The words make sentences, but the sentences don't make sense.
Flight of ideas. A succession of multiple associations so that thoughts seem to move abruptly from idea to idea; often (but not invariably) expressed through rapid, pressured speech.
Neologism. The invention of new words or phrases or the use of conventional words in idiosyncratic ways.
Perseveration. Repetition out of context of words, phrases, or ideas.
Tangentiality. In response to a question, the patient gives a reply that is appropriate to the general topic without actually answering the question. Example:
Doctor: "Have you had any trouble sleeping lately?"
Patient: "I usually sleep in my bed, but now I'm sleeping on the sofa."
Thought blocking. A sudden disruption of thought or a break in the flow of ideas.

degeneration (Wilson's disease); and *jaundice* and a *sense of imminent doom* are associated with *pancreatic carcinoma.*

Table 9.5 gives some examples of medical problems that may present as psychiatric symptoms.

Answers 9.29–9.33

9.29 The answer is A

9.30 The answer is A

9.31 The answer is B

9.32 The answer is A

9.33 The answer is B

The serotonin metabolite 5-hydroxyindoleacetic acid (5-HIAA) is *elevated* in the urine of patients with *carcinoid tumors,* at times in patients who take *phenothiazine medications,* and in persons who eat foods high in L-tryptophan, the chemical precursor of serotonin (for example, walnuts, *bananas*, and avocados). The amount of 5-HIAA in cerebrospinal fluid is *decreased* in some persons who display *aggressive behavior* and in some *suicidal patients* who have committed suicide in particularly violent ways.

Answers 9.34–9.38

9.34 The answer is D

9.35 The answer is E

9.36 The answer is A

9.37 The answer is B

9.38 The answer is C

See Table 9.6.

10

Signs and Symptoms in Psychiatry

Signs are observations and objective findings elicited by the clinician. Symptoms are the subjective experiences described by the patient. A syndrome is a group of signs and symptoms that together make up a recognizable condition. There are hundreds of terms used to describe the signs and symptoms of psychiatric illness, and students of psychiatry are encouraged to familiarize themselves with as many as possible. The language of psychiatry is precise, and this allows clinicians to articulate their observations reliably.

In psychiatry, the presentation of signs and symptoms is not always straightforward. A patient may insist that nothing is wrong (that there are no symptoms), when it is obvious to most observers that certain behaviors or ways of thinking are bizarre, damaging, or disruptive. These might be defined as ego-syntonic symptoms. Ego-dystonic symptoms are those of which the patient is aware and that are experienced as uncomfortable or unacceptable. Another complicating factor is that a clinician may not be able to literally observe or to hear a described symptom (such as an auditory hallucination), and may have to depend on indirect evidence (for example, a patient's preoccupation or distraction) to diagnose it.

In psychiatry there are few if any pathognomonic signs and symptoms. Human behavior is too complex for this. Complicating matters further, medical conditions can frequently present initially with psychiatric signs and symptoms, and psychiatric conditions with medical ones. Medical pathology can underlie apparent psychiatric symptomatology and psychiatric syndromes can be expressed in physical terms. The skilled clinician must know when to have a heightened level of suspicion that a condition may not be what it first appears to be and must know concretely how to differentiate between them.

Students should study the questions and answers below for a useful review of these topics.

HELPFUL HINTS

The student should be able to define and categorize the signs and symptoms and other terms listed below.

- affect and mood
- aggression
- agnosias
- anxiety
- aphasic disturbances
- cerea flexibilitas
- coma
- *déjà entendu*
- *déjà pensé*
- *déjà vu*
- delirium
- delusion
- dementia
- depersonalization
- disorientation
- distractibility
- disturbances in speech
- disturbances in the form and the content of thought
- disturbances of conation
- disturbances of consciousness and attention
- disturbances of intelligence
- disturbances of memory
- disturbances of perception, both those caused by brain diseases and those associated with psychological phenomena
- *folie à deux*
- hypnosis
- illusions
- insight and judgment
- *jamais vu*
- noesis
- panic
- phobias
- pseudodementia
- stereotypy
- synesthesia

QUESTIONS

Directions

Each of the questions or incomplete statements below is followed by five suggested responses or completions. Select the *one* that is *best* in each case.

10.1 Sundowning

A. usually occurs in the young
B. is associated with stupor
C. occurs usually as a function of mania
D. is a result of overmedication
E. is associated with akathisia

10.2 Which of the following is a paramnesia?

A. *Jamais vu*
B. Eidetic images
C. Repression

D. Screen memories
E. Lethologica

10.3 A psychiatric patient who, although coherent, never gets to the point has a disturbance in the form of thought called

A. word salad
B. circumstantiality
C. tangentiality
D. verbigeration
E. blocking

10.4 Perceptual disturbances include all of the following *except*

A. hallucinations
B. hypnagogic experiences
C. echolalia
D. depersonalization
E. derealization

10.5 Physiological disturbances associated with mood include

A. hyperphagia
B. anorexia
C. hypersomnia
D. diurnal variation
E. all of the above

10.6 Loss of normal speech melody is known as

A. stuttering
B. stammering
C. aphonia
D. dysprosody
E. dyslexia

10.7 Stereotypy is

A. temporary loss of muscle tone and weakness precipitated by a variety of emotional states
B. pathological imitation of movements of one person by another
C. ingrained, habitual involuntary movement
D. repetitive fixed pattern of physical action or speech
E. subjective feeling of muscular tension and restlessness secondary to antipsychotic or other medication

10.8 Disturbances of attention include

A. hypervigilance
B. twilight state
C. somnolence
D. sundowning
E. all of the above

10.9 Asking a patient to interpret a proverb is used as a way of assessing

A. judgment
B. impulse control
C. abstract thinking
D. insight
E. intelligence

10.10 Alexithymia is

A. an unpleasant mood
B. a loss of interest in and withdrawal from pleasurable activities
C. an inability to describe or to be aware of emotions or mood
D. a normal range of mood, implying absence of depressed or elevated emotional state
E. a state in which a person is easily annoyed and provoked to anger

10.11 Primary process thinking is

A. a form of magical thinking
B. similar to that of the preoperational phase in children
C. normally found in dreams
D. dereistic
E. all of the above

Directions

Each group of questions below consists of lettered headings followed by a list of numbered phrases or statements. For each numbered phrase or statement, select the *one* lettered heading that is most associated with it. Each lettered heading may be selected once, more than once, or not at all.

Questions 10.12–10.16

A. Stimulagnosia
B. Anosognosia
C. Apraxia
D. Astereognosis
E. Adiadochokinesia

10.12 Inability to carry out specific tasks
10.13 Inability to perform rapid alternating movements
10.14 Inability to comprehend more than one element of a visual scene at a time
10.15 Inability to recognize objects by touch
10.16 Inability to recognize one's own neurological deficit

Questions 10.17–10.21

A. Loosening of associations
B. Flight of ideas
C. Clang association
D. Blocking
E. Neologism

10.17 "I was gigglifying, not just tempifying; you know what I mean."
10.18 "I was grocery training; but, when I ride the grocery, I drive the food everywhere on top of lollipops."
10.19 "Cain and Abel—they were cannibals. You see brothers kill brothers—that is laudable. If you ask me, though, never name your son Huxtibal. OK."
10.20 Patient: "I never wanted." Physician: "Go on. What were you saying?" Patient: "I don't know."
10.21 "Tired, mired, schmired, wired."

Questions 10.22–10.26

A. Narcolepsy
B. Cataplexy
C. Restless legs syndrome
D. Klein-Levin syndrome
E. Nocturnal myoclonus

10.22 Peculiar feelings during sleep, causing an irresistible need to move around
10.23 Periods of sleepiness, alternating with confusion, hunger, and sexual activity
10.24 Sudden attacks of generalized muscle weakness, leading to physical collapse while alert
10.25 Sudden attacks of irresistible sleepiness
10.26 Repetitive jerking of the legs during sleep, waking patients as well as their partners

Questions 10.27–10.30

A. Cluster A
B. Cluster B
C. Cluster C

10.27 Borderline personality disorder
10.28 Paranoid personality disorder
10.29 Obsessive-compulsive personality disorder
10.30 Schizoid personality disorder

Questions 10.31–10.35

A. Haptic hallucinations
B. Olfactory hallucinations
C. Ictal hallucinations
D. Autoscopic hallucinations
E. Migrainous hallucinations

10.31 Most are simple visual hallucinations of geometric patterns, but phenomena such as micropsia and macropsia may occur
10.32 Hallucinations of one's own physical self
10.33 Involve the sense of smell and are most often associated with organic brain disease or psychotic depression
10.34 Occur as part of seizure activity, and are typically brief and stereotyped
10.35 Formication

Questions 10.36–10.38

A. Registration
B. Retention
C. Recall

10.36 Capacity to return previously stored memories to consciousness
10.37 Capacity to add new material to memory
10.38 Capacity to hold memories in storage

Questions 10.39–10.42

A. *Déjà vu*
B. *Déjà entendu*
C. *Déjà pensé*
D. *Jamais vu*
E. Confabulation

10.39 Illusion of auditory recognition
10.40 Regarding a new thought as a repetition of a previous thought
10.41 Feeling of unfamiliarity with a familiar situation
10.42 Regarding a new situation as a repetition of a previous experience

Questions 10.43–10.46

A. Synesthesia
B. Paramnesia
C. Hypermnesia
D. Eidetic images
E. Lethologica

10.43 Exaggerated degree of retention and recall
10.44 Temporary inability to remember a name
10.45 Confusion of facts and fantasies
10.46 Sensations that accompany sensations of another modality

Questions 10.47–10.49

A. Information variance
B. Criterion variance
C. Observation bias
D. Validity

10.47 Discrepancies in psychiatric evaluation caused by differences in the patient's status or in information imparted by the patient from examination to examination
10.48 Discrepancies caused by differences in perceiving and interpreting the patient's responses to questions within the interview
10.49 Discrepancies caused by differences in the observer's definition of the symptoms or signs in question

Questions 10.50–10.53

A. Anxiety
B. Ambivalence
C. Guilt
D. Abreaction

10.50 Coexistence of two opposing impulses
10.51 Emotional discharge after recalling a painful experience
10.52 Feeling of apprehension
10.53 Emotion resulting from doing something perceived as wrong

Questions 10.54–10.58

A. Ophidiophobia
B. Triskaidekaphobia
C. Acrophobia
D. Amathophobia
E. Gatophobia

10.54 Fear of heights
10.55 Fear of cats
10.56 Fear of the number 13
10.57 Fear of snakes
10.58 Fear of dust

Questions 10.59–10.63

A. Capgras's syndrome
B. Frégoli's phenomenon
C. Clérambault's syndrome
D. Delusion of doubles
E. Delusional jealousy

10.59 Patients believe that another person has been physically transformed into themselves
10.60 Strangers are identified as familiar persons in the patient's life
10.61 False belief that someone (usually of higher status or authority) is erotically attached to the patient
10.62 Patient believes that someone close to him or her has been replaced by an exact double
10.63 False belief about a spouse's infidelity

Questions 10.64–10.68

A. Broca's aphasia
B. Syntactical aphasia
C. Coprophasia
D. Amnestic aphasia
E. Wernicke's aphasia

10.64 Difficulty finding the correct name for an object.
10.65 Spontaneous but incoherent speech
10.66 Inability to arrange words in proper sequence
10.67 Understanding remains but speech is grossly impaired
10.68 Involuntary obscene language

ANSWERS

10.1 The answer is D
Sundowning or sundowner's syndrome is *the result of being overly sedated with medications. It occurs in older people* and usually occurs at night. It is characterized by drowsiness, confusion, ataxia, and falling. *It has no association with mania. Stupor is a disturbance of consciousness that is defined by a lack of reaction to and unawareness of one's surroundings; this is not true of sundowning.*

10.2 The answer is A
Paramnesias are the falsification of memory by distortion of recall. *Jamais vu* is the false feeling of unfamiliarity with a real situation that the person has experienced and, like confabulation, déjà vu and false memory, is an example of a paramnesia. *Eidetic images* are visual memories of almost hallucinatory vividness. *Repression* is a defense mechanism characterized by unconscious forgetting of unacceptable ideas. *A screen memory* is a consciously tolerable memory that covers a painful memory. *Lethologica* is the temporary inability to remember a name or proper noun.

10.3 The answer is C
Tangentiality is the inability to have a goal-directed association of thoughts. The patient never gets from the desired point to the desired goal. *Word salad* is an incoherent mixture of words and phrases. *Circumstantiality* is indirect speech that is delayed in reaching the point but eventually gets there. Circumstantiality is characterized by an overinclusion of details and parenthetical remarks. *Verbigeration* is a meaningless repetition of specific words or phrases. *Blocking* is an abrupt interruption in the train of thinking before a thought or idea is finished. After a brief pause, the person indicates no recall of what was being said or what was going to be said. It is also known as thought deprivation.

10.4 The answer is C
A disturbance in perception is a disturbance in the mental process by which data—intellectual, sensory, and emotional—are organized. Through perception, people are capable of making sense out of the many stimuli that bombard them. Perceptual disturbances do not include *echolalia,* which is the repetition of another's words or phrases. Echolalia is a disturbance of thought form and communication. Examples of perceptual disturbances are *hallucinations,* which are false sensory perceptions without concrete external stimuli. Common hallucinations involve sights or sounds, although any of the senses may be involved, and *hypnagogic experiences,* which are hallucinations that occur just before falling asleep. Other disturbances of perception include *depersonalization,* which is the sensation of unreality concerning oneself or one's environment, and *derealization,* which is the feeling of changed reality or the feeling that one's surroundings have changed.

10.5 The answer is E (all)
Physiological disturbances associated with mood are signs of somatic (usually autonomic) dysfunction, most often associated with depression (also called vegetative signs). They include:

Anorexia: loss of or decrease in appetite.
Hyperphagia: increase in appetite and intake of food.
Insomnia: lack of or diminished ability to sleep.

a. Initial: difficulty in falling asleep.
b. Middle: difficulty in sleeping through the night without waking up and difficulty in going back to sleep.
c. Terminal: early morning awakening.

Hypersomnia: excessive sleeping.
Diurnal variation: mood is regularly worse in the morning, immediately after awakening, and improves as the day progresses.
Diminished libido: decreased sexual interest, drive, and performance (increased libido is often associated with manic states).
Constipation: inability to defecate or difficulty in defecating.
Fatigue: a feeling of weariness, sleepiness, or irritability following a period of mental or bodily activity.
Pica: craving and eating of nonfood substances, such as paint and clay.
Pseudocyesis: rare condition in which a nonpregnant patient has the signs and symptoms of pregnancy.
Bulimia: insatiable hunger and voracious eating; seen in bulimia nervosa and atypical depression.

10.6 The answer is D

Loss of normal speech melody is known as *dysprosody*. A disturbance in speech inflection and rhythm results in a monotonous and halting speech pattern, which occasionally suggests a foreign accent. It can be the result of a brain disease, such as Parkinson's disease, or it can be a psychological defensive mechanism (seen in some people with schizophrenia). As a psychological device, it can serve the function of maintaining a safe distance in social encounters.

Stuttering is a speech disorder characterized by repetitions or prolongations of sound syllables and words and by hesitations or pauses that disrupt the flow of speech. It is also known as *stammering*. *Aphonia* is a loss of one's voice. *Dyslexia* is a specific learning disability involving a reading impairment that is unrelated to the person's intelligence.

10.7 The answer is D

Motor behavior is that aspect of the psyche that includes impulses, motivations, wishes, drives, instincts, and cravings, as expressed by a person's behavior or motor activity.

Stereotypy is a *repetitive fixed pattern* of physical action or speech.

Echopraxia is a *pathological imitation* of movements of one person by another.

Cataplexy is *a temporary loss* of muscle tone and weakness precipitated by a variety of emotional states.

Mannerism is an *ingrained, habitual* involuntary movement.

Akathisia is a subjective feeling of muscular tension secondary to antipsychotic or other medication, which can cause *restlessness*, pacing, and repeated sitting and standing; can be mistaken for psychotic agitation.

10.8 The answer is A

Attention is the amount of effort exerted in focusing on certain portions of an experience; ability to sustain a focus on one activity; and ability to concentrate. Examples of disturbances of attention include:

Hypervigilance: excessive attention and focus on all internal and external stimuli, usually secondary to delusional or paranoid states.

Selective inattention: blocking out only those things that generate anxiety.

Distractibility: inability to concentrate attention; state in which attention is drawn to unimportant or irrelevant external stimuli.

Trance: focused attention and altered consciousness, usually seen in hypnosis, dissociative disorders, and ecstatic religious experiences.

Apperception is perception modified by a person's own emotions and thoughts; sensorium is the state of cognitive functioning of the special senses (sometimes used as a synonym for consciousness); disturbances of consciousness are most often associated with brain pathology. Examples include:

Twilight state: disturbed consciousness with hallucinations.

Somnolence: abnormal drowsiness.

Sundowning: syndrome in older people that usually occurs at night and is characterized by drowsiness, confusion, ataxia, and falling as the result of being overly sedated with medications; also called sundowner's syndrome.

10.9 The answer is C

Asking a patient to interpret a proverb is generally used as a way of assessing whether the person has the capacity for abstract thought. *Abstract thinking*, as opposed to concrete thinking, is characterized primarily by the ability to shift voluntarily from one aspect of a situation to another, to keep in mind simultaneously various aspects of a situation, and to think symbolically. Concrete thinking is characterized by an inability to conceptualize beyond immediate experience or beyond actual things and events. Psychopathologically, it is most characteristic of persons with schizophrenia or organic brain disorders.

Judgment, the patient's ability to comprehend the meaning of events and to appreciate the consequences of actions, is often tested by asking how the patient would act in certain standard circumstances; for example, if the patient smelled smoke in a crowded movie theater. *Impulse control* is the ability to control acting on a wish to discharge energy in a manner that is, at the moment, felt to be dangerous, inappropriate, or otherwise ill-advised. *Insight* is a conscious understanding of forces that have led to a particular feeling, action, or situation. *Intelligence* is the capacity for learning, recalling, integrating, and applying knowledge and experience.

10.10 The answer is C

Mood is a pervasive and sustained emotion, subjectively experienced and reported by a patient and observed by others; examples include depression, elation, and anger.

Euthymic mood is a normal range of mood, implying absence of depressed or elevated mood.

Alexithymia is a person's inability to describe, or difficulty in describing or being aware of, emotions or mood.

Irritable mood is a state in which a person is easily annoyed and provoked to anger. Anhedonia is a loss of interest in and withdrawal from all regular and pleasurable activities, often associated with depression.

10.11 The answer is E (all)

Thinking is the goal-directed flow of ideas, symbols, and associations initiated by a problem or task and leading toward a reality-oriented conclusion; when a logical sequence occurs, thinking is normal; parapraxis (an unconsciously motivated lapse from logic also called a Freudian slip) is considered part of normal thinking. Disturbances in the form of process of thinking include dereism, a form of mental activity not concordant with logic or experience; *magical thinking*, a form of *dereistic thought*; thinking similar to that of the *preoperational phase in children* (Jean Piaget), in which thoughts, words, or actions assume power (for example, to cause or prevent events); and primary process thinking, which is a general term for thinking that is dereistic, illogical, magical and is normally found in *dreams*, abnormally in psychosis.

Answers 10.12–10.16

10.12 The answer is C

10.13 The answer is E

10.14 The answer is A

10.15 The answer is D

10.16 The answer is B

Simultagnosia is the inability to comprehend more than one element of a visual scene at a time or to integrate the parts into a whole. *Anosognosia*, or the ignorance of illness, is a person's inability to recognize a neurological deficit as occurring to him- or herself. *Apraxias* refer to the inability to carry our specific tasks. *Astereognosis* is the inability to recognize objects by touch. *Adiadochokinesia* is the inability to perform rapid alternating movements.

Answers 10.17–10.21

10.17 The answer is E

10.18 The answer is A

10.19 The answer is B

10.20 The answer is D

10.21 The answer is C

All the lettered responses are examples of specific disturbances in form of thought. *Neologisms* are new words created by the patient, often by combining syllables of other words, for idiosyncratic psychological reasons. *Loosening of associations* is a flow of thoughts in which ideas shift from one subject to another in completely unrelated ways. When the condition is severe, the patient's speech may be incoherent. *Flight of ideas* is a rapid, continuous verbalization or play on words that produces a constant shifting from one idea to another; the ideas tend to be connected, and when the condition is not severe, a listener may be able to follow them; the thought disorder is most characteristic of someone in a manic state. *Blocking* is an abrupt interruption in a train of thinking before a thought or idea is finished; after a brief pause, the person indicates no recall of what was being said or what was going to be said. The condition is also known as thought deprivation. A person who is using *clang association* uses an association of words similar in sound but not in meaning; the words used have no logical connections and may include examples of rhyming and punning.

Answers 10.22–10.26

10.22 The answer is C

10.23 The answer is D

10.24 The answer is B

10.25 The answer is A

10.26 The answer is E

In *narcolepsy*, the patient has *sudden attacks of irresistible sleepiness,* a symptom that may be part of a broader syndrome that includes *cataplexy* (*sudden attacks of generalized muscle weakness leading to physical collapse* in the presence of alert consciousness).

Periodic hypersomnia occurs in the *Klein-Levin syndrome,* a condition that typically affects young men, in which *periods of sleepiness alternate with confusional states, ravenous hunger, and protracted sexual activity.*

Sensory symptoms during sleep, typically described by patients as peculiar feelings in their *legs, causing an irresistible need to move* around, are characteristic of *restless legs syndrome.* The motor abnormality of *repetitive myoclonic jerking of the legs, awakening both patients and their partners,* is known as *nocturnal myoclonus.*

Answers 10.27–10.30

10.27 The answer is B

10.28 The answer is A

10.29 The answer is C

10.30 The answer is A

The DSM-IV-TR uses a categorical approach to personality. The large overlap among the DSM personality disorders and the clustering of these personality disorders into three broad groups imply a lack of clear boundaries to the currently defined categories. The three DSM-IV-TR clusters describe odd or eccentric types (*Cluster A*); dramatic, emotional, and erratic types (*Cluster B*); and anxious and fearful types (*Cluster C*).

The odd or eccentric group includes *paranoid, schizoid,* and schizotypal personality disorders. Patients with these personality disorders have the core traits of being interpersonally distant and emotionally constricted. People with paranoid personality disorder are quick to feel slighted and jealous, carry grudges, and expect to be exploited and harmed by others. People with schizoid personality disorder lack friendships or close relationships with others and are indifferent to praise or criticism by others. People with schizotypal personality disorder display odd beliefs, engage in odd and eccentric gestures and practices, and exhibit odd speech.

The dramatic, emotional, and erratic group includes *borderline,* histrionic, narcissistic, and antisocial personality disorders. Patients with these personality disorders characteristically have chaotic lives, emotions, and relationships. People with borderline personality disorder are impulsive, unpredictable, angry, temperamental, unstable in relationships, compulsively interpersonal, and self-damaging with regard to sex, money, and substance use. People with histrionic personality disorder are attention-seeking, exhibitionistic, seductive, and self-indulgent; exhibit exaggerated expressions of emotions; and are overconcerned with physical appearance. People with narcissistic personality disorder tend to be hypersensitive to criticism, exploitative of others, egocentric with an inflated sense of self-importance, feel entitled to special treatment, and demand constant attention. People with antisocial personality disorder are described almost exclusively in behavioral rather than affective or relational terms. They commit truancy, lie, steal, start fights, break rules, are unable to sustain work or school, and shirk day-to-day responsibilities.

The anxious and fearful group includes patients with avoidant, dependent, and *obsessive-compulsive* personality disorders. Patients with these disorders are characterized by constricting behaviors that serve to limit risks. People with avoidant personality disorder avoid relationships, people with dependent personality disorder avoid being responsible for decisions, and people with obsessive-compulsive personality disorder use rigid rules that preclude new behaviors. People with avoidant personality disorders are hypersensitive to rejection and are reluctant to enter close relationships in spite of strong desires for affection. Those with dependent personality disorders show excessive reliance on others to make major life decisions, stay trapped in abusive relationships for fear of being alone, have difficulty initiating projects on their own, and constantly seek reassurance and praise. Individuals with obsessive-compulsive personality disorders exhibit restricted expressions of warmth, tenderness, and generosity, and also exhibit stubbornness with a need to be right and to control decisions; indecisive at times, they often apply rules and morals too rigidly, to the point of being inflexible.

Answers 10.31–10.35

10.31 The answer is E

10.32 The answer is D

10.33 The answer is B

10.34 The answer is C

10.35 The answer is A

Hallucinations are perceptions that occur in the absence of corresponding sensory stimuli. Phenomenologically, hallucinations are ordinarily subjectively indistinguishable from normal perceptions. Hallucinations are often experienced as being private, so that others are not able to see or hear the same perceptions. The patient's explanation for this is typically delusional. Hallucinations can affect any sensory system and sometimes occur in several concurrently.

Autoscopic hallucinations are *hallucinations of one's own physical self.* Such hallucinations may stimulate the delusion that one has a double (*Doppelgänger*). Reports of near-death out-of-body experiences in which individuals see themselves rising to the ceiling and looking down at themselves in a hospital bed may be autoscopic hallucinations. In *Lilliputian hallucinations,* the individual sees figures in very reduced size, like midgets or dwarfs. They may be related to the perceptual distortions of *macropsia* and *micropsia,* respectively, the perceptions of objects as much bigger or smaller than they actually are.

Haptic hallucinations involve touch. Simple haptic hallucinations, such as the feeling that *bugs are crawling over one's skin (formication)* are common in alcohol withdrawal syndromes and in cocaine intoxication. When unkempt and physically neglectful patients complain of these sensations, they may be caused by the presence of real physical stimuli such as lice. Some tactile hallucinations, having sexual intercourse with God, for example, are highly suggestive of schizophrenia, but may also occur in tertiary syphilis and other conditions, and may in fact be stimulated by local genital irritation. *Olfactory* and gustatory *hallucinations, involving smell and taste* respectively, have most often been associated with organic brain disease, particularly with the uncinate fits of complex partial seizures. Olfactory hallucinations may also be seen in psychotic depression, typically as odors of decay, rotting, or death.

Ictal hallucinations, occurring as *part of seizure activity,* are typically brief, lasting only seconds to minutes, and stereotyped. They may be simple images—such as flashes of light—or elaborate ones, such as visual recollections of past experiences. During the hallucinations the patient ordinarily experiences altered consciousness or a twilight sleep.

Migrainous hallucinations are reported by about 50 percent of patients with migraines. Most are simple *visual hallucinations of geometric patterns, but fully formed visual hallucinations, sometimes with micropsia and macropsia,* may also occur. This complex has been called the *Alice in Wonderland syndrome* after Lewis Carroll's descriptions of the world in *Through the Looking Glass,* which mirrored some of his own migrainous experiences. In turn, these phenomena closely resemble visual hallucinations induced by psychedelic drugs such as mescaline.

Answers 10.36–10.38

10.36 The answer is C

10.37 The answer is A

10.38 The answer is B

Memory functions have been divided into three stages: registration, retention, and recall. *Registration or acquisition refers to the capacity to add new material to memory.* The material may be sensory, perceptual, or conceptual and may come from the environment or from within the person. In order for new material to be acquired, the person must attend to the information presented; it must then be processed or cortically organized. *Retention* is the *ability to hold memories in storage.* Large numbers of neurons are thought to be involved in the storage of a specific memory, and it is believed that reverberating circuits are formed in which memory traces are held by means of changes in proteins or synaptic connectivity, or both. *Recall is the capacity to return previously stored memories to consciousness.*

Registration and short-term memory retention are usually impaired in disorders that affect vigilance and attention, such as head trauma, delirium, intoxication, psychosis, spontaneous or induced seizures, anxiety, depression, and fatigue. A variety of other metabolic and structural brain disturbances can affect short-term memory as well, particularly lesions affecting the mammillary bodies, hippocampus, fornix, and closely associated areas. Patients with impaired attention and concentration who are able to demonstrate immediate recall may not be able to retain or recollect these items from short-term memory. Benzodiazepine use has been associated with working memory difficulties, especially in the elderly. Some short-acting high-potency benzodiazepines used as sleeping pills may be particularly troublesome in this regard.

The retention of memories is impaired in posttraumatic amnesia as well as in a number of cognitive disorders, such as dementia of the Alzheimer's type and the Wernicke-Korsakoff syndrome. The latter, which ordinarily results from the chronic thiamine deficiency seen with alcoholism, is associated with pathological alterations in the mammillary bodies and thalamus.

Disturbances in recall can occur even when memories have been registered and are in storage. Research has shown that memories are not passively retrieved but are actively reconstructed. Each act of recollection requires an act of putting the memory together, not simply lifting it ready made from a file. Because memories are often retrieved for specific purposes to meet the individual's particular needs and agendas, this act of reconstruction is often subject to the introduction of distortions and falsification. As a result, memories may fail to truly represent past events. At times, failure to recall may signify that the memory traces themselves have disappeared and are no longer retrievable. However, difficulties in recall can occur separately, as in the everyday event of forgetting the name of a person or object, only to spontaneously remember it hours or days later.

Answers 10.39–10.42

10.39 The answer is B

10.40 The answer is C

10.41 The answer is D

10.42 The answer is A

Déjà vu is *regarding a new situation as a repetition of a previous experience. Déjà entendu* is an *illusion of auditory recognition. Déjà pensé* is *regarding a new thought as a repetition of a previous thought. Jamais vu* is a *feeling of unfamiliarity with a familiar situation. Confabulation* is the *unconscious filling in of memory* by imagining experiences that have no basis in fact.

Answers 10.43–10.46

10.43 The answer is C

10.44 The answer is E

10.45 The answer is B

10.46 The answer is A

In *synesthesia* the patient experiences *sensations that accompany sensations of another modality;* for example, an auditory sensation is accompanied by or triggers a visual sensation, or a sound is experienced as being seen or accompanied by a visual experience. *Paramnesia* is a *confusion of facts and fantasies;* it leads to a falsification of memory with the distortion of real events by fantasies. *Hypermnesia* is an *exaggerated degree of retention and recall* or an ability to remember material that ordinarily is not retrievable. *Eidetic images,* also known as primary memory images, are *visual memories* of almost hallucinatory vividness. *Lethologica* is the *temporary inability to remember a name* or a proper noun.

Answers 10.47–10.49

10.47 The answer is A

10.48 The answer is C

10.49 The answer is B

Among the core difficulties in psychiatric evaluation has been that multiple observers may note different symptoms or interpret signs differently when interviewing the same patient. *These discrepancies may be caused by differences in the patient's status or in* information imparted by the patient from examination to examination, in the *observers' definitions of the symptoms or signs* in question, and *differences in perceiving and interpreting the patient's responses* to general presentation or *questions within* the interview. These three types of reliability problems are called *information variance, criterion variance,* and *observation bias.*

Although good interrater reliability can be achieved for most symptoms of Axis I disorders, this may not hold true for personality disorders or for some specific symptoms. Furthermore, good interrater reliability may occur consistently only under optimal circumstances and may not be as common in clinical practice.

Even when simply responding to direct questions about symptoms, patients may answer differently depending on the interviewer's manner, how the questions are asked, their personal sense of trust or safety, whether they have answered these questions before, the amount of cuing that may signal the desired response, fatigue, or a host of other variables.

Most clinicians still rely heavily on their own clinical intuition and subjective responses to patients as part of a diagnostic assessment. Unfortunately, whether accurate or not, these clinical judgments are often based on unconscious assumptions, comparisons with other patients not well remembered, or distortions based on the clinician's own personal experiences. When the basis for these intuitions can be identified and described clearly, they may prove to be reliable and valid. However, intuitions are often wrong—simple trust in intuition alone is not sufficient. Thus, a clinician's sense that a patient is angry and potentially violent may result from the patient's subtle (but verifiable) body language and tone of voice—or it may represent a countertransference distortion that is not prompted by any observable patient behavior.

Often, clinicians too quickly label behaviors as inappropriate when they fail to appreciate and understand contextual or cultural considerations. Appropriateness depends heavily on context, and definitions of what is proper in a given context may also be highly subjective. Appropriate behavior or clothing in some parts of California may be inappropriate in Boston. A low intensity of emotional expression leading to a clinical description of "constricted affect" may reflect cultural norms or a psychopathological state.

Validity reflects that a designated disorder is actually what is described.

Answers 10.50–10.53

10.50 The answer is B

10.51 The answer is D

10.52 The answer is A

10.53 The answer is C

Anxiety is a *feeling of apprehension* caused by anticipation of danger, which may be internal or external. *Ambivalence* is the *coexistence of two opposing impulses* toward the same thing in the same person at the same time. *Guilt* is an *emotion resulting from doing something perceived as wrong. Abreaction* is an *emotional discharge after recalling a painful experience.*

Answers 10.54–10.58

10.54 The answer is C

10.55 The answer is E

10.56 The answer is B

10.57 The answer is A

10.58 The answer is D
Phobias are irrational fears. In an effort to reduce the intense anxiety attached to phobic objects and situations, patients do their best to avoid the feared stimuli. Thus, phobias consist both of the fears and the avoidance components. The fear itself may include all the symptoms of extreme anxiety, up to and including panic. In *specific phobias,* persistent, irrational fears are provoked by specific stimuli. Table 10.1 lists some specific phobias. Common specific phobias include *fear of dust*, excreta, *snakes*, spiders, *heights*, and blood.

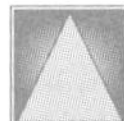

Table 10.1
Specific Phobias

Acrophobia	Fear of heights
Agoraphobia	Fear of open spaces
Amathophobia	Fear of dust
Apiphobia	Fear of bees
Astrapophobia	Fear of lightning
Blennophobia	Fear of slime
Claustrophobia	Fear of enclosed spaces
Cynophobia	Fear of dogs
Decidophobia	Fear of making decisions
Electrophobia	Fear of electricity
Eremophobia	Fear of being alone
Gamophobia	Fear of marriage
Gatophobia	Fear of cats
Gephyrophobia	Fear of crossing bridges
Gynophobia	Fear of women
Hydrophobia	Fear of water
Kakorrhaphiophobia	Fear of failure
Katagelophobia	Fear of ridicule
Keraunophobia	Fear of thunder
Musophobia	Fear of mice
Nyctophobia	Fear of night
Ochlophobia	Fear of crowds
Odynophobia	Fear of pain
Ophidiophobia	Fear of snakes
Pnigerophobia	Fear of smothering
Pyrophobia	Fear of fire
Scholionophobia	Fear of school
Sciophobia	Fear of shadows
Spheksophobia	Fear of wasps
Technophobia	Fear of technology
Thalassophobia	Fear of the ocean
Triskaidekaphobia	Fear of number 13
Tropophobia	Fear of moving or making changes

Answers 10.59–10.60

10.59 The answer is D

10.60 The answer is B

10.61 The answer is C

10.62 The answer is A

10.63 The answer is E
Delusions are fixed, false beliefs, strongly held and immutable in the face of refuting evidence, that are not consonant with the person's education, social, and cultural background.

Delusions of misidentification are prominently reported because of their inherently intriguing nature. In *Capgras's syndrome*, the patient believes that someone close to him has been replaced by an exact double. In *Frégoli's phenomenon, strangers are identified as familiar persons in the patient's life.* In the *delusion of doubles, patients believe that another person has been physically transformed into themselves.* In *Clérambault's syndrome,* patients believe that a person is erotically attached to them, when in fact they are not. *Delusional jealousy* is a false belief about a spouse's infidelity.

Answers 10.64–10.68

10.64 The answer is D

10.65 The answer is E

10.66 The answer is B

10.67 The answer is A

10.68 The answer is C
Broca's, nonfluent and expressive aphasia are motor aphasias in which there is a disturbance of speech caused by a cognitive disorder in which understanding remains, but the ability to speak is grossly impaired, with halting, laborious and inaccurate speech. In a *syntactical* aphasia, there is an inability to arrange words in proper sequence. In *coprophasia*, there is the involuntary use of vulgar language, seen in Tourette's disorder and some patients with schizophrenia. Nominal aphasias, also termed *amnestic aphasias* or anomies, result in difficulty finding the correct name for an object. *Wernicke's aphasia* is a sensory, fluent, or receptive aphasia in which there is an organic loss of ability to comprehend the meaning of words; speech is fluid and spontaneous, but incoherent and nonsensical.

11 Classification in Psychiatry and Psychiatric Rating Scales

Advances in psychiatry are greatly shaped by its system of disease classification. Systems of classification for psychiatric diagnoses help distinguish one diagnosis from the other, so that clinicians can provide the most appropriate and effective treatment. They delineate a language common to all health care providers, so that all involved are treating and managing the same condition. They also provide a system to explore the still unknown etiology of mental disorders.

The 10th revision of *International Statistical Classification of Diseases and Related Health Problems* (ICD-10) is the official classification system used in Europe and many other parts of the world, developed by the World Health Organization. The text revision of the fourth edition of *Diagnostic and Statistical Manual of Mental Disorders* (DSM-IV-TR), developed by the American Psychiatric Association, is the official coding system used in the United States. It describes the manifestations of mental disorder in terms of its associated features; age, culture, and gender-related features; prevalence, incidence, and risk; course; complications; predisposing factors; familial pattern; and differential diagnosis. It is a multiaxial system that evaluated patients along several variables and contains five axes.

Psychiatric rating scales, or instruments, provide a way to quantify aspects of a patient's psyche, behavior, and relationships with other people and society. Many rating scales successfully measure carefully chosen features of well-formulated concepts. Psychiatrists who do not use these scales are left with only their clinical impressions, which does not allow for reliable comparison. Without these scales, quantitative data in psychiatry are crude. In order to ready any research article critically, a familiarity with these classification systems and rating instruments is essential.

HELPFUL HINTS

The student should be able to define the terms below, especially the diagnostic categories.

- age of onset
- agoraphobia
- alcohol delirium
- amnestic disorders
- associated and essential features
- atheoretical
- bipolar I disorder
- body dysmorphic disorder
- classification
- clinical syndromes
- cognitive disorders
- competence
- complications
- conversion disorder
- course
- delusional disorder
- dementia precox
- depersonalization disorder
- depressive disorders
- descriptive approach
- diagnostic criteria
- differential diagnosis
- disability determination
- dissociative disorders
- dissociative fugue
- dissociative identity disorder
- DSM-IV-TR
- dysthymic disorder
- ego-dystonic and ego-syntonic
- familial pattern
- general medical conditions
- generalized anxiety disorder
- Global Assessment of Functioning Scale
- gross social norms
- highest level of functioning
- hypochondriasis
- ICD-10
- impairment
- Emil Kraepelin
- mood disorders
- multiaxial system
- obsessive-compulsive disorder
- panic disorder
- paraphilias
- partial and full remission
- personality disorders
- pervasive developmental disorders
- phobias
- posttraumatic stress disorder
- predictive validity
- predisposing factors
- premenstrual dysphoric disorder
- prevalence
- psychological factors affecting medical condition
- psychosis
- psychosocial and environmental stressors
- reality testing
- residual type
- schizophrenia
- severity-of-stress rating
- sex ratio
- sexual dysfunctions
- somatization disorder
- somatoform disorders
- validity and reliability

CLASSIFICATION IN PSYCHIATRY

QUESTIONS

Directions

Each of the incomplete statements below is followed by five suggested completions. Select the *one* that is *best* in each case.

11.1 Which of the following about the multiaxial diagnostic classification is *true*?

A. Axis III lists only the physical disorders that are causative of the patient's mental disorder.
B. Axis II consists of personality disorders only.
C. It is a causation-driven diagnostic system.
D. Axis IV stressors are evaluated based on the clinician's assessment of the stress that an average person with similar socio-cultural values and circumstances would experience from the psychosocial stressors.
E. Axis I precludes disorders diagnosed in infancy, childhood or adolescence.

11.2 DSM-IV-TR

A. uses the term disorders because most of the entities lack the features necessary to warrant the term disease
B. never specifies cause
C. officially employs the term psychopathy as a disorder
D. is not compatible with ICD-10
E. none of the above

11.3 DSM-IV-TR

A. strives to be neutral or atheoretical with regard to etiology
B. provides specific diagnostic criteria that tend to increase the reliability of clinicians
C. makes no mention of management or treatment
D. provides explicit rules to be used in making a diagnosis when the clinical information is insufficient
E. all of the above

11.4 "Not otherwise specified categories" (NOS) of DSM-IV-TR may be used when

A. the symptoms are below the threshold for a specific disorder
B. there is an atypical presentation
C. the symptom pattern causes significant distress but has not been included in the DSM-IV-TR classification
D. the cause is uncertain
E. all of the above

11.5 True statements about DSM-IV-TR include

A. Axis I and Axis II comprise the entire classification of mental disorders.
B. Many patients have one or more disorders on both Axis I and Axis II.
C. The habitual use of a particular defense mechanism can be indicated on Axis II.
D. On Axis III, the identified physical condition may be causative, interactive, and effect, or unrelated to the mental state.
E. All of the above

11.6 Dementia in Alzheimer's disease may be characterized by each of the following terms *except*

A. mixed type
B. atypical type
C. of acute onset
D. with late onset
E. with early onset

11.7 The DSM-IV-TR definition of a mental disorder includes all of the following *except*

A. significant distress
B. significantly increased morbidity
C. deviant behaviors that are primarily between the individual and society
D. not merely expectable responses to particular events
E. significant disability

Directions

Each set of lettered headings below is followed by a list of numbered phrases or statements. For each numbered phrase or statement select the *one* lettered heading that is most closely associated with it. Each lettered heading may be selected once, more than once, or not at all.

Questions 11.8–11.13

A. Axis I
B. Axis II
C. Axis III
D. Axis IV
E. Axis V

11.8 Alcohol abuse
11.9 Threat of job loss
11.10 Frequent use of denial
11.11 Mood disorder due to hypothyroidism, with depressive features
11.12 GAF = 45 (on admission), GAF = 65 (at discharge)
11.13 Mental retardation

ANSWERS

11.1 The answer is D

Axis IV codes the psychosocial and environmental problems that contribute significantly to the development or exacerbation of the current disorder. The evaluation of the stressors is *based on the clinician's assessment of the stress that an average person with similar values and circumstances would experience.* This judgment is based on the amount of change that the stressor causes in the person's life, the degree to which the event is desired and under the person's control, and the number of stressors. *Axis I* consists of clinical disorders and other conditions that may be a focus of clinical attention. It *includes disorders first diagnosed in infancy, childhood, or adolescence,* excluding *mental retardation, which is coded on Axis II, together with personality disorders. Axis III* lists any physical disorder or general medical condition that is present in addition to the mental disorder. *The physical condition may be causative, the result of the mental disorder or unrelated to the mental disorder.* This approach to diagnosis attempts to describe the manifestations of the mental disorders and is *atheoretical with regard to causes.*

11.2 The answer is A

As with DSM-I and -II, the development of DSM-III was coordinated with the development of ICD-9 and published in 1980 by the APA. It represented a return to a descriptive system of diagnosis based on explicit operational diagnostic criteria, theoretically neutral, and multiaxial in format. DSM-III-R (1987) and DSM-IV-TR (1994) along with DSM-IV-TR (2000) refined the diagnostic categories based on available empirical data and proceeded to make the current diagnostic system compatible with that of the latest revision of ICD-10 system.

As late as the end of the 19th century, the adjective *psychopathic* meant psychopathological and applied to any form of mental disorder. However, Koch, Gross, Morel, and others were narrowing the concept to apply to less severe forms of pathology that would eventually evolve into the contemporary concepts of personality disorders.

Psychopathic personality became a subclass of the larger group of abnormal personalities. In the conceptualization of discordant adaptation, Eugen Khan used the term *psychopathic* to designate these conditions as complex states that lay intermediately between mental health and illness. Although Sigmund Freud was less interested in the issue, other psychodynamic and psychoanalytic writers like Daniel Stern and Wilhelm Reich contributed significantly to the understanding of character pathology. Carl Gustav Jung reinvigorated views of personality by shifting the focus away from archaic views of stereotyped behavioral forms to the contemporary perspective of combinations of dimensions and typologies. Erne Kretschmer proposed typology based on biological speculation that followed Kraepelin's approach to the psychoses. These perspectives led incrementally to the current concepts of personality disorder that, like the current nosological paradigm, are primarily descriptive and directed towards neurobiological explanatory hypotheses. Although *psychopathy* does not appear in the current official nosology, a residue of the concept is retained in DSM-IV-TR's antisocial personality disorder and ICD-10's dissocial personality disorder.

The official diagnostic nomenclature in *DSM-IV-TR uses the term disorder because most of the entities lack the features necessary to warrant the term disease. Cause is not specified except for cases of posttraumatic stress disorder, mental disorders due to a general medical condition, and substance-induced mental disorders.* Other than some of the dementias, even these disorders lack a specified mechanism; most psychiatric illnesses and many medical illnesses are not diseases in the strict sense of the word.

11.3 The answer is E (all)

DSM-IV-TR is the current classification of mental disorders; it is used by mental health professionals of all disciplines and is cited in insurance reimbursement, disability deliberations, statistical determinations, and forensic matters. Although there has been substantial criticism of each consecutive version of the DSM, DSM-IV-TR is the official nomenclature and is used throughout the land.

Specified diagnostic criteria are provided for each mental disorder. Those criteria include a list of features and, in most cases, how many must be present for the diagnosis to be made. The use of specific criteria *tends to increase the reliability of the diagnostic process among clinicians.*

DSM-IV-TR also systematically describes each disorder in terms of its associated features: specific age-, culture-, and gender-related aspects; prevalence, incidence, and predisposing factors; course; complications; familial pattern; and differential diagnosis. In cases where many of the specific disorders share common features, that information is included in the introduction to the entire section. Laboratory findings and associated physical examination signs and symptoms are described when relevant. DSM-IV-TR explicitly states that it is not a textbook. *No mention is made of causal theories, management, or treatment*; nor are the controversial issues surrounding particular diagnostic categories discussed.

DSM-IV-TR *provides explicit rules to be used when the information is insufficient* (diagnosis to be deferred or provisional) or the patient's clinical presentation and history do not meet the required criteria of a prototypical category (atypical type, residual, or not otherwise specified).

11.4 The answer is E (all)

Each diagnosis has a "not otherwise specified" category. According to DSM-IV-TR, an NOS diagnosis may be appropriate either *when the symptoms are below the diagnostic threshold* for one of the specific disorders or when there is an *atypical or mixed presentation.* It is similarly applicable if the *symptom pattern has not been included in the DSM-IV-TR classification but it causes clinically significant distress* or impairment of functioning, or the *cause is uncertain.*

11.5 The answer is E (all)

DSM-IV-TR is a multiaxial system that comprises five axes and evaluates the patient along each. *Axis I and Axis II comprise the entire classification of mental disorders*: 17 major groupings, more than 300 specific disorders, and almost 400 categories. In many instances, the patient has *one or more disorders on both Axes I and II.* For example, a patient may have major depressive disorder noted on Axis I and borderline and narcissistic personality disorders on Axis II. In general, multiple diagnoses on each axis are encouraged.

Axis II consists of personality disorders and mental retardation. The *habitual use of a particular defense mechanism can be indicated on Axis II.*

Axis III lists any physical disorder or general medical condition that is present in addition to the mental disorder. The identified physical condition may be causative (e.g., hepatic failure causing delirium), interactive (e.g., gastritis secondary to alcohol dependence), and effect (e.g., dementia and human immunodeficiency virus [HIV]–related pneumonia), or unrelated to the mental disorder. When a medical condition is causally related to a mental disorder, a mental disorder due to a general condition is listed on Axis I and the general medical condition is listed on both Axes I and III.

11.6 The answer is C

Acute onset refers to vascular dementia, not to dementia in Alzheimer's disease, which has a slow onset. The other four types—*mixed, atypical, with late onset*, and *with early onset*—all refer to dementia in Alzheimer's disease.

11.7 The answer is C

Mental disorders must be considered a manifestation of a behavioral, psychological, or biological dysfunction in the individual. *Neither deviant behavior nor conflicts that are primarily between the individual and society are mental disorders unless the deviance or conflict is a symptom of a dysfunction in the individual.* They are conceptualized as *clinically significant behavioral or psychological syndromes* or patterns that occur in an individual and that are associated with present *distress or disability* or with significantly *increased risk of suffering death, pain, disability, or an important loss of freedom*. The syndromes *must not be an expectable and culturally sanctioned response to a particular event.*

Answers 11.8–11.13

11.8 The answer is A

11.9 The answer is D

11.10 The answer is B

11.11 The answer is C

11.12 The answer is E

11.13 The answer is B

DSM-IV-TR uses a multiaxial scheme of classification consisting of five axes, each of which covers a different aspect of functioning. Each axis should be covered for each diagnosis. *Axis I* consists of all clinical syndromes as well as other conditions that may be a focus of clinical syndromes and other conditions that may be a focus of clinical attention. Examples include schizophrenia, mood disorders, and *alcohol abuse*. *Axis II* consists of personality disorders, *mental retardation,* and *frequent use of a defense mechanism such as denial*. *Axis III* consists of general medical conditions. The condition may be causative (for example, *hypothyroidism causing depression*), secondary (e.g., acquired immune deficiency syndrome [AIDS] as a result of a substance-related disorder), or unrelated. *Axis IV* consists of psychosocial and environmental problems that are related to the current mental disorder. Examples include divorce, *threat of job loss*, and inadequate health insurance. *Axis V* is a global assessment in which the clinician evaluates the highest level of functioning by the patient in the past year. The *Global Assessment of Functioning (GAF)* Scale is a 100-point scale, with 100 representing the highest level of functioning in all areas.

PSYCHIATRIC RATING SCALES

QUESTIONS

Directions

Each of the questions or incomplete statements below is followed by five suggested responses or completions. Select the *one* that is *best* in each case.

11.14 The global assessment of function

A. is recorded on Axis IV of a multiaxial evaluation
B. is assessed by a 50-point global assessment of functioning scale
C. bears no relation to prognosis
D. is a composite of social, occupational, and psychological functioning
E. included impairment due to physical limitations

11.15 The Social and Occupational Functioning Assessment Scale (SOFAS)

A. is scored independently from the person's psychological symptoms
B. does not include impairment in functioning that is caused by a general medical condition
C. may not be used to rate functioning at the time of the evaluation
D. may not be used to rate functioning of a past period
E. is included on Axis III

11.16 Which of the following scales is *not* used to rate a mood disorder?

A. Montgomer-Asberg Scale
B. Patterns of Individual Change Scale
C. Beck Depression Inventory
D. Hamilton Rating Scale
E. Raskin Depression Rating Scale

11.17 In the Scale for the Assessment of Negative Symptoms (SANS), which of the following is assessed?

A. Vocal inflection
B. Sexual activity
C. Impersistence at work
D. Social inattentiveness
E. All of the above

11.18 Which of the following is *true* of the Defensive Functioning Scale?

A. Suppression is measured on the "disavowal level."
B. Idealization is measured in the "major image-distorting level."
C. Splitting is measured in the "minor image-distorting level."
D. Apathetic withdrawal is measured on the "action level."
E. Sublimation is measured on the "mental inhibitions level."

11.19 The Hamilton Anxiety Rating Scale

A. is a ten-item scale
B. includes an item on mood
C. addresses suicidality
D. is exclusively history-based
E. excludes somatic symptoms

Directions

Each set of lettered headings below is followed by a list of numbered phrases or statements. For each numbered phrase or statement select the *one* lettered heading that is most closely associated with it. Each lettered heading may be selected once, more than once, or not at all.

Questions 11.20–11.23

A. Brief Psychiatric Rating Scale
B. Hamilton Rating Scale
C. Yale-Brown Scale
D. Social and Occupational Functioning Assessment Scale
E. None of the above

11.20 Obsessive-compulsive symptoms
11.21 Psychotic disorders
11.22 Depression and anxiety
11.23 Abnormal involuntary movements

ANSWERS

11.14 The answer is D

The Global Assessment of Functioning (GAF) Scale is considered a *composite of three major areas: social functioning, occupational functioning, and psychological functioning.* It is documented on *Axis V*, and is a *100-point scale*, based on a continuum of mental health and illness. It is *specifically not designed to include impairment in functioning due to physical or environmental limitations.* People with a *high level of functioning before an episode of illness generally have a better prognosis than those who had a low level of functioning.*

11.15 The answer is A

The Social and Occupational Functioning Assessment Scale (SOFAS) is a new scale included in a DSM-IV-TR appendix. The scale differs from the Global Assessment of Functioning (GAF) Scale in that it focuses only on the person's level of social and occupational functioning. *It is scored independent of the severity of the person's psychological symptoms.* And, unlike the GAF scale, the SOFAS may include *impairment in functioning* that is caused by a general *medical condition.* The SOFAS may be used to rate functioning at the time of the evaluation, or *it may be used to rate functioning of a past period. The SOFAS is included on Axis V, not Axis III.*

11.16 The answer is B

The Patterns of Individual Change Scale (PICS) is used in the assessment of quality of life. All the other scales listed are rating scales used for mood disorders.

11.17 The answer is E (all)

The Scale for the Assessment of Negative Symptoms (SANS) has five main categories: affective blunting, alogia, avolition-apathy, anhedonia-asociality, and attention. In the affective blunting category, *vocal inflection,* eye contact, facial expression, spontaneous movements, expressive gestures, and affective responsivity are measured. The avolition-apathy category measures *impersistence at work* or school, grooming, and physical anergia. The anhedonia-asocialty category looks at *sexual activity,* recreational interests, ability to feel intimacy, and relationships with peers and friends. The attention category assesses *social inattentiveness* and inattentiveness during the mental status examination. Another scale, used extensively for both positive and negative symptoms is called the Positive and Negative Syndrome Scale (PANSS).

11.18 The answer is D

The *"action level" is characterized by defensive functioning that deals with internal or external stressors by action or withdrawal, like apathetic withdrawal. Suppression and sublimation are rated on the "high adaptive level,"* the level of defensive functioning that results in the optimal adaptation in the handling of stressors. *Idealization is rated on the "minor image-distorting" level,* the level characterized by distortion in the image of self, body, or others that may be employed to regulate self-esteem. *Splitting is rated on the "major image-distorting level,"* the level characterized by gross distortion or misattribution of the image of self or others.

11.19 he answer is B

The Hamilton Anxiety Rating Scale addresses *depressed mood,* focusing on loss of interest, lack of pleasure in hobbies, depression, early wakening, and diurnal swing. It is a *fourteen-item scale* that includes assessment of *sensory, cardiovascular, respiratory, gastrointestinal, genitourinary, and autonomic* symptoms. It includes an assessment of *behavior at the time of interview,* focusing on fidgeting, restlessness, tremor, furrowed brow, strained face, sighing, facial pallor, swallowing, belching, brisk tendon jerks, dilated pupils, and exophthalmos. There is *no item dedicated to assessing suicidal ideation or intent.*

Answers 11.20–11.23

11.20 The answer is C

11.21 The answer is A

11.22 The answer is B

11.23 The answer is E

Psychiatric rating scales, also called rating instruments, provide a way to quantify aspects of a patient's psyche, behavior, and relationships with individuals and society. The measurement of pathology in these areas of a person's life may initially seem to be less straightforward than is the measurement of pathology—hypertension, for example—by other medical specialists. Nevertheless, many psychiatric rating scales are able to measure carefully chosen features of well-formulated concepts. Moreover, psychiatrists who do not use these rating scales are left with only their clinical impressions, which are difficult to record in a manner that allows for reliable future comparison and communication. Without psychiatric rating scales, quantitative data in psychiatry are crude (for example, length of hospitalization or other treatment, discharge and readmission to hospital, length of relationships or employment, and presence of legal troubles).

Rating scales can be specific or comprehensive, and they can measure both internally experienced variables (e.g., mood) and externally observable variables (e.g., behavior). Specific scales measure discrete thoughts, moods, or behaviors, such as *obsessive thoughts* and temper tantrums; comprehensive scales measure broad abstractions, such as *depression* and anxiety. Well-known rating scales include the *Hamilton Rating Scale for depression and anxiety and the Yale-Brown Scale for obsessive-compulsive symptoms.*

Classic items from the mental status examination are the most frequently assessed items on rating scales. These items include *thought disorders*, *mood disturbances*, and gross behaviors (i.e., the Brief Psychiatric Rating Scale). Another type of information covered by rating scales is the assessment of adverse effects from psychotherapeutic drugs. *Social adjustments* (e.g., *occupational success* and quality of relationships with the SOFAS) and psychoanalytic concepts (e.g., ego strength and defense mechanisms) are also measured by some rating scales, although the reliability and the validity of such scales are lowered by the absence of agreed-on norms, the high level of inference required on some items, and the lack of independence between measures.

Other characteristics of rating scales include the time covered, the level of judgment required, and the method of recording answers. The time covered by a rating scale must be specified, and the rate must adhere to this period. For example, a particular rating scale may rate a 5-minute observation period, a week-long period, or a patient's entire life.

The most reliable rating scales require a limited amount of judgment or inference on the part of the rater. Whatever the level of judgment required, clear definitions of the answer scale, preferably with clinical examples, should be provided by the developer of the scale and should be read by the rater.

The actual answer given may be recorded as either a dichotomous variable (for example, true or false, present or absent) or a continuous variable. Continuous items may ask the rater to choose a term to describe severity (absent, slight, mild, moderate, severe, or extreme) or frequency (never, rarely, occasionally, often, very often, or always). Although many psychiatric symptoms are thought of as existing in dichotomous states—for example, the presence or absence of delusions—most experienced clinicians know that the world is not so simple.

12

Delirium, Dementia, and Amnestic and Other Cognitive Disorders and Mental Disorders Due to a General Medical Condition

In the text revision of the fourth edition of Diagnostic Statistical Manual of Mental Disorders (DSM-IV-TR) three groups of disorders—delirium, dementia, and the amnestic disorders—are characterized by the primary symptom common to all the disorders, which is an impairment in cognition (as in memory, language, or attention). Although DSM-IV-TR acknowledges that other psychiatric disorders can exhibit some cognitive impairment as a symptom, cognitive impairment is the cardinal symptom in delirium, dementia, and the amnestic disorders. Within each of these diagnostic categories, DSM-IV-TR delimits specific types.

Dementia is also characterized by marked cognitive deficits, but unlike delirium, these deficits occur in the context of a clear sensorium. The deficits include impairments in intelligence, learning and memory, language, problem solving, orientation, perception, attention and concentration, judgment, and social skills. The clinical work-up of etiology is crucial. Clinicians need to be especially familiar with dementias of the Alzheimer's type as well as vascular dementias. Knowledge of the course and prognosis of both these dementia types is essential. Principles of treatment, and perhaps most importantly, long-term management of people with these disorders, must be learned in order to most effectively assist patients and their families.

Amnestic disorders are characterized by memory impairments that are associated with significant deficits in social or occupational functioning. The amnestic disorders are causally related to general medical conditions, such as head trauma. This characteristic distinguishes them from the dissociative disorders involving memory impairments.

The questions and answers below can test knowledge of the subject.

HELPFUL HINTS

The student should be able to define the signs, symptoms, and syndromes listed below.

- abstract attitude
- Addison's disease
- AIP
- ALS
- amnestic disorders
- anxiety disorder due to a general medical condition
- auditory, olfactory, and visual hallucinations
- beclouded dementia
- beriberi
- black-patch
- catastrophic reaction
- cognitive disorders
- confabulation
- cretinism
- Creutzfeldt-Jakob disease
- Cushing's syndrome
- delirium
- delusional disorder
- dementia
- dementia of the Alzheimer's type
- diabetic ketoacidosis
- dissociative amnesia
- Down's syndrome
- dysarthria
- epilepsy
- general paresis
- granulovacuolar degeneration
- Huntington's disease
- hypnagogic and hypnopompic hallucinations
- hypoglycemic, hepatic, and uremic encephalopathy
- intellectual functions
- interictal
- intoxication and withdrawal
- intracranial neoplasms
- Korsakoff's syndrome
- kuru
- Lilliputian hallucinations
- manifestations
- memory
- mood disorder due to a general medical condition
- multiple sclerosis
- myxedema
- neurofibrillary tangles
- normal aging
- normal pressure hydrocephalus
- orientation
- parkinsonism
- partial versus generalized seizures
- pellagra
- pernicious anemia

- personality change due to a general medical condition
- Pick's disease
- postoperative
- prion disease
- pseudobulbar palsy
- pseudodementia
- retrograde versus anterograde amnesia
- senile plaques
- short-term versus long-term memory loss
- SLE
- sundowner syndrome
- tactile or haptic hallucinations
- TIA
- transient global amnesia
- vascular dementia
- vertebrobasilar disease

QUESTIONS

Directions

Each of the questions or incomplete statements below is followed by five suggested responses or completions. Select the *one* that is *best* in each case.

12.1 Factors that predispose to delirium include all of the following *except*

A. Use of bladder catheter
B. Age older than 60
C. Vision impairment
D. Smoking history
E. Abnormal glucose level

12.2 Which of the following statements about delirium is *true*?

A. Male gender is an independent risk factor.
B. Few hospitalized medically ill patients develop delirium.
C. It is independent of age.
D. It has no bearing on overall patient prognosis.
E. Post-cardiotomy patients rarely develop delirium.

12.3 The most common cause of delirium within 3 days post-operatively in a 40-year-old man with a history of alcohol dependence is

A. stress of surgery
B. postoperative pain
C. pain medication
D. infection
E. delirium tremens

12.4 Which of the following is a prion disease?

A. Creutzfeldt-Jakob disease
B. Fatal familial insomnia
C. Variant Creutzfeldt-Jakob disease
D. Kuru
E. All of the above

12.5 Which clinical features may be associated with delirium?

A. Disorganized thought processes
B. Illusions
C. Mood alterations
D. Hallucinations
E. All of the above

12.6 Dementia with Lewy bodies

A. is a clinical diagnosis
B. is the second most prevalent dementia subtype
C. is commonly associated with visual hallucinations
D. is associated with pronounced psychomotor impairment
E. all of the above

12.7 Which of the following drugs is best used to treat acute delirium?

A. chlorpromazine (Thorazine)
B. diazepam (Valium)
C. haloperidol (Haldol)
D. amobarbital (Amytal)
E. physostigmine salicylate (Antilirium)

12.8 In delirium

A. epinephrine is hypothesized to be the major neurotransmitter involved
B. the major pathway implicated is the dorsal tegmental pathway
C. the electroencephalogram (EEG) usually shows diffuse background quickening
D. there is hyperactivity in the nucleus accumbens
E. the level of consciousness is preserved

12.9 Alzheimer's dementia is

A. linked to chromosome 7
B. a clinical diagnosis
C. associated with hypoactive levels of acetylcholine
D. associated with pathognomonic neurofibrillary tangles
E. more common in men

12.10 Mr. E is 68 years old and married with two children. His wife reports changes in his memory and behavior over the last 9 years. She reports that he frequently forgets his keys, goes into the house to get something and then forgets what he wants, and that he has changed from an outgoing pleasant person, to one who avoids conversation. She says that he seems hostile at times for no apparent reason. Mr. E is in good general health, taking no medications, and his alcohol consumption is limited to two to three beers a day.

What may you observe on examination of Mr. E?

A. Paranoid delusions
B. Pathological crying
C. A grasp reflex
D. Poor hygiene
E. All of the above

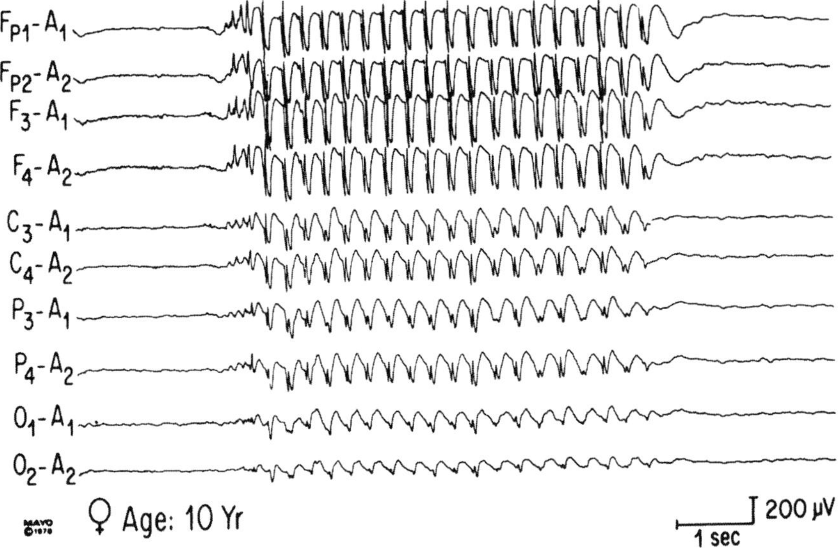

FIGURE 12.1
Electroencephalogram (EEG).

12.11 In the case described above, what is the most likely diagnosis other than dementia for Mr. E?

A. Major depression
B. Chronic paranoid schizophrenia
C. Normal aging
D. Delirium
E. Factitious disorder

12.12 Which of the following would be consistent with the progression of Mr. E's illness?

A. Increased agitation
B. Frequent nighttime pacing
C. Physical threats toward his wife
D. Urinary incontinence
E. All of the above

12.13 The EEG shown in Figure 12.1 is an example of

A. partial seizure
B. grand mal epilepsy
C. petit mal epilepsy or absence seizure
D. psychomotor epilepsy
E. none of the above

12.14 True statements about the epidemiology of dementia include all of the following *except*

A. The estimated prevalence in a population over 65 years is consistently reported to be about 5 percent.
B. Dementia of Alzheimer's type is the most common dementing disorder in North America, Scandinavia, and Europe.
C. The risk for vascular dementia is six times greater than that for Alzheimer's among people older than 75 years.
D. There appears to be a higher rate of vascular dementia in men, and a higher rate of Alzheimer's in women.
E. In geriatric psychiatric populations, Alzheimer's is much more common than vascular dementia.

12.15 Delirium

A. has an insidious onset
B. rarely has associated neurological symptoms
C. generally has an underlying cause residing in the central nervous system
D. may be successfully treated with lithium
E. generally causes a diffuse slowing of brain activity

12.16 Of the following cognitive functions, the one most likely to be difficult to evaluate and interpret on formal testing is

A. memory
B. visuospatial and constructional ability
C. reading and writing
D. abstraction
E. calculations

12.17 True statements about Alzheimer's disease include all of the following *except*

A. Age at onset is earlier in patients with a family history of the disease.
B. There is clear phenomenological separation between early-onset and late-onset cases.
C. The early-onset type may have a more rapidly progressive course.
D. No features of the physical examination or laboratory evaluation are pathognomonic.
E. Brain-imaging studies are used to exclude other identifiable causes.

12.18 Creutzfeldt-Jakob disease is characterized by

A. rapid deterioration

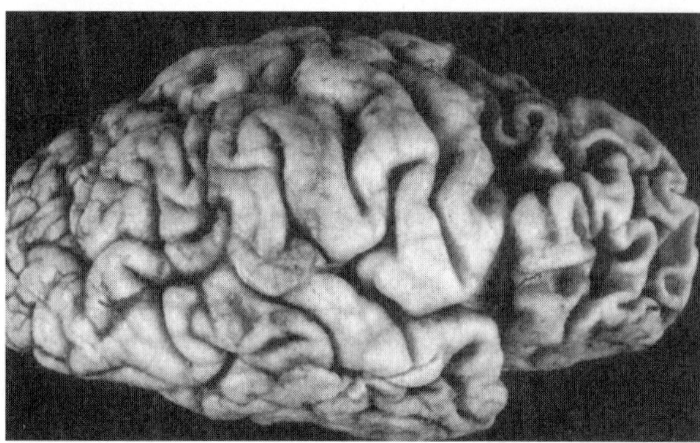

FIGURE 12.2

Pick's disease gross pathology. This demonstrates the marked frontal and temporal atrophy seen in frontotemporal dementias, such as Pick's disease. (Courtesy of Dashyant Purohit, M.D., Associate Professor, Department of Neuropathology, Mount Sinai School of Medicine, New York, NY.)

B. myoclonus
C. diffuse, symmetric, rhythmic slow waves in EEG
D. postmortem definitive diagnosis
E. all of the above

12.19 Amnestic disorders

A. are invariably persistent, lasting at least a month
B. are defined by a better memory for remote events than recent ones
C. do not typically impair the ability to immediately repeat a sequential string of information (e.g., digit span)
D. typically have a gradual onset
E. none of the above

12.20 The brain depicted in Figure 12.2 shows frontal and temporal atrophy associated with frontotemporal dementia. Which of the following statements is *true*?

A. Progressive nonfluent aphasia is a frontotemporal dementia.
B. Pick's disease has its own separate diagnostic criteria in DSM-IV-TR.
C. Frontotemporal dementia is more likely to affect older populations.
D. Pick bodies are found in all the frontotemporal dementias.
E. Genetic linkage to chromosome 9 has been found in frontotemporal dementia.

12.21 Amnestic disorders

A. may be diagnosed in the context of delirium
B. may be diagnosed in the context of dementia
C. are secondary syndromes caused by primary etiologies
D. are most often due to nutritional deficiencies related to chronic alcohol dependence
E. none of the above

12.22 True statements about vascular etiologies of dementia include

A. Together they comprise the second most common cause of dementia.
B. It is believed that tissue damage in infarction underlies vascular dementia.
C. The most common cause of cerebral infarction is thromboembolism from a large vessel plaque.
D. Approximately 15 percent of cerebrovascular disease is due to cerebral hemorrhage related to hypertension.
E. All of the above

12.23 Frontal lobe degeneration is associated with

A. disinhibition
B. social misconduct
C. lack of insight
D. apathy
E. all of the above

12.24 Which of the following is a *true* statement about Parkinson's disease?

A. It is a prototype of a cortical degenerative disease.
B. It cannot be distinguished from parkinsonian syndromes that arise from a variety of causes.
C. It is the result of the degeneration of the substantia nigra, globus pallidus, putamen, and caudate.
D. The only cells affected are those containing dopamine.
E. Dementia is more common in early-onset disease.

12.25 Risk factors for the development of delirium include

A. increased severity of physical illness
B. older age
C. preexisting dementia
D. the use of anticholinergics
E. all of the above

12.26 BSE is associated with all of the following *except*

A. Spongiform vacuolization
B. Neuronal loss
C. Astrocyte proliferation in the cerebral cortex
D. Amyloid plaques
E. "Bulls-Eye" rash on the thigh

12.27 Clinical characteristics of vascular dementia

A. are the same regardless of the area of infarction
B. are the same regardless of the number of infarctions
C. are the same regardless of the type of vasculature involved
D. are the same regardless of whether or not deficits accumulate or resolve quickly after small strokes
E. none of the above

12.28 Features supportive of the diagnosis of dementia with Lewy bodies include

A. recurrent visual hallucinations that are typically well formed and detailed
B. fluctuating cognition with profound variations in attention and alertness

C. spontaneous motor features of parkinsonism
D. neuroleptic sensitivity
E. all of the above

12.29 Vascular dementia

A. is more common in women
B. is primarily a large vessel disease
C. is not associated with fundoscopic abnormalities
D. includes Binswanger's disease
E. is not associated with hypertension

12.30 Transient global amnesia

A. is more common in women
B. has a characteristically abnormal EEG pattern
C. is associated with loss of self identity
D. has been linked to vascular instability
E. is more common in young people

12.31 Huntington's disease

A. is linked to the long arm of chromosome 4
B. affects men only
C. is associated with "boxcar" ventricles on brain scanning
D. shows striatal hypermetabolism on positron emission tomography (PET)
E. is not usually associated with emotional symptoms

Directions

Each group of questions below consists of lettered headings followed by a list of numbered phrases or statements. For each numbered phrase or statement, select the *one* lettered heading that is most closely associated with it. Each lettered heading may be used once, more than once, or not at all.

Questions 12.32–12.36

A. Creutzfeldt-Jakob disease
B. Normal-pressure hydrocephalus
C. Neurosyphilis
D. Huntington's disease
E. Multiple sclerosis

12.32 Death occurring 15 to 20 years after the onset of the disease, with suicide being common
12.33 Slow virus, with death occurring within 2 years of the diagnosis
12.34 Manic syndrome with neurological signs in up to 20 percent of cases
12.35 Treatment of choice being a shunt
12.36 More prevalent in cold and temperate climates than in the tropics and subtropics

Questions 12.37–12.40

A. Lead poisoning
B. Manganese madness
C. Mercury poisoning
D. Thallium intoxication
E. None of the above

12.37 Alopecia
12.38 Succimer (Chemet)
12.39 Mad Hatter syndrome
12.40 Masked facies

Directions

Each set of lettered headings below is followed by a list of numbered phrases. For each numbered phrase, select

A. if the item is associated with A only
B. if the item is associated with B only
C. if the item is associated with both A and B
D. if the item is associated with neither A nor B

Questions 12.41–12.47

A. Cortical dementia
B. Subcortical dementia

12.41 Huntington's chorea
12.42 Alzheimer's disease
12.43 Early decline in calculation, naming, and copying skills
12.44 Fine and gross motor movements are generally preserved until later in the disease process
12.45 Language is relatively spared
12.46 Presenting symptoms more likely to be a personality change or mood disturbance
12.47 Presenting symptoms more often reflect cognitive impairment

Questions 12.48–12.53

A. Delirium
B. Dementia

12.48 Hallucinations
12.49 Sundowning
12.50 Catastrophic reaction
12.51 High mortality rate
12.52 Decreased acetylcholine activity
12.53 Insight present

ANSWERS

12.1 The answer is B

There are numerous factors that increase a patient's risk for delirium (Table 12-1). These range from extremes of age to the number of medications taken. For example, pharamcokinetic and pharmacodynamic changes specific to the young and the old contribute to the increased risk as in both populations. In one study of elderly hospitalized patients, the risk of delirium was higher if the patients had *vision impairment*, more severe medical illness, cognitive impairment, or an elevated blood urea nitrogen (BUN) to creatinine ratio. Other studies of ICU patients suggested that hypertension, abnormal total bilirubin, *smoking history*, epidural use, morphine, and intravenous (IV) dopamine were associated with delirium. *Being older than 70, not 60*, is a predisposing factor to delirium.

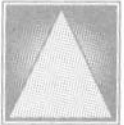

Table 12.1
Factors That Predispose Patients to Delirium

Vision impairment	Hypertension	Use of bladder catheter
Medical illnesses (severity and quantity)	Chronic obstructive pulmonary disease	Preoperative cognitive impairment
Cognitive impairment	Alcohol abuse	Functional limitations
Older than 70 years of age	Smoking history	History of delirium
Any iatrogenic event	Abnormal sodium level	Abnormal potassium, sodium, or glucose test
Use of physical restraints	Abnormal glucose level	Preoperative use of benzodiazepines
Malnutrition	Abnormal bilirubin level	Preoperative use of narcotic analgesics
More than three medications added	Blood urea nitrogen to creatinine ratio >18	Epidural use

12.2 The answer is A

Male gender is an independent risk factor for delirium, according to DSM-IV-TR. The point of prevalence in the general population is 0.4 percent for people 18 years and older, and 1.1 percent for people 55 years and older. *About 10 to 30 percent of medically ill patients who are hospitalized exhibit delirium. Advanced age* is a major risk factor for its development, and approximately 30 to 40 percent of hospitalized patients older than 65 have an episode of delirium. *The highest rate of delirium is found in post-cardiotomy patients, which is more than 90 percent.* Delirium is a poor prognostic sign. Rates of institutionalization are increased threefold for patients 65 years and older who exhibit delirium while in the hospital, and the one year mortality rate for patients who have an episode of delirium may be as high as 50 percent.

12.3 The answer is E

The most common cause of delirium in this case is *delirium tremens* (called alcohol withdrawal delirium in DSM-IV-TR). It is a medical emergency that results in mortality in about 20 percent of cases if left untreated. It occurs within 1 week after the person stops drinking. It usually develops on the third hospital day in a patient admitted for an unrelated condition (such as surgery) who has no access to alcohol and stops drinking suddenly. Another less common cause of postoperative delirium is *stress*, especially in major procedures such as cardiac or transplantation surgery. *Pain, pain medication*, and *infection* must also be considered in the postoperative period.

12.4 The answer is E (all)

Prion disease is a group of related disorders caused by a transmissible infectious protein known as a prion. Included in this group are Creutzfeldt-Jakob disease (CJD), Gerstmann-Straussler syndrome (GSS), fatal familial insomnia (FFI), and kuru. A variant of CJD (vCJD), also called "mad cow disease," appeared in 1995 in the United Kingdom and is attributed to the transmission of bovine spongiform encephalopathy (BSE) from cattle to humans.

12.5 The answer is E (all)

The core features of delirium include altered consciousness, altered attention, impaired cognition, rapid onset, brief duration, and unpredictable fluctuations in severity. Associated features that are often present include *disorganized thought processes*, perceptual disturbances such as *illusions* and *hallucinations*, psychomotor hyperactivity and hypoactivity, disruptions of the sleep-wake cycle, *mood alterations*, and other manifestations of altered neurological function, like autonomic instability.

12.6 The answer is E (all)

Dementia with Lewy bodies is the preferred term that encompasses several conditions, including senile dementia of Lewy body type, Lewy body variant of Alzheimer's disease, Lewy body dementia, diffuse Lewy body disease, and cortical Lewy body disease. *It is a clinical diagnosis*, based on progressive dementia with parkinsonism and a fluctuation in the level of attention and the severity of the cognitive deficits. *Visual hallucinations are a common feature. Dementia with Lewy bodies may be the second most prevalent dementia subtype. Patients with it have pronounced visuospatial deficits and psychomotor impairments.* Figure 12.3 shows cortical Lewy bodies.

12.7 The answer is C

Of the drugs listed, the best choice is *haloperidol (Haldol)*, a butyrophenone. Depending on the patient's age, weight, and physical condition, the initial dose may range from 0.5 to 10 mg intramuscularly, repeated in an hour if the patient remains agitated. As soon as the patient is calm, oral medication in liquid concentrate or tablet form should begin. Two daily oral doses should suffice, with two-thirds of the dose being given at bedtime. To achieve the same therapeutic effect, the clinician should give an oral dose about 1.5 times higher than a parenteral dose. The effective total daily dosage of haloperidol may range from 5 to 50 mg for the majority of delirious patients. The patient's

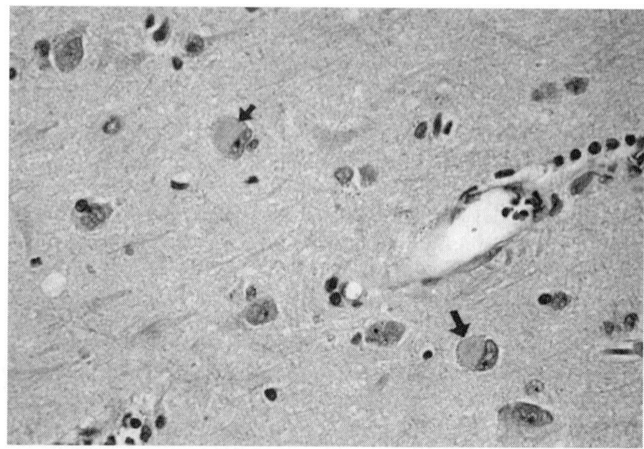

FIGURE 12.3

Cortical Lewy bodies (*arrows*), seen with hematoxylin and eosin staining. Lewy bodies are weekly eosinophilic, spherical, cytoplasmic inclusions. (Courtesy of Dashyant Purohit, M.D., Associate Professor, Department of Neuropathology, Mount Sinai School of Medicine, New York, NY.)

response should always be closely monitored for possible side effects.

Phenothiazines, such as *chlorpromazine (Thorazine)*, should be avoided in delirious patients because those drugs are associated with significant anticholinergic activity. *Benzodiazepines* with long half-lives, such as *diazepam (Valium)*, and barbiturates, such as *amobarbital (Amytal)*, should be avoided unless they are being used as part of the treatment for the underlying disorder (for example, alcohol withdrawal). Sedatives can increase cognitive disorganization in delirious patients. When the delirium is due to anticholinergic toxicity, the use of *physostigmine salicylate (Antilirium)* may be indicated; but it is not the first drug to be used in an acute delirium in which the cause has not been determined.

12.8 The answer is B

The reticular formation of the brainstem is the principal area regulating attention and arousal; *the major pathway implicated is the dorsal tegmental pathway*, which projects from the mesencephalic reticular formation to the tectum and thalamus. The major neurotransmitter hypothesized to be involved is acetylcholine, *not epinephrine*. In delirium *there is no hyperactivity in the nucleus accumbens*. The *EEG characteristically shows a generalized slowing of activity*. A core feature of delirium is *altered consciousness*.

12.9 The answer is C

The neurotransmitters that are most often implicated in the pathophysiological condition of Alzheimer's disease are *acetylcholine and norepinephrine, both of which are hypoactive in the disease*. The disease has shown *linkage to chromosomes 1, 14, and 21, not chromosome 7*. Although it is commonly diagnosed in the clinical setting after other causes of dementia have been excluded, *the final diagnosis of Alzheimer's disease requires a neuropathological examination of the brain*. The classic gross neuroanatomical observation of the brain from patients with this disease is diffuse atrophy. The classic microscopic findings are senile plaques, neuronal loss, synaptic loss, and granulovascular degeneration of the neurons. *Neurofibrillary tangles are not unique to Alzheimer's disease*, but also occur in Down syndrome, dementia pugilistica, Parkinson-dementia complex of Guam, and the brains of normal people as they age. *The risk factors for developing Alzheimer's dementia include being female*, having a first-degree relative with the disorder, and having a history of head injury or Down syndrome.

12.10 The answer is E (all)

An estimated 20 to 30 percent of patients with dementia have hallucinations, and *30 to 40 percent have delusions, primarily of a paranoid or persecutory nature*. They may exhibit *pathological laughter or crying* with no apparent provocation. *Primitive reflexes, such as the grasp*, snout, suck, tonic-foot, and palmomental reflexes may be present. Patients with dementia often have disregard for the conventional rules of social conduct and demonstrate coarse language, inappropriate jokes, *and neglect of personal appearance and hygiene*.

12.11 The answer is A

Although all of the diagnoses listed should be considered in the differential diagnosis of dementia, the cognitive impairment associated with depression is often the most difficult to distinguish from the symptoms of dementia. *The clinical picture is often referred to as pseudodementia, or depression-related cognitive dysfunction* (Table 12.2). Although *schizophrenia* may be associated with some acquired intellectual impairment, its symptoms are much less severe than are the related symptoms of psychosis and thought disorder seen in dementia. *Aging* is not necessarily associated with any significant cognitive decline. Minor memory problems can occur as a normal part of aging, but these do not interfere significantly with a person's social or occupational behavior. *Delirium* has a rapid onset, brief duration, fluctuating cognitive impairment, nocturnal exacerbations, and prominent disturbances in attention and perception. People who attempt to simulate memory loss, as *in factitious disorder*, do so in an erratic and inconsistent manner. In true dementia, memory for time and place is lost before memory for persons, and recent memory is lost before remote memory.

12.12 The answer is E (all)

The classic course of dementia is an onset in the patient's 50s or 60s, with gradual deterioration over 5 to 10 years, leading eventually to death. The average survival expectation for patients with dementia of the Alzheimer's type is 8 years. Progression of the disease involves *increased agitation*, frequent emotional outbursts, with poor sleep, *night pacing*, and wandering. In the terminal phases of dementia, patients become empty shells of their former selves, profoundly disoriented, amnestic, and *incontinent of urine and feces*.

12.13 The answer is C

Petit mal epilepsy or absence seizure is associated with a characteristic generalized, bilaterally synchronous, 3-hertz spike-and-wave pattern in the electroencephalogram (EEG) and is often easily induced by hyperventilation. Petit mal epilepsy occurs predominantly in children. It usually consists of simple absence attacks lasting 5 to 10 seconds, during which the patient has an abrupt alteration in awareness and responsiveness and an interruption in motor activity. The child often has a blank stare associated with an upward deviation of the eyes and some mild twitching movements of the eyes, eyelids, face, or extremities. Petit mal epilepsy is usually a fairly benign seizure disorder, often resolving after adolescence.

A *partial seizure* (also known as jacksonian epilepsy) is a type of epilepsy characterized by recurrent episodes of focal motor seizures. It begins with localized tonic or clonic contraction, increases in severity, spreads progressively through the entire body, and terminates in a generalized convulsion with loss of consciousness. *Grand mal epilepsy* is the major form of epilepsy. Gross tonic-clonic convulsive seizures are accompanied by loss of consciousness and, often, incontinence of stool or urine. *Psychomotor epilepsy* is a type of epilepsy characterized by recurrent behavior disturbances. Complex hallucinations or illusions, frequently gustatory or olfactory, often herald the onset of the seizure, which typically involves a state of impaired consciousness resembling a dream, during which paramnestic phenomena, such as *déjà vu* and *jamais vu,* are experienced, and the patient exhibits repetitive, automatic, or semipurposeful behaviors. In rare instances, violent behavior may be prominent. The EEG reveals a localized seizure focus in the temporal lobe.

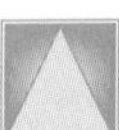

Table 12.2
Major Clinical Features Differentiating Pseudodementia from Dementia

Pseudodementia	Dementia
Clinical course and history	
Family always aware of dysfunction and its severity	Family often unaware of dysfunction and its severity
Onset can be dated with some precision	Onset can be dated only within broad limits
Symptoms of short duration before medical help is sought	Symptoms usually of long duration before medical help is sought
Rapid progression of symptoms after onset	Slow progression of symptoms throughout course
History of previous psychiatric dysfunction common	History of previous psychiatric dysfunction unusual
Complaints and clinical behavior	
Patients usually complain much of cognitive loss	Patients usually complain little of cognitive loss
Patients' complaints of cognitive dysfunction usually detailed	Patients' complaints of cognitive dysfunction usually vague
Patients emphasize disability	Patients conceal disability
Patients highlight failures	Patients delight in accomplishments, however trivial
Patients make little effort to perform even simple tasks	Patients struggle to perform tasks
	Patients rely on notes, calendars, etc., to keep up
Patients usually communicate strong sense of distress	Patients often appear unconcerned
Affective change often pervasive	Affect labile and shallow
Loss of social skills often early and prominent	Social skills often retained
Behavior often incongruent with severity of cognitive dysfunction	Behavior usually compatible with severity of cognitive dysfunction
Nocturnal accentuation of dysfunction uncommon	Nocturnal accentuation of dysfunction common
Clinical features related to memory, cognitive, and intellectual dysfunctions	
Attention and concentration often well preserved	Attention and concentration usually faulty
"Don't know" answers typical	Near-miss answers frequent
On tests of orientation, patients often give "don't know" answers	On tests of orientation, patients often mistake unusual for usual
Memory loss for recent and remote events usually severe	Memory loss for recent events usually more severe than for remote events
Memory gaps for specific periods or events common	Memory gaps for specific periods unusual[a]
Marked variability in performance on tasks of similar difficulty	Consistently poor performance on tasks of similar difficulty

[a] Except when caused by delirium, trauma, seizures, etc.

Reprinted with permission from Wells CE. Pseudodementia. *Am J. Psychiatry.* 1979:36:898.

12.14 The answer is C

The prevalence of dementia rises exponentially with age. *The estimated prevalence* of moderate to severe dementia in a population aged 65 years or older is consistently reported at *approximately 5 percent.* Within that age group the exponential curve is pronounced so that the prevalence in the subgroup aged 65 to 69 years is 1.5 to 2 percent; in the subgroup aged 75 to 79 years, it is 5.5 to 6.5 percent; and in the subgroup aged 85 to 89 years, it is 20 to 22 percent. *Dementia of the Alzheimer's type is the most common dementing* disorder in clinical and neuropathological prevalence studies reported from North America, Scandinavia, and Europe. Prevalence studies from Russia and Japan show vascular dementia to be more common in those countries. It remains unclear whether those apparent clinical differences reflect true etiological distinctions or inconsistent uses of diagnostic criteria. Dementia of the Alzheimer's type becomes more common with increasing age; among persons older than 75 years, *the risk is six times greater than the risk for vascular dementia.* There is a suggestion of *higher rates of dementia of the Alzheimer's type in females and higher rates of vascular dementia in males. In geriatric psychiatric patient samples, dementia of the Alzheimer's type is a much more common etiology (50 to 70 percent) than vascular dementia (15 to 25 percent).*

Studies of the incidence of dementia have been plagued by widely differing methodology and results. Again, there is an exponential increase in incidence with age, although some reports have noted a leveling off starting around age 75 years.

12.15 The answer is E

Delirium *generally causes a diffuse slowing of brain activity* on the EEG, which may be useful in differentiating delirium from depression and psychosis. The EEG of a delirious patient sometimes shows focal areas of hyperactivity. In rare cases, differentiating delirium related to epilepsy from delirium related to other causes may be difficult. In general, *delirium has a sudden, not insidious, onset.* Patients with delirium *commonly (not rarely) have associated neurological* symptoms, including dysphasia, tremor, asterixis, incoordination, and urinary incontinence. Delirium does not generally have an underlying cause residing in the central nervous system. Delirium has many causes, all of which result in a similar pattern of symptoms relating to the patient's level of consciousness and cognitive impairment. *Most of the causes of delirium lie outside the central nervous system*—for example, renal and hepatic failures. Delirium *cannot be successfully treated with lithium (Eskalith).* Patients with variable lithium serum concentrations may be at risk for delirium.

12.16 The answer is D

When testing cognitive functions the clinician should evaluate *memory*; *visuospatial and constructional abilities*; *reading and writing*, and *mathematical abilities. Abstraction ability* is also valuable to assess, although a patient's performance on tasks, such as proverb interpretation, may be difficult to evaluate when abnormal. Proverb interpretation may be a useful bedside projective test in some patients, but the specific interpretation may result from a variety of factors, such as poor education, low intelligence, and failure to understand the concept of proverbs, as well as a broad array of primary and secondary psychopathological disturbances. Although testing similarities are also education-sensitive, similarities may be more easily understood by patients.

12.17 The answer is B

Alzheimer's disease is the prototype of a cortical degenerative disease. Alzheimer's original description in 1906 detailed most of the familiar clinical and neuropathological features. Of note, his patient suffered from paranoia in addition to cognitive decline. Currently, the diagnosis of Alzheimer's disease requires neuropathological confirmation, but the diagnosis is used clinically for cases identified antemortem. *Age at onset is earlier in patients with a family history of the disease.* Despite some data to suggest distinctive age-related clinical patterns, *no phenomenological separation between early-onset and late-onset cases has been found consistently* enough for age to substitute for detailed clinical description; however, *early-onset dementia of the Alzheimer's type may have a more rapidly progressive course.* A major component of the presenting symptoms is usually subjective complaints of memory difficulty, language impairment ("I can't find the word"), and dyspraxia (e.g., difficulty driving). Diagnosis at this juncture is primarily based on exclusion of other possible etiologies for dementia. *No features of the physical examination or laboratory evaluation are pathognomonic for dementia of the Alzheimer's type.* Some studies have apparently discriminated patients with dementia of the Alzheimer's type from patients with dementia of other etiologies and from normal controls by using techniques such as EEG, magnetic resonance imaging (MRI), and single photon emission computed tomography (SPECT). These studies have been difficult to replicate consistently, and at present, *brain-imaging studies are best used to exclude other identifiable causes.* Indeed, available technological diagnostic methods have not proved more sensitive and specific than astute clinical evaluation in comparisons of patients with dementia of the Alzheimer's type and healthy control subjects. PET holds promise but currently is too expensive for routine clinical diagnostic use.

12.18 The answer is E (all)

Creutzfeldt-Jakob disease is an infection that causes a rapidly progressive cortical-pattern dementia. The infectious agent, a *prion,* is a subviral replicative protein that is now known to cause a variety of so-called spongiform diseases in animals and humans. The 1998 Nobel Prize for Medicine was awarded to Stanley Prusiner for his work describing this novel biological entity. The age at onset of Creutzfeldt-Jakob disease is usually in the sixth or seventh decade, although onset can occur at any age. The incidence is 1 in 1,000,000. The clinical symptoms vary with progression of the illness and depend on the regions of the brain that become involved. Patients may present initially with nonspecific symptoms, including lethargy, depression, and fatigue. Within weeks, however, more fulminant symptoms develop, including progressive cortical-pattern dementia, myoclonus, and pyramidal and extrapyramidal signs. Although blood, CSF, and imaging studies are unremarkable, the *EEG can demonstrate a characteristic pattern of diffuse, symmetric, rhythmic slow waves. A presentation with rapid deterioration, myoclonus, and the characteristic EEG pattern* should raise suspicion of Creutzfeldt-Jakob disease. The *definitive diagnosis is made by postmortem microscopic examination,* which demonstrates spongiform neural degeneration and gliosis throughout the cortical and subcortical gray matter; white matter tracts are usually spared. Prion disease can incubate for decades before the emergence of clinical symptoms and subsequent rapid progression. Reported routes of transmission include invasive body contacts, such as direct tissue transplantation (e.g., corneal transplants) or hormonal extracts (e.g., human growth hormone, before synthetic supplies were developed). Familial patterns have also been reported, which suggests that there may be genetic susceptibility to infection or vertical transmission of the disease agent. No antiviral agents have been shown to be effective in retarding or slowing disease progress, although amantadine (Symmetrel) has been reported occasionally to have had some success. Death usually ensues within 6 months to 2 years of onset. During the past several years, a pathologically similar condition, bovine spongiform encephalopathy, has been described. Diagnosed primarily in the United Kingdom, this disease underscores the effects of modern animal husbandry methods on the amplification of rare diseases and the continuing threat of xenobiotic transmission of these to humans.

12.19 The answer is C

For some forms of amnestic disorder, events from the *remote past may be better remembered than more recent events.* However, such a gradient of recall is not present uniformly among individuals with amnestic disorders. *Typically, the ability to immediately repeat a sequential string of information (e.g., a digit span) is not impaired* in amnestic disorder; when such impairment is evident, it suggests the presence of attentional dysfunction that may be indicative of delirium. Amnestic disorders *may be transient, lasting for several hours to a few days, as in transient global amnesia, or persistent, lasting at least 1 month.* In the context of a newly developed but unresolved memory impairment, the term *provisional* should be added to a diagnosis of transient amnesia.

Transient global amnesia is a form of transient amnestic disorder associated with episodes that are characterized by a dense, transitory inability to learn new information (i.e., to form sustained memories), with a variable (ultimately shrinking on recovery) inability to recall events that occurred during the duration of the disturbance. The episode is followed by restoration to a completely intact cognitive state. There are no data to suggest that the memory impairment is associated with disturbed or abnormal behavior beyond the mild confusion or perplexity that may be manifest during the episode.

Depending on the cause of the disorder, the *onset of amnesia may be sudden or gradual.* Head trauma, vascular events, or specific types of neurotoxic exposure (e.g., carbon monoxide poisoning) may lead to acute mental status changes. Prolonged substance abuse, chronic neurotoxic exposure, or sustained nutritional deficiency exemplifies conditions that may lead to an insidious memory decline, eventually causing a clinically definable cognitive impairment.

Amnestic disorder may develop as a result of alcohol dependence associated with dietary and vitamin deficiency. Alternatively, it may be the primary clinical deficit arising from traumatic head injury and may present as the major feature of a postconcussional state. When memory dysfunction exceeds other features of a postconcussional syndrome, it is preferable to diagnose the condition as amnestic disorder due to head trauma.

12.20 The answer is A

Frontotemporal dementia is a term that encompasses several variant forms of dementia, and includes Pick's disease, *primary progressive aphasia*, semantic dementia, and corticobasal degeneration. The DSM-IV-TR lists dementia due to Pick's disease within the category of dementia due to other general medical conditions; *there are no separate diagnostic criteria for Pick's disease or other frontotemporal dementias. Frontotemporal dementia is more likely to affect younger populations*, and the age of onset ranges between 35 and 75 years of age. The etiology remains unclear, but, in some cases, *genetic linkage to chromosome 17, not 9, has been found.* Frontotemporal dementia is typically characterized by asymmetrical focal atrophy of the frontotemporal regions. There is underlying neuronal loss, gliosis, and subsequent spongiform change in the affected cortices. Pick's cells are pathognomonic in Pick's disease, and they appear swollen and stain pink on H and E stain.

12.21 The answer is C

The essential feature of amnestic disorders is the acquired impaired ability to learn and recall new information, coupled variably with the inability to recall previously learned knowledge or past events. The impairment must be sufficiently severe to compromise personal, social, or occupational functioning. The diagnosis is not made if the memory impairment exists in the context of reduced ability to maintain and shift attention, as encountered in *delirium*, or in association with significant functional problems due to the compromise of multiple intellectual abilities, as seen in *dementia. Amnestic disorders are secondary syndromes caused by systemic medical or primary cerebral diseases, substance-use disorders, or medication adverse effects*, as evidenced by findings from clinical history, physical examination, or laboratory examination.

The number of individuals given amnestic diagnoses due to nutritional deficiency, often related to *chronic alcohol dependence*, has declined. In contrast, traumatic causes have increased dramatically during recent decades.

12.22 The answer is E (all)

Cerebrovascular diseases together comprise the second most common cause of dementia. This category of dementia was referred to in the past as arteriosclerotic dementia, reflecting the belief that vascular insufficiency was responsible for the cognitive degeneration. That has now been supplanted by the belief that *tissue damage or infarction underlies the vascular dementias.* Cerebral infarction can be the result of a number of processes, of which *thromboembolism from a large vessel plaque* or cardiothrombus is the most common. Anoxia due to cardiac arrest, hypotension, anemia, or sleep apnea can also produce ischemia and infarction. *Cerebral hemorrhage related to hypertension or an arteriovenous malformation accounts for approximately 15 percent of cerebrovascular disease.*

12.23 The answer is E (all)

In recent years several authors have sought to distinguish dementias of the frontal lobe from other disorders. The uncertain status of dementias of the frontal lobe as distinct clinical and neuropathological entities has not yet warranted their formal inclusion in DSM-IV-TR or ICD-10. They are described as cortical dementias that are found in as many as 10 to 20 percent of cases in some neuropathological series. Age at onset is apparently between 50 and 60 years for the majority, but the reported range is broad—20 to 80 years. The early clinical features of frontal lobe dementias are typified by damage to the frontal lobes and include prominent changes in personality and behavior. *The personality changes include disinhibition, social misconduct, and lack of insight; these changes progress to apathy, mutism, and repetitive behaviors.*

Neuropsychological testing in patients suspected of having dementia of frontal lobe origin may demonstrate disproportionate impairment in tasks related to frontal lobe function, such as deficiency in abstract thinking, attentional shifting, or set formation. Structural neuroimaging, such as computed tomography (CT) or MRI, may reveal prominent atrophy of the frontal lobe, especially early in the disease process. Functional neuroimaging may prove more reliable for distinguishing dementia of frontal lobe origin from dementia of the Alzheimer's type. Regional cerebral blood flow studies using radioactively labeled xenon and SPECT studies have demonstrated disproportionate decreases in blood flow, radio tracer uptake, and glucose metabolism in the frontal lobes in patients with suspected or autopsy-confirmed frontal lobe dementia.

At present, the definitive diagnosis of any degenerative dementia rests on postmortem neuropathological examination. Only one type of frontal lobe dementia, Pick's disease, is associated with distinctive histopathological abnormalities that allow for certain diagnosis. Swollen neurons known as Pick bodies define the disorder neuropathologically. Demyelination and gliosis of the frontal lobe white matter may also be found. Other frontal lobe dementias have been referred to as dementia of the frontal lobe type or frontal lobe degeneration of non-Alzheimer's type. They have been distinguished from Alzheimer's disease by their marked gross morphological involvement of frontal and anterior temporal lobes, with relative sparing of the postcentral and temporoparietal areas mostly affected in Alzheimer's disease, and by the absence of amyloid plaques and neurofibrillary tangles microscopically. The lack of positive neuropathological inclusion criteria leaves many of these clinical conditions as disease entities of uncertain status, defined histopathologically by the absence of specific features. Whenever the hallmark findings of Alzheimer's disease are present, that diagnosis has been applied, irrespective of prior clinical findings. Thus, there are no data available to determine how many clinically diagnosed cases of frontal lobe dementia have been recast as Alzheimer's disease after death.

Of the potentially multiple forms of dementia associated with progressive frontal lobe dysfunction, only one type can be distinguished from Alzheimer's disease neuropathologically; the others show no defining postmortem signs. They may also be difficult to distinguish clinically in life. In the early stages of disease, the predominance of behavioral and personality disturbance, the presence of primitive reflexes, and neuropsychological and neuroimaging evidence of disproportionate frontal lobe involvement can help with a more confident premortem diagnosis of frontal lobe dementia. Some authors have assumed that there are many variants of dementia of frontal lobe origin that cannot be distinguished from each other clinically; at present, only Pick's disease has definitive neuropathological features.

12.24 The answer is C

Described by James Parkinson in 1817, Parkinson's disease is *a prototype of a subcortical, not cortical, degenerative disease.* It is idiopathic *and must be distinguished from parkinsonian syndromes that arise from a variety of causes.*

Parkinson's disease is the result of the degeneration of subcortical structures, *primarily the substantia nigra but also the globus pallidus, putamen, and caudate. Cells containing dopamine* are *predominantly affected, although serotonergic and other systems are disrupted as well.* Just as the appellation "cortical pattern" is pseudoanatomical, so in subcortical Parkinson's disease there can be significant degeneration of cortical structures. The parkinsonian syndrome manifests with structural damage that reflects the underlying process or insult. Medication-induced parkinsonism presumably involves only a dysfunction of the basal ganglia structures, without any obvious pathoanatomical abnormality. The typical age at the onset of Parkinson's disease is between 50 and 60 years but may vary widely with the onset sometimes occurring 1 to 2 decades earlier. The clinical course is chronic and progressive with severe disability attained after approximately 10 years. A smaller proportion of patients have a more rapidly progressive disease, and a yet smaller group has a slowly progressive disorder in which deterioration plateaus or remains minimal for two to three decades.

In general, subcortical diseases are thought to impinge on the three Ms—movement, mentation, and mood. In Parkinson's disease, all three of these areas are affected, although not always uniformly. The movement abnormalities are characterized by the triad of tremor, rigidity, and bradykinesia. The tremor and rigidity can be unilateral or bilateral. Bradykinesia is manifested by slowness in the initiation and execution of movement. The typical presentation, with a mask-like facies, minimal blink, and monotonic speech, is a concomitant of the rigidity and slowness of movement. Other prominent characteristics include postural changes such as chin-to-chest flexion and gait abnormalities. The gait is characteristically slow and shuffling, and the patient has difficulty turning (en bloc turning) and trouble initiating and stopping walking. Seborrhea, sialorrhea, excessive fatigue, and constipation are also common.

Mentation or cognition in Parkinson's disease is an area of controversy. Most patients complain of slowed thinking, sometimes called bradyphrenia. In general, approximately 20 to 30 percent of patients with Parkinson's disease are found to have *dementia with the likelihood greater in those with late-onset disease (after 70 years).* Approximately 40 percent of nondemented patients with Parkinson's disease, however, demonstrate some neuropsychological impairment in most studies. The impairments are primarily in visuospatial capacities, as measured by copying, tracing, and tracking tasks, and in the shifting of cognitive sets, as measured by the Wisconsin Card Sorting Test or the Stroop Test. Such deficits have been noted in the absence of cognitive-based functional decline or other evidence of cognitive impairment. Controversy has emerged over whether these two patterns represent a single continuum of dementia integral to the process of Parkinson's disease or are two separate processes indicative of two distinct diseases. Neuropathologically, cases intermediate between Parkinson's disease and Alzheimer's disease exist, with the characteristic microscopic features of the latter and Lewy bodies in the substantia nigra suggesting the former. There is no clear line of division as yet between a process resembling dementia of the Alzheimer's type on which abnormal parkinsonian movements are superimposed and a clinical presentation of Parkinson's disease in which the patient slowly develops a global progressive dementia.

12.25 The answer is E (all)

There have been relatively few studies of the incidence and prevalence of delirium. Little is known about the epidemiology of delirium in community or other nonpatient, noninstitutionalized populations. An estimated 10 to 15 percent of general medical inpatients are delirious at any given time, and studies indicate that as many as 30 to 50 percent of acutely ill geriatric patients become delirious at some point during their hospital stay. Rates of delirium in psychiatric and nursing home populations are not well established but are clearly substantial. Risk factors for the development of delirium include *increased severity of physical illness, older age, baseline cognitive impairment (e.g., due to dementia),* and *use of anticholinergics.*

Delirium is frequently unrecognized by treating physicians. Because of its wide array of associated symptoms, it may be detected but misdiagnosed as depression, schizophrenia, or another psychiatric disorder. Delirium is a frequent cause for psychiatric consultation in the general hospital but often is not recognized as such by the referring physician.

12.26 The answer is E

BSE is also known as subacute spongiform encephalopathy because of shared neuropathological changes that consist of (1) *spongiform vacuolization,* (2) *neuronal loss,* and (3) *astrocyte proliferation in the cerebral cortex. Amyloid plaques* may or may not be present. A characteristic *bull's eye rash* is found at the site of a tick bite and is not associated with BSE.

12.27 The answer is E (none)

The clinical characteristics of a vascular dementia depend on the area of infarction. As such, there is a wide variability in the possible presenting features of a vascular dementia. *Single infarctions may result in the discrete loss of one particular function* (e.g., language) without dementia per se. *However, some strategically located infarctions can affect more than one domain of cognitive function* and mimic the clinical picture of a global dementia. An example is the angular gyrus syndrome that can occur with large posterior lesions in the dominant hemisphere. It has been characterized as manifesting with alexia with agraphia, aphasia, constructional disturbances, and Gerstmann syndrome (acalculia, agraphia, right-left disorientation, and finger agnosia). Although the findings are similar to those of dementia of the Alzheimer's type, angular gyrus syndrome can be distinguished by its abrupt onset; the presence of focal neurological, EEG, and imaging abnormalities; and preservation of memory and ideomotor praxis.

Vascular dementia is more commonly associated with multiple infarctions. The infarctions may take the form of numerous large infarctions accompanied by widespread cognitive and motor deficits. Tiny, deep infarctions, *lacunae,* result from disease of the small arteries that usually involves subcortical structures, such as the basal ganglia, thalamus, and internal capsule. The neurological and cognitive *deficits may resolve quickly after each of the small strokes; however, the deficits may accumulate*, leading to a persisting functional and intellectual decline. In the past a stepwise pattern of deterioration was described for that type of vascular dementia, but it was dropped from the DSM-IV-TR criteria, as no specific pattern of deterioration has been reliably demonstrated for vascular dementias. Similarly, the description of patchy deficits has been deleted, in light of the *marked variability in presentation of vascular dementia, depending on the type of vasculature and the site and extent of infarction.*

12.28 The answer is E (all)

Since the late 1980s research has revealed that, beyond dementia of the Alzheimer's type and vascular dementia, a common cause of progressive dementia may be related to the presence of Lewy bodies in the brainstem and cerebral cortex. Lewy bodies—intracytoplasmic, spherical, eosinophilic neuronal inclusion bodies—are scattered through the brainstem, subcortical nuclei, limbic cortex (cingulate, entorhinal, amygdala), and neocortex (temporal, frontal, parietal). Parkinson's disease, in contrast, manifests Lewy bodies in subcortical nuclei, in addition to degeneration of dopamine cell bodies in substantia nigra. Table 12.3 lists the pathological features of dementia with Lewy bodies; Table 12.4 includes recently developed consensus guidelines for clinical diagnosis. Neuropsychiatric features, including *visual hallucinations*, delusions, fluctuating attention, and executive or managerial *cognitive deficits*, are prominent; although not specific, mood disturbances are common.

12.29 The answer is D

Binswanger's disease, or subcortical arteriosclerotic encephalopathy, is characterized by the presence of many small infarction of the white matter that spare the cortical regions. MRI has revealed that this condition is more common than previously thought. Vascular dementia is *most common in men*, especially those with *preexisting hypertension* or other cardiovascular risk factors. *Fundoscopic changes are common. It affects primarily small and medium sized vessels*, which undergo infarction and produce multiple parenchymal lesions spread over wide areas of the brain.

12.30 The answer is D

Transient global amnesia is a syndrome characterized by the sudden onset of a profound anterograde amnesia and a graded retrograde amnesia for the past weeks or months. There is an association with migraine in about 15 percent of cases, leading to etiologic speculation of *vascular instability. It occurs in men more than women, and typically after age 50. The patient is generally able to recall his or her own identity* and that of relatives or close associates, but is not able to retain his or her immediate context even when explained to the patient repeatedly. There is no disturbance of consciousness and no detectable seizure activity on electroencephalogram obtained during the event.

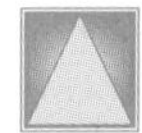

Table 12.3
Pathological Features Associated with Dementia with Lewy Bodies

Essential for diagnosis
- Lewy bodies

Associated but not essential
- Lewy-related neurites
- Plaques (all morphological types)
- Neurofibrillary tangles
- Regional neuronal loss—especially brainstem (substantia nigra and locus ceruleus) and nucleus basalis of Meynert
- Microvacuolation (spongiform change) and synapse loss
- Neurochemical abnormalities and neurotransmitter deficits

Reprinted with permission from McKeith IG, Galasko D, Kosaka K, et al. For the Consortium on Dementia with Lewy Bodies. *Neurology.* 1996;47:1113.

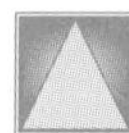

Table 12.4
Consensus Criteria for the Clinical Diagnosis of Probable and Possible Dementia with Lewy Bodies

1. The central feature required for a diagnosis of dementia with Lewy bodies is progressive cognitive decline of sufficient magnitude to interfere with normal social or occupational function. Prominent or persistent memory impairment may not necessarily occur in the early stages but is usually evident with progression. Deficits on tests of attention and of frontal-subcortical skills and visuospatial ability may be especially prominent.
2. Two of the following core features are essential for a diagnosis of probable dementia with Lewy bodies, and one is essential for possible dementia with Lewy bodies:
   a. Fluctuating cognition with profound variations in attention and alertness
   b. Recurrent visual hallucinations that are typically well formed and detailed
   c. Spontaneous motor features of parkinsonism
3. Features supportive of the diagnosis are:
   a. Repeated falls
   b. Syncope
   c. Transient loss of consciousness
   d. Neuroleptic sensitivity
   e. Systematized delusions
   f. Hallucinations in other modalities
4. A diagnosis of dementia with Lewy bodies is less likely in the presence of
   a. Stroke disease, evident as focal neurologic signs or on brain imaging
   b. Evidence on physical examination and investigation of any physical illness or other brain disorder sufficient to account for the clinical picture

Reprinted with permission from McKeith IG, Galasko D, Kosaka K, et al. For the Consortium on Dementia with Lewy Bodies. *Neurology.* 1996;47:1113.

12.31 The answer is C

In Huntington's disease, CT and MRI scans show caudate atrophy and characteristic, *"boxcar" ventricles*. Functional imaging, such as PET, *may show striatal hypometabolism*. It is transmitted by a single autosomal dominant gene found on *the short arm of chromosome 4*. It is usually diagnosed in the late 30s or early 40s, *and affects men and women equally*. Emotional symptoms often appear early and include irritability, depression or psychosis.

Answers 12.32–12.36

12.32 The answer is D

12.33 The answer is A

12.34 The answer is C

12.35 The answer is B

12.36 The answer is E

Huntington's disease, inherited in an autosomal dominant pattern, leads to major atrophy of the brain with extensive degeneration of the caudate nucleus. The onset is usually insidious and most commonly begins in late middle life. The course is one of gradual progression; *death occurs 15 to 20 years after the onset* of the disease, and *suicide* is common.

Creutzfeldt-Jakob disease is a rare degenerative brain disease caused by a *slow virus*, with death occurring within 2 years of the diagnosis. A CT scan shows cerebellar and cortical atrophy.

Neurosyphilis (also known as general paresis) is a chronic dementia and psychosis caused by the tertiary form of syphilis that affects the brain. The presenting symptoms include a *manic syndrome* with neurological signs in up to 20 percent of cases.

Normal pressure hydrocephalus is associated with enlarged ventricles and normal cerebrospinal fluid (CSF) pressure. The characteristic signs include dementia, a gait disturbance, and urinary incontinence. *The treatment of choice is a shunt* of the CSF from the ventricular space to either the atrium or the peritoneal space. Reversal of the dementia and associated signs is sometimes dramatic after treatment.

Multiple sclerosis is characterized by diffuse multifocal lesions in the white matter of the central nervous system (CNS). Its clinical course is characterized by exacerbations and remissions. It has no known specific cause, although research has focused on slow viral infections and autoimmune disturbances. Multiple sclerosis is much *more prevalent in cold and temperate climates* than in the tropics and subtropics, is *more* common in women than in men, and is predominantly a disease of young adults.

Answers 12.37–12.40

12.37 The answer is D

12.38 The answer is A

12.39 The answer is C

12.40 The answer is B

In acute *mercury poisoning*, the central nervous system symptoms of lethargy and restlessness may occur, but the primary symptoms are secondary to severe gastrointestinal irritation, with bloody stools, diarrhea, and vomiting leading to circulatory collapse because of dehydration. *Mad Hatter syndrome*, named for the *Mad Hatter* in *Alice's Adventures in Wonderland*, is a parody of the madness resulting from the inhalation of mercury nitrate vapors; mercury nitrate was used in the past in the processing of felt hats.

Early intoxication with manganese produces *manganese madness*, with symptoms of headache, irritability, joint pains, and somnolence. Lesions involving the basal ganglia and pyramidal system result in gait impairment, rigidity, monotonous or whispering speech, tremors of the extremities and tongue, *masked facies (manganese mask)*, micrographia, dystonia, dysarthria, and loss of equilibrium.

Thallium intoxication initially causes severe pains in the legs, as well as diarrhea and vomiting. Within a week, delirium, convulsions, cranial nerve palsies, blindness, choreiform movements, and coma may occur. Behavioral changes include paranoid thinking and depression, with suicidal tendencies. *Alopecia* is a common and important diagnostic clue.

Chronic *lead poisoning* occurs when the amount of lead ingested exceeds the ability to eliminate it. Toxic symptoms appear after several months. Treatment should be instituted as rapidly as possible, even without laboratory confirmation, because of the high mortality. The treatment of choice to facilitate lead excretion is the oral administration of *succimer (Chemet).*

Answers 12.41–12.47

12.41 The answer is B

12.42 The answer is A

12.43 The answer is A

12.44 The answer is A

12.45 The answer is B

12.46 The answer is B

12.47 The answer is A

Degenerative CNS diseases can be distinguished clinically from one another by the relative impairment and sparing of various cognitive and behavioral functions. *Two basic clinical patterns of dementia have been characterized clinically: cortical and subcortical.*

The *cortical pattern* of dementia is characterized by impairments in memory (primarily a storage and recall deficit) and gnostic-practice abilities (primarily involving language, visuospatial abilities, calculation, and motor praxis). Executive or managerial functions such as organization, judgment, abstraction, emotional control or modulation, and insight and social judgment are similarly affected. *Fine and gross motor movements are generally preserved until later in the disease course.* Personality often remains intact or displays subtle variations, with patients becoming more passive or less spontaneous, or becoming coarse and crude in their interactions. With disease progression the changes in personality become more common and pronounced. Affective expression is generally preserved, although again a coarsening may be noted in the form of emotional lability. Early in the disease, patients frequently discern and express dismay about their intellectual decline.

The subcortical pattern is characterized by a generalized slowing of mental processing. *Specific cognitive skills, such as calculation, naming, or copying are less affected initially, in contrast to their early decline in the cortical degenerative processes.* Verbal and visual memory impairment may be present early in the course, although such impairment more often takes the form of forgetfulness or a failure of retrieval that is initially amenable to prompting, in contrast to the more severe recall deficits of cortical dementia. Patients also show deficits in learning new motor movements or complex psychomotor procedures. Planning and organizational skills are disrupted. Abnormal movements are common and manifest as a slowing and awkwardness in normal movement or as the intrusion of such extraneous movements as chorea or tremor. *In contrast to the early impairment of language function in cortical disease, language is relatively spared,* although the motor production of speech may be abnormal. The personality change is often marked, with striking patterns of apathy, inertia, and diminished spontaneity. Mood disorders, including major depression and mania, occur frequently. The presenting symptoms in subcortical degenerative processes may be those of a *personality change or a mood disorder* at a time when cognitive impairment or motor dysfunction is not yet obvious. *In the cortical processes, by contrast, the presenting symptoms more often reflect cognitive impairment,* particularly memory and language dysfunction. As the dementia and the degenerative process progress, the clinical presentations of cortical and subcortical diseases become nearly indistinguishable from one another.

The term *subcortical dementia* was first used to describe the cognitive and behavioral deficits seen in patients with *Huntington's disease.* A similar clinical pattern was soon described for other subcortical diseases, such as progressive supranuclear palsy and Parkinson's disease. Although the term was initially used in reference to a clinical picture that could be localized to the subcortex, *subcortical dementia* is now considered a pseudoanatomical designation. It is clear from imaging and neuropathological studies that cortical dementia (e.g., *dementia of the Alzheimer's* type) is not restricted pathologically to the cortex; major affected cholinergic fiber pathways are subcortical in origin. Subcortical diseases similarly affect regions outside the subcortex, especially the frontal lobes, because of the brain's robust frontal-subcortical connections. Moreover, failure of subcortical nuclei that directly receive cortical efferent pathways can lead to clinical symptoms whose cerebral level of origin cannot be differentiated. Nonetheless, the cortical-subcortical distinction has been of clinical utility in defining patterns of cognitive, behavioral, mood, personality, and motor impairment, especially in the early stages of the degenerative disease process.

Answers 12.48–12.53

12.48 The answer is C

12.49 The answer is C

12.50 The answer is B

12.51 The answer is A

12.52 The answer is C

12.53 The answer is D

The differentiation between delirium and dementia can be difficult. Several clinical features help in the differentiation. In contrast to the sudden onset of delirium, dementia usually has an insidious onset. Although both conditions include cognitive impairment, the changes in dementia are relatively stable over time and do not fluctuate over the course of a day, for example. A patient with dementia is usually alert; a patient with delirium has episodes of clouding of consciousness. Both delirium and dementia are reversible, although delirium has a better chance of reversing if treatment is timely. *Insight,* defined as the awareness that one is mentally ill, is absent in both conditions. *Hallucinations* can occur in both conditions and must be differentiated from those that occur in schizophrenia. In general, the hallucinations of schizophrenic patients are more constant and better formed than are the hallucinations of delirious patients. *Sundowning* is observed in both demented and delirious patients. Sundowning is characterized by drowsiness, confusion, ataxia, and accidental falls just about bedtime. Kurt Goldstein described a *catastrophic reaction* in demented patients; it is marked by agitation secondary to the subjective awareness of one's intellectual deficits under stressful circumstances. The presence of delirium is a bad prognostic sign. Patients with delirium have a *high mortality rate.* The 3-month mortality rate of patients who have an episode of delirium is estimated to be 23 to 33 percent; the 1-year mortality rate may be as high as 50 percent. The major neurotransmitter hypothesized to be involved in delirium and dementia is acetylcholine. Several types of studies of delirium and dementia have shown a correlation between *decreased acetylcholine activity* in the brain and both delirium and dementia.

13 Neuropsychiatric Aspects of Human Immunodeficiency Virus (HIV) Infection and Acquired Immune Deficiency Syndrome (AIDS)

AIDS and HIV-related disorders have profoundly altered health care throughout the world. The World Health Organization estimates that worldwide, 2.5 million adults and 1 million children have AIDS, and about 30 million people are infected with HIV.

At least 50 percent of people with AIDS have neuropsychiatric complications, such as HIV encephalopathy. There is an extensive array of disease processes that can affect the brain of a patient with HIV, and there are multiple psychiatric syndromes, from adjustment disorders to mood disorders to substance abuse disorders and suicide with which the psychiatrist must be familiar. Similarly, the pharmacotherapies used in the management and treatment of HIV disease and AIDS may directly affect the brain or interact with the medications used by the psychiatrist to treat the associated psychiatric syndromes.

Psychiatrists must be familiar with counseling patients about their risk factors for the disease, and the importance of HIV testing. Confidentiality issues are key in this matter. Psychotherapy plays an important role in working with this patient population, and the psychiatrist must be familiar with the range of approaches that may be appropriate for these patients: supportive, cognitive, behavioral, or psychodynamic, both as individual treatments or in groups.

The student should study the questions and answers below for a useful review of this topic.

HELPFUL HINTS

The following terms should be known by the student.

- AIDS dementia complex
- AIDS in children
- astrocytes
- AZT
- Candida albicans
- CNS infections
- confidentiality
- ddI
- ELISA
- false-positives
- high-risk groups
- HIV encephalopathy
- HIV-1 and HIV-2
- institutional care
- Kaposi's sarcoma
- neuropsychiatric syndromes
- Pneumocystis carinii pneumonia
- pretest and posttest counseling
- protease inhibitors
- psychopharmacology
- psychotherapy
- retrovirus
- safe sex guidelines
- seropositive
- T4 lymphocytes
- Toxoplasma gondii and Cryptococcus neoformans
- transmission
- tuberculosis
- wasting syndrome
- Western blot analysis
- worried well

QUESTIONS

Directions

Each of the questions or incomplete statements below is followed by five suggested responses or completions. Select the *one* that is *best* in each case.

13.1 All of the following tasks should be done in pretest HIV counseling *except*?

A. Explore past reactions to severe stress
B. Discuss why the test is necessary
C. Explore high risk behaviors
D. Avoid discussion of a positive result
E. Document discussions in the chart

13.2 Which of the following about the pharmacotherapy of HIV disease is *true*?

A. Two protease inhibitors and one reverse transcriptase is indicated.
B. Protease inhibitors are metabolized primarily in the kidney.
C. Zidovudine penetrates the blood-brain barrier well.
D. A two-agent therapy is indicated in health care workers who have been pricked by a needle from an HIV-infected patient.
E. White matter signal abnormalities on MRI in patients who are HIV positive are permanent and not responsive to anti-HIV pharmacotherapy.

13.3 In persons infected by HIV

A. seroconversion usually occurs 2 weeks after infection
B. the estimated length of time from infection to the development of AIDS is 5 years
C. 10 percent have neuropsychiatric complications
D. the T4-lymphocyte count usually falls to abnormal levels during the asymptomatic period
E. the majority are infected by HIV type 2 (HIV-2)

13.4 True statements about the association of suicide and HIV disease include

A. Studies suggest that patients with advanced HIV disease have a 30-fold risk of committing suicide compared to matched seronegative persons.
B. Some reports indicate that high-risk seronegative persons have an elevated lifetime prevalence of suicidal ideation and attempt compared to community controls.
C. Psychiatric disorder is strongly implicated in suicidal ideation and attempted suicide.
D. HIV-infected adolescents are at a particularly high risk for suicide.
E. All of the above

13.5 True statements associated with the treatment of delirium in HIV illness include

A. There is no increased incidence of extrapyramidal symptoms associated with high-potency typical agents in advanced HIV illness.
B. Patients with underlying HIV-associated dementia do not appear to be at higher risk for medication-induced movement disorders.
C. The use of benzodiazepines alone appears to be effective in delirious states.
D. Symptoms of delirium in HIV illness can be managed effectively with low-potency antipsychotics such as chlorpromazine.
E. None of the above

13.6 Mania in people with AIDS

A. may have a rate of up to ten times the general population rates
B. may be precipitated by steroids, zidovudine, and ganciclovir
C. is associated with personal or family history of bipolar I disorder, if the onset is early in HIV illness
D. is associated with a higher prevalence of comorbid dementia if the onset is late in the course of HIV illness, and there is no personal or family history of mood disorders
E. all of the above

13.7 In a test for HIV

A. Assays usually detect the presence of viral proteins.
B. The enzyme-linked immunosorbent assay (ELISA) is used to confirm positive test results of the Western blot analysis.
C. The results cannot be shared with other members of a medical treatment team.
D. Pretest counseling should not inquire why a person desires HIV testing.
E. A person may have a true-negative result, even if the person is infected by HIV.

13.8 Neuropathic pain related to HIV

A. is generally more effectively treated with SSRIs than with tricyclic antidepressants
B. is rarely effectively treated with opioid analgesics
C. is not effectively managed with anticonvulsants such as phenytoin (Dilantin) or carbamazepine (Tegretol)
D. should not be treated with acetaminophen (Tylenol), because it may diminish the metabolism of zidovudine
E. all of the above

13.9 Diseases affecting the central nervous system (CNS) in patients with AIDS include

A. atypical aseptic meningitis
B. *Candida albicans* abscess
C. primary CNS lymphoma
D. cerebrovascular infarction
E. all of the above

13.10 Psychotic symptoms associated with HIV infection

A. are usually early-stage complications
B. are rare
C. most often take the form of persecutory, grandiose, or somatic delusions
D. rarely are associated with bizarre behavior
E. are also associated with frequent and specific neurological findings

13.11 Mild neurocognitive deficits associated with HIV infection

A. include attentional problems, slowing of information processing, and deficiencies in learning
B. do not suggest selective involvement of subcortical structures
C. are often characterized by confabulatory responses on formal memory testing
D. do not occur independently of depression or anxiety
E. are rarely associated with difficulties in abstract reasoning

13.12 Potential complications in the treatment of mania in patients with AIDS include

A. Lithium and antipsychotic medications may be poorly tolerated by individuals with HIV-related neurocognitive disorders.
B. Valproate is usually poorly tolerated by individuals with evidence of brain atrophy on MRI.
C. The gastrointestinal disturbances associated with AIDS (e.g., vomiting and diarrhea) rarely affect lithium absorption or excretion.
D. Carbamazepine may increase serum concentrations of protease inhibitors.
E. Protease inhibitors increase valproate concentrations.

13.13 Clinical symptoms associated with HIV encephalopathy diagnosis include all of the following *except*

A. early-onset aphasia
B. mood and personality changes
C. hyperreflexia and paraparesis
D. psychomotor slowing
E. problems with memory and concentration

13.14 Protease inhibitors can increase plasma levels of all of the following *except*

A. bupropion
B. fluoxetine
C. alprazolam and zolpidem
D. nefazodone
E. valproate

13.15 Which of the following is *true*?

A. All patients infected with HIV experience a brief flu-like syndrome shortly after becoming infected
B. In the United States, the median duration of the asymptomatic stages is twenty years
C. During the asymptomatic period, the T4 cell count remains stable
D. The most common infection with HIV-infected persons with AIDS is Pneumocystis carinii pneumonia
E. HIV-associated dementia has no impact on prognosis

Directions

The group of questions below consists of lettered headings followed by a list of numbered words or statements. For each numbered word or statement, select the *one* lettered heading most closely associated with it. Each lettered heading may be selected once, more than once, or not at all.

Questions 13.16–13.20

A. Nucleoside reverse transcriptase inhibitor
B. Nonnucleoside reverse transcriptase inhibitor
C. Protease inhibitor
D. All of the above
E. None of the above

13.16 Stavudine
13.17 Ritonavir
13.18 Nevirapine
13.19 AZT
13.20 3TC

ANSWERS

13.1 The answer is D

Pretest counseling *should include a discussion of the meaning of a positive test result with a clarification of any distortions.* The counselor should be sure to discuss how being seropositive can potentially affect social status, like health and life insurance, and explore the patient's potential reactions to a positive result, taking appropriate necessary steps to intervene in a potentially catastrophic reactions, like "I will kill myself if I'm positive". A discussion of *why the test is necessary* and an *exploration of high risk behaviors* are indicated, as in *exploration of past reactions* to severe stress. The discussion should also include the meaning of a negative result and the confidentiality issues relevant to the testing situation. All discussion *should be documented* in the chart.

13.2 The answer is C

High-dosage *ziduvodine monotherapy can ameliorate HIV-associated neurocognitive impairment because it penetrates the blood-brain barrier well.* Since the introduction of protease inhibitors and combination antiretroviral therapy, ziduvodine monotherapy is no longer an option of treatment, but remains an important component of combination regimes. Current recommendations are that treatment should be initiated with triple therapy, that is, a combination of two reverse transcriptase inhibitors and one protease inhibitor. *Triple therapy* may also be used for people who have had an unexpected sexual encounter with a potentially infected partner, and *in health care workers who have been pricked by a needle from an infected patient*. Protease inhibitors are metabolized in the liver, by the hepatic cytochrome P450 oxidase system and can therefore increase levels of certain psychotropic drugs that are similarly metabolized. Clinical improvement, including enhanced performance on standardized neuropsychological testing and of the pattern and severity of white matter signal abnormalities on MRI, can be seen within 2 to 3 months of beginning therapy.

13.3 The answer is D

The T4-lymphocyte count usually falls to abnormal levels during the asymptomatic period of HIV infection. The normal values are greater than 1,000/mm^3 and grossly abnormal values can be fewer than 200/mm^3.

Seroconversion is the change after infection with HIV from a negative HIV antibody test result to a positive HIV antibody test result. *Seroconversion usually occurs 6 to 12 weeks after infection.* In rare cases, seroconversion can take 6 to 12 months. The estimated length of *time from infection to the development of AIDS is 8 to 11 years*, although that time is gradually increasing because of the early implementation of treatment. *At least 50 percent* of HIV-infected patients *have neuropsychiatric complications,* which may be the first signs of the disease in about 10 percent of patients. At least two types of HIV have been identified, HIV type 1 (HIV-1) and HIV type 2 (HIV-2). *The majority* of HIV-positive patients *are infected by HIV-1*. However, HIV-2 infection seems to be increasing in Africa.

13.4 The answer is E (all)

Studies based on coroners' reports suggest that *patients with advanced HIV disease have a 30-fold risk of committing suicide* compared to seronegative persons matched for age and social position. Some survey reports indicate that seronegative persons who are in a high-risk group for HIV infection, as well as seropositive persons at all stages of HIV infection, have *an elevated lifetime prevalence of suicidal ideation and suicide attempt* compared with community controls. It is important to note that both sources of data suggest that *psychiatric disorder is strongly implicated in suicide, attempted suicide, and suicidal ideation.* Psychological autopsies from coroners' cases have identified psychiatric histories in almost 50 percent of the cases. Suicide attempt and suicidal ideation are correlated with histories of major depressive disorder or substance-related disorders, and in over half of the cases, these suicidal behaviors commenced before the likely date of seroconversion. Conflicts about sexual orientation may be associated with suicide attempts by adolescents. This, together with the increase in HIV infection in adolescents, may place *HIV-infected youths at particularly high risk.* Suicide rates in women are not noted to be elevated, but the epidemic is now just starting to affect large numbers of women, and their greater vulnerability to major depressive disorder may mean that women are at increased risk. Advances in therapy may heighten hope and reduce the risk of suicide. However, those whose hopes are first raised but who then do not respond to or cannot tolerate these agents may require psychotherapeutic intervention. Thus, while debate over the distinction between suicide and the right to choose death or to refuse unwanted treatment are important issues, it is imperative that persons expressing suicidal behaviors or ideas be examined for a major psychiatric disorder and be offered appropriate treatment.

13.5 The answer is D

Symptoms of delirium in HIV illness can be managed effectively with modest dosages of either low-potency antipsychotic agents, such as chlorpromazine at 10 to 25 mg once to three times daily, or with high-potency agents, such as haloperidol (Haldol) at 0.25 mg to 5 mg once to three times daily, or with atypical serotonin-dopamine agonists, including risperidone (Risperdal) at 0.5 mg to 2 mg daily, or olanzapine (Zyprexa) at 10 mg daily. There may well be *an increased incidence of extrapyramidal symptoms* associated with high-potency typical agents in advanced HIV illness, and *patients with underlying HIV-associated dementia appear to be at higher risk for medication-induced movement disorders.* For patients who do not respond to low-dosage oral therapy, excellent results have been reported with intravenous haloperidol given in individual boluses ranging from up to 2 to 10 mg every hour. Some clinicians have also had good results with a combination of intravenous haloperidol and lorazepam, with an average daily intravenous dose of less than 50 mg of haloperidol and 10 mg of lorazepam. In general, no serious adverse effects have been noted with those more aggressive intravenous regimens, although nearly one-half of the patients treated may have extrapyramidal symptoms and extreme care must be utilized.

Benzodiazepines alone (e.g., lorazepam) do not appear to be effective in delirious states and they may accentuate confusion.

13.6 The answer is E (all)

Mood disorders with manic features, with or without hallucinations, delusions, or a disorder of thought process can complicate any stage of HIV infection, but most commonly occur in late-stage disease complicated by neurocognitive impairment.

Precise estimates of prevalence or incidence of mania are not available but may approach 1 percent. *Some evidence suggests the rate in AIDS is up to ten times the general population rates.*

In non–HIV-infected patients, mood disorders with manic features are noted to occur at therapeutic dosages of many medications and in a wide variety of neurological conditions, such as cerebrovascular disorder, meningitis, and tumor, and these sources can also be causative in HIV illness. *Steroids, zidovudine, and ganciclovir are the most frequently reported iatrogenic causes.* There are two typical onsets of mania in HIV. *Manic states with onset early in HIV are associated with personal or family history of bipolar I disorder.* Manic syndromes in persons without previous personal or family history of mood disorder usually have their *onset late in the course of HIV illness and have a higher prevalence of comorbid dementia*; in these cases the etiology is presumed to be related to the pathophysiology of HIV infection of the CNS.

13.7 The answer is E

A person may have a true negative result, even if the person is infected by HIV, if the test takes place after infection but before seroconversion. *Assays do not usually detect the presence of viral proteins. The enzyme-linked immunosorbent assay (ELISA) is not used to confirm positive test results of the Western blot analysis.* Rather, the ELISA is used as an initial screening test because it is less expensive than the Western blot analysis and more easily used to screen a large number of samples. The ELISA is sensitive and reasonably specific; although it is unlikely to report a false-negative result, it may indicate a false-positive result. For that reason, positive results from an ELISA are confirmed by using the more expensive and cumbersome Western blot analysis, which is sensitive and specific.

Confidentiality is a key issue in serum testing. No persons should be given HIV tests without their prior knowledge and consent, although various jurisdictions and organizations (for example, the military) now require HIV testing for all their inhabitants or members. *The results can be shared with other members of a medical treatment team* but should be provided to no one else.

Any person who wants to be screened should probably be tested, although *pretest counseling should inquire why a person desires HIV testing* to detect unspoken concerns and motivations that may merit psychotherapeutic intervention. Table 13.1 lists general guidelines for HIV testing and counseling.

13.8 The answer is D

Pain probably remains the most underrecognized and undertreated symptom in HIV disease, as it is in other life-threatening illnesses, such as cancer. Undertreatment of pain is especially prevalent in injection drug users. The etiology and pathogenesis of pain in HIV-related disorders is just beginning to be understood. Psychiatric disorders may complicate persisting pain, and, because no one specialty addresses pain syndromes, patient care is often fragmented between anesthesiologists, neurologists, internists, and psychiatrists.

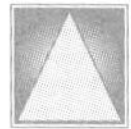

Table 13.1
Pretest HIV Counseling

1. Discuss the meaning of a positive result and clarify distortions (e.g., the test detects exposure to the AIDS virus; it is not a test for AIDS).
2. Discuss the meaning of a negative result (e.g., seroconversion requires time, recent high-risk behavior may require follow-up testing).
3. Be available to discuss the patient's fears and concerns (unrealistic fears may require appropriate psychological intervention).
4. Discuss why the test is necessary (not all patients will admit to high-risk behaviors).
5. Explore the patient's potential reactions to a positive result (e.g. "I'll kill myself if I'm positive"). Take appropriate necessary steps to intervene in a potentially catastrophic reaction.
6. Explore past reactions to severe stresses.
7. Discuss the confidentiality issues relevant to the testing situation (e.g., is it an anonymous or nonanonymous setting?). Inform the patient of other possible testing options where the counseling and testing can be done completely anonymously (e.g., where the result is not made a permanent part of a hospital chart). Discuss who has access to the test results.
8. Discuss with the patient how being seropositive can potentially affect social status (e.g., health and life insurance coverage, employment, housing).
9. Explore high-risk behaviors and recommend risk-reducing interventions.
10. Document discussions in chart.
11. Allow the patient time to ask questions.

Reprinted with permission from Rosse RB, Giese AA, Deutsch SI, Morihisa JM. *Laboratory and Diagnostic Testing in Psychiatry*. Washington, DC: American Psychiatric Press; 1989:55.

Neuropathic pain related to HIV usually presents as a persisting, painful sensorimotor neuropathy with dysesthesia, stocking-glove sensory loss, diminished distal reflexes, and distal weakness. Similarly, postherpetic neuralgia (herpes zoster radiculitis) may involve pain of the face or trunk. Treatment of neuropathic pain syndromes is usually with low-dosage tricyclic antidepressant agents, such as desipramine or nortriptyline at 10 to 25 mg a day. The typical steady-state dosage is 50 mg a day, although some patients require higher amounts (75 to 100 mg daily). A response will often ensue within 1 to 2 weeks, but 4 to 6 weeks of treatment may be necessary before response occurs or another tricyclic agent is chosen. In general, *tricyclic antidepressants are more effective than SSRIs* for chronic neuropathic pain. *Opioid analgesics* are also useful. *Anticonvulsants* such as phenytoin (Dilantin) or carbamazepine, at usual therapeutic concentrations required for seizure management, may also be effective. Postherpetic neuralgia may likewise be treated with topical capsaicin (Dolorac) and may respond to clonazepam at 1 to 5 mg daily.

Chronic headache may appear as a residual symptom from acute aseptic meningitis in seroconversion illness or as an effect of zidovudine (which may persist after drug discontinuation). It is known that imipramine, desipramine, amitriptyline, and nortriptyline can be effective in treating migraine and mixed migraine–tension headache syndromes in non-HIV populations, and there is speculation that persisting headache following aseptic meningitis may also respond to low-dosage regimens of these agents (e.g., nortriptyline or desipramine at 10 to 25 mg daily with increases up to 75 mg).

Among the rheumatological disorders are arthralgias, myalgias, and arthritides involving large joints of the leg. HIV-related arthralgias may respond to nonsteroidal antiinflammatory agents, although *acetaminophen (Tylenol) should be avoided* because it may diminish the metabolism of zidovudine. HIV may also be associated with a polymyositis, which involves pain, weakness, and elevated CPK, along with changes on electromyography indicating a myopathic process. Long-term administration of zidovudine may also produce a myositis that persists when the medication is discontinued. Psychopharmacological interventions are not of demonstrated efficacy in these states.

Multidisciplinary pain-treatment approaches, which employ coordinated efforts of experts in various disciplines, may be as useful in chronic HIV-related pain as they are in chronic, non-HIV pain syndromes. Such approaches employ education about the nature of persisting pain, activity scheduling, self-monitoring and relaxation training, and cognitive therapies to reduce disability related to pain.

Finally, studies of acute postoperative pain and chronic cancer pain generally indicate that for those conditions in which opiate analgesia is indicated, those medications are often underprescribed, or irrationally prescribed, in subtherapeutic doses at too extended an interval. The clinician should always be alert to that possibility in advanced HIV disease.

13.9 The answer is E (all)

Most of the infections secondary to HIV involvement of the central nervous system (CNS) are viral or fungal. *Atypical aseptic meningitis,* Candida albicans *abscess, primary CNS lymphoma,* and *cerebrovascular infarction* can all affect a patient with AIDS.

13.10 The answer is C

Psychotic symptoms are usually later-stage complications of HIV infection. They require immediate medical and neurological evaluation and often require management with antipsychotic medications. Whereas psychotic symptoms can obviously occur in deliria or can reflect neurological or primary psychiatric disorders or iatrogenic origins, there is also considerable interest in new-onset psychosis, wherein these etiologies do not seem to be present (e.g., psychotic disorder due to HIV disease).

Prevalence estimates vary widely depending on methodology: large-scale surveys find a prevalence of new-onset psychosis at less than 0.5 percent whereas chart review methods find frequencies ranging from 3 to 15 percent in persons for whom obvious causes (e.g., delirium) have been excluded. Thus, *psychotic symptoms may be uncommon, but not rare in* HIV-infected populations.

The clinical presentation in new-onset psychosis is extremely variable. The most prevalent symptom seems to be *delusions* (occurring in almost 90 percent of the cases in some series) with *persecutory*, *grandiose*, or *somatic* components. Persecutory themes can be quite elaborate, with patients proclaiming messianic themes or believing that they have been accorded superhuman powers by God. Somatic delusions may include being shot through with electricity or lasers. Delusions of thought insertion, thought broadcasting, and of passivity and control are also described. Most patients experience auditory hallucinations, with perhaps one-half of those also experiencing visual hallucinations. A majority of series also report disorders of thought process, including looseness of associations or frankly disorganized thinking. Disturbances of mood commonly coexist, with anxiety being the most prevalent symptom, followed by depressed mood, euphoria, or irritability, and mixed depressed and euphoric states. Lability, flatness, and inappropriate laughter or anger are also described; *bizarre behavior is commonplace.* There are reports of persons eating dirt to conquer their fear of germs, and one patient painted himself and his entire apartment, including furniture and appliances, with green paint in an effort to "celebrate life."

Bedside examination reveals impairment in memory or other cognitive functions in perhaps one-third of patients; more comprehensive and formal neuropsychological assessment would be likely to detect neurocognitive difficulties in a larger proportion of the cases, but many psychotic individuals are unable to complete such examinations.

Neurological findings are infrequent and nonspecific, usually consisting of ataxia, mild increases in motor tone, hyperreflexia, and tremor, but bizarre grimacing and posturing can also be present. Cerebrospinal fluid is generally unremarkable except for the mild pleocytosis common to HIV infection. Diffuse cortical slowing has been reported in about one-half of patients on whom an electroencephalogram (EEG) was performed. Computed tomography (CT) and magnetic resonance (MR) scans reveal nonspecific cerebral atrophy in about one-half of the cases; rarely, focal abnormalities are evident, suggesting tumor, opportunistic infection, or vascular etiology.

13.11 The answer is A

A person experiencing mild neurocognitve disorder associated with HIV infection will typically have some difficulty concentrating, may experience unusual fatigability when engaged in demanding mental tasks, may feel subjectively slowed down, and may notice *difficulty in remembering*. Such persons may say that they are not as sharp or as quick as they once were.

Such a set of presenting complaints, especially in younger individuals who may be struggling to accept their seropositive status, may lead the clinician to conclude *that anxiety, depression*, or hypochondriasis is responsible. Although affective features are occasionally the best explanation for such complaints, that is not generally the case. Rather, comprehensive neuropsychological testing may reveal that the individual does indeed have difficulties with speeded information processing, divided attention, and sustained effortful processing as well as deficiencies in learning and recalling new information.

Some individuals with mild neurocognitive disorder also have difficulties with tasks involving problem solving and *abstract reasoning*, and there may also be slowing of simple motor performance (e.g., speed of finger tapping). Verbal skills are less affected, although there may be some decrement in fluency (e.g., quickly reciting as many animals as possible or as many words beginning with a particular letter as possible).

These neuropsychological findings, which emphasize *attentional problems, slowing of information processing*, and *deficiencies in learning*, are reminiscent of neuropsychological patterns seen in patients with so-called subcortical dementias (e.g., Huntington's disease and Parkinson's disease). Fine-grained analysis of memory breakdown in HIV-infected persons also confirms a subcortical pattern. For example, persons with HIV-associated cognitive disorders have difficulty recalling words from a list, but do not make intrusion errors (i.e., *confabulatory responses*) the way patients with cortical dementias (e.g., dementia of the Alzheimer's type) tend to do. Neuropsychological features that suggest *selective involvement of subcortical structures* are consistent with neuropathological findings. It is important to stress that these mild neurocognitive deficits occur independently of depression, anxiety, and other non-HIV sources of cognitive deficit.

13.12 The answer is A

For immediate control of manic excitement up to 10 mg of clonazepam (Klonopin) daily is effective in many instances although the risk for disinhibition or delirium must always be monitored. If psychotic features are present, low doses of antipsychotic agents, such as risperidone at 0.5 to 2 mg daily, olanzapine up to 10 mg daily, chlorpromazine at 25 to 150 mg daily, or haloperidol at 0.5 to 5 mg daily, may be employed. For longer-term management lithium is effective but may not be as well tolerated as is carbamazepine and valproate (depakene). For example, *in some studies lithium and antipsychotic medications are poorly tolerated* by individuals with HIV-associated neurocognitive disorders, especially if brain MRI abnormalities are present (e.g., atrophy), whereas *valproate* (dosage range, 750 to 1,750 mg daily; plasma concentration >50 μg per mL) is more successful. Good control is usually possible within 7 days, and treatment gains have been maintained for up to 4-year follow-up. Lithium has been used to treat patients who develop manic syndromes as an adverse effect of zidovudine, with good control of symptoms, which allows a patient to continue antiretroviral therapy. It may be that valproic acid and carbamazepine would be effective in these iatrogenic manias.

In HIV-infected patients treated with lithium for the control of bipolar I disorder care must be taken to monitor lithium concentrations closely, especially if the patient has significant *gastrointestinal disturbances* (e.g., vomiting and diarrhea) that may affect lithium absorption and excretion. *Carbamazepine may reduce serum concentrations of protease inhibitors, and these agents themselves may lower valproate concentrations.*

13.13 The answer is A

HIV encephalopathy is a subacute encephalitis that results in a progressive subcortical dementia without focal neurological signs. The major differentiating feature between subcortical dementia and cortical dementia is the absence of classical cortical symptoms (for example, *aphasia*) until late in the illness. Patients with HIV encephalitis or their friends usually notice *subtle mood and personality changes, problems with memory and concentration*, and some *psychomotor slowing*. The presence of motor symptoms may also suggest a diagnosis of HIV encephalopathy. Motor symptoms associated with subcortical dementia include *hyperreflexia*, spastic or ataxic gait, *paraparesis*, and increased muscle tone.

13.14 The answer is E

A growing list of agents that act at different points of viral replication has raised for the first time the hope that HIV can be permanently suppressed or actually eradicated from the body. At the time of this writing, the active agents were in two general classes: the reverse transcriptase inhibitors and the protease inhibitors. The reverse transcriptase inhibitors are further subdivided into the nucleoside reverse transcriptase inhibitor group and the nonnucleoside reverse transcriptase inhibitors.

The antiretroviral agents have many adverse effects, too numerous to describe. Of importance to psychiatrists is that protease inhibitors are metabolized by the hepatic cytochrome P 450 oxidase system and can, therefore, increase levels of certain psychotropic drugs that are similarly metabolized. These include *bupropion* (Wellbutrin), meperidine (Demerol), various benzodiazepines, and selective serotonin reuptake inhibitors (SSRIs). Therefore, prescribing psychotropic drugs to persons taking protease inhibitors must be done with caution.

All protease inhibitors will increase psychotropic drug concentrations if the major route of metabolism of the psychotropic agent is the CYP 3A system. If the CYP 2D6 system is the primary route of metabolism (e.g., tricyclic medications, SSRIs), ritonavir (Norvir) will specifically inhibit their metabolism. Thus the protease inhibitors may inhibit the metabolism of many antidepressants and antipsychotic agents as well as benzodiazepines. For example, plasma concentrations of *alprazolam* (Xanax), midazolam (Versed), triazolam (Ilalcion), and *zolpidem* (Ambien) may be increased and dosage reduction and careful monitoring may be required to prevent oversedation or other toxic effects. Protease inhibitors have been reported to increase concentrations of bupropion, *nefazodone* (Serzone), and *fluoxetine* (Prozac) to toxic levels and to increase desipramine plasma concentrations by 100 to 150 percent. Drug interactions with antipsychotic agents are less well studied, but here ritonavir particularly may increase concentrations. Concentrations of methadone and meperidine are also reported to be elevated. Additionally, concentrations of some drugs of abuse such as methylenedioxymethamphetamine (MDMA) may be increased. In turn, protease inhibitors may induce the metabolism of valproate (*Depakene*) and of lorazepam (Ativan) and lead to *lower plasma concentrations.*

Some psychotropic medications may induce metabolism of protease inhibitors. Carbamazepine and phenobarbital may reduce serum concentrations of protease inhibitors. The clinical relevance of this potential interaction is not clear, but use of an alternate mood stabilizer may be indicated. Interactions with lithium (Eskalith) and gabapentin (Neurontin) have not been reported.

Finally, psychotropic drugs may reduce the metabolism of some protease inhibitors, with an increase of protease inhibitor adverse effects; this has been reported with *nefazodone* and fluoxetine.

13.15 The answer is D

The most common infection in HIV-infected people who have AIDS is *Pneumocystis carinii pneumonia*, which is characterized by a chronic, nonproductive cough and dynspnea, sometimes severe enough to result in hypoxemia and its resultant cognitive effects. About 30 percent of people infected with HIV *experience a flulike syndrome* 3 to 6 weeks after becoming infected, but most never notice any symptoms immediately or shortly after their infection. In the United States, the median duration of the asymptomatic stages is *10 years (not 20 years)*, although nonspecific symptoms, like lymphadenopathy, chronic diarrhea, weight loss, malaise fatigue, fever and night sweats, may invariably appear. During the asymptomatic period *the T4 cell count almost always declines* from normal values of $>1000/mm^3$ to grossly abnormal values of $<200/mm^3$. The development of *dementia is generally a poor prognostic sign*; 50 to 75 percent of patients with dementia die within 6 months.

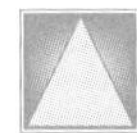

Table 13.2
Antiretroviral Agents

Generic Name	Trade Name	Usual Abbreviation
Nucleoside reverse transcriptase inhibitors		
Zidovudine	Retrovir	AZT or ZDV
Didanosine	Videx	ddI
Zalcitabine	Hivid	ddC
Stavudine	Zerit	d4T
Lamivudine	Epivir	3TC
Abacavir	Ziagen	
Nonnucleoside reverse transcriptase inhibitors		
Nevirapine	Viramune	
Delavirdine	Rescriptor	
Efavirenz	Sustiva	
Protease inhibitors		
Saquinavir	Invirase	
Ritonavir	Norvir	
Indinavir	Crixivan	
Nelfinavir	Viracept	

Answers 13.16–13.20

13.16 The answer is A

13.17 The answer is C

13.18 The answer is B

13.19 The answer is A

13.20 The answer is A

A growing list of agents that act at different points in viral replication has raised for the first time the hope that HIV might be permanently suppressed or actually eradicated from the body. At the time of this writing, the active agents were in two general classes: reverse transcriptase inhibitors and protease inhibitors. The reverse transcriptase inhibitors are further subdivided into the nucleoside reverse transcriptase inhibitor group and the nonnucleoside reverse transcriptase inhibitors. In addition to the new nucleoside reverse transcriptase inhibitors, nonnucleoside reverse transcriptase inhibitors, and protease inhibitors, other classes of drugs are under investigation. These include agents that interfere with HIV cell binding and fusion inhibitors (e.g. enfurvitide [Fuzeon]), the action of HIV integrase, and certain HIV genes such as gag, among others. Table 13.2 lists some of the available agents in these three categories.

14 Substance-Related Disorders

The phenomenon of substance abuse has many implications for brain research and for clinical psychiatry. Some substances can affect both internally perceived mental states, such as mood, and externally observable activities, such as behavior. Substances can cause neuropsychiatric symptoms indistinguishable from those of common psychiatric disorders with no known causes (e.g. schizophrenia and mood disorders), and thus primary psychiatric disorders and disorders involving the use of substances are possibly related. The study of brain-altering chemicals can provide important clues regarding how the brain functions in both normal and abnormal states.

Diagnosing a psychiatric disorder in the context of substance abuse can be complicated. A careful and detailed chronological history of symptom development and its relationship to substance use is critical to clarifying diagnoses. Although a primary diagnosis may be unclear at times, what does seem clear is that substance abuse worsens the course, prognosis, and presentation of any preexisting psychiatric disorder. The schizophrenic patient abusing crack, or the depressed patient abusing cocaine or benzodiazepines, will undoubtedly be more impaired that the patient who is not. In fact, most experienced clinicians will agree that effectively treating any psychiatric disorder in the context of ongoing substance abuse is not possible.

Clinicians need to be clear about the definitions of many terms relating to substance use, including addiction, dependence, abuse, tolerance, cross-tolerance, intoxication, and withdrawal. Each substance-related disorder also has its own definition, epidemiology, and clinical features, and skilled clinicians must be knowledgeable about each one.

The student should study the questions and answers below for a useful review of these disorders.

HELPFUL HINTS

The student should know each of the terms below

- AA
- abuse
- addiction
- AIDS
- Al-Anon
- alcohol delirium
- alcohol psychotic disorder
- alcohol withdrawal
- amotivational syndrome
- anabolic
- anabolic steroids
- anticholinergic side effects
- arylcyclohexylamine
- belladonna alkaloids
- binge drinking
- blackouts
- caffeine
- cocaine delirium
- cocaine intoxication and withdrawal
- cocaine psychotic disorder
- codependence
- comorbidity
- cross-tolerance
- DEA
- delta alcohol dependence
- dementia
- dispositional tolerance
- disulfiram
- DMT
- DOM
- DPT
- drug-seeking behavior
- DSM-IV-TR course modifiers
- DTS
- dual diagnosis
- fetal alcohol syndrome
- flashback
- freebase
- gamma alcohol dependence
- hallucinogen
- hallucinogen persisting perception disorder
- idiosyncratic alcohol intoxication
- illicit drug use
- inhalant intoxication
- ketamine
- Korsakoff's and Wernicke's syndromes
- LAMM
- LSD
- MDMA
- methadone withdrawal
- miosis
- misuse
- MPTP-induced parkinsonism
- mydriasis
- nicotine receptor
- NIDA
- nitrous oxide
- opiate
- opioid
- opioid antagonists
- opioid intoxication
- opioid withdrawal
- pathological alcohol use
- patterns of pathological use
- PCP
- persisting amnestic disorder

- persisting dementia
- physical dependence
- psychedelics
- psychoactive
- psychological dependence
- RFLP
- "roid" rage
- sedative-hypnotic-anxiolytic
- STP alcohol intoxication; blood levels
- substance abuse
- substance dependence
- sympathomimetic signs
- THC
- tolerance
- type I alcoholism
- type II alcoholism
- volatile hydrocarbons
- WHO
- WHO definitions
- Withdrawal

QUESTIONS

Directions

Each of the questions or incomplete statements below is followed by five suggested responses or completions. Select the *one* that is *best* in each case.

14.1 Which of the following is *not* a component of acute nicotine intoxication?

A. Bizarre dreams
B. Lability of mood
C. Cardiac arrhythmias
D. Tachycardia
E. Visual hallucinations

14.2 Mouth ulceration is associated with which of the following types of withdrawal?

A. Cocaine
B. Opioids
C. Nicotine
D. Alcohol
E. Benzodiazepines

14.3 Laboratory tests useful in making the diagnosis of alcohol abuse or dependence include

A. GGT
B. MCV
C. triglycerides
D. all of the above
E. none of the above

14.4 Which of the following is *not* a DSM-IV-TR course specifier for substance dependence remission?

A. Early full remission
B. Sustained partial remission
C. Remission on agonist therapy
D. Remission in a controlled environment
E. None of the above

14.5 Cocaine

A. competitively blocks dopamine reuptake by the dopamine transporter
B. does not lead to physiological dependence
C. induces psychotic disorders
D. has been used by 40 percent of the United States population since 1991
E. is no longer used as a local anesthetic

14.6 You are called for a consult on a 42-year-old woman with alcohol dependence who is complaining of persisting severe depressive symptoms despite 5 days of abstinence. In the initial stage of the interview, she noted that she had "always been depressed" and believed that she "drank to cope with the depression." Her current complaint included a prominent sadness that had persisted for several weeks, difficulties concentrating, initial and terminal insomnia, and a feeling of hopelessness and guilt.

What is the most appropriate next step to distinguish between alcohol-induced depression and an independent major depressive episode?

A. Trial of electroconvulsive therapy (ECT)
B. Chronological history
C. Proton emission tomography (PET) scan
D. Intensive psychotherapy
E. Antidepressant treatment

14.7 Which of the following atypical substances is also known to produce symptoms of intoxication?

A. Catnip
B. Betel nut
C. Kava
D. Benadryl
E. All of the above

14.8 Which of the following drugs is an opioid antagonist?

A. naloxone
B. naltrexone
C. nalorphine
D. apomorphine
E. all of the above

14.9 Which of the following statements regarding alcohol's effect on sleep is *not* true?

A. Alcohol can significantly impair sleep patterns
B. Alcohol increases rapid eye movement (REM) sleep
C. Heavy drinkers often awaken at night and have difficulty going back to sleep
D. Alcohol use tends to inhibit stage 4 sleep
E. Alcoholics tend to have more dreams earlier in the night

14.10 The single photon emission computed tomography (SPECT) image in Figure 14.1 shows multifocal areas of hypoperfusion in a patient with chronic substance abuse. The patient's ischemic cerebrovascular disorder is most likely precipitated by which of the following substances?

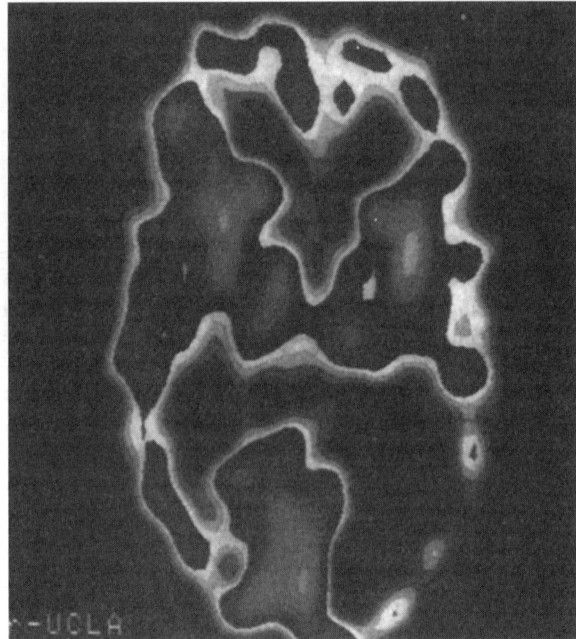

FIGURE 14.1

Reprinted with permission from Kaplan HI, Sadock BJ, eds. *Comprehensive Textbook of Psychiatry*, 6th ed. Baltimore: Williams & Wilkins; 1995:268.

A. phencyclidine (PCP)
B. cocaine
C. heroin
D. cannabis
E. barbiturates

14.11 Inhalant use most often correlates with which of the following comorbid conditions?

A. Conduct disorder
B. Major depression
C. Borderline personality disorder
D. Schizophrenia
E. Manic episode

14.12 Amphetamines and cocaine are similar in

A. their mechanisms of action at the cellular level
B. their duration of action
C. their metabolic pathways
D. the induction of paranoia and production of major cardiovascular toxicities
E. all of the above

14.13 Which of the following is *not* a therapeutic effect for which cannabinoids are commonly used?

A. Relief of nausea and vomiting
B. Appetite stimulant
C. Weight loss
D. Reduced muscle spasticity
E. Decreased intraocular pressure

14.14 Minor signs and symptoms of the benzodiazepine discontinuation syndrome commonly include

A. grand mal seizures
B. psychosis
C. nightmares
D. hyperpyrexia
E. death

14.15 Which of the following is contraindicated for the treatment of acute disulfiram (Antabuse) overdose?

A. Gastric lavage
B. Activated charcoal
C. Syrup of ipecac
D. Hemodialysis
E. Decontamination

14.16 Acute PCP intoxication is *not* treated with

A. diazepam (Valium)
B. cranberry juice
C. phentolamine (Regitine)
D. phenothiazines
E. all of the above

14.17 Which of the following is *not* a therapeutic indication for use of anabolic-androgenic steroids?

A. Male hypogonadism
B. Hyperthyroidism
C. Hereditary angioedema
D. Anemia
E. Osteoporosis

14.18 DSM-IV-TR states specifically that the diagnosis of dependence can be applied to every class of substances *except*

A. nicotine
B. caffeine
C. anabolic steroids
D. nitrous oxide
E. none of the above

14.19 Ms. E is a 32-year-old single, white woman employed full time at a local factory. She is a smoker, and occasionally has flares of her asthma. She typically drinks four to five mugs of coffee each day and prefers to drink it without cream, milk, or sugar. She estimates that 5 minutes usually elapse between the time she gets up in the morning and the time she has her first cup of coffee. She spaces her mugs over the course of the day, with her last mug either after lunch or with dinner. Physicians had recommended she cut down or stop her coffee use because of complaints of mild indigestion, and she abruptly stops her caffeine intake as a result of these recommendations.

Which of the following statements regarding caffeine is *true*?

A. The rate of caffeine elimination is increased by smoking.

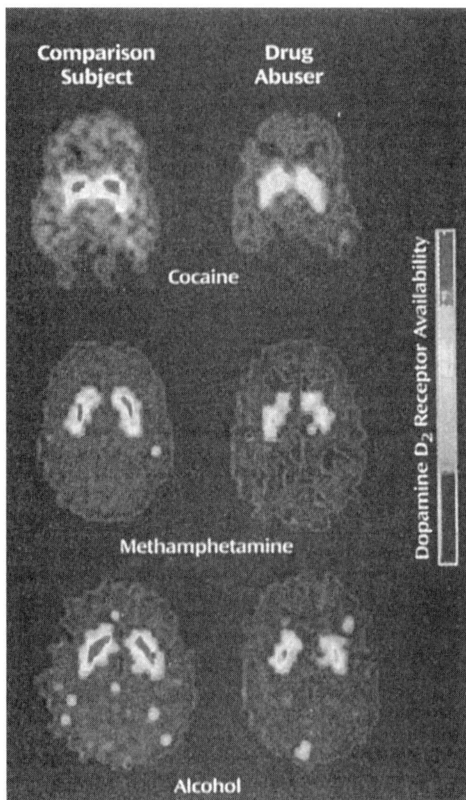

FIGURE 14.2

B. Caffeine's effects on the body include bronchoconstriction.
C. Caffeine is slowly absorbed and metabolized by the kidney.
D. Caffeine increases the metabolism of the antipsychotic clozapine.
E. Caffeine metabolism is markedly increased at the end of pregnancy.

14.20 The above patient would most likely experience all of the following due to her abruptly stopping caffeine intake *except*?

A. Irritability
B. Insomnia
C. Decreased concentration
D. Headache
E. Muscle aches

14.21 The image in Figure 14.2 shows decreased dopamine type 2 (D_2) receptor binding in the striatum in drug users compared to normal control subjects. Which of the following types of substance withdrawal is this pattern *not* typical of?

A. Cocaine
B. Methamphetamine
C. Opioids
D. Alcohol
E. All of the above

14.22 In distinguishing schizophrenia from amphetamine-induced toxic psychosis, the presence of which of the following is most helpful?

A. paranoid delusions
B. auditory hallucinations
C. clear consciousness
D. tactile or visual hallucinations
E. intact orientation

14.23 Which of the following statements regarding cancer and alcohol use is *correct*?

A. Cancer may be due to the immunosuppressive effects of ethanol
B. Cancer is the second leading cause of premature death in alcoholics
C. Increases in breast cancer have been noted with just two drinks per day
D. Alcohol can be directly linked to cancers of mucus membranes
E. All of the above

14.24 Which of the following most accurately represents the percentage of 8th graders who have experimented at least once with inhalants?

A. 1 percent
B. 5 percent
C. 15 percent
D. 30 percent
E. 50 percent

Directions

Each set of lettered headings below is followed by a list of numbered words or phrases. For each numbered word or phrase, select

A. if the item is associated with A only
B. if the item is associated with B only
C. if the item is associated with both A and B
D. if the item is associated with neither A nor B

Questions 14.25–14.29

A. Alcohol dehydrogenase
B. Aldehyde dehydrogenase

14.25 Involved in alcohol metabolism
14.26 Converts alcohol into acetaldehyde
14.27 Inhibited by disulfiram (Antabuse)
14.28 Converts acetaldehyde into acetic acid
14.29 Decreased in Asian people

Questions 14.30–14.34

A. Benzodiazepines
B. Barbiturates

14.30 Cause rapid eye movement (REM)–sleep suppression

14.31 Have symptoms of withdrawal that usually appear within 3 days
14.32 Are associated with high suicide potential when used alone
14.33 Are clinically used as muscle relaxants
14.34 Are antipsychotics

Directions

Each group of questions below consists of lettered headings followed by a list of numbered words or statements. For each numbered word or statement, select the *one* lettered heading most closely associated with it. Each lettered heading may be selected once, more than once, or not at all.

Questions 14.35–14.41

A. γ-Aminobutyric acid (GABA) receptor system
B. Opioid receptor system
C. Glutamate receptor system
D. Adenosine receptor system
E. Acetylcholine receptor system

14.35 Ethanol
14.36 Phenobarbital
14.37 Diazepam
14.38 Heroin
14.39 PCP
14.40 Caffeine
14.41 Nicotine

Questions 14.42–14.46

A. Cocaine
B. Amphetamines
C. Marijuana
D. PCP
E. LSD

14.42 Horizontal and vertical nystagmus
14.43 Injected conjunctiva
14.44 Atrophic nasal mucosa
14.45 Amotivational syndrome
14.46 Colorful hallucinations

ANSWERS

14.1 The answer is E

Nicotine is a highly toxic alkaloid. Doses of 60 mg in an adult are fatal secondary to respiratory paralysis; doses of 0.5 mg are delivered by smoking an average cigarette. Acute intoxication due to nicotine is evidenced by dysfunctional behavior or perceptual abnormalities, as well as physical signs that are often attributed to sympathetic activation. The behavioral abnormalities include insomnia, *bizarre dreams*, *labile mood*, derealization, and interference with personal functioning. Physically, nicotine intoxication can lead to nausea, vomiting, sweating, *tachycardia*, and *cardiac arrhythmias. Visual hallucinations have not been noted* to be an effect of nicotine intoxication.

14.2 The answer is C

The development of mouth ulcers and dry mouth *has been noted as a sign of chronic tobacco use* and may occur acutely during withdrawal. The DSM-IV-TR does not have a diagnostic category for nicotine intoxication, but does have a diagnostic category for nicotine withdrawal. Withdrawal symptoms can develop within 2 hours of smoking the last cigarette, generally peak in the first 24 to 48 hours, and can last for weeks or months. The common symptoms include an intense craving for nicotine, tension, irritability, difficulty concentrating, drowsiness and paradoxical trouble sleeping, decreased heart rate and blood pressure, increased appetite and weight gain, decreased motor performance, and increased muscle tension.

14.3 The answer is D (all)

Establishing the diagnosis for alcohol abuse or dependence centers on obtaining from the patient and a resource person a history of the patient's life problems and the possible role played by alcohol. Up to one third of all psychiatric patients are likely to have an alcohol problem that either caused or exacerbated the presenting clinical condition.

The process of identification can also be facilitated by a series of blood tests, outlined in Table 14.1. Those state markers of heavy drinking reflect physiological alterations likely to be observed if the patient regularly ingests four or more drinks a day over many days or weeks. One of the most sensitive and specific of the markers (perhaps 60 to 80 percent sensitivity and specificity) is a level of 30 or more units per liter of *γ-glutamyltransferase (GGT)*, an enzyme that aids in the transport of amino acids and that is found in most areas of the body. Because this enzyme is likely to return to normal levels after 2 to 4 weeks of abstinence, even 20 percent increases in enzyme levels above those observed after 4 weeks of abstinence can be useful in identifying patients who have returned to drinking after treatment. Equally impressive results have been reported for the measure of a deglycosylated form of the protein transferrin, known as carbohydrate-deficient transferrin (CDT). Using a commercially available assay, CDTect, and employing a cutoff of 20 mg/L, this test has both a sensitivity and a specificity of 65 to 80 percent for the identification of the heavy consumption of alcohol (e.g., five to eight drinks per day for a week); these figures might be slightly lower for women. With a

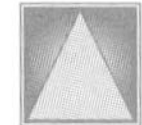

Table 14.1
State Markers of Heavy Drinking Useful in Screening for Alcoholism

Test	Relevant Range of Results
γ-Glutamyltransferase (GGT)	>30 U/L
Carbohydrate-deficient transferrin (CDT)	>20 mg/L
Mean corpuscular volume (MCV)	>91 μm^3
Uric acid	>6.4 mg/dL for men >5.0 mg/dL for women
Serum glutamic-oxaloacetic transaminase (aspartate aminotransferase) (SGOT [AST])	>45 IU/L
Serum glutamic-pyruvic transaminase (alanine aminotransferase) (SGPT [ALT])	>45 IU/L
Triglycerides	>160 mg/dL

biological half-life of about 16 days, this test can also be useful in monitoring abstinence in alcoholics. It appears that patients not identified by higher GGT values might still have elevations in CDT so that both tests should be used for identification and abstinence-monitoring functions in alcoholics.

The *MCV blood test*, with perhaps 70 percent sensitivity and specificity, is a state marker when the size of the red blood cell is 91 or more cubic micrometers. The 120-day life span of the red cell does not allow the test to be used as an indicator of a return to drinking after about 1 month of abstinence. Other tests that can be helpful in identifying patients who are regularly consuming heavy doses of alcohol include those for high-normal concentrations of uric acid (greater than 6.4 mg/dL, with a range that depends on the sex of the person); mild elevations in the usual liver function tests, including asparatate aminotransferase and alanine aminotransferase; and elevated levels of *triglycerides* or LDL cholesterol.

14.4 The answer is E (none)

The DSM-IV-TR specifiers for remission require a period of at least 1 month, after a period of active dependence, during which no criteria of dependence are present. If a patient has not met any criteria for dependence for at least 1 month but fewer than 12 months, the course specifier is *early full remission*. If the period during which no criteria of dependence are met exceeds 12 months, the specifier of *sustained full remission* can be used. If the full criteria for dependence or abuse have not been met for less than 1 year, but one or more criteria have been present, *early partial remission* may be designated. If the period exceeds 12 months, *sustained partial remission* may be used. Two additional remission specifiers should be used when appropriate: *on agonist therapy* (includes partial agonists) and *in a controlled environment*. Thus, a heroin-dependent patient or client successfully enrolled in a methadone maintenance program for 12 months is described as in remission on agonist therapy, as are those maintained successfully on buprenorphine, a partial agonist.

The DSM-IV-TR does not use the term "in recovery" to describe any part of the course of remission from substance use disorders. It is a term commonly used among patients who are currently abstinent while participating in 12-step programs. Many professionals who are interacting with such patients also use it. Individuals who were formerly dependent on drugs or alcohol and have been stably abstinent for many years may also refer to themselves as being "in recovery," typically to convey the idea that they are vulnerable to relapse.

14.5 The answer is A

Cocaine *competitively blocks dopamine reuptake by the dopamine transporter.* This primary pharmacodynamic effect is believed to be related to cocaine's behavioral effects, including elation, euphoria, heightened self-esteem, and perceived improvement on mental and physical tasks. Cocaine *does lead to physiological dependence,* although cocaine withdrawal is mild compared with the effects of withdrawal from opiates and opioids. A psychological dependence on cocaine can develop after a single use because of its potency as a positive reinforcer of behavior. *Cocaine-induced psychotic disorders are most common in intravenous (IV) users and crack users, not in those who snort cocaine.* The National Institute of Drug Abuse (NIDA) reported that cocaine *has been used by 12 percent, not 40 percent, of the United States population since 1991.* The highest use was in the 18- to 25-year-old age group; 18 percent of them had used cocaine at least once, and 2 percent were current users. In that age group, 3.8 percent had used crack at least once. Although cocaine use is highest among the unemployed, cocaine is also used by highly educated persons in high socioeconomic groups. Cocaine use among males is twice as frequent as cocaine use among females.

Despite its reputation as the most addictive commonly abused substance and one of the most dangerous, cocaine does have some important medical applications. Cocaine *is still used as a local anesthetic,* especially for eye, nose, and throat surgery, for which its vasoconstrictive effects are helpful.

14.6 The answer is B

In an effort to distinguish between an alcohol-induced mood disorder and an independent major depressive episode, *a timeline-based chronological history* should be obtained. This should focus on the age of onset of this patient's alcohol dependence, periods of abstinence that extended for several months or more since the onset of dependence, and the ages of occurrence of clear major depressive episodes lasting several weeks or more at a time.

Heavy intake of alcohol over several days results in many of the symptoms observed in major depressive disorder, but the intense sadness markedly improves within days to 1 month of abstinence. Eighty percent of alcoholic patients report histories of intense depression, including 30 to 40 percent who were depressed for 2 or more weeks at a time. However, when information from patients and resource people was carefully evaluated, only 5 percent of alcoholic men and 10 percent of alcoholic women ever had depressions that met the criteria for major depressive disorder when they had not been drinking heavily.

Clinical data reveal that when even severe depression develops in alcoholic people, they are likely to improve fairly rapidly without *medications or intensive psychotherapy* aimed at the depressive symptoms. A recent study of almost 200 alcoholic men found that, although 40 percent had severe levels of depression after 1 week of abstinence, these symptoms markedly improved in all but 5 percent after 3 additional weeks of sobriety. At the end of several weeks to 1 month, most alcoholic patients are left with mood swings or intermittent symptoms of sadness that can resemble cyclothymic disorder or dysthymic disorder. *ECT* is indicated only in depression resistant to all other treatments.

14.7 The answer is E

Many atypical substances are capable of producing mild intoxication. These include *catnip*, which can produce states similar to those observed with marijuana and which in high doses is reported to result in lysergic acid diethylamide–type perceptions; *betel nut*, which is chewed in many cultures to produce a mild euphoria; and *kava* (a substance derived from the South Pacific pepper plant), which produces sedation, incoordination, weight loss, mild forms of hepatitis, and lung abnormalities. In addition, individuals can develop dependence and impairment through repeated self-administration of over-the-counter and prescription drugs, including cortisol, antiparkinsonian agents that have anticholinergic properties, and antihistamines (*such as Benadryl*).

14.8 The answer is E (all)

Opioid antagonists block or antagonize the effects of opiates and opioids. Unlike methadone, they do not in themselves exert narcotic effects and do not cause dependence. The antagonists include the following drugs: *naloxone,* which is used in the treatment of opiate and opioid overdose because it reverses the effects of narcotics; *naltrexone,* which is the longest-acting (72 hours) antagonist; *nalorphine,* levallorphan, and *apomorphine*.

14.9 The answer is B

Alcohol intoxication can help a person fall asleep more quickly, but if the intake in an evening is more than one or two drinks, the *sleep pattern can be significantly impaired*. Most heavy drinkers awaken after several hours and can have problems falling back asleep. Alcohol also tends to *depress rapid eye movements (REMs)* and *inhibit stage 4 sleep* and, thus, is likely to be associated with frequent alternations between sleep stages (sleep fragmentation) and with *more dreams late in the night* as the blood alcohol level falls. Exaggerated forms of similar problems are seen in alcoholics in whom sleep stages might not return to normal for 3 or more months after abstinence.

14.10 The answer is B

The development of an ischemic cerebrovascular disorder is *an adverse effect of cocaine abuse.* The most common cerebrovascular diseases associated with cocaine use are nonhemorrhagic cerebral infarctions. When hemorrhagic infarctions do occur, they can include subarachnoid hemorrhages. Other adverse effects of cocaine use include seizures, myocardial infarction, and arrhythmias.

14.11 The answer is A

Multiple factors contribute to the etiology of inhalant-related disorders. In addition to multiple extrinsic factors, at least one intrinsic factor contributes to inhalant problems. A risk-taking propensity may lead some people to the at-the-brink excitement and danger of inhalant intoxication. People with *adolescent conduct disorder* or adult antisocial personality disorder are prone to taking extreme risks, and many inhalant users have those disorders. Several studies suggest an association of inhalant use and conduct problems. Among youths in grades 7 through 12, inhalant users (compared with others who used no drugs or who used only cannabis or alcohol) had many characteristics suggesting conduct disorder. They accepted cheating more readily, admitted to more stealing, perceived less objection to drug use from their families, liked school less, and reported more sadness, tension, anger, and a feeling of being blamed by others. In addition, school surveys showed that solvent users were more likely to be involved with other drugs. Similarly, among youths referred to court-mandated education for minor alcohol offenses, those who also had used inhalants reported fewer school honors and more expulsions, truancy, academic failures, criminal offenses, running away, and associations with troubled peers as well as many more drug and alcohol problems. More of them also had mothers or siblings with alcohol- or drug-related problems. Some families are burdened by antisocial personality disorder and substance dependence in the adults and by conduct disorder and substance use disorders (often including inhalant abuse or dependence) in the adolescent children, and there is growing evidence that genetics play a role in these familial disorders.

14.12 The answer is D

The reinforcing and toxic effects of amphetamines and amphetamine-like drugs play an important role in the genesis of amphetamine dependence and other amphetamine-related disorders. Amphetamines produce subjective effects very similar, if not identical, to those produced by cocaine. Both categories of drugs can produce a sense of alertness, euphoria, and well-being. Performance impaired by fatigue is usually improved. There may be decreased hunger and decreased need for sleep. Patterns of toxicity are also similar, although not identical. Both the amphetamines and cocaine *can induce paranoia*, suspiciousness, and overt psychosis that can be difficult to distinguish from paranoid-type schizophrenia; both *can produce major cardiovascular toxicities.* However, the *amphetamines and cocaine differ distinctly in their mechanisms of action at the cellular level*, their *duration of action*, and their *metabolic pathways.*

Although amphetamines inhibit reuptake of monoamines to a small degree, their major action is the release of monoamines from storage sites in axon terminals, which in turn increases monoamine concentrations in the synaptic cleft. The release of dopamine in the nucleus accumbens and related structures is thought to account for their reinforcing and mood-elevating effects; the release of norepinephrine is probably responsible for the cardiovascular effects. In contrast to cocaine, which binds to neurotransporters and inhibits reuptake of the neurotransmitters released into the synapse, amphetamine-like drugs are taken into the neurons where they are transported into the neurotransmitter storage vesicles. By changing the internal environment of the vesicles, the drugs cause the neurotransmitters to leak out into the cytoplasm and into the synaptic cleft. The dopamine released into the cytoplasm may undergo oxidation, which results in the production of several highly toxic and reactive chemicals (oxygen radicals, peroxides, and hydroxylquinones). Some of the neuronal toxicity of methamphetamine is due, therefore, not to the drug per se, but to the intracellular accumulation of dopamine.

Amphetamine and methamphetamine are extensively metabolized in the liver, but much of what is ingested is excreted unchanged in the urine. The half-lives of amphetamine and methamphetamine (weak bases) are considerably shortened when the urine is acidic. The half-life of amphetamine after therapeutic doses ranges from 7 to 19 hours and that of methamphetamine appears slightly longer. Thus, after toxic dosage, resolution of symptoms may take far longer (up to several days) with amphetamines than with cocaine, depending on the pH of the urine.

14.13 The answer is C

When cannabinoids and cannabis are advocated for medical uses, it is primarily to relieve symptoms rather than to cure underlying diseases. The conditions for which cannabis is most commonly advocated are for symptomatic *relief of nausea and vomiting* caused by cancer chemotherapy, appetite loss in AIDS, and *muscle spasticity* and chronic pain in neurological disorders. Cannabis and THC has also been documented to *reduce intraocular pressure* by 25 percent, a therapeutic effect that may be useful in the treatment of glaucoma. THC has been shown to *stimulate appetite* and assist with weight gain (*not weight loss*) in AIDS patients in short-term trials.

14.14 The answer is C

Studies in the early 1960s by Leo Hollister established that abrupt discontinuation of high doses of chlordiazepoxide or diazepam could lead to a withdrawal syndrome.

The American Psychiatric Association's *Task Force Report on Benzodiazepine Dependence, Toxicity, and Abuse* defined withdrawal as a true abstinence syndrome consisting of "new signs and symptoms and worsening of preexisting symptoms following drug discontinuance that were not part of the disorder for which the drugs were originally prescribed." Many authorities have taken issue with that definition of withdrawal and prefer to distinguish withdrawal only from recurrence, not from rebound symptoms, viewing the true abstinence syndrome as consisting of rebound symptoms plus new signs and symptoms.

The signs and symptoms of the benzodiazepine discontinuation syndrome (Table 14.2) have been classified as major or minor, like those of the alcohol withdrawal syndrome. According to that classification, minor symptoms include anxiety, insomnia, and *nightmares*. Major symptoms (which are extremely rare) include *grand mal seizures*, *psychosis*, *hyperpyrexia*, and death.

The discontinuance syndrome may also be divided into symptoms of rebound, recurrence, and withdrawal. *Rebound symptoms* are symptoms for which the benzodiazepine was originally prescribed that return in a more severe form than they had before treatment. They have a rapid onset following termination of therapy and a brief duration. *Recurrence* refers to return of the original symptoms at or below their original intensity. The pattern and course of these symptoms will reflect the anxiety disorder for which treatment was originally instituted.

The temporal sequence of symptom development is not well established, but upon the abrupt cessation of benzodiazepines with short elimination half-lives, symptoms may appear within 24 hours and peak at 48 hours. Symptoms arising from abrupt discontinuation of benzodiazepines with long half-lives may not peak until 2 weeks later. Although some investigators suggest that a subgroup of patients had withdrawal syndromes that lasted for many months, no medical or scientific evidence validates the existence of such a syndrome. Prolonged symptoms are almost certainly attributable to recurrence of the original anxiety or progression of the anxiety disorder itself.

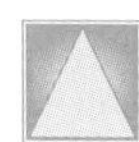

Table 14.2
Signs and Symptoms of the Benzodiazepine Discontinuation Syndrome

The following signs and symptoms may be seen when benzodiazepine therapy is discontinued; they reflect the return of the original anxiety symptoms (recurrence), worsening of the original anxiety symptoms (rebound), or emergence of new symptoms (true withdrawal)

Disturbances of mood and cognition:
- Anxiety, apprehension, dysphoria, pessimism, irritability, obsessive rumination, paranoid ideation

Disturbances of sleep:
- Insomnia, altered sleep–wake cycle, daytime drowsiness

Physical signs and symptoms:
- Tachycardia, elevated blood pressure, hyperreflexia, muscle tension, agitation—motor restlessness, tremor, myoclonus, muscle and joint pain, nausea, coryza, diaphoresis, ataxia, tinnitus, grand mal seizures

Perceptual disturbances:
- Hyperacusis, depersonalization, blurred vision, illusions, hallucinations

14.15 The answer is C

Disulfiram (Antabuse) is used to ensure abstinence in the treatment of alcohol dependence. Its main effect is to produce a rapid and violently unpleasant reaction in a person who ingests even a small amount of alcohol while taking disulfiram. Disulfiram is an aldehyde dehydrogenase inhibitor that interferes with the metabolism of alcohol and produces a marked increase in blood acetaldehyde levels, as it prevents the conversion of acetaldehyde to acetyl coenzyme A. The accumulation of acetaldehyde, which may be tenfold more than normal, leads to many unpleasant effects, including nausea, throbbing headache, vomiting, hypertension, flushing, sweating, thirst, dyspnea, chest pain, vertigo, and blurred vision.

No specific antidote is available for treatment of acute disulfiram overdose. *Using ipecac syrup is contraindicated* as this syrup contains ethanol and could precipitate a disulfiramethanol reaction. Emesis is also not recommended as this may delay the administration of *activated charcoal*, worsen nausea and vomiting, and increase the risk of pulmonary aspiration by an unprotected airway if seizures and coma suddenly supercede. The use of activated charcoal in multiple doses may be beneficial as it increases the rate of elimination of disulfiram. *Gastric lavage* may be useful in cases of massive alcohol ingestion. *Neither decontamination nor hemodialysis* are likely to be beneficial once the reaction begins, however, they are not contraindicated.

14.16 The answer is D

Phenothiazines are not used in the treatment of acute PCP intoxication because they have anticholinergic effects that may potentiate the adverse effects of PCP, such as seizures. *Diazepam (Valium)* is useful in reducing agitation. If agitation is severe, however, the antipsychotic haloperidol (Haldol) may have to be used. *Cranberry juice* is used to acidify the urine and to promote the elimination of the drug. Ammonium chloride or ascorbic acid also serves the same purpose. *Phentolamine (Regitine)* is a hypotensive agent that may be needed to deal with severe hypertensive crises produced by PCP.

14.17 The answer is B

The anabolic steroids are a family of drugs comprising the natural male hormone testosterone and a group of more than 50 synthetic analogs of testosterone, synthesized over the last 60 years. These drugs all exhibit various degrees of anabolic (muscle building) and androgenic (masculinizing) effects. Thus, they should more correctly be called anabolic-androgenic steroids (AAS). Note that it is important not to confuse the AAS (testosterone-like hormones) with corticosteroids (cortisol-like hormones such as hydrocortisone and prednisone). Corticosteroids have no muscle-building properties and, hence, little abuse potential. AAS, by contrast, have only limited legitimate medical applications. However, AAS are widely used illicitly, especially by boys and young men seeking to gain increased muscle mass and strength either for athletic purposes or simply to improve personal appearance.

AAS are primarily indicated for testosterone deficiency (*male hypogonadism*), *hereditary angioedema* (a congenital skin disorder), and some uncommon forms of *anemia* caused by bone marrow or renal failure. In women, they are given, although not as first-choice agents, for metastatic breast cancer, *osteoporosis*, endometriosis, and adjunctive treatment of menopausal symptoms. In men, they have also been used experimentally as a male contraceptive and for treating major depressive disorder and sexual disorders in eugonadal men. Recently, they have been used to treat wasting syndromes associated with acquired immune deficiency syndrome (AIDS). Controlled studies have also suggested that testosterone has antidepressant effects in some HIV-infected men with major depressive disorder, and is also a supplementary (augmentation) treatment in some depressed men with low endogenous testosterone levels who are refractory to conventional antidepressants. *AAS have not been used in the treatment of hyperthyroidism.*

14.18 The answer is B

The DSM-IV-TR section dealing with substance dependence and substance abuse presents descriptions of the clinical phenomena associated with the use of 11 designated classes of pharmacological agents: alcohol, amphetamines or similarly acting agents; *caffeine*; cannabis; cocaine; hallucinogens; inhalants; *nicotine*; opioids; PCP or similar agents; and sedatives, hypnotics, and anxiolytics. A residual twelfth category includes a variety of agents, such as *anabolic steroids* and *nitrous oxide*, that are not in the 11 designated classes.

DSM-III-R, DSM-IV-TR, and ICD-10 formulations for substance abuse and dependence closely follow the concepts and terminology developed in 1980 by an International Working Group sponsored by the World Health Organization (WHO) and the Alcohol, Drug Abuse, and Mental Health Administration (ADAMHA) of the United States, which defined substance dependence as follows:

> A syndrome manifested by a behavioral pattern in which the use of a given psychoactive drug, or class of drugs, is given a much higher priority than other behaviors that once had higher value. The term "syndrome" is taken to mean no more than a clustering of phenomena so that not all the components need always be present or not always present with the same intensity. . . . The dependence syndrome is not absolute, but is a quantitative phenomenon that exists in different degrees. The intensity of the syndrome is measured by the behaviors that are elicited in relation to using the drug and by the other behaviors that are secondary to drug use. . . . No sharp cut-off point can be identified for distinguishing drug dependence from non-dependent but recurrent drug use. At the extreme, the dependence syndrome is associated with "compulsive drug-using behavior."

That central notion is continued in DSM-IV-TR, which states

> The essential feature of dependence is a cluster of cognitive, behavioral, and physiological symptoms indicating that the individual continues substance use despite significant substance-related problems.

In addition to requiring the clustering of three criteria in a 12-month period, DSM-IV-TR includes a few other qualifications. *It states specifically that the diagnosis of dependence can be applied to every class of substances except caffeine.* That point is admittedly controversial, and some researchers believe, on the basis of the same DSM-IV-TR generic criteria, that caffeine produces a distinct form of dependence, although it is relatively benign for most persons.

14.19 The answer is A

Caffeine is a methylxanthine, as are theobromine (found in chocolate) and theophylline (typically used in the treatment of asthma). Caffeine is well absorbed from the gastrointestinal (GI) tract, with peak plasma concentrations typically occurring within 1 hour after ingestion. *Caffeine is readily distributed throughout the body and is metabolized by the liver.* Although there are several metabolic pathways for caffeine, it is primarily metabolized by the P450 1A2 system, and it is frequently used as a metabolic probe to assess this system's activity. The half-life of caffeine is approximately 5 hours, with large individual differences. *The rate of caffeine elimination is increased by smoking*, oral contraceptive steroids, cimetidine, and fluvoxamine (Luvox). *Caffeine inhibits the metabolism of the antipsychotic clozapine* (Clozaril) and the bronchodilator theophylline (Theo-Dur) to an extent that might be clinically significant. *Caffeine metabolism is markedly slowed at the end of pregnancy.*

Caffeine exerts effects throughout the body, including *bronchodilation* (hence the therapeutic application of caffeine and theophylline in the treatment of asthma); modest increases in blood pressure (which are reduced in caffeine-tolerant individuals); increased production of urine; increases in gastric acid secretion; and increases in plasma epinephrine, norepinephrine, renin, and free fatty acids. Centrally, caffeine affects turnover or levels of various neurotransmitters, and it functions as a central nervous system (CNS) stimulant.

14.20 The answer is B

In spite of the fact that DSM-IV-TR does not include a diagnosis of caffeine withdrawal, several well-controlled studies indicate that caffeine withdrawal is a real phenomenon. The appearance of withdrawal symptoms reflects the tolerance and physiological dependence that develop with continued caffeine use. Several epidemiological studies have reported symptoms of caffeine withdrawal in 50 to 75 percent of all caffeine users studied. The most common symptoms are *headache* and *fatigue*; other symptoms include anxiety, *irritability*, mild depressive symptoms, impaired psychomotor performance, nausea, vomiting, craving for caffeine, and *muscle aches* and stiffness. The number and severity of the withdrawal symptoms are correlated with the amount of caffeine ingested and the abruptness of the withdrawal. Caffeine withdrawal symptoms have their onset at 12 to 24 hours after the last dose; the symptoms peak in 24 to 48 hours and resolve within 1 week. *Insomnia is a symptom of caffeine intoxication, not withdrawal.*

14.21 The answer is C

It has been found repeatedly that there are perfusion deficits in brains of cocaine-dependent subjects recently withdrawn from *cocaine*. This deficit is probably not related to tolerance or withdrawal, but several other findings probably are. Many (but not all) studies using positron emission tomography (PET) and SPECT to examine the brains of cocaine-dependent subjects have found a decreased number of dopamine transporters in the striatum, a finding consistent with postmortem studies. Within a few days of withdrawal, cocaine abusers show higher than normal cerebral metabolic rates in orbitofrontal cortex and basal ganglia that correlate with craving. At 1 to 4 weeks and at 3 to 4 months postwithdrawal, cocaine abusers have lower metabolic rates in the frontal cortex that correlate with symptoms of depression and decreased availability of D_2 receptors that correlates with decreased cerebral metabolic rates and years of cocaine use. These findings were similar in studies of patients after alcohol and amphetamine withdrawal. *Opioid withdrawal has not been associated with decreased dopamine binding in the striatum.*

14.22 The answer is D

Amphetamine-induced toxic psychosis can be exceedingly difficult to differentiate from schizophrenia and other psychotic disorders characterized by hallucinations or delusions. *Paranoid delusions* occur in about 80 percent of patients, and *hallucinations* in 60 to 70 percent. *Consciousness is clear* and *disorientation is uncommon. The presence of vivid visual or tactile hallucinations should raise suspicion of a drug-induced disorder.* In areas and populations where amphetamine use is common it may be necessary to provide only a provisional diagnosis until the patient can be observed and drug test results are obtained. Even then, there may be difficulties because in some urban areas a high percentage of persons with established diagnoses of schizophrenia also use amphetamines or cocaine. Typically, symptoms of amphetamine psychosis remit within a week, but in a small proportion of patients, psychosis may last for more than a month.

14.23 The answer is E

High rates of most cancers are seen in alcoholic people, especially those of the head, neck, esophagus, stomach, liver, colon, lungs, and breast tissue. An enhanced risk for breast malignancies might be seen *with as few as two drinks per day*, especially in women with family histories of this disease. The association with cancer probably reflects *alcohol-related immune system suppression* and the *direct effects of ethanol on mucosal membranes*. The heightened rates of malignant tumors in alcoholic people remain significant even when the possible effects of smoking and poor nutrition are considered, and this is the *second leading cause of premature death* in alcohol-dependent men and women.

14.24 The answer is C

According to the National Institute on Drug Abuse's annual survey of school students, the lifetime use of inhalants has increased significantly among 8th-graders, from *15.8* percent in 2003 to *17.3* percent in 2004, continuing an upward trend in use noted among 8th-graders last year, after several years of decline. Since 2001, there appears to be a gradual decline among 8th-graders in the perceived risk of using inhalants. It is also notable that the percentage of eighth-graders who reported using inhalants at least once was significantly higher than that for marijuana or any other drugs addressed in the survey.

Answers 14.25–14.29

14.25 The answer is C

14.26 The answer is A

14.27 The answer is B

14.28 The answer is B

14.29 The answer is C

Alcohol is metabolized by two enzymes: *alcohol dehydrogenase* (ADH) and *aldehyde dehydrogenase. ADH catalyzes the conversion of alcohol into acetaldehyde*, which is a toxic compound, and *aldehyde dehydrogenase catalyzes the conversion of acetaldehyde into acetic acid.* Aldehyde dehydrogenase is *inhibited by disulfiram (Antabuse)*, often used in the treatment of alcohol-related disorders. Some studies have shown that women have a lower ADH blood content than do men; this fact may account for women's tendency to become more intoxicated than do men after drinking the same amount of alcohol. The decreased function of *alcohol-metabolizing enzymes in some Asian people* can also lead to easy intoxication and toxic symptoms.

About 90 percent of absorbed alcohol is metabolized through oxidation in the liver; the remaining 10 percent is excreted unchanged by the kidney and the lungs. The rate of oxidation by the liver is constant and independent of the body's energy requirements. The body is capable of metabolizing at 15 mg/dLan hour, the range of 10 to 34 mg/dLan hour. Stated another way, the average person oxidizes three-fourths of an ounce of 40 percent (80 proof) alcohol in an hour. In people with a history of alcohol consumption, an up-regulation of the necessary enzymes results in fast metabolism of alcohol.

Answers 14.30–14.34

14.30 The answer is B

14.31 The answer is C

14.32 The answer is B

14.33 The answer is A

14.34 The answer is D

Barbiturates *cause rapid eye movement (REM) sleep suppression.* An abrupt withdrawal of a barbiturate will cause a marked increase or rebound in REM sleep. *Symptoms of withdrawal* from both benzodiazepines and barbiturates *usually appear within 3 days.* Barbiturates have a *high suicide potential.* Virtually no cases of successful suicide have occurred in patients taking benzodiazepines by themselves. In addition to treating anxiety, benzodiazepines are used in alcohol detoxification, for anesthetic induction, *as muscle relaxants,* and as anticonvulsants. *Neither* benzodiazepines nor barbiturates *are antipsychotics.*

Answers 14.35–14.41

14.35 The answer is A

14.36 The answer is A

14.37 The answer is A

14.38 The answer is B

14.39 The answer is C

14.40 The answer is D

14.41 The answer is E

Ethanol acts on the GABA receptor system and has effects on noradrenergic neurons in the locus ceruleus and on the dopaminergic neurons of the ventral tegmental area. Barbiturates, such as *phenobarbital*, also act primarily on the GABA system, specifically on the GABA receptor complex, which includes a binding site for the inhibitory amino acid GABA, a regulatory site that binds benzodiazepines, and a chloride ion channel. The binding of the barbiturate results in the facilitation of chloride ion influx into the neuron, making the neuron more negatively charged and less likely to be stimulated.

Diazepam (Valium), a benzodiazepine, affects the GABA receptor complex by binding to the site for benzodiazepines. When diazepam or another benzodiazepine binds to that site, the chloride ions flow through the channel, resulting in inhibition of the neuron. The benzodiazepine antagonist flumazenil (Mazicon) reverses the effects of benzodiazepines.

Opiates such as *heroin* bind to specific sites in the brain labeled opioid receptors. Changes in the number or the sensitivity of the opiate receptors may occur as the result of continuous exposure to an opiate, producing dependence on the substance. The activity of adrenergic neurons in the locus ceruleus also decreases with long-term use.

PCP binds to specific receptor sites located in the ion channel associated with the receptor for glutamate, an excitatory amino acid. Tolerance to PCP does not occur.

The leading theory regarding a mechanism of action for *caffeine* involves antagonism of the adenosine receptors. Adenosine appears to function as a neuromodulator, possibly as a neurotransmitter in the brain. Caffeine may also affect dopaminergic systems and adrenergic systems.

Nicotine is believed to exert its effects on the central nervous system through the nicotinic receptors, one subclass of *acetylcholine receptors*. Nicotine affects the nicotinic receptors in the receptor-gated ion channels of the receptor system.

Answers 14.42–14.46

14.42 The answer is D

14.43 The answer is C

14.44 The answer is A

14.45 The answer is C

14.46 The answer is E

A common *adverse effect associated with cocaine use is nasal congestion; serious inflammation, swelling, bleeding, and ulceration of the nasal mucosa can also occur*. Long-term use of cocaine can also lead to perforation of the nasal septa. Freebasing and smoking crack can damage the bronchial passages and the lungs. The IV use of cocaine can result in infection, embolisms, and the transmission of HIV. The major complications of cocaine use are cerebrovascular (infarctions), epileptic, and cardiac (MI and arrhythmias). About two thirds of these acute toxic effects occur within 1 hour of intoxication.

The most common *physical effects of cannabis are dilation of the conjunctival vessels* (injected or red eyes) and mild tachycardia. At high doses, orthostatic hypotension may appear. Increased appetite and dry mouth are also common effects of cannabis intoxication. Traditionally, *amotivational syndrome* has been associated with long-term heavy use and has been characterized by a person's unwillingness to persist in a task, be it at school, work, or in any setting that requires prolonged attention or tenacity. Persons are described as becoming apathetic and anergic, usually gaining weight, and appearing slothful.

People who have just taken PCP are frequently uncommunicative, appear to be oblivious, and report active fantasy production. They experience speedy feelings, euphoria, bodily warmth, tingling, peaceful floating sensations, and occasionally feelings of depersonalization. Hypertension, hyperthermia, and *vertical or horizontal nystagmus are common effects of PCP*. The short-term effects last 3 to 6 hours and sometimes give way to a mild depression, irritability, paranoia, and occasionally belligerent and aggressive behavior.

With hallucinogen use, such as LSD, perceptions become unusually brilliant and intense. Colors and textures seem richer than in the past, contours sharpened, music more emotionally profound, and smells and tastes heightened. Synthesthesia is common; colors may be heard or sounds seen.

15 Schizophrenia

Schizophrenia is a clinical syndrome of variable but profoundly disruptive psychopathology. It affects cognition, emotion, perception and other aspects of behavior. Although the expression of these manifestations varies across patients and over time, the effect of the illness is always severe and is usually long lasting. Schizophrenia affects just less than 1 percent of the world's population, and in the United States, has a financial cost that is estimated to exceed that of all cancers combined.

Schizophrenia is found in all societies and geographical areas. There is a slightly greater incidence in men than in women, and a greater incidence in urban versus rural areas. The illness is more severe in developed versus developing countries. Patients with schizophrenia are at increased risk for substance abuse, especially nicotine dependence. They are also at increased risk for suicidal and assaultive behavior. Approximately 10 percent of patients with schizophrenia commit suicide.

The etiology of schizophrenia is not yet known. There is considerable evidence that genetic factors make a robust contribution to the etiology. The presence of a proband with schizophrenia significantly increases the prevalence of this disorder among biological relatives.

Eight linkage sites have been identified, and specific candidate genes have been implicated. A number of potential environmental factors have also been identified that may contribute to the development of schizophrenia. These include gestational and birth complications, exposure to influenza epidemics or maternal starvation during pregnancy, Rhesus factor incompatibility, and an excess of winter births.

A central conceptual issue is whether schizophrenia is a neurodevelopmental or a neurodegenerative disorder. Both may be true, because the schizophrenia syndrome probably represents more than one disease process. The illness usually plateaus within the first 5 to 10 years of psychosis and does not manifest progressive deterioration throughout the course of life. The neuropathological investigation of the illness seems clearer. Although most studies have failed to document the presence of gliosis, the absence of gliosis does not preclude a neurodegenerative process. The preponderance of post mortem evidence is consistent with the neurodevelopmental hypothesis. This is further supported by neuropsychological, cognitive psychological, and neuroimaging findings.

Over the last 25 years, there has been a gradual evolution from conceptualizing schizophrenia as a disorder that involves discrete areas of the brain to a perspective that views it as a disorder of brain neural circuits. These models posit that a structural or functional lesion disrupts the functional capacity of the entire circuit. Major biochemical hypotheses involve dopamine, noradrenaline, serotonin, acetylcholine, glutamate and several neuromodulatory peptides or their receptors. The dopamine hypothesis is the most prominent and enduring hypothesis.

Issues relating to the reliability and validity of schizophrenia diagnoses have become more conceptual and theoretical since the development of the diagnostic system implemented in the American Psychiatric Association's third edition of the *Diagnostic and Statistical Manual of Mental Disorders* (DSM-III). The DSM approach is now the accepted diagnostic system in North America and throughout the international research community. The use of this approach has led to the reliable and consistent differential diagnosis of schizophrenia. The close connection of diagnosis and drug treatment is the dominant paradigm in drug development and is essential in registration studies seeking US Food and Drug Administration (FDA) approval of new drugs and new indications.

There is a large body of literature and scientific data regarding the pharmacological and psychosocial and rehabilitation of patients with schizophrenia. The antipsychotic drugs used to treat schizophrenia have a wide variety of pharmacological properties, but all share the capacity to antagonize postsynaptic dopamine receptors in the brain. Psychosocial and rehabilitative interventions are essential components of the comprehensive treatment of patients with schizophrenia. These include cognitive behavior therapy, supportive educationally oriented psychotherapy, family therapy and education programs, social and living skills training, supported employment programs, and supervised residential living arrangements.

Our field is at the beginning of a new century of opportunity for major breakthroughs in the treatment and prevention of schizophrenia. New paradigms providing heuristic advantage in the classification of psychopathological phenomena provide a means of addressing the problem of syndromic heterogeneity. Multidisciplinary work has become critical. Challenges in our understanding of this illness remain equally great. The complexity of this most distinctively human disease syndrome assures that the conquest of schizophrenia will be one of medicine's most difficult challenges.

Students should test their knowledge by addressing the following questions and answers.

HELPFUL HINTS

The following names and terms, including the schizophrenic signs and symptoms listed, should be studied and the definitions learned.

- antipsychotics
- autistic disorder
- Gregory Bateson
- Eugen Bleuler
- *bouffée délirante*
- brain imaging—CT, PET, MRI
- catatonic type
- deinstitutionalization
- delusions
- dementia precox
- disorganized type
- dopamine hypothesis
- double bind
- downward-drift hypothesis
- ECT
- ego boundaries
- electrophysiology—EEG
- expressed emotion
- first-rank symptoms
- flat affect and blunted affect
- forme fruste
- fundamental and accessory symptoms
- genetic hypothesis
- hallucinations
- impulse control, suicide, and homicide
- Karl Jaspers
- Karl Kahlbaum
- Emil Kraepelin
- Gabriel Langfeldt
- mesocortical and mesolimbic tracts
- Adolf Meyer
- Benedict Morel
- neurotransmitters and neurodegeneration
- orientation, memory, judgment, and insight
- paranoia
- paranoid type
- paraphrenia
- positive and negative symptoms
- projective testing
- psychoanalytic and learning theories
- psychoimmunology and psychoendocrinology
- psychosocial treatments
- residual type
- RFLPs
- schizoaffective disorder
- Kurt Schneider
- seasonality of birth
- serotonin hypothesis
- social causation hypothesis
- soft signs
- stress–diathesis model
- Harry Stack Sullivan
- tardive dyskinesia
- the four As
- thought disorders
- undifferentiated type

QUESTIONS

Directions

Each of the questions or incomplete statements below is followed by five suggested responses or completions. Select the *one* that is *best* in each case.

15.1 Which of the following is *not* typically associated with catatonia?

A. mutism
B. verbigeration
C. stereotypies
D. mannerisms
E. waxy flexibility

15.2 Late-onset schizophrenia

A. is clinically distinguishable from schizophrenia.
B. is more common in men.
C. has an onset after age 60.
D. is associated with a preponderance of paranoid symptoms.
E. results in poorer response to antipsychotic medications.

15.3 True statements about eye movement dysfunction in schizophrenia include

A. Eye movement dysfunction is independent of drug treatment
B. Eye movement dysfunction is seen in first degree probands
C. Eye movement dysfunction is associated with a frontal lobe pathology
D. Abnormal eye movements occur more often in patients with schizophrenia compared with controls
E. All of the above

Questions 15.4–15.5

15.4 Mr. A is a 22-year-old law student living alone in the school's dormitory. He had hopes to become a federal judge. Over the last 8 months his academic performance has declined, and he is being considered for academic probation. He has become increasingly isolated and withdrawn, and the girl he was dating broke off their relationship. He believes that she had been replaced by a look-alike from a distant planet, and that his fellow law students are conspiring against him. He believes that they snort and sneeze whenever he enters the classroom. He reports getting distracting "signals" from the television set, and that he hears voices of "the devil" calling to him. He called his father and asked for his help. Distressed, his father, himself a lawyer, brought him to the psychiatric emergency room for an evaluation. Physical examination was normal, and laboratory tests, including head computed tomography (CT) scan and urine toxicology, were negative.

Which of the following psychiatric conditions is the most likely diagnosis?

A. brief psychotic disorder
B. schizophreniform disorder
C. delusional disorder
D. schizophrenia, paranoid type
E. malingering

15.5 Mr. C was admitted to a psychiatric unit for acute management of his symptoms. On risperidone 2 mg per day, by day 6 he was noted to be less isolated, and was less troubled by the hallucinations. On day 7, he was found in the bathroom, trying to tie a bed-sheet around his neck in an attempt to kill himself. Risk factors for suicide in this patient include:

A. his age
B. his sex
C. his overly high ambitions
D. an improvement in his condition
E. all of the above

15.6 Persons in the United States who develop schizophrenia are more likely to

A. have been born abroad
B. have been born in the months from January to April
C. have been born in the months from July to September
D. have been exposed to the para-influenza virus
E. none of the above

15.7 Which of the following is *true* of brain-imaging technologies in the study of schizophrenia?

A. CT is used more than magnetic resonance imaging (MRI) in schizophrenia research because its resolution is superior to that of MRI
B. The abnormalities reported in CT studies of patients with schizophrenia are specific for the pathophysiological processes underlying the disease
C. In studies of monozygotic twins discordant for schizophrenia, MRI studies have shown that the cerebral ventricles in the affected twins are larger than in the non-affected twins
D. PET studies have shown almost no impairment of brain areas after psychological test stimulation
E. fMRI has shown no differences in the brains of patients with schizophrenia compared with controls

15.8 The negative symptoms of schizophrenia include all of the following *except*

A. alogia
B. affective flattening
C. avolition
D. aggressivity
E. inattentiveness

15.9 False statements comparing the Serotonin-Dopamine Antagonists (SDAs) with Dopamine Receptor Antagonists include all of the following *except*

A. The SDAs produce more extrapyramidal symptoms than the dopamine receptor antagonists
B. The SDAs are less effective than the dopamine receptor antagonists for positive symptoms of schizophrenia
C. The SDAs produce more neurological adverse effects than dopamine receptor antagonists
D. The SDAs affect both serotonin and glutamate receptors
E. Dopamine receptor antagonists remain the first choice of treatment for schizophrenia

15.10 Appropriate psychosocial therapies in the management and treatment of schizophrenia include

A. social skills training
B. case management
C. individual psychotherapy
D. group therapy
E. all of the above

15.11 Clozapine (Clozaril)

A. causes significant increases in prolactin levels
B. is associated with a 10 to 20 percent incidence of agranulocytosis
C. requires monthly monitoring of blood chemistry
D. has been associated with few, if any, extrapyramidal side effects
E. is believed to exert its therapeutic effect mainly by blocking dopamine receptors

15.12 Which of the following statements best describes a characteristic of the epidemiology of schizophrenia?

A. Schizophrenia patients occupy about 50 percent of all hospital beds.
B. Some regions of the world have an unusually high prevalence of schizophrenia.
C. Female patients with schizophrenia are more likely to commit suicide than are male patients.
D. In the northern hemisphere, schizophrenia occurs more often among people born from July to September than in those born in the other months.
E. Reproduction rates among people with schizophrenia are typically higher than those among the general population.

15.13 Investigations into the cause of schizophrenia have revealed that

A. no significant abnormalities appear in the evoked potentials in schizophrenic patients
B. a monozygotic twin reared by adoptive parents has schizophrenia at the same rate as his/her twin raised by biological parents
C. a specific family pattern plays a causative role in the development of schizophrenia
D. the efficacy and potency of most antipsychotics correlate with their ability to act primarily as antagonists of the dopamine type 1 (D_1) receptor
E. a particular defective chromosomal site has been found in all schizophrenic patients

15.14 Epidemiological studies of schizophrenia have found all of the following *except*

A. Hospital records suggest that the incidence of schizophrenia in the United States has remained unchanged for the past 100 years.
B. The peak age of onset for schizophrenia is the same for men and women.

C. Schizophrenia is equally prevalent among men and women.
D. Approximately 50 percent of schizophrenic patients attempt suicide at least once in their lifetimes.
E. The lifetime prevalence is usually between 1 and 1.5 percent of the population.

15.15 All of the following statements are factors with an increased risk of schizophrenia *except*

A. having a schizophrenic family member
B. having a history of temporal lobe epilepsy
C. having low levels of monoamine oxidase, type B, in blood platelets
D. having previously attempted suicide
E. having a deviant course of personality maturation and development

15.16 A schizophrenic patient who states that he feels his brain burning is most likely experiencing a

A. delusional feeling
B. gustatory hallucination
C. cenesthetic hallucination
D. haptic hallucination
E. hypnopompic hallucination

15.17 The majority of CT studies of patients with schizophrenia have reported

A. enlarged lateral and third ventricles in 10 to 50 percent of patients
B. cortical atrophy in 10 to 35 percent of patients
C. atrophy of the cerebellar vermis
D. findings that are not artifacts of treatment
E. all of the above

15.18 In general, pooled studies show concordance rates for schizophrenia in monozygotic twins of

A. 0.1 percent
B. 5 percent
C. 25 percent
D. 40 percent
E. 50 percent

15.19 Features weighing toward a good prognosis in schizophrenia include all of the following *except*

A. depression
B. a family history of mood disorders
C. paranoid features
D. undifferentiated or disorganized features
E. an undulating course

15.20 Electrophysiological studies of persons with schizophrenia show

A. decreased alpha activity
B. spikes in the limbic area that correlate with psychotic behavior
C. increased frontal lobe slow-wave activity
D. increased parietal lobe fast-wave activity
E. all of the above

15.21 With regard to the ventricular size in schizophrenia, which of the following statements is *true*?

A. Ventricular enlargement is a pathognomonic finding in schizophrenia.
B. Ventricular changes in schizophrenia are likely to be specific for the pathophysiological processes underlying this disorder.
C. Patients with schizophrenia invariably demonstrate significant enlargement of the lateral ventricles.
D. All of the above
E. None of the above

15.22 MRI studies of schizophrenics have found evidence for

A. increased cortical gray matter
B. increased volume of the amygdala
C. increased volume of basal ganglia nuclei
D. increased temporal cortex gray matter
E. increased volume of the hippocampus

15.23 Prefrontal cortex and limbic system hypotheses are the predominant neuroanatomical theories of schizophrenia because of the demonstration of

A. decreased volume of prefrontal gray or white matter
B. prefrontal cortical interneuron abnormalities
C. disturbed prefrontal metabolism and blood flow
D. disarray or abnormal migration of hippocampal neurons
E. all of the above

15.24 The rationale for the role of excess dopamine in schizophrenia is based on observations that

A. Dopaminergic drugs can induce paranoid psychosis.
B. Drugs that block postsynaptic dopamine receptors reduce symptoms of schizophrenia.
C. Metabolic alterations in limbic anatomy are consistent with a disturbance in dopamine metabolism.
D. Increased concentrations of dopamine have been found in the amygdalas in postmortem brains of schizophrenic patients.
E. All of the above

15.25 Possible risk factors for the development of schizophrenia include

A. birth during winter months
B. increased number of birth complications
C. social class
D. recent immigration status
E. all of the above

15.26 True statements about structural brain abnormalities in patients with schizophrenia include

A. abnormalities are present from birth
B. cortical involvement is multifocal rather than diffuse

C. abnormalities are present in a minority of patients
D. abnormalities have not been correlated with cognitive deficits
E. none of the above

15.27 True statements about hypothesized neurobiological models of schizophrenia include

A. Genes function in part by increasing vulnerability to environmental factors.
B. Environmental factors increase risk by producing subtle brain damage.
C. The apparent lack of gliosis in postmortem studies implicates in utero factors.
D. As the prefrontal cortex matures, behavioral and cognitive sequelae of subtle structural deficits become manifest.
E. All of the above

15.28 In simple deteriorative disorder

A. hallucinations are common.
B. delusions are common.
C. homelessness is common.
D. early diagnosis is common.
E. All of the above

15.29 Childhood schizophrenia

A. is not diagnosed using the same symptoms as are used for adult schizophrenia
B. tends to have an abrupt onset
C. tends to have a chronic course
D. tends to have a better prognosis that adult schizophrenia
E. all of the above

15.30 True statements about violence and schizophrenia include all of the following *except*

A. Patients with schizophrenia are more violent as a group than the general population.
B. Patients with disorganized schizophrenia are at much greater risk to commit violence than those with paranoid schizophrenia.
C. Command hallucinations do not appear to play a particularly important role in violence.
D. Violence in a hospital setting can result from undiagnosed neuroleptic-induced acute akathisia.
E. It is more difficult to prevent most schizophrenic homicides compared to the general population.

15.31 Mr. G, a 36-year-old man, is admitted to a psychiatric unit after having been brought to the emergency department by police. As he was walking past a hotel in the central part of the city, he saw a man and woman standing on the sidewalk about to take a photograph of a building across the street. Thinking that they were going to take his picture, he grabbed the camera, smashed it on the ground, and pulled out all the film. He explained his actions by saying the photograph would be used to control him and that it is illegal to take another person's photograph.

Mr. G has a history of multiple hospitalizations dating back to age 14. During the hospitalizations, his symptoms have been well-controlled with a variety of typical and atypical antipsychotic medications. Once discharged he begins drinking four to five beers a day, neglects getting prescriptions refilled, and stops medication when his supply runs out. He made two prior suicide attempts, both by hanging, in which he suffered no serious medical sequelae. He reports numerous blackouts from drinking, but he has never had seizures or DTs. He does not use illicit drugs.

Mr. G dropped out of high school in the 11th grade. He worked a number of short-term, unskilled jobs before going on public assistance at age 21. He lives alone, is estranged from his family, and has no friends. On examination, Mr. G is lying motionless. He makes good eye contact and says, "I'm trying not to move." He fears that if he moves he may die. He currently hears voices saying, "Be good," "Get the dog," and "He's the one." He also sees shapes, which he describes as colored letters dancing in front of his eyes. He talks about being monitored by hidden cameras and microphones everywhere he goes in the city. He is alert and oriented. He can recall three out of three objects after 5 minutes. Concentration is impaired.

Which of the following is the most likely diagnosis for the case described above?

A. Schizophrenia, catatonic type
B. Schizophrenia, undifferentiated type
C. Schizophrenia, paranoid type
D. Delusional disorder
E. Schizoaffective disorder

15.32 Which of the following interventions is most likely to prevent relapse in the case above?

A. Vocational rehabilitation
B. Increased socialization
C. Use of a long-term depot antipsychotic
D. Alcohol counseling
E. Use of an atypical antipsychotic

Directions

Each group of questions consists of lettered headings followed by a list of numbered words or statements. For each numbered word or statement, select the one lettered heading that is most closely associated with it. Each lettered heading may be selected once, more than once, or not at all.

Questions 15.33–15.36

A. Eugen Bleuler
B. Emil Kraepelin

15.33 Latinized the term démence précoce
15.34 Classified patients as being afflicted with manic-depressive psychoses, dementia precox, or paranoia
15.35 Coined the term schizophrenia

15.36 Described the four As of schizophrenia—associations, autism, affect, and ambivalence

Questions 15.37–15.42

A. Schneiderian first-rank symptom
B. Schneiderian second-rank symptom

15.37 Sudden delusional ideas
15.38 Perplexity
15.39 Audible thoughts
15.40 Voices commenting
15.41 Thought withdrawal
15.42 The experience of having one's thoughts controlled

Questions 15.43–15.47

A. Neologism
B. Echolalia
C. Verbigeration
D. Clang association
E. Loosening of associations

15.43 Loss of logical relations between thoughts
15.44 Creation of a new expression or word
15.45 Repetition of interviewer's words when answering a question
15.46 Words associated by sound rather than meaning
15.47 Use of words in stereotypically repetitive fashion

Questions 15.48–15.52

A. Echopraxia
B. Negativism
C. Anhedonia
D. Stereotypies
E. Mutism

15.48 Functional inhibition of speech
15.49 Imitation of movements
15.50 Repetitive, often bizarre, speech or behavior
15.51 Unwillingness to cooperate without apparent reason
15.52 Diminution in ability to experience pleasure

ANSWERS

15.1 The answer is B

Verbigeration is a specific disorder in the form of thought. It is the meaningless repetition of specific words or phrases, and is not associated with catatonia.

The catatonic type of schizophrenia, which was common several decades ago, has become rare in Europe and North America. The classic feature of the catatonic type is a marked disturbance in motor function; this disturbance may involve stupor, negativism, rigidity, excitement, or posturing. Sometimes, the patient shows rapid alteration between extremes of excitement and stupor. Associated features include *stereotypies*, *mannerisms* and *waxy flexibility*, or *cerea flexibilitas*. *Stereotypies* are repetitive fixed patterns of physical action or speech. *Mannerisms* are ingrained, habitual involuntary movements. Finally, *waxy flexibility* or *cerea flexibilitas* is a condition in which a person can be molded into a position and then maintained, or when an examiner moves the person's limb, the limb feels as if it were made of wax; this is another term for catatonia.

15.2 The answer is D

Late-onset schizophrenia is *clinically indistinguishable* from schizophrenia but has an *onset after age 45*. This condition tends to *appear more frequently in women* and also tends to be *characterized by a predominance of paranoid symptoms*. The prognosis is favorable, and *these patients usually do well on antipsychotic medication*.

15.3 The answer is E (all)

The inability to follow a moving visual target accurately is the defining basis for the disorders of smooth visual pursuit and disinhibition of saccadic eye movements seen in patients with schizophrenia. Eye movement dysfunction may be a trait marker for schizophrenia; it is *independent of drug treatment and clinical state* and is also *seen in first-degree relatives of pro-bands with schizophrenia*. Various studies have reported *abnormal eye movements in 50 to 85 percent of patients with schizophrenia,* compared with about 25 percent in psychiatric patients without schizophrenia *and less than 10 percent in non-psychiatrically ill control subjects*. Because eye movement is partly controlled by centers in the frontal lobes, a disorder in eye movement is consistent with *theories that implicate a frontal lobe pathological process* in schizophrenia.

15.4 The answer is D

The presence of hallucinations or delusions is not necessary for a diagnosis of schizophrenia. To make the diagnosis, the patient must demonstrate the presence of two or more of the following: delusions, hallucinations, disorganized speech, grossly disorganized or catatonic behavior, or negative symptoms. Symptoms must persist for at least 6 months (Table 15.1). The *paranoid type of schizophrenia* is characterized by preoccupation with one or more delusions or frequent hallucinations. Classically the paranoid type of schizophrenia is characterized mainly by the presence of delusions of persecution or grandeur.

Brief psychotic disorder is an acute and transient psychotic syndrome. The disorder lasts from 1 day to 1 month, and the symptoms may resemble those of schizophrenia. In addition, the disorder develops in response to a severe psychosocial stressor or group of stressors.

Schizophreniform disorder is similar to schizophrenia except that its symptoms last at least 1 month but less than 6 months. Patients with schizophreniform disorder return to their baseline level of functioning once the disorder has resolved.

Nonbizarre delusions present for at least 1 month without other symptoms of schizophrenia or a mood disorder warrant the diagnosis of *delusional disorder*.

Malingering is characterized by the voluntary production and presentation of false or grossly exaggerated physical or psychological symptoms. The presence of a clearly definable goal is the main factor that differentiates malingering from factitious disorders.

15.5 The answer is E (all)

About 50 percent of all schizophrenic patients attempt suicide and 10 to 15 percent of patients with schizophrenia die by suicide.

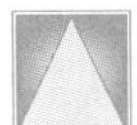

Table 15.1
DSM-IV-TR Diagnostic Criteria for Schizophrenia

A. *Characteristic symptoms:* Two (or more) of the following, each present for a significant portion of time during a 1-month period (or less if successfully treated):
(1) delusions
(2) hallucinations
(3) disorganized speech (e.g., frequent derailment or incoherence)
(4) grossly disorganized or catatonic behavior
(5) negative symptoms, i.e., affective flattening, alogia, or avolition

Note: Only one Criterion A symptom is required if delusions are bizarre or hallucinations consist of a voice keeping up a running commentary on the person's behavior or thoughts, or two or more voices conversing with each other.

B. *Social/occupational dysfunction:* For a significant portion of the time since the onset of the disturbance, one or more major areas of functioning such as work, interpersonal relations, or self-care are markedly below the level achieved prior to the onset (or when the onset is in childhood or adolescence, failure to achieve expected level of interpersonal, academic, or occupational achievement).

C. *Duration:* Continuous signs of the disturbance persist for at least 6 months. This 6-month period must include at least 1 month of symptoms (or less if successfully treated) that meet Criterion A (i.e., active-phase symptoms) and may include periods of prodromal or residual symptoms. During these prodromal or residual periods, the signs of the disturbance may be manifested by only negative symptoms or two or more symptoms listed in Criterion A present in an attenuated form (e.g., odd beliefs, unusual perceptual experiences).

D. *Schizoaffective and mood disorder exclusion:* Schizoaffective disorder and mood disorder with psychotic features have been ruled out because either (1) no major depressive, manic, or mixed episodes have occurred concurrently with the active-phase symptoms; or (2) if mood episodes have occurred during active-phase symptoms, their total duration has been brief relative to the duration of the active and residual periods.

E. *Substance/general medical condition exclusion:* The disturbance is not due to the direct physiological effects of a substance (e.g., a drug of abuse, a medication) or a general medical condition.

F. *Relationship to a pervasive developmental disorder:* If there is a history of autistic disorder or another pervasive developmental disorder, the additional diagnosis of schizophrenia is made only if prominent delusions or hallucinations are also present for at least a month (or less if successfully treated).

Classification of longitudinal course (can be applied only after at least 1 year has elapsed since the initial onset of active-phase symptoms):

Episodic with interepisode residual symptoms (episodes are defined by the reemergence of prominent psychotic symptoms); also *specify* if: **with prominent negative symptoms**
Episodic with no interepisode residual symptoms
Continuous (prominent psychotic symptoms are present throughout the period of observation); also *specify* if: **with prominent negative symptoms**
Single episode in partial remission: also *specify* if: **with prominent negative symptoms**
Single episode in full remission
Other or unspecified pattern

From American Psychiatric Association, *Diagnostic and Statistical Manual of Mental Disorders.* 4th ed. Text rev. Washington, DC: American Psychiatric Association; copyright 2000, with permission.

The risk factors for suicide in this case are the patient's *male sex*, college education, *young age*, and *overly high ambitions*. Suicide is also associated with his *improvement*, because the patient now has an awareness of his illness and an increased motivation to act on it.

15.6 The answer is B

Persons who develop schizophrenia are more likely to have been born in the winter and early spring. In the Northern Hemisphere, including the United States, *persons with schizophrenia are more often born in the months from January to April.* In the Southern Hemisphere, persons with schizophrenia are more often born in the months from July to September. *There are no data to suggest that being born abroad is a risk factor for developing schizophrenia.* Some studies show that *the frequency of schizophrenia is increased following exposure to influenza.*

15.7 The answer is C

MRI studies demonstrate that in monozygotic twins who are discordant for schizophrenia, *virtually all the affected twins have larger cerebral ventricles than their non-affected twins.* MRI is used in schizophrenia research because its *resolution is superior to that with CT.* The abnormalities reported in CT studies of patients with schizophrenia have also been reported in other neuropsychiatric conditions, and *are unlikely to be specific for the patho-physiological processes underlying schizophrenia.* PET studies have shown evidence of impaired activation of certain brain areas after psychological test stimulation in schizophrenics. *fMRI has shown differences in sensori-motor cortex activation and a decreased blood flow to the occipital lobes in patients with schizophrenia.*

15.8 The answer is D

The negative symptoms of schizophrenia include *affective flattening* or blunting, poverty of speech (*alogia*) or speech content, blocking, poor grooming, lack of motivation (*avolition*), anhedonia or asociality, and *social inattentiveness. Aggressive or agitated behavior* is considered more to be a positive symptom of schizophrenia.

15.9 The answer is C

The SDAs affect both serotonin and glutamate receptors. However, the SDAs produce minimal or no extrapyramidal symptoms and interact with different subtypes of dopamine receptors than do the standard antipsychotics. They also produce fewer neurological adverse effects and *are effective in treating negative symptoms of schizophrenia. They are at least as effective as haloperidone for positive symptoms*, and are uniquely effective for the negative symptoms. *These drugs have replaced the dopamine receptor antagonists as the drug of first choice for the treatment of schizophrenia.*

15.10 The answer is E (all)

Psychosocial therapies include a variety of methods to increase social abilities, self-sufficiency, practical skills and interpersonal communication in schizophrenia patients. The goal is to enable persons who are severely ill to develop social and vocational skills for independent living. *Social skills training*, also referred to as behavioral skills therapy can be directly supportive and useful to the patient along with pharmacological treatment. Because a variety of professionals with specialized skills are involved in a treatment program, it is helpful to have one person, *the case manager* coordinate the care. Studies on the effects of *individual psychotherapy* in the treatment of schizophrenia have provided data that the therapy is helpful and that the effects are additive to those of pharmacological treatment. *Group therapy* in patients with schizophrenia is effective in reducing social isolation, and when led in a supportive manner, is most helpful.

15.11 The answer is D

Clozapine (Clozaril) *has been associated with few, if any, extrapyramidal side effects* or tardive dyskinesia. It is an antipsychotic medication that is appropriate in the treatment of schizophrenic patients who have not responded to first-line dopamine receptor antagonists or who have tardive dyskinesia. It *is not an appropriate first-line drug for the treatment of schizophrenia.* Clozapine *has been associated with a 1 to 2 percent (not 10 to 20 percent) incidence of agranulocytosis* and thus *requires weekly, not monthly, monitoring of blood chemistries.* Clozapine *is believed to exert its therapeutic effect* by blocking serotonin type 2 (5-HT_2) and, secondarily, dopamine receptors.

15.12 The answer is B

An important epidemiological factor in schizophrenia is that *some regions of the world have an unusually high prevalence* of the disorder. Certain researchers have interpreted this geographic inequity as supporting an infectious cause for schizophrenia, whereas others emphasize genetic or social factors.

Schizophrenic patients occupy 50 percent of mental hospital beds, not of all hospital beds.

Female patients with schizophrenia are no more likely to commit suicide than are male patients; the risk factors are equal.

There is a difference in prevalence of schizophrenia according to season, but *in the northern hemisphere, schizophrenia occurs more often among people* born from January to April, not from July to September. The latter time range refers to seasonal preference for the disorder in the southern hemisphere. *Reproduction rates among people with schizophrenia* have been rising in recent years because of newly introduced medications and changes in laws and policies about hospitalization and community-based care. *The fertility rate among people with schizophrenia, however, is only approaching the rate for the general population and does not exceed it.*

15.13 The answer is B

The cause of schizophrenia is not known. However, a wide range of genetic studies strongly suggest a genetic component to the inheritance of schizophrenia. Monozygotic twins have the highest concordance rate for schizophrenia. *The studies of adopted monozygotic twins show that twins who are reared by adoptive parents have schizophrenia at the same rate as their twin siblings raised by their biological parents.* That finding suggests that the genetic influence outweighs the environmental influence. In further support of the genetic basis is the observation that the more severe the schizophrenia, the more likely the twins are to be concordant for the disorder.

Nevertheless, *a particular genetic defect has not been found in all schizophrenic patients.* Many associations between particular chromosomal sites and schizophrenia have been reported in the literature since the widespread application of the techniques of molecular biology. More than half of the chromosomes have been associated with schizophrenia in those various reports, but the long arms of chromosomes 5, 11, 18, and 22; the short arms of chromosomes 6, 8, and 19; and the X chromosome have been the most commonly reported. At this time, the literature is best summarized as indicating a potentially heterogeneous genetic basis for schizophrenia.

The research literature also reports that *a large number of abnormalities appear in the evoked potentials in schizophrenic patients.* The P300, so far the most studied, is defined as a large positive evoked-potential wave that occurs about 300 milliseconds after a sensory stimulus is detected. The major source of the P300 wave may be in the limbic system structures of the medial temporal lobes. In schizophrenic patients the P300 has been reported to be statistically smaller and later than in comparison groups.

Except for the serotonin-dopamine antagonists, *the efficacy and the potency of most antipsychotics correlate* with their ability to act as antagonists of the dopamine type 2 (D_2) (not type 1) receptor.

No well-controlled evidence indicates that any specific family pattern plays a causative role in the development of schizophrenia. Some schizophrenic patients do come from dysfunctional families, just as many persons who are not psychiatrically ill come from dysfunctional families.

15.14 The answer is B

Men have an earlier onset of schizophrenia than do women. The peak ages of onset for men are 25 to 35. However, *schizophrenia is equally prevalent in men and women.*

Hospital records suggest that the *incidence of schizophrenia in the United States has probably remained unchanged for the past 100 years* and possibly throughout the entire history of the country, despite tremendous socioeconomic and population changes.

Suicide is a common cause of death among schizophrenic patients. *About 50 percent of patients with schizophrenia attempt suicide* at least once in their lifetimes,and 10 to 15 percent of schizophrenic patients die by suicide during a 20-year follow-up period.

The lifetime prevalence of schizophrenia is usually between 1 and 1.5 percent of the population. Consistent with that range, the National Institute of Mental Health (NIMH)-sponsored Epidemiologic Catchment Area (ECA) study reported a lifetime prevalence of 1.3 percent.

15.15 The answer is D

Having previously attempted suicide does not increase the risk for developing schizophrenia, although at least 50 percent of schizophrenic patients attempt suicide once in their lifetimes. *Having a schizophrenic family member,* especially having one or two schizophrenic parents or a monozygotic twin who is schizophrenic, *increases the risk for schizophrenia.* Other risk factors include the following: (1) having lived through a difficult obstetrical delivery, presumably with trauma to the brain; (2) having, for unknown reasons, *a deviant course of personality maturation and development* that has produced an excessively shy, daydreaming, withdrawn, friendless child; an excessively compliant, good, or dependent child; a child with idiosyncratic thought processes; a child who is particularly sensitive to separation; a child who is destructive, violent, incorrigible, and prone to truancy; or an anhedonic child; (3) having a parent who has paranoid attitudes and formal disturbances of thinking; (4) *having low levels of monoamine oxidase, type B, in the blood platelets;* (5) having abnormal pursuit eye movements; (6) having taken a variety of drugs—particularly lysergic acid diethylamide (LSD), amphetamines, cannabis, cocaine, and phencyclidine; and (7) *having a history of temporal lobe epilepsy,* Huntington's disease, homocystinuria, folic acid deficiency, and the adult form of metachromatic leukodystrophy.

None of those risk factors invariably occurs in schizophrenic patients; they may occur in various combinations. The vast majority of people who ingest psychotomimetic drugs do not become schizophrenic. Not every schizophrenic patient has abnormal pursuit eye movements, and some well relatives of schizophrenic patients may also have abnormal pursuit eye movements.

15.16 The answer is C

A person with schizophrenia often experiences a *cenesthetic hallucination,* a sensation of an altered state in body organs without any special receptor apparatus to explain the sensation—for example, *a burning sensation in the brain,* a pushing sensation in the abdominal blood vessels, or a cutting sensation in the bone marrow.

A *delusional feeling* is a feeling of false belief, based on an incorrect inference about external reality. A *gustatory hallucination* involves primarily taste. A tactile or *haptic hallucination* involves the sense of touch (for example, formication—the feeling of bugs crawling under the skin). A *hypnopompic hallucination* is a hallucination that occurs as one awakes. Neither hallucinations nor delusions are pathognomonic of schizophrenia; they may occur in other disorders.

15.17 The answer is E (all)

The majority of CT studies of patients with schizophrenia have reported *enlarged lateral and third ventricles in* 10 to 50 percent of patients and *cortical atrophy* in 10 to 35 percent of patients. Controlled studies have also revealed *atrophy of the cerebellar vermis,* decreased radiodensity of brain parenchyma, and reversals of the normal brain asymmetries. Those *findings are not artifacts of treatment* and are not progressive or reversible. The enlargement of the ventricles seems to be present at the time of diagnosis, before the use of medication. Some studies have correlated the presence of CT scan findings with the presence of negative or deficit symptoms (for example, social isolation), neuropsychological impairment, frequent motor side effects from antipsychotics, and a poor premorbid adjustment.

15.18 The answer is E

In general, pooled studies show *concordance rates of about 50 percent* in monozygotic twins. This is the most robust finding pointing to a genetic etiologic component to the disorder.

15.19 The answer is D

Poor prognostic features in schizophrenia include a family history of schizophrenia; poor premorbid social, sexual, and work histories; and *undifferentiated or disorganized features.* Features weighting toward a good prognosis in schizophrenia include mood symptoms (especially *depression*), *a family history of mood disorders, paranoid features,* and *an undulating course.*

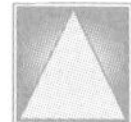

Table 15.2
Features Weighting toward Good to Poor Prognosis in Schizophrenia

Good Prognosis	Poor Prognosis
Late onset	Young onset
Obvious precipitating factors	No precipitating factors
Acute onset	Insidious onset
Good premorbid social, sexual, and work histories	Poor premorbid social, sexual, and work histories
Mood disorder symptoms (especially depressive disorders)	Withdrawn, autistic behavior
Married	Single, divorced, or widowed
Family history of mood disorders	Family history of schizophrenia
Good support systems	Poor support systems
Positive symptoms	Negative symptoms
	Neurological signs and symptoms
	History of perinatal trauma
	No remissions in 3 years
	Many relapses
	History of assaultiveness

Table 15.2 presents a summary of the factors used to assess prognosis in schizophrenia.

15.20 The answer is E (all)

Electrophysiological studies of schizophrenia patients include electroencephalogram (EEG) studies. Those studies indicate a higher than usual number of patients with abnormal recordings, increased sensitivity (for example, frequent spike activity) to activation procedures (for example, sleep deprivation), *decreased alpha activity,* increased theta and delta activity, possibly more epileptiform activity, and possibly more left-sided abnormalities. Evoked potential studies have generally shown increased amplitude of early components and decreased amplitude of late components. That difference may indicate that although schizophrenia patients are more sensitive to sensory stimulation than other persons, they compensate for that increased sensitivity by blunting their processing of the information at higher cortical levels.

Other central nervous system (CNS) electrophysiological investigations include depth electrodes and quantitative EEG (QEEG). One study reported that schizophrenic patients showed *spikes in the limbic area that correlate with psychotic behavior*; however, no control subjects were examined. QEEG studies of schizophrenia show *increased frontal lobe slow-wave activity* and *increased parietal lobe fast-wave activity.*

15.21 The answer is E (none)

MRI studies have consistently shown that the brains of many schizophrenic patients have *lateral* and *third ventricular enlargement* and some degree of reduction in cortical volume. Those findings can be interpreted as consistent with the presence of less than usual brain tissue in affected patients; whether that decrease is due to abnormal development or to degeneration remains undetermined.

However, the abnormalities reported in MRI studies of schizophrenic patients have also been reported in other neuropsychiatric conditions, including mood disorders, alcohol-related disorders, and dementias. Thus, those *changes are not likely to be pathognomonic for the pathological processes underlying schizophrenia.* Although the *enlarged ventricles* in schizophrenic patients can be shown when groups of patients and controls are used, the difference between affected and unaffected persons is variable and usually small.

One of the most important MRI studies examined monozygotic twins who were discordant with schizophrenia. The study found that virtually all of the affected twins had larger cerebral ventricles than did the nonaffected twins, although most of the affected twins had cerebral ventricles within a normal range.

15.22 The answer is C

Studies employing MRI have found evidence in schizophrenic patients for *decreased (not increased) cortical gray matter, especially in the temporal cortex,* decreased volume of limbic system structures (e.g., *the amygdala, hippocampus,* and parahippocampus), and *increased volume of basal ganglia nuclei.* These findings are consistent with the findings of neuropathological examinations of postmortem tissue, including ultrastructural examination, which in some cases indicates cell loss, misalignment of cells, altered intracellular structure, and protein expression, or gliosis.

15.23 The answer is E (all)

Prefrontal cortex and limbic system hypotheses are the predominant neuroanatomical theories of schizophrenia. The demonstration of *decreased volumes of prefrontal gray or white matter, prefrontal cortical interneuron abnormalities, disturbed prefrontal metabolism and blood flow*, decreased volumes of hippocampal and entorhinal cortex, and *disarray or abnormal migration of hippocampal* and entorhinal *neurons* provide strong support for the involvement of these brain regions in the pathophysiology of schizophrenia. In the context of neural circuit hypotheses linking the prefrontal cortex and limbic system, studies demonstrating a relation between hippocampal morphological abnormalities and disturbances in prefrontal cortex metabolism or function are particularly interesting.

15.24 The answer is E (all)

The hyperdopaminergic hypothesis of schizophrenia arose from two sets of observations of drug action relating to the dopaminergic system. *Drugs that increase dopamine system activity,* such as D-amphetamine, cocaine, levodopa (Larodopa), and methylphenidate (Ritalin), *can induce a paranoid psychosis* that is similar to some aspects of schizophrenia. Substantial evidence supports the *role of postsynaptic dopamine blockade* as an initiating factor in a cascade of events responsible for the mode of therapeutic action of antipsychotic drugs.

However, despite the compelling evidence for the role of dopamine in schizophrenia, testing the hypothesis has proven problematic. Clinical studies across a broad range of indices of dopamine metabolism have been characterized by marked variability in results. The most decisive clinical testing of the hypothesis has been at the level of observed drug action and symptom manipulation. Studies aimed at measuring abnormal concentrations of dopamine or its metabolites in blood, urine, and spinal fluid are confronted by problems that are almost insurmountable. In large fluid compartments, alterations in dopamine metabolism associated with schizophrenia will represent only a minor contribution to the particular index of dopamine metabolism; spinal fluid necessarily provides a summation of total brain activity, most of which is not considered germane to schizophrenia, and blood and urine provide even more indirect indices.

Functional imaging studies provide indirect evidence of dopamine involvement through the examination of metabolic rates in brain regions where dopamine is an important neurotransmitter. For example, data confirming *metabolic alterations in limbic anatomy are consistent with a disturbance in dopamine metabolism,* but it is not possible to determine the extent to which this reflects an alteration of dopamine biochemistry versus an alteration of any one of a number of interacting neurotransmitter and neuromodulatory systems. A more informative approach for assessing abnormal dopamine metabolism in patients with schizophrenia is to infuse subjects with an indirect dopamine agonist and then to determine the extent to which radioligand occupancy of postsynaptic dopamine receptors is reduced by competition with the increased endogenous dopamine. The comparison of preinfusion and postinfusion radioligand occupancy provides an index of dopamine release and reuptake rates. PET studies of dopamine receptor distribution and the density of receptor expression may offer an alternative approach for documenting the dopamine hypothesis. The observation of an increased quantity of dopamine type 2 (D_2) receptors in the caudate nucleus of drug-free schizophrenic patients is an example of this approach, but replication has been difficult. The extension of this approach to other dopamine receptor types is an important new direction of research.

Finally, there is the potential for the relatively precise biochemical study of dopamine in postmortem tissue, but here, as with the use of body fluids, sources of artifact and imprecision have been difficult to manage.

Despite these methodological limitations, postmortem studies have reported differences between schizophrenic and control brains. For example, *increased concentration of dopamine has been found in the left amygdala* (a limbic system structure) in the postmortem brains of patients with schizophrenia. This finding has been replicated and, since it is lateralized, is not likely to be an artifact. There has also been a report of an increase in D_2 postsynaptic receptors in postmortem tissue of schizophrenic patients whose medical records provided a diagnosis of schizophrenia but did not reveal neuroleptic drug use. These results suggest that the increase in binding (receptor) number is not secondary to neuroleptic drugs. The investigation of receptor abnormalities has been extended to other dopamine receptor types, and an increase of D_4 receptors in the entorhinal cortex, independent of antipsychotic use, has been reported.

15.25 The answer is E (all)

Studies have shown *that a disproportionate number of persons with schizophrenia are born during winter months* (seasonal excess of approximately 10 percent); which, together with a birth pattern in their nonschizophrenic siblings that is similar to that seen in the general population, suggests the presence of a seasonal factor. Proposed explanations for this seasonal effect include deleterious environmental factors in the winter (such as temperature, nutritional deficiencies, infectious agents); a genetic factor in those with a propensity for schizophrenia that protects against infection and other insults and thus increases the likelihood of survival; and more frequent conception in the spring and summer by the parents of persons with schizophrenia.

Although no experimental testing has been conducted, studies appear to favor the harmful-effects hypothesis that schizophrenia involves infectious agents, but the other hypotheses have not been ruled out conclusively. Although some studies in the southern hemisphere confirm a higher birth rate for schizophrenic persons in winter than in other seasons, further study of that hypothesis is needed. There are a number of methodological problems with previous studies. If there are statistically significant increases of schizophrenic births during the southern hemisphere winter, environmental factors should be favored over sociocultural ones. Whether winter- and summer-born persons with schizophrenia differ is not clear, but that would not necessarily be expected if the causative agent is active all year but more active in the colder months.

When compared with controls, persons with schizophrenia as a group, and especially male infants, experience a greater number of birth complications. Some studies have also reported a relationship between perinatal complications and early onset of disease, negative symptoms, and poorer prognosis. The crucial factor appears to be transient perinatal hypoxia, although not all infants so affected later develop a psychiatric disorder. There is, however, a general trend toward psychopathology in persons who have suffered obstetrical complications; such events appear to increase the vulnerability to development of schizophrenia and probably are not a specific cause. Some have proposed that complications at birth may be the result of preexisting fetal neurodevelopmental abnormalities or a vulnerability to such abnormalities. No prospective studies have been done, and retrospective case control studies may be biased if informants interviewed about a relative with schizophrenia try harder to remember birth complications than do informants reporting on healthy controls. Obstetrical records often refer only to severe complications.

Social class can be specified in various ways using some combinations of income, occupation, education, and place of residence. In previous studies *the prevalence and number of newly identified cases of schizophrenia have been reported to be higher among members of the lower than the upper social classes.* Two different explanations have been proposed. One explanation is that socioenvironmental factors found at lower socioeconomic levels are a cause of schizophrenia (social causation theory). Those factors include more life event stressors, increased exposure to environmental and occupational hazards and infectious agents, poorer prenatal care, and fewer support resources if stress does occur.

The other explanation is that lower socioeconomic status is a consequence of the disorder (social selection or drift theory). The insidious onset of inherited schizophrenia is believed to preclude elevating one's status or to cause a downward drift in status. Prospective studies have shown that persons with schizophrenia have less upward mobility from generation to generation than do the general population and that there is downward drift after the onset of symptoms. Many continue to argue this unsettled question, but a recent study strongly suggests that social drift processes are more important than social causation.

A higher risk for schizophrenia among recent immigrants than in native populations has been reported, but no study to date has confirmed that immigration stress leads to schizophrenia. Indeed, the ECA study found a low prevalence of schizophrenia among Mexican-Americans followed in Los Angeles, most of whom were immigrants. The generally reported increased prevalence of schizophrenia among immigrants could result from selection (i.e., persons with schizophrenia may be more likely to leave their families); from the failure to control for such other factors as social class, age, and sex; or from the failure to compare immigrant patients to nonimmigrant controls from the same homeland. These methodological issues limit any conclusions that can be drawn from existing reports.

15.26 The answer is E (none)

Structural abnormalities in schizophrenia, such as enlarged ventricles and reduced cortical volume, are a prominent feature. *It is unclear whether cortical involvement is multifocal or diffuse.* Temporal and frontal lobe regions are certainly involved. These abnormalities are present very early in the illness. *It is too early to say, however, whether they are present from birth or develop at a later stage. Structural abnormalities may be present in a majority of patients,* although the exact percentage is unknown. The prevalence is most apparent when compared to ideally matched genetic controls. Structural abnormalities are *correlated to some degree with clinical aspects of the illness, such as cognitive deficits.* A key issue remains unresolved: what neurobiological processes account for these enigmatic changes?

15.27 The answer is E (all)

The essential neurobiological features of schizophrenia may place some constraints on plausible pathophysiological processes. First, there is a major genetic contribution. *Many genes* are likely to be involved and these *may function in part by increasing vulnerability to the deleterious effects of environmental factors. Several environmental factors have been hypothesized to increase the risk of schizophrenia, perhaps by producing subtle brain damage.* Structural abnormalities have played an important role in placing theoretical constraints on mechanisms. Since they are present from early in the illness and do not appear to progress, they may predate the onset of illness. Neuropathological data and studies of obstetric and perinatal complications support the idea that an early lesion may account for structural changes. *The apparent lack of gliosis in postmortem studies is particularly critical and implicates in utero factors.* Structural and functional neuroimaging, as well as neuropsychological data and animal studies present converging evidence for the importance of frontal and temporal regions. Finally, altered dopamine and glutamate neurotransmission is likely to play a part in the expression of psychotic symptoms.

The neurodevelopmental model can account for many of these findings. In short, some process (genetic or environmental) produces damage to selected brain areas early in life. Temporal lobe regions such as the hippocampus may be particularly vulnerable. Secondary functional abnormalities develop later. *As the prefrontal cortex matures in late adolescence, the behavioral and cognitive sequelae of subtle structural deficits become manifest.* One result is hypofrontality and cognitive impairment. Alterations in limbic and prefrontal function then produce downstream, secondary alterations in subcortical dopamine, glutamate, and other neurotransmitter systems. Dopamine dysfunction, in particular, may lead to positive psychotic symptoms. The feasibility of this model has received substantial validation from animal studies showing the delayed behavioral and neurobiological effects of minor damage to the hippocampus in neonatal rats. Observations that children at risk for schizophrenia have a number of subtle neuropsychiatric abnormalities, such as deficits in attention, motor control, and social interactions, also support the neurodevelopmental model.

15.28 The answer is C

The DSM-IV-TR diagnosis of simple deteriorative disorder (simple schizophrenia) is characterized by a gradual, insidious loss of drive, interest, ambition, and initiative. *Hallucinations and delusions are uncommon, and if those symptoms do occur, they do not persist.* Patients with simple deteriorative disorder withdraw from contact with other people, tend to stay in their rooms, avoid meeting or eating with other members of the family, stop working, and stop seeing friends. If they are still in school, their marks drop to a low level, even if they were consistently high in the past.

These patients avoid going out into the street during the day but may go for long walks alone at 2:00 or 3:00 A.M. They tend to sleep until noon or later, after staying up alone most of the night. During the early stages of the illness, they may have many somatic complaints, variously described as fatigue, nervousness, neurosis, psychosomatic disease, and laziness. *Patients are often treated for a year or more before the correct diagnosis is made. In many cases, patients with simple deteriorative disorder later become homeless.* They become increasingly shallow in their emotional responses and are quite content to drift aimlessly through life as long as they are left alone.

Although patients appear to be indifferent to their environment, they may react with sudden rage to persistent nagging by family members. The immediate reason for admission of patients with simple schizophrenia to a hospital is often an outburst of violence directed against their mothers or fathers for a trivial reason.

Patients with simple deteriorative disorder may resemble personalities of the schizoid type. The distinguishing feature is the disorder makes its appearance at some time during or after puberty and from then on goes on to definite deterioration; personality deviations usually start earlier and remain the same over the years.

To meet the ICD-10 diagnostic criteria for simple schizophrenia, the individual must show over a period of at least 1 year all of the following manifestations: (1) a significant and consistent change in the overall quality of some aspect of personal behavior such as loss of drive and interest; (2) gradual appearance and deepening of negative symptoms such as marked apathy; and (3) a marked decline in social, scholastic, or occupational performance.

15.29 The answer is C

Recent studies have established that *the diagnosis of childhood schizophrenia may be based on the same symptoms used for adult schizophrenia.* What characterizes childhood schizophrenia is not the nature but the dramatic intensity of its symptoms. *Its onset is usually insidious, its course tends to be chronic, and the prognosis is mostly unfavorable.* Briefly, it resembles the typical kraepelinian case of dementia precox. What gives childhood schizophrenia unique importance for research is the observation that anatomical features of the brain that are often associated with adult-onset schizophrenia (e.g., enlarged ventricles) are also present in this early-onset form of the disease. Neurobiological studies of children with schizophrenia may therefore provide significant clues to the developmental pathogenesis of adult-onset schizophrenia.

15.30 The answer is B

Patients with schizophrenia are more violent as a group than the general population. This is particularly a problem for patients with the paranoid type who may act quite suddenly and impulsively on a delusional idea. *Patients with paranoia tend to be intelligent and capable of forming plans; therefore, they represent a much greater risk than individuals who are disorganized and cannot plan an effective attack. Despite earlier beliefs, command hallucinations do not appear to play a particularly important role in violence.* Violence between patients in hospitals frequently results from the attacking patient's mistaken belief that another patient is behaving in a threatening way or getting physically too close. *Studies have revealed that violence in a hospital setting can result from undiagnosed neuroleptic-induced acute akathisia.* Persistently violent inpatients often do well in special treatment units that provide a more structured program and a less crowded environment. The patients who fail to respond to this kind of care usually show neurological signs in addition to their diagnosis.

Unfortunately, it is exceedingly difficult to prevent most schizophrenic homicides, because there is usually no clear warning. Most of the homicides come as a horrifying surprise. Patients who are known to be paranoid with homicidal tendencies should not, as a rule, be allowed to move about freely as long as they retain their delusions and their aggressive tension.

15.31 The answer is B

15.32 The answer is D

Mr. G has a long-standing illness characterized by periods of hallucinations and delusions. He is socially isolated and not working. *The most likely diagnosis is schizophrenia.* There is no description of current or past mood symptoms that would make a diagnosis of schizoaffective disorder reasonable, and the presence of prominent hallucinations is inconsistent with a diagnosis of delusional disorder. The designation of the subtype of schizophrenia is based on the current episode. Although Mr. G attempt not to move superficially resembles catatonia, his openly discussing with the examiner his reasons for remaining still is most uncharacteristic of the catatonic subtype. The continued presence of delusions and auditory and visual hallucinations *makes the diagnosis of an undifferentiated subtype more appropriate.*

Mr. G is lucky in having a good response to many different antipsychotics. There is no reason to suppose that an atypical agent will help him more than conventional antipsychotics. His multiple relapses result from his failure to fill prescriptions because of his drinking, and a long-acting depot medication is not likely to disturb that pattern. It is probable that he would get an injection, start drinking, and not go for his next injection. *Alcohol counseling is, therefore, of the greatest importance* in giving him some stability and freedom from the ongoing cycle of relapse and rehospitalization. Vocational counseling and increased socialization may help, but only if his drinking is brought under control.

Answers 15.33–15.36

15.33 The answer is B

15.34 The answer is B

15.35 The answer is A

15.36 The answer is A
Emil Kraepelin (1856–1926) *latinized the term* démence précoce *to dementia precox*, a term that emphasized a distinct cognitive process (dementia) and the early onset (precox) that is characteristic of the disorder. Kraepelin *classified patients as being afflicted with manic-depressive psychoses, dementia precox, or paranoia.*

Eugen Bleuler (1857–1939) *coined the term "schizophrenia"* and *described the four As of schizophrenia: Associations* are loose; ideas have *autistic* qualities with meanings only the patient can understand; *affect* is restricted or flat; and the patient has conscious *ambivalent* feelings about almost everything.

Answers 15.37–15.42

15.37 The answer is B

15.38 The answer is B

15.39 The answer is A

15.40 The answer is A

15.41 The answer is A

15.42 The answer is A
Kurt Schneider (1887–1967) described a number of *first-rank symptoms* of schizophrenia that are considered of pragmatic value in making the diagnosis of schizophrenia, although they are not specific to the disease. The symptoms include *audible thoughts* (hearing one's thoughts aloud); *voices* or auditory hallucinations *commenting* on the patient's behavior; *thought withdrawal* (the removal of the patient's thoughts by others); and *the experience of having one's thoughts controlled.* Schneider pointed out that schizophrenia can be diagnosed by second-rank symptoms when accompanied by a typical clinical presentation. *Second-rank symptoms* include *sudden delusional ideas, perplexity*, and feelings of emotional impoverishment. Schneider's diagnostic criteria for schizophrenia are listed in Table 15.3.

Answers 15.43–15.47

15.43 The answer is E

15.44 The answer is A

15.45 The answer is B

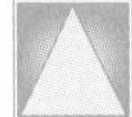

Table 15.3
Kurt Schneider's Diagnostic Criteria for Schizophrenia

1. First-rank symptoms
   a. Audible thoughts
   b. Voices arguing or discussing or both
   c. Voices commenting
   d. Somatic passivity experiences
   e. Thought withdrawal and other experiences of influenced thought
   f. Thought broadcasting
   g. Delusional perceptions
   h. All other experiences involving volition, made affects, and made impulses
2. Second-rank symptoms
   a. Other disorders of perception
   b. Sudden delusional ideas
   c. Perplexity
   d. Depressive and euphoric mood changes
   e. Feelings of emotional impoverishment
   f. ". . . and several others as well"

15.46 The answer is D

15.47 The answer is C
Occasionally, patients with schizophrenia *create a completely new expression, a neologism*, when they need to express a concept for which no ordinary word exists.

A woman with schizophrenia who had been hospitalized for several years kept repeating (in an otherwise quite rational conversation) the word "polamolalittersjitterstittersleelitla." Her psychiatrist asked her to spell it out, and she proceeded to explain the meaning of the various components, which she insisted were to be used as one word. "Polamolalitters" was intended to recall the disease poliomyelitis, because the patient wanted to indicate that she felt she was suffering from a serious disease affecting her nervous system; the component "litters" stood for untidiness or messiness, the way she felt inside; "jitterstitters" reflected her inner nervousness and lack of ease; "leelita" was a reference to the French *le lit là* (that bed there), meaning that she both depended on and felt handicapped by her illness. That single neologistic production thus enabled the patient to express—in a condensed, autistic manner—information about her preoccupations and apprehensions that otherwise would have taken a whole paragraph to explain in common language.

It is assumed that the disorders of language reflect an underlying disorder of thinking. A variety of features have been reported by clinicians for the last 100 years as characteristic of this syndrome. These include the loss of the logical relations between antecedent and subsequent associations that is termed *loosening of associations.* Words can be combined on the basis of sound rather than on meaning called *clang association. Verbigeration* involves the use of words in a stereotypically repetitive fashion. This rare symptom is found almost exclusively in chronic and very regressed patients with schizophrenia. It consists of the senseless repetition of the same words or phrases, and it may go on for days. Like neologisms and echolalia, verbigeration is a rare symptom today and is almost restricted to long-term institutionalized schizophrenia patients. Many psychiatrists working with schizophrenia patients in the community may never encounter these manifestations of deterioration.

Echolalia involves the repetition of the examiner's words.

Examiner: How did you sleep last night?

Patient: I slept well last night.

Examiner: Can you tell me the name of your head nurse?

Patient: The name of my head nurse is Miss Brown.

Echolalia seems to signal two facts, patients are aware of some shortcomings in their ideation and they are striving to maintain active rapport with the interviewer. They act much like someone learning a new language who answers the teacher's questions with as many of the teacher's words in the strange language as they can possibly manage.

Thought blocking involves the sudden and inexplicable blocking of thoughts manifested by the patient's inability to speak.

Loosening of associations is based on the late 19th century association theory. According to association theory language is determined by purpose. This purposefulness is often lost in schizophrenic speech. A sentence completion test illustrates the point. The sentence to be completed was "The man fell on the street. . . ." The patient's response was "because of World War I." Although the thought of falling might be associated with falling in combat, it was an inappropriate association for the stimulus.

It can be helpful to look at disorders of association as disorders of the word and disorders of the sentence. Disorders of the word range from loss of symbolic meaning of the word, as in clang associations, to inability to maintain the correct semantic context for a word, to approximate use of words, to the creation of new words. Disorders of the sentence include associative failures and failures of system placement. Most words have multiple meanings. Even a simple question such as "Where is your husband?" must be answered in terms of the frame of reference. In one context, the question might ask for the physical location of the husband, and in another context it might ask for his identification in his graduating class picture. An example of system shifting was reported by Silvano Arieti. Commenting on the Japanese attack on Pearl Harbor, a patient said, "The next time they may attack Diamond Harbor or Emerald Harbor." The patient had lost the contextual system of Pearl Harbor as a geographical military base and had substituted a contextual system in which pearls are precious stones.

Answers 15.48–15.52

15.48 The answer is E

15.49 The answer is A

15.50 The answer is D

15.51 The answer is B

15.52 The answer is C

The motor symptom *echopraxia* is analogous to echolalia in the verbal sphere. It is the *imitation of movements* and gestures of the person the patient is observing.

Negativism refers to a patient's *unwillingness to cooperate without any apparent reason* for that lack of cooperation. It does not appear to be related to fatigue, depression, suspicion, or anger. Negativism may even take the form of unwillingness to follow a request for a physical movement. It can become so severe that the patient will do the opposite of what is asked. For example, when asked to raise an arm, he or she may lower it.

Anhedonia is a particularly distressing symptom. Sandor Rado, M. D. considered anhedonia to be a cardinal feature of schizophrenia. There is frequently a *diminution in the patient's ability to experience pleasure* and, in some severe cases, even to imagine a pleasant feeling. Patients may not meet the criteria for the diagnosis of clinical depression but will describe an emotional emptiness or barrenness. Anhedonia can become unbearable enough to contribute to a suicide attempt.

Stereotyped behavior is primarily seen in patients with chronic schizophrenia, including those in the community. *At times it may take a motoric form and be expressed in a repetitive pattern of walking or pacing*. It may also be demonstrated in repetitive strange gestures, which may or may not have a magical meaning to the patient. Finally, *in language one can have the repetition of phrases or comments for long periods*. This is separate from perseveration and distinct from verbigeration. Interestingly, when schizophrenia patients are engaged psychosocially, this symptom tends to diminish. It appears to be a consequence of psychosocial isolation.

Functional inhibition of speech and vocalization may last for hours or days, but before the use of modern treatment methods, it often lasted for years in patients with catatonic schizophrenia. Many of these patients tend to be monosyllabic and answer questions as briefly as possible. They attempt to restrict contact with the interviewer without being altogether uncooperative.

16

Other Psychotic Disorders

The disorders in this chapter occur less frequently than schizophrenia but can have profound short term or long-term psychosocial consequences. As a group, they are more poorly understood than schizophrenia, and can be difficult to distinguish from other forms of psychosis.

Brief psychotic disorder is a psychotic condition involving the sudden onset of psychotic symptoms which lasts one day or more, but less than one month. Remission is full, and the individual returns to the premorbid level of functioning. Schizophreniform disorder is conceptualized as a variant of schizophrenia. Patients with this condition are floridly psychotic, with a prodromal, active and residual phase between one and six months. If the duration of illness extends beyond six months, the diagnosis might be changed to schizophrenia. Risk factors include unemployment, residence in a metropolitan area, low income, being separated, widowed or divorced, young age, low education, living with non relatives, obstetric and early neonatal complications, childhood emotional problems and cannabis use.

Delusional disorders, once referred to as paranoid disorders, are diagnosed when the individual reports non-bizarre delusions for more than one month without prominent hallucinations, and with a relative preservation of functioning. Non-bizarre delusions are plausible, understandable, and derive from ordinary life experience. The course appears to be less chronic, with less associated deterioration in functioning than the course of schizophrenic patients. Shared psychotic disorder, commonly referred to as a folie a deux, refers to the condition in which two individuals with a close and generally long-term relationship, share the same delusional belief, although it may involve more than two individuals, including entire families.

Schizoaffective disorder combines the symptoms of mood disorders and schizophrenia. It may be a neurodevelopmental disorder, and gender differences parallel those seen in mood disorders. While almost 85 percent of women experience some type of mood disturbance during the postpartum period, postpartum psychosis is rare. The student should be familiar with it because infanticide may occur. Hormonal hypotheses have been posited to explain its etiology, which remains unknown however.

Knowledge of the culture-bound syndromes is increasingly important. The growing wave of immigration from developing countries to the United States over the past few decades has meant that doctors in the United States need to acquire a basic understanding of the formulations of health and illness in the culture from which their patients come. The course of these syndromes is generally favorable, and most present as self-limiting episodes after stressful.

The student should study the questions and answers below for a useful review of these disorders.

HELPFUL HINTS

Students should know the psychotic syndromes and other terms listed here.

- age of onset
- amok
- antipsychotic drugs:
  - clozapine
  - dopamine receptor antagonists
- Arctic hysteria
- atypical psychoses
- autoscopic psychosis
- *bouffée délirante*
- brief psychotic disorder
- Norman Cameron
- Capgras's syndrome
- Clérambault's syndrome
- conjugal paranoia
- Cotard's syndrome
- course
- culture-bound syndromes
- Cushing's syndrome
- delusional disorder
- delusions
- denial
- differential diagnosis
- double insanity
- EEG and CT scan
- erotomania
- Fregoli's syndrome
- Ganser's syndrome
- good-prognosis schizophrenia
- heutoscopy
- homicide
- ICD-10
- incidence
- inclusion and exclusion criteria
- *koro*
- Gabriel Langfeldt
- lifetime prevalence
- limbic system and basal ganglia
- lithium
- lycanthropy
- marital status
- mental status examination
- mood-congruent and –incongruent psychotic features
- neuroendocrine function
- neurological conditions
- neuropsychological testing
- nihilistic delusion
- paranoia
- paranoid
- pseudocommunity
- paranoid states
- paraphrenia
- *piblokto*
- postpartum blues

- postpartum psychosis
- postpsychotic depressive disorder of schizophrenia
- prognostic variables
- projection
- pseudocommunity
- psychodynamic formulation
- psychosis of association
- psychotherapy
- psychotic disorder not otherwise specified
- reaction formation
- reduplicative paramnesia
- schizoaffective disorder
- schizophreniform disorder
- Daniel Paul Schreber
- SES
- shared psychotic disorder
- significant stressor
- simple schizophrenia
- suicidal incidence
- *suk-yeong*
- TRH stimulation test
- wihtigo psychosis

QUESTIONS

Directions

Each of the questions or incomplete statements below is followed by five suggested responses or completions. Select the *one* that is *best* in each case.

16.1 Attaque de nervios:

A. is most common in Puerto Ricans
B. usually has no precipitating stressful event
C. usually features a sense of being out of control
D. is usually associated with acute fear
E. usually results in a deteriorating course

16.2 The postpartum blues

A. occur in up to 50 percent of women after childbirth
B. are self-limited
C. begin shortly after childbirth and lessens in severity over the course of a week
D. are considered to be normal
E. all of the above

16.3 Postpartum psychosis

A. occurs more commonly in multigravida women
B. is rarely correlated with perinatal complications
C. almost always begins within eight weeks of delivery
D. usually occurs abruptly, with no prodromal psychotic symptoms
E. is essentially an episode of a psychotic disorder

16.4 Erotomania, the delusional disorder in which the person makes repeated efforts to contact the object of the delusion, through letter, phone call, and stalking, is also referred to as

A. Cotard's syndrome
B. Clérambault's syndrome
C. Fregoli's syndrome
D. Ganser's syndrome
E. Capgras's syndrome

16.5 A 40-year-old single unemployed man is referred by his primary care physician because of repeated consultations related to his complaint of hair loss. Multiple dermatologists had evaluated the patient, found no pathology, and told him that the minimal hair loss was normal, but he refused to accept their judgment and demanded further consultations. He told one of them "everything else about me is fine. This needs to be corrected for completeness." He had become increasingly indebted financially to pay for consultations with out-of network providers.

The most likely diagnosis in this man is:

A. delusional disorder, somatic type
B. hypochondriasis
C. body dysmorphic disorder
D. paranoid schizophrenia
E. psychotic depression

16.6 All of the following are true statements about postpartum psychosis *except*

A. The risk is increased if the patient had a recent mood disorder.
B. Hallucinations involve voices telling the patient to kill her baby.
C. It is found in 1 to 2 per 1,000 deliveries.
D. Generally, it is not considered a psychiatric emergency.
E. Delusional material may involve the idea that the baby is dead.

16.7 In schizoaffective disorder, all of the following variables indicate a poor prognosis *except*

A. depressive type
B. no precipitating factor
C. a predominance of psychotic symptoms
D. bipolar type
E. early onset

16.8 A 17-year-old high school junior was brought to the emergency room by her distraught mother, who was at a loss to understand her daughter's behavior. Two days earlier, the patient's father had been buried: he had died of a sudden myocardial infarction earlier in the week. The patient had become wildly agitated at the cemetery, screaming uncontrollably and needing to be restrained by relatives. She was inconsolable at home, sat rocking in a corner, and talked about a devil that had come to claim her soul. Before her father's death, her mother reported, she was a "typical teenager, popular, a very good student, but sometimes prone to overreacting." The girl had no previous psychiatric history.

The most likely diagnosis is:

A. grief
B. brief psychotic disorder

C. schizophrenia
D. substance intoxication
E. delusional disorder

16.9 True statements concerning the treatment of shared psychotic disorder include all of the following *except*

A. Recovery rates have been reported to be as low as 10 percent.
B. The submissive person commonly requires treatment with antipsychotic drugs.
C. Psychotherapy for nondelusional members of the patient's family should be undertaken.
D. Separation of the submissive person from the dominant person is the primary intervention.
E. The submissive person and the dominant person usually move back together after treatment.

16.10 Most studies of normal pregnant women indicate that the percentage who report the "blues" in the early postpartum period is about

A. 10 percent
B. 25 percent
C. 50 percent
D. 75 percent
E. 100 percent

16.11 All of the following are associated with a good prognosis in a brief psychotic disorder *except*

A. Sudden onset of symptoms
B. No affective symptoms
C. Confusion during psychosis
D. Severe precipitating stressor
E. Few premorbid schizoid traits

16.12 The differential diagnosis of brief psychotic disorder includes

A. substance-induced psychotic disorder
B. psychotic disorder due to a general medical condition
C. severe personality disorders
D. malingering
E. all of the above

16.13 Delusional disorder

A. is less common than schizophrenia
B. is caused by frontal lobe lesions
C. is an early stage of schizophrenia
D. usually begins by age 20
E. is more common in men than in women

16.14 The best-documented risk factor for delusional disorder is

A. sensory impairment
B. recent immigration
C. advanced age
D. family history
E. social isolation

16.15 Evidence that suggests delusional disorder is a separate entity from schizophrenia or mood disorders includes

A. epidemiological data
B. family or genetic studies
C. natural history of the disorder
D. premorbid personality data
E. all of the above

16.16 Delusional disorder may include

A. tactile hallucinations
B. olfactory hallucinations
C. auditory hallucinations
D. visual hallucinations
E. all of the above

16.17 True statements about patients with delusional disorder, erotomanic type, include:

A. they exhibit what has been called "paradoxical conduct"
B. the course of the disorder is invariably chronic
C. separation from the love object is usually not an effective treatment
D. women predominate in forensic populations
E. all of the above

16.18 Of the following somatic treatments for delusional disorder, which is considered the *least* likely to be successful?

A. dopamine receptor antagonists
B. serotonin-dopamine antagonists
C. selective serotonin reuptake inhibitors
D. electroconvulsive treatment
E. all of the above are considered equally effective

16.19 Puerperal psychosis

A. has a prevalence of 10 to 15 percent
B. usually does not occur until 2 to 3 months postpartum
C. usually has insidious onset
D. is most likely to occur in patients with a previous history of the disorder
E. all of the above

16.20 Which of the following statements is *true* about brief psychotic disorder?

A. Approximately 10 percent of patients diagnosed retain the diagnosis.
B. Fifty percent of the cases evolve into either schizophrenia or major mood disorder.
C. There are clear distinguishing features between brief psychotic disorder and acute-onset schizophrenia on initial presentation.
D. Poor prognosis is associated with emotional turmoil
E. None of the above

16.21 Ms. R, a 24-year-old woman, is brought to an emergency room by her father with a chief complaint, "I have bugs all over my body and in my hair. They're making me weaker." Two weeks earlier, the apartment Ms. R shares with a roommate flooded after a pipe burst. Following the flood, the apartment was infested with insects. At one point, Ms. R had insects crawling in an open wound on her arm. The apartment was cleaned and fumigated, but Ms. R persisted in believing bugs were everywhere. She washed herself with alcohol several times a day and avoided seeing friends and family because of her fear that the infestation would spread to others. She believed that a cocoon was being spread over her body and that insects were crawling over her internal organs. She spent most of the last 3 days immersed in a bathtub of water. Her roommate became alarmed and called her father, who brought her to the emergency room. She denies sleep or appetite changes, and has not experienced auditory or visual hallucinations.

Ms. R had a history of outpatient treatment for anorexia nervosa and a major depressive episode. When she was 16 she became withdrawn, tearful, preoccupied with death, had difficulty sleeping, and lost 10 pounds. She was treated with individual psychotherapy and citalopram pharmacotherapy. All symptoms of depression resolved within a month and she had no recurrence. When she was 19, coinciding with a brief modeling career, she began a severe diet, exercised intensively, and lost 25 pounds. Her menses ceased for 6 months. She resumed psychotherapy but not medication. Her modeling career ended abruptly when the agency representing her went out of business. She began a romantic relationship and went back to school. Gradually, she lost interest in dieting, her weight stabilized, and menses returned. She experimented with cocaine around that time, but claims not to have used illicit drugs for over 4 years. She drinks no more than one or two glasses of wine a week. She has been working as an administrative assistant for a recording studio and was going to work regularly and working without difficulties until the day of the flood and the infestation. She has not returned to work since.

Her blood pressure is 115/75, heart rate 70, and temperature 37°C. She weighs 125 pounds and is 5 feet 6 inches tall. Physical examination is unremarkable. Routine laboratory studies, including liver function tests, are within normal limits. A urine toxicology screen is negative. She appears apprehensive. She describes feeling bugs crawling on her skin and she believes that insects have entered her body and are slowly enveloping her in a cocoon. She denies auditory hallucinations. Her thoughts are logical and goal-directed. She is alert and oriented.

Which of the following is the most likely diagnosis?

A. Schizophrenia
B. Cocaine-induced psychotic disorder
C. Major depression with psychotic symptoms
D. Delusional disorder
E. Brief psychotic episode

16.22 The patient's belief in the case above that insects were crawling on her arm is called

A. dyskinesia
B. illusion
C. formication
D. paresthesia
E. none of the above

Directions

Each group of questions below consists of lettered headings followed by a list of numbered words or statements. For each numbered word or statement, select the *one* lettered heading that is most closely associated with it. Each lettered heading may be selected once, more than once, or not at all.

Questions 16.23–16.27

A. Delusions of guilt
B. Delusions secondary to perceptual disturbances
C. Grandiose delusions
D. Bizarre delusions of being controlled
E. Delusions of jealousy

16.23 Delusional disorder
16.24 Schizophrenia
16.25 Mania
16.26 Depressive disorders
16.27 Cognitive disorders

Questions 16.28–16.32

A. Paranoid personality disorder
B. Delusional disorder
C. Schizophrenia
D. Manic episode
E. Major depressive episode

16.28 Psychomotor retardation
16.29 Thought broadcasting
16.30 Easy distractibility with an elevated, expansive, or irritable mood
16.31 Nonbizarre persecutory or grandiose delusions
16.32 Suspiciousness and mistrust of people, without psychotic symptoms

Questions 16.33–16.37

A. Cortical impairment
B. Subcortical impairment

16.33 Simple, transient delusions
16.34 Persecutory delusions
16.35 Elaborate and systematic delusions
16.36 Delusions with strong affective components
16.37 Delusions associated with Alzheimer's disease

ANSWERS

16.1 The answer is C

A general feature of attaque de nervios *is a sense of being out of control*. Attaque de nervios is reported in Latinos from throughout the Caribbean, and is *not most common among Puerto Ricans*.

It also occurs in South America and Mediterranean countries. *It frequently occurs as a direct result of a stressful event* relating to the family. It most closely resembles a panic attack, but unlike panic attacks, *it is associated with a precipitating event*. Panic attacks occur spontaneously. Persons may experience amnesia for what occurred during the attack, but they otherwise return rapidly to their usual level of functioning.

16.2 The answer is E (all)

The so-called postpartum blues is *a normal condition* that occurs in up *to 50 percent of women after childbirth*. Postpartum blues is *self-limited*, lasts only a few days, and is characterized by tearfulness, fatigue, anxiety and irritability that *begin shortly after childbirth and lessen in severity over the course of a week*.

16.3 The answer is C

The symptoms of postpartum psychosis most *often begins within eight weeks of the delivery*. About 50 to 60 percent of affected women with postpartum psychosis have just had *their first child*, and in that group, *half of the newborns have perinatal complications*. The onset of florid psychotic symptoms is *usually preceded by prodromal signs*, such as insomnia, restlessness, agitation, lability of mood, and mild cognitive deficits. The most robust data indicate that *postpartum psychosis is related to a mood disorder*, usually a bipolar disorder. Relatives of those with postpartum psychosis have an incidence of mood disorders that is similar to the incidence in relatives of persons with mood disorders.

16.4 The answer is B

Erotomania, the delusional disorder in which the person makes repeated efforts to contact the object of the delusion, through letters, phone calls, gifts, visits, surveillance, and even stalking, is also called *Clérambault's syndrome*. Most patients with erotomania are women. In forensic samples in which harm is done to another person, most are men. In *Cotard's syndrome*, patients may believe that they have lost everything: possessions, strength, and even bodily organs. *Fregoli's syndrome* is the delusion that a persecutor is taking on a variety of faces, like an actor. *Ganser's syndrome* is the voluntary production of severe psychiatric symptoms, sometimes described as the giving of approximate answers. *Capgras's syndrome* is the delusion that familiar people have been replaced by identical impostors.

16.5 The answer is A

Delusional disorder with somatic delusions has been called monosymptomatic hypochondriacal psychosis. The condition differs from other conditions with hypochondriacal symptoms in the degree of reality impairment. In delusional disorder the delusion is fixed, unarguable and presented intensely, because the patient is totally convinced of the physical nature of the disorder. In contrast, persons with *hypochondriasis* often admit that their fear if illness is largely groundless. Patients with *body dysmorphic disorder* have a pervasive subjective feeling of ugliness of some aspect of their appearance despite a normal or nearly normal appearance. They also strongly believe that they are unattractive or repulsive, which this patient does not. The patient has no hallucinations, with no significant social or occupation dysfunction, making *paranoid schizophrenia* unlikely. In the absence of mood symptoms (loss of appetite, change in sleep, *depressed mood*) there is no data to support a diagnosis of a mood disorder.

16.6 The answer is D

Postpartum psychosis is found in 1 to 2 per 1,000 deliveries. The risk is increased if the patient or the patient's mother had a previous postpartum illness or mood disorder. The symptoms are usually experienced within days of delivery and almost always within the first 8 weeks after giving birth. The patient begins to complain of insomnia, restlessness, and fatigue, and she shows lability of mood with tearfulness. Later symptoms include suspiciousness, confusion, incoherence, irrational statements, and obsessive concerns about the baby's health. *Delusional material may involve the idea that the baby is dead* or defective. The birth may be denied, or ideas of persecution, influence, or perversity may be expressed. *Hallucinations may involve voices telling the patient to kill her baby. Postpartum psychosis is a psychiatric emergency*. In one study, 5 percent of patients killed themselves, and 4 percent killed the baby. Postpartum psychosis is not to be confused with postpartum "blues."

16.7 The answer is D

The course and the prognosis of schizoaffective disorder are variable. As a group, patients with this disorder have a prognosis intermediate between patients with schizophrenia and patients with mood disorders. Schizoaffective disorder, *bipolar type*, typically has a better prognosis. A poor prognosis is associated with the *depressive type* of schizoaffective disorder. A poor prognosis is also associated with the following variables: *no precipitating factor, a predominance of psychotic symptoms, early* or insidious *onset*, a poor premorbid history, and a positive family history of schizophrenia.

16.8 The answer is B

The sudden onset of a florid psychotic episode immediately after a marked psychosocial stressor, such as the death of a loved one, in the absence of increasing psychopathology before the stressor indicates the diagnosis of *brief psychotic disorder*. Grief is an expected and normal reaction to the loss of a loved one. The girl's reaction, however, was not only more severe than would be expected (wildly agitated, screaming) but also involved psychotic symptoms (the devil). Typically, the psychotic symptoms in brief psychotic disorder last for more than a day but no more than a month. In *schizophrenia* the symptoms last for at least 6 months. *Substance intoxication* can mimic brief psychotic disorder, but the case presented shows no evidence of substance use. *Delusional disorder* presents with nonbizarre delusions of at least 1 month's duration, with otherwise relatively normal behavior.

16.9 The answer is C

Psychotherapy for nondelusional *members of the patient's family is usually not necessary.* Clinical reports vary, but the prognosis is guarded—recovery rates have been reported to be *as low as 10 percent.* The *submissive person often requires treatment with antipsychotic drugs,* as does the dominant person. *Separation* of the submissive person from the dominant person is the primary intervention. The submissive person and the dominant person usually *move back together after treatment.*

16.10 The answer is C

Postpartum psychosis should not be confused with postpartum "blues," a normal condition that *occurs in about 50 percent of women after childbirth*. The "blues" are self-limited, last only a few days, and are characterized by tearfulness, fatigue, anxiety, and irritability that begin shortly after childbirth and lessen in severity each day postpartum. Postpartum psychosis is characterized by agitation, severe depression, and thoughts of infanticide.

16.11 The answer is B

Good prognostic features for brief psychotic disorders include: good premorbid adjustment, *few premorbid schizoid traits, a severe precipitating stressor*, the *sudden onset of symptoms, affective symptoms, confusion and perplexity during psychosis*, little affective blunting, a short duration of symptoms, and the absence of schizophrenic relatives.

16.12 The answer is E (all)

Sharing rapid onset of symptoms, brief psychotic disorder must be differentiated from *substance-induced psychotic disorders* and *psychotic disorders due to a general medical condition*. A thorough medical evaluation, including a physical examination, laboratory studies, and brain imaging, will help rule out many of those conditions. With only cross-sectional information, brief psychotic disorder is difficult to differentiate from other types of functional psychosis.

The relationship between brief psychotic disorder and both schizophrenia and affective disorders remains uncertain. DSM-IV-TR has made the distinction between brief psychotic disorder and schizophreniform disorder clearer by now requiring a full month of psychotic symptoms for the latter. If psychotic symptoms are present longer than 1 month, the diagnoses of schizophreniform disorder, schizoaffective disorder, schizophrenia, mood disorders with psychotic features, delusional disorder, and psychotic disorder not otherwise specified need to be entertained. If psychotic symptoms of sudden onset are present for less than a month in response to an obvious stressor, the diagnosis of brief psychotic disorder is strongly suggested. Other diagnoses to differentiate include factitious disorder, *malingering, and severe personality disorders,* with consequent transient psychosis possible.

16.13 The answer is A

Delusional disorder *is less common than schizophrenia.* Its prevalence in the United States is estimated to be 0.03 percent—in contrast with schizophrenia, 1 percent, and mood disorders, 5 percent.

The neuropsychiatric approach to delusional disorder derives from the observation that delusions are a common symptom in many neurological conditions, particularly those involving the limbic system and the basal ganglia. *No evidence indicates that the disorder is caused by frontal lobe lesions.* Long-term follow-up of patients with delusional disorder has found that their diagnoses are rarely revised as schizophrenia or mood disorders; hence, delusional disorder *is not an early stage of schizophrenia* or mood disorders. Moreover, delusional disorder has a later onset than does schizophrenia or mood disorders. The mean age of onset is 40 years; the disorder *does not usually begin by age 20.* The disorder *is slightly more common in women than in men.*

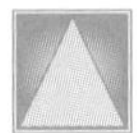

Table 16.1
Risk Factors Associated with Delusional Disorder

Advanced age
Sensory impairment/isolation
Family history
Social isolation
Personality features (e.g., unusual interpersonal sensitivity)
Recent immigration

16.14 The answer is D

The cause of delusional disorder is unknown. The epidemiological and clinical literature suggests that certain risk factors may be relevant to etiology and deserve further research elaboration. These risk factors are found in Table 16.1. Whether they are risk predictors or simply characteristics or markers of the disorder, is unknown. *Familial psychiatric disorder,* including delusional disorder, is the *best-documented risk factor at present.*

16.15 The answer is E (all)

An issue that is central to attributing causation is whether delusional disorder represents a separate group of conditions or is an atypical form of schizophrenic and mood disorders. The relevant data come from a limited number of studies and are inconclusive. *Epidemiology data suggest that delusional disorder is a separate condition;* it is far less prevalent than schizophrenic or mood disorders; age of onset is later than in schizophrenia, although men tend to experience the illness at earlier ages than women; and the sex ratio is different from that of mood disorder, which occurs disproportionately among women. Findings *from family or genetic studies* also support the theory that delusional disorder is a distinct entity. If delusional disorder is simply an unusual form of schizophrenic or mood disorders, the incidence of these latter conditions in family studies of delusional disorder patient probands should be higher than that of the general population. However, this has not been a consistent finding. A recent study concluded that patients with delusional disorder are more likely to have family members who show suspiciousness, jealousy, secretiveness, even paranoid illness, than families of controls. Other investigative efforts have found paranoid personality disorder and avoidant personality disorder to be more common in the relatives of patients with delusional disorder than in the relatives of controls or of schizophrenic patients. A recent study documented modest evidence for an increased risk of alcoholism among the relatives of patients with delusional disorder as compared to probands with schizophrenia, probands with psychotic disorder not otherwise specified, and probands with schizophreniform disorder.

Investigations into *patient's natural history* also lend support to the suggestion that delusional disorder is a distinct category: age of onset appears to be later than in schizophrenia and outcome generally is better for delusional disorder patients than for schizophrenia patients. Although fraught with methodological shortcomings, *premorbid personality data* indicate that schizophrenia patients and patients with delusional disorder differ early in life. The former are more likely to be introverted, schizoid, and submissive; the latter extroverted, dominant, and hypersensitive. Delusional disorder patients may have below-average intelligence. Precipitating factors, especially related to social isolation, conflicts of conscience, and immigration, are more closely associated to delusional disorder than schizophrenia. These characteristics support the view that environmental factors may play an important etiological role. Clinical characteristics such as greater intensity of delusions, uncommon occurrence of negative symptoms, and possible association with cerebrovascular disorder in late-onset cases also suggest differences from late-onset schizophrenia. Recent observations of successful treatment with pimozide (Orap) in several subtypes of delusional disorders suggest the possibility of a common pathogenetic mechanism in these disorders. Follow-up studies indicate that the diagnosis of delusional disorder remains fairly stable: only a small proportion of cases (3 to 22 percent) are diagnosed as having schizophrenia, and even fewer (6 percent) are diagnosed as having a mood disorder. Outcome in terms of hospitalization and occupational adjustment is markedly more favorable for delusional disorder than for schizophrenia. When social or occupational functioning is poor in delusional disorder, it generally occurs as the result of the delusional beliefs themselves, not because of cognitive impairment or negative symptoms.

The evidence argues in favor of the distinctiveness of delusional disorder, but it is likely that at least some patients diagnosed as having delusional disorder will develop schizophrenia or mood disorders. Hence, current clinical criteria have limitations and need improvement, which may be possible with the use of laboratory techniques or more specified clinical definitions. Furthermore, the data suggest that delusional disorder is relatively chronic and is probably biologically distinct from other psychotic disorders.

16.16 The answer is E (all)

Generally in delusional disorders, the patient's delusions are well systematized and have been developed logically. The person *may experience auditory or visual hallucinations,* but these are not prominent features. *Tactile or olfactory hallucinations* may be present and prominent if they are related to the delusional content or theme; examples are the sensation of being infested by bugs or parasites, associated with delusions of infestation; and the belief that one's body odor is foul, associated with somatic delusions. The person's behavioral and emotional responses to the delusion appear to be appropriate. Impairment of functioning is not marked and personality deterioration is minimal, if it occurs at all. General behavior is neither obviously odd nor bizarre.

16.17 The answer is A

Patients with erotomania have delusions of secret lovers. Most frequently the patient is a woman, but men are also susceptible to the delusion. The patient believes that a suitor, usually more socially prominent than herself, is in love with her. The delusion becomes the central focus of the patient's existence and the onset can be sudden.

Erotomania, the *psychose passionelle,* is also referred to as Clérambault's syndrome to emphasize its occurrence in different disorders. Besides being the key symptom in some cases of delusional disorder, it is known to occur in schizophrenia, mood disorder, and other organic disorders. There is no mention of erotomania in DSM-III: the condition was termed *atypical psychosis.* DSM-III-R reinstated the condition, and it remains in DSM-IV-TR.

Patients with erotomania frequently show certain characteristics: they are generally but not exclusively women, may be considered unattractive in appearance, are in low-level jobs, and lead withdrawn, lonely lives, being single and having few sexual contacts. They select secret lovers who are substantially different from themselves. *They exhibit what has been called "paradoxical conduct,"* the delusional phenomenon of interpreting all denials of love, no matter how clear, as secret affirmations of love. The *course may be chronic, recurrent, or brief. Separation from the love object may be the only satisfactory means of intervention.* Although men are less commonly afflicted by this condition than women, they may be more aggressive and possibly violent in their pursuit of love. Hence, *in forensic populations men with this condition predominate.* The object of aggression may not be the loved individual but companions or protectors of the love object who are viewed as trying to come between the lovers. The tendency toward violence among men with erotomania may lead initially to police rather than psychiatric contact. In certain cases resentment and rage in response to an absence of reaction from all forms of love communication may escalate to a point that the love object is in danger.

16.18 The answer is D

Delusional disorder is a psychotic disorder by definition, and the natural presumption has been that the condition would respond to antipsychotic medication. Because controlled studies are limited and the disorder is uncommon, the results required to support this practice empirically have been only partially obtained.

The disparate findings in the recent literature on delusional disorder treatment have been summarized recently, with several qualifications. Of approximately 1,000 articles published since 1961, the majority since 1980, 257 cases of delusional disorder (consistent with DSM-IV-TR criteria), of which 209 provided sufficient treatment detail to make comparison, were assessed. Overall treatment results indicated that 80.8 percent of cases either recovered fully or partially. Pimozide (the most frequently reported treatment) produced full recovery in 68.5 percent and partial recovery in 22.4 percent of cases treated, whereas there was full recovery in 22.6 percent and partial recovery in 45.3 percent of cases treated with *dopamine-receptor antagonists* that are typical neuroleptic agents (e.g., thioridazine [Mellaril], haloperidol [Haldol], chlorpromazine [Thorazine], loxapine [Loxitane], perphenazine [Trilafon], and others). The remaining cases were noncompliant with any treatment. There were no specific conclusions drawn regarding treatment with *selective serotonin reuptake inhibitors (SSRIs),* although a number of such reports have been published.

The results of treatment with the *serotonin-dopamine antagonists* (i.e., clozapine [Clozaril], risperidone [Risperdal], olanzapine [Zyprexa], and others) is preliminary. Unfortunately, systematic case series will develop slowly, but these early results suggest that the atypical neuroleptic agents may add to the available treatment options.

The impression is growing that antipsychotic drugs are effective, and a trial, especially with pimozide or a serotonin-dopamine antagonist, is warranted. Certainly, trials of antipsychotic medication make sense when the agitation, apprehension, and anxiety that accompany delusions are prominent.

Delusional disorders *respond less well generally to electroconvulsive treatment* than do major mood disorders with psychotic features. Some cases may respond to SSRIs, especially cases of body dysmorphic disorder with delusional concerns. Dopamine-receptor antagonists (particularly pimozide), serotonin-dopamine antagonists, and selective serotonin reuptake inhibitors are pharmacological agents with reports of successful use in delusional disorder.

16.19 The answer is D

Puerperal psychosis is the most severe form of postpartum psychiatric illness. In contrast to postpartum blues and depression, puerperal psychosis is a *rare event that occurs in approximately 1 to 2 per 1,000 women after childbirth*. Its presentation is often dramatic, with onset of psychosis as early as the first 48 to 72 hours postpartum. *Most women with puerperal psychosis develop symptoms within the first 2 to 4 weeks after delivery.*

In women with this disorder, psychotic symptoms and disorganized behavior are prominent and cause significant dysfunction. Puerperal psychosis *resembles a rapidly evolving affective psychosis* with restlessness, irritability, and insomnia. Women with this disorder may exhibit a rapidly shifting depressed or elated mood, disorientation or depersonalization, and disorganized behavior. Delusional beliefs often center on the infant and include delusions that the child may be defective or dying, that the infant has special powers, or that the child is either Satan or God. Auditory hallucinations that instruct the mother to harm or kill herself or her infant are sometimes reported. Although most believe that this illness is indistinguishable from an affective (or manic) psychosis, some have argued that puerperal psychosis may be clinically distinct in that it is more commonly associated with confusion and delirium than nonpuerperal psychotic mood disorder.

Although it has been difficult to identify specific demographic and psychosocial variables that consistently predict risk for postpartum illness, there is a well-defined association between all types of postpartum psychiatric illness and a personal history of mood disorder (Table 16.2). *At highest risk are women with a history of postpartum psychosis; up to 70 percent of women who have had one episode of puerperal psychosis will experience another episode following a subsequent pregnancy.* Similarly, women with histories of postpartum depression are at significant risk, with rates of postpartum depression recurrence as high as 50 percent. Women with bipolar disorders also appear to be particularly vulnerable during the postpartum period, with rates of bipolar relapse ranging from 20 to 50 percent.

16.20 The answer is B

The course of brief psychotic disorder is found in the diagnostic criteria of DSM-IV-TR. It is a psychotic episode that lasts more than 1 day but less than 1 month, with eventual return to premorbid level of functioning. *Approximately 50 percent patients diagnosed with brief psychotic disorder retain this diagnosis; the other 50 percent will evolve into either schizophrenia or a major affective disorder.* There are *no apparent distinguishing features* between brief psychotic disorder, acute-onset schizophrenia, and mood disorders with psychotic features on initial presentation. Several prognostic features have been proposed to characterize the illness, but they are inconsistent across studies. The *good prognostic features* are similar to those found in schizophreniform disorder: acute onset of psychotic symptoms, *confusion or emotional turmoil at the height of the psychotic episode,* good premorbid functioning, the presence of affective symptoms, and short duration of symptoms. There is a relative dearth of information on the recurrence of brief psychotic episodes, however, so the course and prognosis of this disorder have not been well characterized.

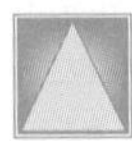

Table 16.2
History of Psychiatric Illness and Risk for Puerperal Relapse

Disorders	Risk of Relapse at Future Pregnancy (%)
Postpartum psychosis	70
Postpartum depression	50
Bipolar I disorder	20–50
Major depressive disorder	30

16.21 The answer is E

Ms. R's symptoms do not appear to be caused by a recurrence of either of the two disorders for which she had previously been treated. Although the delusions in psychotic depression are often somatic, there are no disturbances in appetite, sleep, or mood to suggest that diagnosis. Anorexia nervosa does not include psychotic symptoms (although there is some debate about whether the characteristic disturbance of body image—seeing oneself as fat rather than emaciated—should be considered delusional). More important, she is at normal weight, and a diagnosis of anorexia is not correct. The history and mental status examination strongly suggest that she has both delusions and tactile hallucinations of insects crawling on her skin. More focused questioning would help to clarify this point. Delusional disorders do not include prominent hallucinations, and the delusional belief must be nonbizarre—that is, something that could happen in everyday life. The belief of body infestation is arguably nonbizarre, but the beliefs that insects are crawling inside her and that she is being wrapped in a cocoon are bizarre by any measure. Schizophrenia requires the presence of symptoms for 6 months. Her psychotic symptoms have been present for only 2 weeks *and are best described, at least provisionally, as a brief psychotic episode*. By definition, in a brief psychotic episode symptoms are present for more than a day but less than a month. She was working well and was symptom-free up until the time of the flood and the real invasion of insects in the apartment. It appears that those events triggered the brief psychotic episode, but this can only be an item of conjecture and is unlikely to affect treatment.

It is essential to rule out a medical or drug-related cause. We are not given information about her current medical history, but her unremarkable physical examination and normal laboratory studies make a medical cause less likely.

16.22 The answer is C

Formication is a tactile hallucination involving the sensation that tiny insects are crawling over the skin. It is most commonly encountered in cocaine addiction and in delirium tremens.

Dyskinesia is defined as difficulty performing voluntary movements, as in extrapyramidal disorders.

An *illusion* is defined as the perceptual misinterpretation of a real external stimulus.

Paresthesia is an abnormal spontaneous tactile sensation, such as a burning, tingling, or pins-and-needles sensation.

Answers 16.23–16.27

16.23 The answer is E

16.24 The answer is D

16.25 The answer is C

16.26 The answer is A

16.27 The answer is B

In *delusional disorder, delusions of jealousy* are most commonly found. In *schizophrenia, bizarre delusions* may occur, for instance of being controlled by outside persons or forces and delusions of persecution. *Grandiose delusions* are most often seen in *mania* but can be observed in other psychotic disorder as well. In *depressive disorders, delusions of guilt* are especially characteristic. In *cognitive disorders,* such as dementia, *delusions secondary to perceptual disturbances* are most often evident.

Answers 16.28–16.32

16.28 The answer is E

16.29 The answer is C

16.30 The answer is D

16.31 The answer is B

16.32 The answer is A

Psychomotor retardation is a general slowing of mental and physical activity. It is often a sign of a *major depressive episode,* which is characterized by feelings of sadness, loneliness, despair, low self-esteem, and self-reproach. *Thought broadcasting* is the feeling that one's thoughts are being broadcast or projected into the environment. Such feelings are encountered in *schizophrenia*.

A patient in a *manic episode* is *easily distracted, with an elevated, expansive, or irritable mood* with pressured speech and hyperactivity.

Delusional disorder is characterized by nonbizarre *persecutory or grandiose delusions* and related disturbances in mood, thought, and behavior.

The essential feature of *paranoid personality disorder* is a long-standing *suspiciousness and mistrust of people without the presence of psychotic symptoms.* Patients with this disorder are hypersensitive and continually alert for environmental clues that will validate their original prejudicial ideas.

Answers 16.33–16.37

16.33 The answer is A

16.34 The answer is A

16.35 The answer is B

16.36 The answer is B

16.37 The answer is A

As in most psychiatric conditions, there is no evidence of localized brain pathology to correlate with clinical psychopathology in patients with delusional disorder. These patients seldom die early and show no consistent abnormalities on neurological examination. Delusions can complicate many disorders and virtually all brain disorders. Certain disorders produce delusions at rates greater than that expected in the general population: for example, epilepsy (especially of the temporal lobe), degenerative dementias (dementia of the Alzheimer's type and vascular dementia), cerebrovascular disease, extrapyramidal disorders, and traumatic brain injury.

Although many types of delusions have been reported in patients with brain disorders, there appear to be particular connections between delusion phenomenology and certain kinds of brain dysfunction. For example, patients with *more severe cortical impairment tend to experience simpler, transient, persecutory delusions*. This type of delusional experience is characteristic of conditions such as *Alzheimer's disease,* dementia, and metabolic encephalopathy that are also associated with significant cognitive disturbance. *More complex (i.e., elaborate and systematic) delusional experiences* tend to be more chronic, intensely held, resistant to treatment, and associated with neurological conditions producing less intellectual impairment and *strong affective components.* Those features occur in patients with neurological lesions involving the limbic system or *subcortical* nuclei rather than cortical areas. That, coupled with the observation of response of some patients to drug treatment, such as pimozide and other medications, provides a rational basis on which to hypothesize the presence of subcortical pathology, possibly involving systems subserving temporolimbic areas. Available evidence suggests that if there is a lesion, it will be subtle.

17 Mood Disorders

Mood disorders encompass a large group of psychiatric disorders in which pathological moods and related vegetative and psychomotor disturbances dominate the clinical picture. Known in previous editions of the *Diagnostic and Statistical Manual of Mental Disorders* as *affective disorders*, the term *mood disorders* is preferred today because it refers to sustained emotional states, not merely to the external (affective) expression of the present emotional state. Mood disorders are best considered as syndromes (rather than discrete diseases) consisting of a cluster of signs and symptoms, sustained over a period of weeks to months, that represent a marked departure from a person's habitual functioning and tend to recur, often in periodic or cyclical fashion.

Mood disorders can sometimes be difficult to diagnose, given the subjective nature of the symptoms. All people have normal periods of feeling either blue or elated, and most of these obviously are not diagnosable as disorders. A mood disorder is characterized by the intensity, duration, and severity of the symptoms. People with mood disorders cannot control their symptoms, the most severe of which are psychotic. Symptoms interfere with normal thought process and content, and cognitive, speech, and social functioning. Many people with depressive disorders unfortunately go untreated, as their symptoms are minimized or misinterpreted. People with bipolar disorders are more often treated, as their symptoms more frequently are bizarre or disruptive enough to bring them to medical and psychiatric attention.

Mood disorders are caused by a complex interplay of biological and psychological factors. Biologic theories involve the role of the biogenic amines, in particular dysfunction in the norepinephrine, serotonin, dopamine, and GABA neurotransmitter systems. Most antidepressant medications involve complex manipulations of these systems. There appears to be dysregulation as well in the adrenal, thyroid, and growth hormone axes, all of which have been implicated in the etiology of mood disorders. Abnormalities in the sleep cycle and in regulation of circadian rhythms have also been studied.

Genetics always play an important role in the etiology of mental disorders, but genetic input is especially relevant in mood disorders. Bipolar I disorder is one of the most genetically determined disorders in psychiatry. However, as with any mental disorder, psychosocial factors play a crucial role in the development, presentation, course, and prognosis of mood disorders. Issues of real and symbolic loss, family relationships and dynamics, environmental stress, and unconscious conflicts all strongly contribute to and determine mood symptoms. Some clinicians believe that these factors are particularly important in the first episodes of mood disorders, but in one form or another they play a role in all episodes.

Skilled clinicians will be knowledgeable about all available treatment modalities, their indications, side effects, limitations, and advantages. They will know how best to combine different treatments, and which treatments are most effective for which disorders, from psychopharmacologic interventions, to the different psychotherapies, to electroconvulsive therapy (ECT).

The student should study the questions and answers below for a useful review of these disorders.

HELPFUL HINTS

The student should know the following terms that relate to mood disorders.

- adrenal axis
- affect
- age-dependent symptoms
- amphetamine
- antipsychotics
- anxiety-blissfulness psychosis
- atypical features
- biogenic amines
- bipolar I disorder
- bipolar II disorder
- carbamazepine
- catatonic features
- clinical management
- cognitive, behavioral, family, and psychoanalytic therapies
- cognitive theories
- cyclothymic disorder
- depression rating scales
- depressive equivalent
- differential diagnosis
- double depression
- dysthymic (early and late onset) disorder
- ECT
- euthymic
- *folie à double forme*
- *folie circulaire*
- *forme fruste*
- GABA
- genetic studies
- GH
- 5-HT
- hypomania
- hypothalamus
- incidence and prevalence
- Karl Kahlbaum
- kindling
- Heinz Kohut
- Emil Kraepelin
- learned helplessness
- LH, FSH

- life events and stress
- lithium
- major depressive disorder
- mania
- MAOIs
- melancholic features
- melatonin
- mild depressive disorder
- mixed episode
- mood
- mood-congruent and incongruent psychotic fear
- neurological, medical, and pharmacological causes of mood disorders
- norepinephrine
- phototherapy
- postpartum onset
- premenstrual dysphoric disorder
- premorbid factors
- pseudodementia
- rapid cycling
- REM latency, density
- RFLP
- seasonal pattern
- Sex ratios of disorders
- SSRI
- suicide
- T3
- thymoleptics
- TSH, TRH
- vegetative functions
- *Zeitgebers*

QUESTIONS

Directions

Each of the questions or incomplete statements below is followed by five suggested responses or completions. Select the *one* that is *best* in each case.

17.1 Dysthymic Disorder

A. usually begins in adulthood
B. does not respond to anti-depressants
C. presents with symptoms of lack of say in life and preoccupation with inadequacy
D. is usually limited to one or two episodes
E. is characteristically marked by psychomotor agitation or psychomotor retardation

17.2 The person *least* likely to develop major depressive disorder (MDD) in their lifetime is

A. 10-year-old boy diagnosed with dysthymia
B. Identical twin of an MDD patient who committed suicide
C. 12-year-old girl mourning the death of her mother
D. 19-year-old female who was raped 3 weeks ago
E. 60-year-old male with pancreatic cancer

17.3 The defense mechanism most commonly used in depression is

A. projection
B. introjection
C. sublimation
D. undoing
E. altruism

17.4 Which of the following is *not* a change in brain function associated with severe depression?

A. Increased REM sleep
B. Impaired cellular immunity
C. Hypocortisolism
D. Increased glucose metabolism in the amygdala
E. Decreased anterior cerebral blood flow

17.5 Which of the following is *not* part of the DSM-IV-TR criteria for diagnosing atypical depression?

A. Shortening of REM latency
B. Mood reactivity
C. Significant weight gain
D. Hypersomnia
E. Leaden paralysis

17.6 Reactive depression can best be compared to

A. Adjustment Disorder
B. Oppositional Defiant Disorder
C. Conduct Disorder
D. Atypical Depression
E. Schizoaffective Disorder

17.7 L-Tryptophan

A. is the amino acid precursor to dopamine
B. has been used as an adjuvant to both antidepressants and lithium
C. has been used as a stimulant
D. has not been associated with any serious side effects
E. all of the above

17.8 Common features of normal bereavement include

A. Marked psychomotor retardation
B. Mummification
C. Suicidal ideation
D. Guilt of omission
E. All of the above

17.9 Drugs that may precipitate mania include all of the following *except*

A. bromocriptine
B. isoniazid
C. propranolol
D. disulfiram
E. all of the above

17.10 Which of the following statements regarding mood disorders is *false*?

A. Approximately 15 percent of depressed patients will eventually commit suicide.
B. Depressive disorders are more common in women
C. Incidence of depression in younger age groups is increasing
D. Manic forms of mood disorders predominate in men
E. 1 out of 4 patients with an acute depressive episode will have recurrences throughout life

17.11 Which of the following statements regarding hypomanic episodes is *false*?

A. It is characterized by mild elevations of mood
B. Patients often experience increased energy levels
C. It is ego-syntonic
D. It often progresses to manic psychosis
E. It can be mobilized by antidepressant use

17.12 Figure 17.1 depicts the distribution, according to age and sex, of which of the following?

A. incidence of anorexia nervosa
B. prevalence of mood disorders
C. incidence of obsessive-compulsive disorder
D. prevalence of schizophrenia
E. incidence of somatization

17.13 Which of the following statements regarding ECT is *false*?

A. ECT should be used in cases of psychotic depression only
B. Bilateral ECT is somewhat more effective than unilateral ECT
C. Retrograde memory impairment is a common side effect
D. ECT is often used for refractory mood disorders
E. 8 to 12 treatments are usually needed for symptomatic remission

17.14 The most consistent computer tomography (CT) and magnetic resonance imaging (MRI) abnormality observed in depressive disorders is

A. ventricular enlargement
B. increased frequency of hyperintensities in subcortical regions
C. cortical atrophy
D. sulcal widening
E. none of the above

17.15 Which of the following statements regarding rapid cycling bipolar disorder is *true*?

A. More common in men than women
B. Often responds to tricyclic antidepressants
C. Defined as at least 4 episodes per month
D. Alcohol, stimulants, or caffeine use are risk factors
E. Hospitalization of these patients is rare

17.16 All of the following statements regarding Bupropion (Wellbutrin) are true *except*

A. Acts as a dopamine reuptake inhibitor
B. Rapid onset of action
C. No sexual dysfunction or weight gain associated with its use
D. Can be used for smoking cessation
E. Side effects include insomnia and GI distress

17.17 All of the following statements regarding cyclothymic disorder are true *except*

A. Symptoms must be present for at least 2 years
B. Occurs at the same rate in men and women
C. Symptoms may satisfy criteria for major depression
D. Consists of hypomania alternating with depressed mood
E. Lifetime prevalence rate is about 0.4 to 1 percent

17.18 A 35-year-old female has just been diagnosed with major depressive disorder. For the past 8 months, she has suffered from depressed mood, decreased energy and concentration, and loss of interest in previously enjoyed activities. Although she never attempted suicide, she acknowledges that she thought she would probably jump off a local bridge if she ever had the chance. She denies

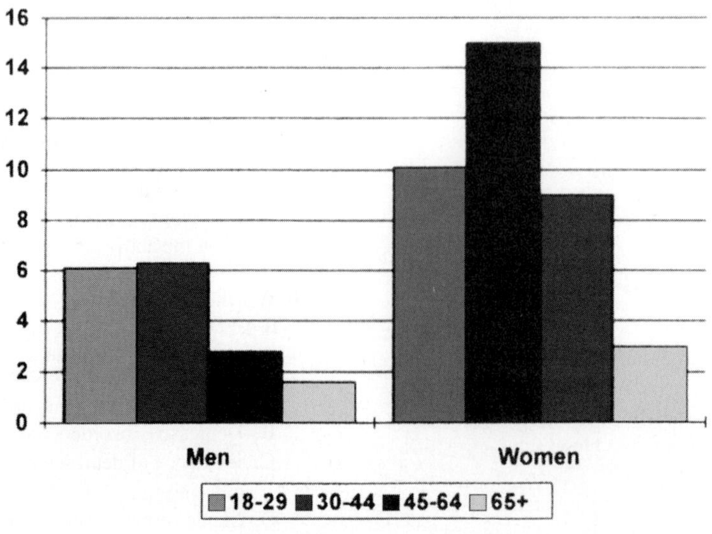

FIGURE 17.1
Data derived from the Epidemiological Catchment Area study.

any history of excessively elevated moods. You decide to start her on antidepressant therapy. Two weeks later, this patient is at greatest risk for

A. Medication noncompliance
B. Suicide completion
C. Manic episode
D. Hypomanic episode
E. Extrapyramidal symptoms

17.19 Which of the following antidepressants would *not* be the best choice for the above patient with a history of suicidal ideation?

A. SSRI
B. MAOI
C. TCA
D. Bupropion (Wellbutrin)
E. Venlafaxine (Effexor)

17.20 Serotonin

A. is an important regulator of sleep, appetite, and libido
B. helps to regulate circadian rhythms
C. permits or facilitates goal-directed motor and consummatory behavior in conjunction with norepinephrine and dopamine
D. stores are increased by transient stress and depleted by chronic stress
E. all of the above

17.21 The *highest* suicide rates are in which of the following age groups?

A. Under age 15
B. 15 to 24 year olds
C. 25 to 44 year olds
D. 45 to 64 year olds
E. Over age 65

17.22 Features of anhedonia may include all of the following *except*

A. Difficulty describing or being aware of emotions
B. Derealization
C. Loss of pleasure
D. Inability to experience normal emotions
E. Withdrawal from interests

17.23 Mirroring, twinship, and idealization are terms associated with

A. Sigmund Freud
B. Melanie Klein
C. Edith Jacobson
D. Heinz Kohut
E. Charles Brenner

17.24 Psychomotor retardation is characterized by all of the following *except*

A. Paucity of spontaneous movements
B. Reduced speech amplitude and flow
C. Indecisiveness
D. Poor concentration
E. Restlessness

17.25 Mr. M is an 87-year-old man who, 6 weeks after coronary artery bypass graft, complicated by pneumonia and renal insufficiency, was admitted to an inpatient rehabilitation service for management of physical deconditioning. Psychiatry was consulted 10 days after admission to rule out depression in the context of persistent low appetite and energy associated with suboptimal participation in rehabilitation. Mr. M reported no prior psychiatric history. He had worked as a chemist until retirement nearly two decades earlier. Laboratory examination revealed a low hematocrit of 21 and moderately elevated blood urea nitrogen of 65. On interview, Mr. M demonstrated psychomotor slowing and bland affect. He denied depression, hopelessness, worthlessness, or suicidal ideation. He expressed a desire to recover from his debilitated state, but acknowledged uncertainty that he was capable of doing so. He also complained of extreme weakness. He stated, "I just don't seem to have an appetite anymore." Cognition largely was intact; there was mild short-term memory deficit.

The most likely diagnosis in this patient is:

A. Major depressive disorder
B. Mood disorder secondary to a general medical condition
C. Dementia
D. Delirium
E. Anxiety disorder with depressed mood

17.26 Double depression is characterized by

A. Two episodes of major depressive disorder per month consistently
B. Superimposed bipolar II disorder and atypical depression
C. Recurrent major depressive disorder superimposed with dysthymic disorder
D. Two family members suffering from major depressive disorder concurrently
E. Recurrent major depressive disorder with current symptoms twice as disabling as usual

17.27 Which of the graphs in Figure 17.2 depicts the prototypical course of double depression?

A. A
B. B
C. C
D. D
E. None of the above

17.28 Which graph in Figure 17.2 depicts the pattern with the best future prognosis?

A. A
B. B
C. C

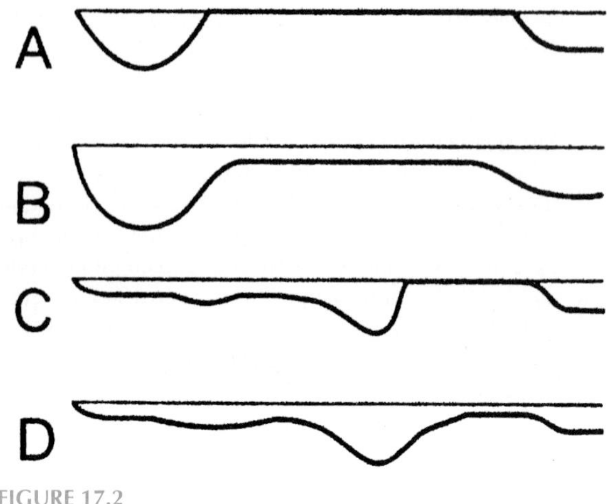

FIGURE 17.2

D. D
E. None of the above

17.29 A 57-year-old female presents to you after being diagnosed with major depressive disorder. She has been depressed ever since the death of her husband 2 years earlier. She has been taking the same antidepressant since her diagnosis 1 year ago, with no relief of her symptoms. She states that she would like your help in ending her life. The best option for your next step is:

A. Respect the patient's wishes as she is of sound mind
B. Seek to more adequately treat her depression
C. Seek family members to make a more informed decision
D. Contact the hospital ethics committee
E. Obtain information from the state regarding physician-assisted suicide laws

17.30 A suicidal patient with chronic depressive disorder presents to your office very frustrated and in tears. He tells you he can't stop thinking about ending his life because he is so depressed. You ask him if he has a plan and he details where he could buy a handgun and where he would go to shoot himself. You fear the patient will carry out this plan because he has not had adequate control of his symptoms since his last antidepressant change 1 month ago. You discuss inpatient hospitalization for medication stabilization, but the patient refuses. You're next step in management of this patient would best be:

A. Admit the patient to the hospital anyway
B. Give the latest antidepressant more time to take affect
C. Change to another class of antidepressant
D. Try to persuade the patient to admit himself to the hospital
E. Initiate psychotherapy to discuss the reasons behind the suicidal thoughts

17.31 The following situations call for a break in doctor-patient confidentiality *except*

A. Patient with bipolar I disorder admits he is homosexual
B. Patient with schizoaffective disorder hallucinates that he can fly
C. Patient with major depressive disorder who is sexually promiscuous contracts syphilis
D. Patient with a delusional disorder thinks his boss is out to get him and threatens to kill her
E. Patient with conduct disorder thrives on the sexual abuse of young children

17.32 A 40-year-old woman presents complaining of depressed mood, insomnia, difficulty concentrating, and decreased interests for the last 2 months. Her symptoms began after discovering her husband was having an extramarital affair. She tells you she feels betrayed and foolish for not realizing what was going on behind her back. She barely eats and has not returned the phone calls of her family and friends. She states "life is just not worth living." What would be the most appropriate next step in her management?

A. Suggest you meet with her husband
B. Prescribe an SSRI
C. Inquire about suicidal thoughts
D. Recommend electroconvulsive therapy
E. Recommend supportive psychotherapy

17.33 A 35-year-old male is being seen in your office for major depressive disorder. He reports feelings of worthlessness, depressed mood, and insomnia for the last 7 months. He also tells you he occasionally hears voices talking about him and telling him to kill himself. You decide to start Risperdal to treat these auditory hallucinations. Risperdal acts by blocking which receptor?

A. Histamine-1 receptors
B. Dopamine-D2 receptors
C. Alpha-1 adrenergic receptors
D. Muscarinic cholinergic receptors
E. None of the above

17.34 Which of the following is the best predictor of likelihood of attempting suicide in future?

A. Gender
B. Alcohol abuse
C. Unemployment
D. Prior suicide attempt
E. Recent divorce

17.35 A 27-year-old patient has been diagnosed with bipolar disorder. Before starting this patient on lithium for mood stabilization, which of the following laboratory tests should be obtained?

A. Thyroid function tests, creatinine, liver function tests
B. Thyroid function tests, complete blood count, pregnancy test
C. Thyroid function tests, liver function tests, pregnancy test
D. Thyroid function tests, creatinine, pregnancy test
E. Thyroid function tests, creatinine, complete blood count

17.36 A 33-year-old female presents to you for evaluation of depressed mood, decreased concentration, and anhedonia for the last month. She has been hesitant to start pharmacotherapy for her symptoms, but finally agrees to try medication. You start her on fluoxetine. Two weeks later, she presents to your office in tears reporting no change in her mood. The most appropriate next step is:

A. Increase dose of fluoxetine
B. Change to another SSRI
C. Discontinue fluoxetine and start amitriptyline
D. Continue fluoxetine and add amitriptyline
E. Continue fluoxetine at same dose

17.37 A young married woman new to your practice suffers from bipolar disorder and has been taking lithium with good effect. She calls you frantic one afternoon because she has just learned she is pregnant and is concerned about the effects of lithium on her child. Which of the following is her child at greatest risk for?

A. Cardiac anomalies
B. Craniofacial defects
C. Neural tube defects
D. Mental retardation
E. Genital anomalies

17.38 A 64-year-old woman with an extensive smoking history has recently been diagnosed with small cell lung cancer. She develops a depressed mood, decreased interests, and difficulty concentrating soon thereafter, as she reports she cannot stop thinking about how worthless her life has been. She eats incessantly and has gained 10 pounds in the last 5 weeks; she also reports increased sleep. You decide to prescribe phenelzine for her symptoms of atypical depression. Which of the following is contraindicated in those patients taking phenelzine?

A. Fluoxetine
B. Valproic Acid
C. Trazodone
D. Lithium
E. Clomipramine

17.39 Ms. S, a 24-year-old woman, is brought for a psychiatric consultation by her mother who complains of bizarre behavior. One month ago Ms. S was fired from her job at a local bookstore because of frequently arriving late and not performing her duties adequately. She states that she fell in love with another employee and tried to get his attention and spend time with him, even though he seemed uninterested. Over the past 3 months she increased her use of alcohol and marijuana to three beers a day and two to three joints per day. Her mother reports a 2-week history of increased energy, eating little, talking a great deal, and interrupting others frequently. A week ago Ms. S reported that her former work colleagues were plotting against her and attempting to control her by broadcasting thoughts into her brain. She did not sleep the last 2 nights. Ms. S has no significant psychiatric or medical history. She takes no medications.

Physical examination reveals a blood pressure of 135/75, heart rate of 84, and a temperature of 37°C. Her conjunctivae are pink and her pupils are equal, 3 mm and reactive to light. Deep tendon reflexes are normal throughout. Urine toxicology reveals the presence of cannabinoids. On mental status testing, her mood is euphoric, her speech is pressured, and she is emotionally labile and irritable. Her thinking is illogical and disorganized. She denies hallucinations. She is alert and oriented to person, place, and time. Immediate recall and recent and remote memory are intact. Throughout the interview she is preoccupied by thoughts of the coworker with whom she has fallen in love.

Ms. S is admitted to a psychiatric unit and treatment is initiated with haloperidol, 10 mg/day, which is increased to 20 mg/day on day 5 because of continued agitation. On day 6 she becomes withdrawn and uncommunicative. She is diffusely rigid with a temperature of 39°C. Her white blood count is 14,300 and her CPK 2,100. Several blood cultures are negative.

Which of the following is the most likely diagnosis at the time of admission?

A. Schizophrenia
B. Delusional disorder, erotomanic type
C. Marijuana-induced psychotic disorder
D. Bipolar disorder
E. Schizoaffective disorder, bipolar type

17.40 Which of the following is the most likely explanation for her behavior on day 6?

A. Worsening psychosis
B. Anticholinergic delirium
C. Neuroleptic malignant syndrome
D. Marijuana-induced delirium
E. Occult infection

17.41 Which of the following pharmacologic approaches is most appropriate on day 6?

A. Increase dose of haloperidol
B. Stop haloperidol and add risperidone
C. Stop haloperidol, add bromocriptine, and seek medical consultation
D. Continue the same dose of haloperidol and add risperidone
E. Continue the same dose of haloperidol and add benztropine

Directions

Each set of lettered headings below is followed by a list of phrases or statements. For each numbered phrase or statement, select:

A. if the item is associated with A only
B. if the item is associated with B only
C. if the item is associated with both A and B
D. if the item is associated with neither A nor B

Questions 17.42–17.45

A. Clozapine
B. Imipramine

17.42 Cardiotoxic
17.43 Causes weight gain
17.44 Acts as an NE partial agonist
17.45 Teratogenic

Directions

Each group of questions consists of lettered headings followed by a list of numbered words or statements. For each numbered word or statement, select the one lettered heading that is most closely associated with it. Each lettered heading may be selected once, more than once, or not at all.

Questions 17.46–17.50

A. Sigmund Freud
B. Adolph Meyer
C. Aaron Beck
D. Emil Kraepelin
E. Martin Seligman

17.46 Depression is a result of aggressive impulses directed against an ambivalently loved internalized object
17.47 Negative cognitive schemata lead to depressive symptoms
17.48 Learned helplessness as a model for depression
17.49 Established manic-depressive illness as a nosological and disease entity
17.50 Coined the term *psychobiology* to emphasize that both psychological and biological facts could cause depression

Questions 17.51–17.54

A. Period effects
B. Age effects
C. Cohort effects
D. All of the above
E. None of the above

17.51 The genetic predisposition to develop major depressive disorder is probably greater during the 30s, and the predisposition to develop bipolar disorder is greatest during the 20s
17.52 The uncertainty of employment among college graduates and the trend to delay marriage during the 1990s
17.53 The association between age and suicide in white males
17.54 People born between 1915 and 1925 exhibit lower suicide rates at all ages than either those born in 1900 or 1940

Questions 17.55–17.58

A. Unipolar depression
B. Bipolar II depression
C. Both
D. Neither

17.55 Never any history of acute mania
17.56 Typically has psychotic features present
17.57 Symptoms of hypomania are present
17.58 Can present with atypical features

Questions 17.59–17.61

A. Light Therapy
B. Electroconvulsive Therapy
C. Tricyclic Antidepressant
D. MAOI Antidepressant

17.59 Depressive Disorder with atypical features
17.60 Refractory Mood Disorder
17.61 Seasonal Affective Disorder

ANSWERS

17.1 The answer is C

Dysthymic disorder *presents with symptoms of lack of say in life and preoccupation with inadequacy*. Most cases of *dysthymic disorder are of early onset and begin in childhood or adolescence*, certainly by the time patients reach their 20s. A late-onset type, much less prevalent and not well characterized clinically, has been identified in middle-aged and geriatric populations, largely through epidemiological studies in the community. The pattern, commonly seen in clinical practice, consists of the baseline dysthymic disorder fluctuating in and out of depressive episodes. The more prototypical patients with dysthymic disorder often complain of having been depressed since birth or feeling depressed all the time. They seem, in the apt words of Kurt Schneider, to view themselves as belonging to an "aristocracy of suffering." Such descriptions of chronic gloominess in the absence of more objective signs of depression earn these patients the label of characterological depression. The description is further reinforced by the fluctuating depressive picture that merges imperceptibly with the patient's habitual self and thus raises uncertainty as to whether dysthymic disorder belongs in Axis I or Axis II. This conceptual uncertainty notwithstanding, given the confluence of data on the efficacy of many classes of antidepressants, *dysthymic patients should not be denied the potential benefit of antidepressants*.

The profile of dysthymic disorder overlaps with that of major depressive disorder but differs from it in that symptoms tend to outnumber signs (more subjective than objective depression). This means that marked disturbances in appetite and libido are uncharacteristic, and *psychomotor agitation or retardation is not observed*. This all translates into a depression with attenuated symptomatology. However, subtle endogenous features are not uncommonly observed: inertia and anhedonia that are characteristically worse in the morning.

17.2 The answer is D

The *19-year-old rape victim* is more likely to develop a variation of post-traumatic stress disorder, which is highest among victims of rape, military combat, and survivors of torture. *Childhood onset of dysthymia* similarly presages extremely high rates of depression and bipolar disorder in adulthood. *Monozygotic twins* have been shown to have a two- to four-fold increase in concordance rates for mood disorders over dizygotic twins, compelling data for the role of genetic factors in mood disorders. *Parental loss before adolescence* is also a well-documented risk factor for adult-onset depression. Medical problems of many types, such as *cancer of the pancreas*, multiple sclerosis, and space-occupying lesions of the brain can produce depression.

17.3 The answer is B

In Sigmund Freud's structural theory, the *introjection* of the lost object into the ego leads to the typical depressive symptoms of a lack of energy available to the ego. The superego, unable to retaliate against the lost object externally, flails out at the psychic representation of the lost object, now internalized in the ego as an introject. When the ego overcomes or merges with the superego, energy previously bound in the depressive symptoms is released, and a mania supervenes with the typical symptoms of excess.

Projection is the unconscious defense mechanism in which a person attributes to another person those generally unconscious ideas, thoughts, feelings, and impulses that are personally undesirable or unacceptable. *Sublimation* is an unconscious defense mechanism in which the energy associated with unacceptable impulses or drives is diverted into personally and socially acceptable channels. *Undoing* is an unconscious defense mechanism by which a person symbolically acts out to reverse something unacceptable that has already been done or against which the ego must defend itself. *Altruism* is regard for and dedication to the welfare of others.

17.4 The answer is C

The changes in brain function associated with severe depression include *increased phasic REM sleep*, poor sleep maintenance, hypercortisolism (not *hypocortisolism*), *impaired cellular immunity*, *reductions in anterior cerebral blood flow* and *increased glucose metabolism in the amygdala*. Such changes suggest consequences of an exaggerated and sustained stress response.

17.5 The answer is A

Nearly two thirds of patients with depressive disorders, whether suffering from typical or atypical symptoms, *exhibit marked shortening of REM latency*, the period from sleep onset to the first REM period. This fact is not specific to atypical depression as are the other choices listed. *Mood reactivity* is characterized by mood elevation in response to something good happening. *Leaden paralysis* (heavy, leaden feelings in one's arms and legs), along with *hypersomnia*, increased appetite, and *significant weight gain*, are also among the features of atypical depression.

17.6 The answer is A

Reactive depression is defined as depression that results from a specific life event. It continues as long as the event is present, and it terminates with the reversal of the event (e.g., return of a lover after a breakup). With interpersonal support, most people can face life's reversals, which explains why reactive depression tends to be self-limiting. Hence, *adjustment disorder* is the more appropriate diagnosis for many cases of reactive depression. *Oppositional defiant disorder* is a recurring pattern of negative, hostile, disobedient, and defiant behavior in a child or adolescent, lasting for at least 6 months without serious violation of the basic rights of others. *Conduct disorder* is a childhood behavioral condition involving a pattern of repetitive and persistent conduct that infringes on the basic rights of others or does not conform to established societal norms or rules that are appropriate for a child of that age. *Atypical depression* is characterized by "reversed vegetative symptoms," which include oversleeping, overeating, rejection sensitivity, and temporary brightening of mood in response to positive events. *Schizoaffective disorder* is a disorder with symptoms of both schizophrenia and manic-depressive disorder.

17.7 The answer is B

L-Tryptophan, the amino acid precursor to serotonin, *has been used as an adjuvant to both antidepressants and lithium* in the treatment of bipolar I disorder. Tyrosine *is the amino acid precursor to dopamine.* L-Tryptophan has also been *used alone as a hypnotic and an antidepressant.* L-Tryptophan and L-tryptophan–containing products have been recalled in the United States because L-tryptophan *has been associated with eosinophilia-myalgia syndrome.* The symptoms include fatigue, myalgia, shortness of breath, rashes, and swelling of the extremities. Congestive heart failure and death can also occur. Although several studies have shown that L-tryptophan is an efficacious adjuvant in the treatment of mood disorders, it should not be used for any purpose until the problem with eosinophilia-myalgia syndrome is resolved. Current evidence points to a contaminant in the manufacturing process.

17.8 The answer is D

Although pathologically depressed patients often experience guilt of commission, typically people experiencing normal bereavement instead feel guilty about not having done certain things that might have saved the life of the deceased (*guilt of omission*). *Marked psychomotor retardation* is usually not observed in normal grief, and *mummification* (keeping deceased's belongings exactly as they were prior to his or her death) can indicate serious psychopathology. Active *suicidal ideation* is also rare in normal grief. Other symptoms of the progression of normal bereavement to a depressive disorder are delusions of worthlessness, psychosis, and a non-reactive mood.

17.9 The answer is C

Propranolol (a β-blocker) is an antihypertensive and may actually cause depressive symptoms. Many pharmacological agents, such as *bromocriptine* (Parlodel), *isoniazid* (Nydrazid), cimetidine (Tagamet), and *disulfiram* (Antabuse), may precipitate mania, as can antidepressant treatment or withdrawal.

17.10 The answer is E

Three (not one) out of four patients with acute depression will experience recurrences, with varying degrees of residual symptoms between episodes. Of note, although depressive disorders are more common in women, more men than women die of suicide due to more lethal methods chosen.

17.11 The answer is D

Hypomania occurring as part of bipolar II disorder *rarely progresses to manic psychosis*, and insight is relatively preserved. Hypomania refers to a distinct period of at least a few days of *mild elevation of mood*, sharpened and positive thinking, and *increased energy levels*, typically without the impairment characteristic of manic episodes. Because hypomania is experienced as a rebound relief from depression, it is often an *ego-syntonic* mood state. Hypomania can also sometimes be *mobilized with antidepressant use*, just as episodes of mania can be precipitated by antidepressants.

17.12 The answer is B

The graph in Figure 17.1 depicts the lifetime *prevalence of mood disorders*. Anorexia nervosa occurs 10 to 20 times more often in females than in males, and the most common age of onset of anorexia nervosa is the mid-teenage years.

Regarding *obsessive-compulsive disorder,* men and women are equally likely to be affected (however, adolescent boys are more commonly affected than adolescent girls). The mean age of onset is about 20 years and about two-thirds of patients have the onset of symptoms before age 25. *Schizophrenia* is equally prevalent among men and women, with the peak ages of onset for men 15 to 25 and women 25 to 35. Women with *somatization disorder* outnumber men 5 to 20 times. Somatization disorder is defined as beginning before age 30; it most often begins during a person's teens.

17.13 The answer is A

Electroconvulsive therapy is effective in *psychotic and nonpsychotic forms of depression*. Usually, *8–12 ECT treatments* are required to achieve symptomatic remission, and this form of therapy has been shown to be effective *even in patients who are refractory* to several different medications. *Bilateral ECT* is somewhat more effective than unilateral therapy, but bilateral ECT also appears to have more cognitive side effects, such as *retrograde memory loss*.

17.14 The answer is B

CAT and MRI scans provide sensitive, noninvasive methods to assess the brain, including cortical and subcortical tracts, as well as white matter lesions. The most consistent abnormality observed in the depressive disorders is *increased frequency of abnormal hyperintensities in subcortical regions,* especially the periventricular area, basal ganglia, and thalamus (Fig. 17.3).

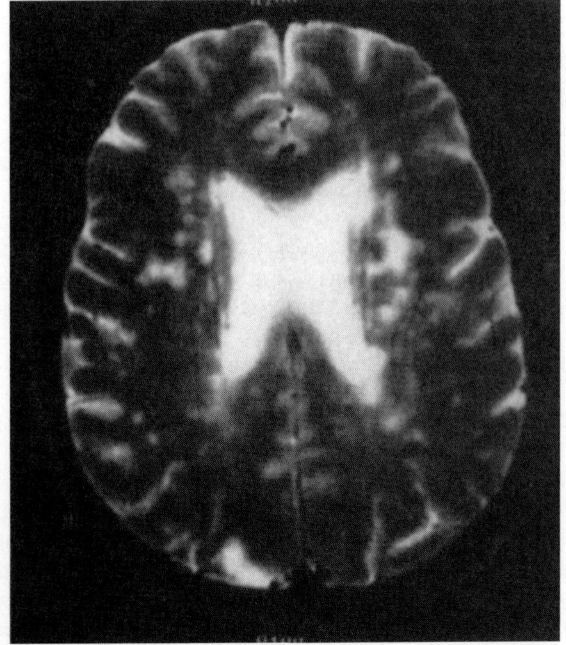

FIGURE 17.3
This MRI scan of a patient with late-onset major depressive disorder illustrates extensive periventricular hyperintensities associated with diffuse cerebrovascular disease.

More common in bipolar I disorder and among the elderly, these hyperintensities appear to reflect the deleterious neurodegenerative effects of recurrent mood episodes. *Ventricular enlargement, cortical atrophy, and sulcal widening* also have been reported in patients with mood disorders as compared to normal controls. In addition to age and illness duration, structural abnormalities are associated with increased illness severity, bipolar status, and increased cortisol levels. Some depressed patients also may have reduced caudate nucleus volumes, suggesting a defect in the mesocorticolimbic system. Cerebrovascular factors often involve subcortical frontal and basal ganglia structures, and appear particularly relevant to late-life depression.

17.15 The answer is D

Among the factors favoring the occurrence of rapid cycling bipolar disorder are *alcohol, stimulant, and caffeine use*. Other factors include female gender, as this subtype is much more common in women than men. Most antidepressants readily induce excited episodes and thus aggravate the rapid cycling pattern. Rapid cycling is defined as the occurrence of at least 4 episodes of depression and hypomania/mania per year (not per month). Hospitalization of these patients is often frequent, in order to stabilize medication and achieve compliance.

17.16 The answer is B

Bupropion acts as a dopamine reuptake inhibitor. It typically takes 1 to 2 weeks for symptomatic effect and *this is not considered a rapid onset of action* even though most antidepressants take 3 to 4 weeks to have an effect. Side effects of Bupropion include insomnia, GI distress, cardiac arrhythmias, and agitation. There is no sexual dysfunction or weight gain associated with Bupropion use. In addition to its use as an antidepressant, it is also useful as a smoking cessation aid.

17.17 The answer is C

Cyclothymia is characterized by at least 2 years of numerous periods with hypomanic symptoms and numerous periods with depressive symptoms that *do not meet criteria for a major depressive episode*. This disorder apparently occurs at the same rate in both men and women, but women seek treatment more often than do men. The lifetime prevalence rate of cyclothymic disorder is 0.4 to 1 percent.

17.18 The answer is B

When antidepressant medications first begin to work, patients tend to report an increase in energy levels before significant improvement in mood symptoms. For this reason, *carrying out suicide plans* is more of a risk during this period. *Medication noncompliance* with effective psychopharmacological treatments during both acute and maintenance therapy is a major cause of morbidity among patients with schizophrenia and disorders with poor insight, not among patients with depression. Although noncompliance is a possibility with any patient, it is not the best choice listed. This patient has nothing in her history to indicate Bipolar disorder as a more appropriate diagnosis, therefore there is no reason to believe *manic or hypomanic episodes* will be precipitated by antidepressant use. *Extrapyramidal symptoms* are a consequence of typical antipsychotic use, not antidepressant use.

17.19 The answer is C

In considering antidepressant use in suicidal or impulsive patients, caution should be taken in using medications that may be lethal in overdose (e.g., *tricyclic antidepressants*) or that may exacerbate disinhibition or cognitive deficits (e.g., benzodiazepines). Therefore, it is not the best idea to prescribe a TCA to this patient. *SSRIs* and *MAOIs* remain better choices given her history and presentation. Care should be taken to avoid precipitating a hypertensive crisis in patients taking MAOIs. *Bupropion* and *Venlafaxine* are other antidepressants that can be used alone or in combination with another medication, and this patient has no contraindications to their use.

17.20 The answer is E (all)

Serotoninergic neurons project from the brainstem dorsal raphe nuclei to the cerebral cortex, hypothalamus, thalamus, basal ganglia, septum, and hippocampus. Serotonin pathways have both inhibitory and facilitatory functions in the brain. For example, much evidence suggests that 5-HT is *an important regulator of sleep, appetite, and libido.* Serotonergic neurons projecting to the suprachiasmatic nucleus of the hypothalamus *help to regulate circadian rhythms* (e.g., sleep–wake cycles, body temperature, and hypothalamic-pituitary-adrenocortical axis function). Serotonin also *permits or facilitates goal-directed motor and consummatory behaviors in conjunction with norepinephrine and dopamine.* Moreover, serotonin inhibits aggressive behavior across mammalian and reptilian species.

There is some evidence that serotonin neurotransmission is partly under genetic control. Nevertheless, acute stress increases serotonin release transiently, whereas *chronic stress eventually will deplete serotonin stores.* Chronic stress may also increase synthesis of 5-HT_{1A} autoreceptors in the dorsal raphe nucleus, which further decrease serotonin transmission. Elevated glucocorticoid levels tend to enhance serotonergic functioning and thus may have significant compensatory effects on chronic stress.

17.21 The answer is E

Suicide is almost twice as frequent in older adults as in the general population. The suicide rate for white men *older than 65 years of age* is five times higher than that of the general population. Aging reduces suicide attempts but increases their lethality. Depression is the most common psychiatric diagnosis in elderly suicide victims, unlike younger adults in whom substance abuse alone or with comorbid mood disorders is the most frequent diagnosis. Older patients with major medical illnesses or a recent loss should be evaluated for depressive symptomatology and suicidal ideation or plans, and aggressive treatment can help prevent their acting on suicidal thoughts. Suicide rates are rising most rapidly in young adults, but *the greatest risk remains in those people over the age of 65.*

17.22 The answer is A

Anhedonia is one of the DSM IV-TR criteria for major depression. Patients with severe depression and anhedonia may complain of being emotionally cut off from others and experience depersonalization in a world that seems strange to them (*derealization*). *Loss of pleasure and withdrawal from previously enjoyable activities* is typical of anhedonia. The impact of the loss of emotional resonance can be so pervasive that patients may denounce values and beliefs that had previously given meaning to their lives (e.g., members of the clergy complain they no longer believe in the Church and have lost God). The *inability of the person with depressive disorder to experience normal emotions* (commonly observed among young depressed patients) differs from the schizophrenic patient's flat affect in that the loss of emotions is itself experienced as painful; that is, the patient suffers immensely from the inability to experience emotions. Anhedonia does not typically include *alexithymia*, which is defined as a person's inability to describe or be aware of one's emotions or mood.

17.23 The answer is D

Heinz Kohut's theory, known as self psychology, rests on the assumption that the developing self has specific needs that must be met by parents to give the child a positive sense of self-esteem and self-cohesion and that similar responses are required from others throughout the course of the life cycle. He *referred to those needs as mirroring, twinship, and idealization.* The *mirroring* responses required by the self are equated with the gleam in the mother's eye when the child exhibitionistically shows off for her. Admiration, validation, and affirmation are responses that are included in the category of mirroring. *Twinship* responses refer to the child's need to be like or identify with significant others. A small boy who is outside playing with his toy lawn mower while his father is mowing the lawn is meeting important psychological needs in asserting his commonality with his father. Finally, the need for *idealization* is an important aspect of the development of the self. Children who grow up with parents they can respect and idealize develop healthy standards of conduct and morality.

Kohut referred to those needs collectively as self-object needs. In other words, the responses demanded from others are required by the self, and the needs of the object as a separate person are not taken into account. The other person serves as an object who meets the needs of the self. Self-object needs essentially refer to certain functions that persons in the environment provide rather than to those persons themselves. Kohut felt that self-object responses continue to be needed throughout life and are as necessary for emotional health as oxygen is for physical health. Within that conceptual framework, depression involves the failure of self-objects in the environment to provide the self of the depressed person with mirroring, twinship, or idealizing responses necessary for the self to feel whole and sustained.

A common finding in depressed patients is profound self-depreciation. *Sigmund Freud,* in his classic 1917 paper "Mourning and Melancholia," attributed that self-reproach to anger turned inward, which he related to object loss, which may or may not be real. A fantasied loss may suffice to trigger a severe depression. Moreover, the patient may actually be unaware of any specific feelings of loss, since the fantasied loss may be entirely unconscious.

Although *Melanie Klein* understood depression as involving the internalized expression of aggression toward loved ones, much as Freud did, the developmental theory on which her view was based is quite different from freudian theory. During the first year of life, Klein believed, the infant progresses from the paranoid-schizoid position to the depressive position. In the first few months of life, according to Klein, the infant projects highly destructive fantasies onto its mother and then becomes terrified of the mother as a sadistic persecutor. That terrifying "bad" mother is kept separate from the loving, nurturing "good" mother through the defense mechanism of splitting. In that manner the infant's blissful feeding experience remains uncontaminated and undisturbed by persecutory fears of attack by the "bad" mother. In the course of normal development, according to Klein, the positive and negative images of the mother are integrated into a more ambivalent view. In other words, the infant recognizes that the "bad" mother it fears and hates is the same mother as the "good" mother it loves and adores. The recognition that one can hurt loved ones is the essence of the depressive position.

Edith Jacobson compared the state of depression to a situation in which the ego is a powerless, helpless child, victimized by the superego, which becomes the equivalent of a sadistic and powerful mother who takes delight in torturing the child. Like Freud, Jacobson assumed that depressed persons have identified with ambivalently regarded lost love objects. The self is experienced as identified with the negative aspects of the object, and ultimately the sadistic qualities of the lost love object are transformed into the cruel superego. Hence, depressed persons feel that they are at the mercy of a sadistic internal tormentor that is unrelenting in its victimization. Jacobson also noted that the boundary between self and object may disappear, resulting in a fusion of the bad self with the bad object.

Some contemporary ego psychologists believe that depression is not truly a psychiatric disorder or illness. Instead, depression is regarded as an affect reflecting conflict and compromise formation. *Charles Brenner,* the principal architect of that view, suggested that concern about such childhood calamities as object loss, loss of love, castration, and punishment are associated with two kinds of unpleasure. One form of unpleasure is anxiety, which involves an anticipated calamity or danger. The other form of unpleasure, depressive affect, involves a calamity that has already happened. That theory of depressive affect differs sharply from the classical views of Freud and Abraham. Brenner pointed out that depression is not always related to object loss or to oral wishes. He also asserted that identification with a lost object is found in some depressed persons but not in all and that anger turned inward is a result of depression, rather than a cause. Depressive affect, in Brenner's view, can be linked to any of the childhood calamities, rather than uniquely to object loss. People can experience depressive affect because they feel unloved, because they feel powerless, or because they feel punished in a variety of ways. In this view, depressive affect is a normal and universal part of the human condition.

17.24 The answer is E

Features such as *restlessness*, agitation, and pressured speech are characteristic of psychomotor agitation, not retardation. Psychomotor retardation, often present in depressed patients, manifests as *paucity of spontaneous movements, reduced speech amplitude and flow*, increased latency of responses, *indecisiveness, poor concentration* and forgetfulness, and overwhelming fatigue. Brain imaging research that has revealed subcortical (extrapyramidal system) disturbances in mood disorders tends to support the centrality of psychomotor dysfunction in these disorders.

17.25 The answer is B

After an extended hospital course, many patients, like this one, demonstrate withdrawn behavior, anorexia, and fatigue, occasionally associated with mild cognitive loss, which do not meet criteria for cognitive or mood disorder, but which are a direct product of resolving medical illness and associated debilitation. The likelihood that a mood disorder is *due to a general medical condition* is increased if a temporal relationship exists between the onset, exacerbation, or remission of the medical condition and the mood disorder. Atypical features (e.g., unusual age of onset, lack of family history, and lack of prior episodes of mood disorder) also raise the likelihood of a medical basis for mood symptoms. Mild short-term memory deficits can be normal with aging and do not necessarily indicate Mr. M is suffering from *dementia*. He also demonstrated largely intact cognition, making *delirium* an unlikely diagnosis. Patients with a diagnosis of *anxiety disorder with depressed mood* primarily exhibit symptoms of anxiety states, such as marked tension, phobias, and panic attacks, all of which predate any depressive symptoms. In addition, anxiety disorders rarely appear for the first time after 40 years of age.

17.26 The answer is C

Double depression is characterized by *recurrent major depressive disorder with antecedent dysthymic disorder* and no period of full remission between the two most recent episodes. This pattern is seen in approximately 20 percent to 25 percent of the persons with major depressive disorder.

17.27 The answer is D

Graph D depicts double depression, which is characterized by recurrent major depressive disorder and antecedent dysthymic disorder with no period of full remission in between the two most recent episodes. *Graph A* is the course of major depressive disorder, recurrent, with no antecedent dysthymic disorder and full remission between episodes. *Graph B* is the course of major depressive disorder, recurrent, with no antecedent dysthymic disorder but with prominent symptoms persisting between episodes (partial remission is attained). *Graph C* is the rare pattern major depressive disorder, recurrent, with antecedent dysthymic disorder but with full interepisodic recovery.

17.28 The answer is A

The course of major depressive disorder, recurrent, with no antecedent dysthymic disorder and a period of full remission between the episodes predicts the best future prognosis. This is depicted in *graph A*.

17.29 The answer is B

Much political and theological heat has been generated in recent years by the debate on physician-assisted suicide. Many of the patients requesting death are depressed and would be likely to respond to psychotherapy or pharmacotherapy, or both. Frequently, they have been inadequately diagnosed or treated. Active depression can be considered a state of incompetence, making such patients unable to make informed decisions for themselves. *Family members or a living will should be consulted only in cases of medical emergencies* in which decisions must be made immediately. *In this case, treating the patient's depression is the best option. It is not necessary to involve the hospital ethics committee* in this decision. Currently, Oregon is the only state that has passed enabling laws regarding physician-assisted suicide.

17.30 The answer is A

Suicidal patients with intent and specific plans should always be taken seriously. For those patients believed to be too much at risk for outpatient therapy or partial hospital programs, *inpatient treatment is required.* Such hospitalization is preferably on a voluntary basis, but, if the patient refuses, involuntary admission is required. The options of *changing antidepressants* and *giving more time for the medication to take effect* are not the best options in this circumstance, although they may be in patients where suicide is less of an acute risk. *Psychotherapy* is also not an option when immediate intervention is needed with actively suicidal patients. Contact with the family and friends of suicidal patients is essential, and maintaining patient confidentiality is not mandatory if divulged material is believed to be necessary to protect the patient's life. There are some patients who appear so imminently and acutely suicidal that the clinician is afraid to let them out of the office. Patients can be admitted to the hospital against their will if they are a danger to themselves or to other people.

17.31 The answer is A

Confidentiality refers to the therapist's responsibility to not release information learned in the course of treatment to third parties. Psychiatrists must maintain confidentiality for two reasons. Confidentiality is an essential ingredient of psychiatric care, as it is a prerequisite for patients to be willing to speak freely to therapists. People would be less likely to go for help and would tend to withhold crucial information if confidentiality was not assured. There is no reason to break doctor-patient confidentiality in situations involving a patient's sexual preference (*homosexuality*), unless there is some threat to patient safety. Confidentiality must give way to the responsibility to protect others when a patient makes a credible threat to harm someone (*the patient threatening to kill his boss*), or acts in a way that could harm himself/herself (*the patient who thinks he can fly*). Reportable diseases (*such as syphilis*) must also be reported to the proper authorities despite the bond of patient confidentiality. Any suspicion of *child abuse* must also be reported to the authorities.

17.32 The answer is C

This patient is suffering from major depression, and will require treatment. Most important at this point however, is *inquiring about the existence of suicidal ideation* and a plan to act on the suicidal thoughts, as these put the patient at high risk for suicide. If she cannot contract for safety, she must be admitted to the hospital for stabilization. *Suggesting a meeting with her husband* does not address the immediate issue of her depression. It may be helpful to recommend marital therapy at a later point in time. *Prescribing an SSRI* is the treatment of choice for major depression, but it is important to establish the patient's level of safety first. Also during the first few weeks of initiating pharmacotherapy, depressed patients should be closely monitored for suicidality as energy levels return. *Electroconvulsive therapy* is more appropriate for treatment of refractory depression and is generally not used as a first line treatment for depression. *Supportive psychotherapy* can often be useful as an adjunct to pharmacotherapy, but is typically insufficient alone for the treatment of depression.

17.33 The answer is B

Psychosis is associated with dopaminergic hyperactivity, and many antipsychotics act by *blocking Dopamine-D2 receptors*. Risperdal is an atypical antipsychotic that acts by this mechanism. These atypical antipsychotics are increasingly preferred because of less incidence of extrapyramidal symptoms compared with typical antipsychotics.

17.34 The answer is D

The strongest indicator of the likelihood of attempting suicide is a *history of previous suicide attempts*. It has been shown that females make more suicidal gestures, but males are more likely to choose lethal methods and thus are more likely to successfully commit suicide. Therefore, male gender is considered more a risk factor for suicide completion. Alcohol or substance abuse, unemployment, recent divorce are all additional risk factors, but are less significant than a history of previous suicide attempts.

17.35 The answer is D

Lithium, used for mood stabilization in patients with bipolar disorder, is known for its low margin of safety, making frequent monitoring necessary. Common side effects include: GI disturbances, nephrotoxicity, hypothyroidism, tremors, leukocytosis, acne, psoriasis flares, hair loss, edema. Due to these effects it is important to get *thyroid function tests* and renal function tests (*creatinine*) before starting any patient on this medication. Lithium is also teratogenic and has been associated with cardiac defects, a *pregnancy test* is necessary prior to lithium therapy.

17.36 The answer is E

All patients prescribed antidepressants should be advised that it may take *4 to 6 weeks for the effects of medication to be realized.* Treatment for less than this amount of time cannot be considered a failure of that medication. Consider increasing the dose of fluoxetine if no effect is noticed in 4 to 6 weeks. *Consider changing to another SSRI once it has been proven the first has failed to show a response.* Tricyclic antidepressants like amitriptyline generally have more side effects and are not a good choice for this patient.

17.37 The answer is A

Lithium exposure in the first trimester of pregnancy is associated with an increased risk of *cardiac malformations*, in particular, of Ebstein's anomaly. This anomaly is due to a defect in the tricuspid valve with the septal and posterior leaflets displaced down into the right ventricle, while the anterior leaflet is malformed and abnormally attached to the RV free wall. This valve often allows blood to regurgitate from the small right ventricle back into the large right atrium. *Neural tube defects* are an effect of folic acid deficiency during early pregnancy.

17.38 The answer is A

Monoamine oxidase inhibitors (MAOI) have been shown to be particularly effective in the treatment of atypical depression. Important side effects of MAOI therapy include hypertensive crisis and serotonin syndrome. Hypertensive crisis can be precipitated when foods rich in tyramine (e.g., wine, cheese) are ingested by someone also taking an MAOI. *Serotonin syndrome* is caused by the interaction of an MAOI with an SSRI, pseudoephedrine, or meperidine. Serotonin syndrome is characterized by hyperthermia, muscle rigidity, and altered mental status. Therefore, *fluoxetine*, an SSRI, is contraindicated in this patient.

17.39 The answer is D

The diagnosis of bipolar disorder best fits the history and symptoms, but it is by no means certain. She presents with a 1-month history of impaired judgment and erratic behavior followed by increased energy, pressured speech, mood lability, and decreased need for sleep, all of which indicate a manic episode. The emergence of paranoid delusions is also consistent with mania, and a single manic episode, with or without major depressive episodes, qualifies for a diagnosis of bipolar disorder. That diagnosis can only be made, however, if it is believed that the symptoms are not the result of a general medical condition or substance use. We know that she has been using increased amounts of marijuana and alcohol, and that she is probably intoxicated with marijuana at the time of admission. Heavy marijuana use in some individuals can cause a psychotic state with paranoid delusions and hallucinations. There are some features, however, that are inconsistent with a purely *marijuana-induced state*, which more typically presents with decreased talkativeness and long response latency than with the pressured speech seen here. In addition, increased energy and activity, and decreased need for sleep, are much more likely in bipolar disorder than in a marijuana psychosis. The delusional belief of her thoughts being controlled by an outside force is strikingly similar to delusions of control that are so often seen in *schizophrenia*, but the prominent mood symptoms and time course (1 month) preclude that diagnosis. The diagnosis of *schizoaffective disorder* would require a 2-week period of psychotic symptoms without prominent mood symptoms, which is not the case here. An *erotomanic delusional belief* is that the patient is loved by another (often famous) person, not as is the case here, which the patient herself is preoccupied with being in love with someone else.

17.40 The answer is C

The events of days 5 and 6 almost certainly represent the *emergence of a neuroleptic malignant syndrome (NMS)*, an idiosyncratic response to antipsychotics (especially high-potency, typical agents) characterized by fever, rigidity, and obtundation. The clinical diagnosis is confirmed, with the typical findings of leukocytosis and greatly increased CPK. *Anticholinergic delirium* includes fever but not the rigidity or laboratory findings. In addition, patients with an anticholinergic delirium are more likely to be agitated than withdrawn.

17.41 The answer is C

Neuroleptic malignant syndrome is a life-threatening medical emergency. *All medications must be stopped*; *switching to an atypical agent such as risperidone will not help her*. Appropriate treatment includes life support, maintaining fluid and electrolyte balance, and decreasing her fever. *Bromocriptine* is a centrally acting dopamine agonist that presumably works by reversing the effects of the antipsychotic-caused dopamine blockade. The treatment of NMS commonly combines bromocriptine with dantrolene, a peripheral muscle relaxant. *Consultation with the medical service* is crucial, as the treatment may be complex.

Answers 17.42–17.45

17.42 The answer is B

17.43 The answer is C

17.44 The answer is D

17.45 The answer is D

Tricyclic antidepressants such as imipramine are known for their *cardiotoxicity* as they prolong cardiac conduction time and can cause a variety of arrhythmias. Also among the substantial side effects of tricyclic antidepressants are *weight gain*, sedation, anticholinergic effects, and orthostatic hypotension. *Weight gain* is also a common adverse effect of clozapine, as well as agranulocytosis therefore weekly blood monitoring is necessary. Neither clozapine nor imipramine act as *norepinephrine partial agonists*, instead, clozapine acts by blockade of serotonin-2a and D2 receptors, while imipramine acts by reducing the reuptake of norepinephrine and serotonin. *There are no known teratogenic effects of clozapine nor imipramine*.

Answers 17.46–17.50

17.46 The answer is A

17.47 The answer is C

17.48 The answer is E

17.49 The answer is D

17.50 The answer is B

Sigmund Freud was initially interested in a psychoneural project for all mental phenomena. Limitations of the brain sciences of the day led him to adopt instead a model that relied on a concept of mental function borrowed from physics. The notion that *depressed affect is derived from retroflexion of aggressive impulses* directed against an ambivalently loved internalized object was actually formulated by his Berlin disciple Karl Abraham and later elaborated by Freud. Abraham and Freud hypothesized that turned-in anger was intended as punishment for the love object that had thwarted the depressed patient's need for dependency and love. Because, in an attempt to prevent the traumatic loss, the object had already been internalized, the patient now became the target of his or her own thanatotic impulses. A central element in those psychic operations was the depressed patient's ambivalence toward the object, which was perceived as a frustrating parent. Aggression directed at a loved object (parent) was therefore attended by considerable guilt. In the extreme, such ambivalence, guilt, and retroflexed anger could lead to suicidal behavior.

Bridging the divide between psyche and soma was the ambition of Swiss-born *Adolf Meyer* (1866–1950), who dominated psychiatry from his chair at Johns Hopkins University during the first half of the 20th century. Meyer *coined the term psychobiology* to emphasize that both psychological and biological factors could enter into the causation of depressive and other mental disorders. Because of the nascent state of brain science during Meyer's time, he was more adept at biography than biology and therefore paid greater attention to psychosocial causation. He preferred the term *depression* (pressed down) to *melancholia* because of its lack of biological connotation. He conceived of depressive states in terms of unspecified constitutional or biological factors interacting with a series of life situations beginning at birth or even at conception. From that viewpoint arose the unique importance accorded personal history in depressive reactions to life events.

The cognitive model, developed by *Aaron Beck* at the University of Pennsylvania, *hypothesizes that thinking along negative lines* (e.g., thinking that one is helpless, unworthy, or useless) is the hallmark of clinical depression. In effect, depression is redefined in terms of a cognitive triad, according to which patients think of themselves as helpless, interpret most events unfavorably vis-à-vis the self, and believe the future to be hopeless. In more recent formulations in academic psychology, these cognitions are said to be characterized by a negative attributional style that is global, internal, and stable and to exist in the form of latent mental schemata that generate biased interpretations of life events.

Emil Kraepelin's (1856–1926) unique contribution was not so much grouping together all the forms of melancholia and mania, but his methodology and painstaking longitudinal observations, *which established manic-depressive illness as a nosological entity and* (he hoped) *a disease entity*. His rationale was that (1) the various forms had a common heredity measured as a function of familial aggregation of homotypic and heterotypic cases; (2) frequent transitions from one form to the other occurred during longitudinal follow-up; (3) a recurrent course with illness-free intervals characterized most cases; (4) the superimposed episodes were commonly opposite to the patient's habitual temperament; that is, mania was superimposed on a depressive temperament and depression was superimposed on a hypomanic temperament; and (5) both depressive and manic features could occur during the same episode (mixed states).

The learned helplessness model is in some ways an experimental analogue of the cognitive model. The model proposes that the depressive posture is learned from past situations in which the person was unable to terminate undesirable contingencies. The model is based on experiments in dogs that were prevented from taking adaptive action to avoid unpleasant electrical shock and subsequently showed no motivation to escape such aversive stimuli, even when escape avenues were readily available. Armed with evidence from many such experiments, a University of Pennsylvania psychologist, *Martin Seligman*, postulated a trait of learned helplessness (a belief that it is futile to initiate personal action to reverse aversive circumstances) formed from the accumulation of past episodes of uncontrollable helplessness.

Answers 17.51–17.54

17.51 The answer is B

17.52 The answer is A

17.53 The answer is B

17.54 The answer is C

Three factors influenced historical trends in the relative prevalence of mood disorders by age: period effects, age effects, and cohort effects.

Period effects are changes in the prevalence of an illness secondary to environmental stressors on the population or particular age groups within the population at a specific period in history. For example, *the uncertainty of employment among college graduates and the trend among younger persons to delay marriage during the 1990s may place young adults at greater risk for depression and suicide* because of economic impairment and lack of affiliative relations.

Age effects are the biological and psychosocial factors that predispose an individual to develop a particular disorder during a specific part of the life cycle. For example, *the genetic predisposition to develop major depressive disorder is probably greatest during the 30s, whereas the predisposition to develop a bipolar disorder is greatest during the 20s.* Age-related changes in the brain, such as increased subcortical hyperintensities on brain magnetic resonance imaging, may also be associated with mood disorders. Perhaps *the most consistently observed age effect relevant to mood disorders that has been observed during the 20th century is the positive association between age and suicide among white males in the United States.*

Cohort effects are the relative differences in rates of illness across different generations. A cohort is usually defined by the year or decade of birth. Persons born in a given year may be at greater risk for an illness, such as major depressive disorder, throughout their lives. Suicide data reveal marked cohort trends throughout the 20th century. *For example, persons currently 75 to 85 years of age (approximately the birth cohorts of 1915–1925) have exhibited lower suicide rates at all ages than either the 1900 or the 1940 birth cohorts.*

Considerable statistical and methodological problems confound sorting out the relative contribution of period, age, and cohort effects upon the prevalence and incidence of mood disorders by age. First, these effects undoubtedly interact. Stressors during a particular period interact with age-related vulnerability. For example, the current high rate of substance abuse among adolescents may reflect both the vulnerability of adolescents to substance abuse, which is an age effect, and the greater availability of drugs to adolescents, a period effect. Second, older persons may not recognize major depressive episodes as such, and so do not report them, thus setting the higher threshold for identifying depression among community-dwelling elders. Yet age does not appear to affect the rate of hospitalization for mood disorders. The more severe cases of major depressive disorder are hospitalized, regardless of age, and the relative cohort differences persist in hospitalization rates.

Most investigators have explained the current data as reflecting a period effect. They argue that the risk for depressive disorders increased dramatically for all ages from about 1965 to 1975 but has since stabilized at a higher incidence. Young persons are more vulnerable to that period effect, however, and therefore carry the greater burden of depressive disorders. A young person who experiences a major depressive episode is likely to exhibit ongoing and severe depressive episodes for many years. Therefore, clinicians can expect to see the current cohort of younger persons endure major depressive disorders for a long time. Despite being the healthiest and most affluent generation of the 20th century, younger persons may be placed at greater risk for major depressive disorders by a variety of environmental risk factors, including increased urbanization, more social isolation and anomie, changes in occupational roles and career trajectories for both men and women, heightened secularization, and expanding geographic mobility.

Answers 17.55–17.58

17.55 The answer is C

17.56 The answer is D

17.57 The answer is B

17.58 The answer is C

Between the extremes of manic-depressive illness defined by at least one acute manic episode, which could be mood-congruent or -incongruent (*bipolar I disorder*), and strictly defined major depressive disorder without any personal or family history of mania (pure *unipolar disorder*), there exists an overlapping group of intermediary forms characterized by recurrent major depressive episodes and hypomania (*bipolar II disorder*). There is never any history of acute mania in either unipolar depression or bipolar II disorder. *Psychotic features* are typically not present in either form of depression. There can be recurrent episodes of major depressive symptoms, as well as *atypical features* in both unipolar and bipolar II forms. *Symptoms of hypomania* are characteristic only of bipolar II disorder.

Answers 17.59–17.61

17.59 The answer is D

17.60 The answer is B

17.61 The answer is A

For those mood disorders with atypical symptoms (hypersomnia, increased appetite, mood reactivity), there is strong evidence that *tricyclic antidepressants are less effective than monoamine oxidase inhibitors for symptomatic relief.* Disorders refractory to several different medications have shown improvement with the use of *electroconvulsive therapy*. Seasonal affective disorder, typically with worsening mood symptoms during the winter months, has been shown to improve with *light therapy* alone or in combination with medication.

18 Anxiety Disorders

Anxiety disorders are among the most prevalent psychiatric conditions in the United States. Further, studies have persistently shown that they produce inordinate morbidity, use of health care services, and functional impairment. Combined with the acknowledgment that many people suffering from anxiety never present for treatment, these facts emphasize the importance of clinical research and exploration of this field. Defining anxiety disorders can be problematic, as there exists a fine line between normal adaptive anxiety and pathologic functioning. The revised fourth edition of the *Diagnostic and Statistical Manual of Mental Disorders* (DSM-IV-TR) attempts to do this by delineating a number of specific anxiety disorders with clear diagnostic criteria. These include panic disorder, agoraphobia, posttraumatic stress disorder (PTSD), and generalized anxiety disorder, among others.

Anxiety disorders, like most psychiatric disorders, are usually the result of a complex interplay of biological, psychological, and psychosocial elements. Treatment of these disorders can be correspondingly complex. Understanding the neuroanatomy and molecular biology of anxiety promises new insights into etiology and more effective treatments in the future. There is currently an array of treatment approaches from the psychoanalytic, to cognitive, to behavioral, to psychopharmacologic. Many times, a combination of these treatments is utilized to best address the multiplicity of etiologic forces.

Another fascinating aspect of anxiety disorders is the exquisite interplay of genetic and experiential factors. Students should also be aware of the role of specific neurotransmitters in the development of anxiety, and the mechanisms of anxiolytic medications.

The student should study the questions and answers below for a useful review of these disorders.

HELPFUL HINTS

The student should know the following names, cases, terms, and acronyms related to anxiety disorders.

- acute stress disorder
- adrenergic
- aggression
- ambivalence
- anticipatory anxiety
- anxiety
- *Aplysia*
- aversive conditioning
- benzodiazepines
- cerebral cortex
- cleanliness
- clomipramine (Anafranil)
- conflict
- counterphobic attitude
- Jacob M. DaCosta
- Charles Darwin
- disorders associated with anxiety
- dopamine
- ego-dystonic
- fear
- Otto Fenichel
- flooding
- Sigmund Freud
- GABA
- generalized anxiety disorder
- hypnosis
- imipramine (Tofranil)
- implosion
- intrapsychic conflict
- isolation
- lactate infusion
- limbic system
- Little Albert
- Little Hans
- locus ceruleus and raphe nuclei
- magical thinking
- MHPG
- mitral valve prolapse
- MMPI, Rorschach
- norepinephrine
- numbing
- obsessive-compulsive disorder (OCD)
- panic attack
- panic disorder
- panicogens
- peripheral manifestations
- PET
- phobias:
    - agoraphobia
    - social
    - specific
- PTSD
- propranolol (Inderal)
- reaction formation
- repression
- secondary gain
- serotonin
- shell shock
- sleep EEG studies
- soldier's heart
- stress
- systematic desensitization
- thought stopping
- time-limited psychotherapy
- trauma
- undoing
- John B. Watson
- Joseph Wolpe

QUESTIONS

Directions

Each of the questions or incomplete statements below is followed by five suggested responses or completions. Select the *one* that is *best* in each case.

18.1 Physiological activity associated with PTSD include all *except*

A. Decreased parasympathetic tone
B. Elevated baseline heart rate
C. Increased circulating thyroxine
D. Excessive sweating
E. Increased blood pressure

18.2 Mr. F sought treatment for symptoms that he developed in the wake of an automobile accident that had occurred approximately 6 weeks before his psychiatric evaluation. While driving to work on a mid-January morning, Mr. F lost control of his car on an icy road. His car swerved out of control into oncoming traffic, collided with another car, and then hit a nearby pedestrian. After referral, Mr. F reported frequent intrusive thoughts about the accident, including nightmares of the event and recurrent intrusive visions of his car slamming into the pedestrian. He reported that he had altered his driving route to work to avoid the scene of the accident and that he found himself switching the TV channel whenever a commercial for snow tires appeared. Mr. F described frequent difficulty falling asleep, poor concentration, and an increased focus on his environment, particularly when he was driving.

Which of the following is the most appropriate diagnosis for this patient?

A. Generalized anxiety disorder
B. Post-traumatic stress disorder
C. Acute stress disorder
D. Adjustment disorder
E. Panic disorder

18.3 Which of the following statements regarding anxiety and gender differences is *true*?

A. Women have greater rates of almost all anxiety disorders.
B. Gender ratios are nearly equal with OCD.
C. No significant difference exists in average age of anxiety onset.
D. Women have a twofold greater lifetime rate of agoraphobia than men.
E. All of the above

18.4 Anxiety disorders

A. are greater among people at lower socioeconomic levels
B. are highest among those with higher levels of education
C. are lowest among homemakers
D. have shown different prevalences with regard to social class but not ethnicity
E. All of the above

18.5 The risk of developing anxiety disorders is enhanced by

A. Eating disorders
B. Depression
C. Substance abuse
D. Allergies
E. All of the above

18.6 Which of the following is *not* typical of the course of panic disorder?

A. Onset is typically in late adolescence or early adulthood
B. Tends to exhibit a fluctuating course
C. Typical patients exhibit a pattern of chronic disability
D. Majority of patients live relatively normal lives
E. All of the above

18.7 Which of the following examples or situations is most likely to cause PTSD?

A. Involvement in an earthquake
B. Being diagnosed with cancer
C. Rape
D. Witnessing a crime
E. Observing a flood

18.8 Which of the following is the most common symptom pattern associated with OCD?

A. Obsession of doubt
B. Obsession of contamination
C. Intrusive thoughts
D. Obsession of symmetry
E. Compulsive hoarding

18.9 Which of the following is *not* a component of the DSM-IV-TR diagnostic criteria for OCD?

A. Obsessions are acknowledged as excessive or unreasonable
B. There are attempts to ignore or suppress compulsive thoughts or impulses
C. Obsessions or compulsions are time consuming, and take more than 1 hour a day
D. Children need not recognize their obsessions are unreasonable
E. The person recognized the obsessional thoughts as a product of outside themselves

18.10 All of the following have been noted through brain imaging in patients with panic disorder *except*

A. Magnetic resonance imaging (MRI) studies have shown pathological involvement of the temporal lobes
B. Generalized cerebral vasoconstriction
C. Right temporal cortical atrophy
D. Increased blood flow to the basal ganglia

E. Positron Tomographic Emission scans have implicated dysregulation of blood flow in panic disorder

18.11 Buspirone acts as a

A. serotonin partial agonist useful in treatment of generalized anxiety disorder
B. dopamine partial agonist useful in the treatment of generalized anxiety disorder
C. serotonin partial agonist useful in the treatment of OCD
D. dopamine partial agonist useful in the treatment of OCD
E. none of the above

18.12 Mr. A was a successful businessman who presented for treatment after a change in his business schedule. Although he had formerly worked largely from an office near his home, a promotion led to a schedule of frequent out-of-town meetings requiring weekly flights. Mr. A reported being "deathly afraid" of flying. Even the thought of getting on an airplane led to thoughts of impending doom in which he envisioned his airplane crashing to the ground. These thoughts were associated with intense fear, palpitations, sweating, clamminess, and stomach upset. Although the thought of flying was terrifying enough, Mr. A became nearly incapacitated when he went to the airport. Immediately before boarding, Mr. A would often have to turn back from the plane, running to the bathroom to vomit. Which of the following is the most appropriate treatment for this patient who has another flight scheduled tomorrow?

A. Lorazepam
B. Paroxetine
C. Beta agonists
D. Exposure therapy
E. None of the above

18.13 Tourette's disorder has been shown to possibly have a familial and genetic relationship with

A. panic disorder
B. social phobia
C. generalized anxiety disorder
D. OCD
E. none of the above

18.14 Unexpected panic attacks are required for the diagnosis of

A. panic disorder
B. social phobia
C. specific phobia
D. generalized anxiety disorder
E. all of the above

18.15 A patient with OCD might exhibit all of the following brain-imaging findings *except*

A. abnormalities in frontal lobes, cingulum, and basal ganglia
B. decreased caudate volumes bilaterally compared with normal controls
C. lower metabolic rates in basal ganglia and white matter than in normal controls
D. longer mean T1 relaxation times in the frontal cortex than normal controls
E. significantly more gray matter and less white matter than normal controls

18.16 Isolated panic attacks without functional disturbances

A. are uncommon
B. occur in less than 2 percent of the population
C. are part of the criteria for diagnostic panic disorder
D. usually involve anticipatory anxiety or phobic avoidance
E. none of the above

18.17 Sigmund Freud postulated that the defense mechanisms necessary in phobias are

A. repression, displacement, and avoidance
B. regression, condensation, and projection
C. regression, repression, and isolation
D. repression, projection, and displacement
E. regression, condensation, and dissociation

18.18 Which of the following choices most accurately describes the role of serotonin in OCD?

A. Serotonergic drugs are an ineffective treatment.
B. Dysregulation of serotonin is involved in the symptom formation.
C. Measures of platelet binding sites of titrated imipramine are abnormally low.
D. Measures of serotonin metabolites in cerebrospinal fluid are abnormally high.
E. None of the above

18.19 Therapy for phobias may include all of the following *except*

A. propranolol (Inderal)
B. systematic desensitization
C. phenelzine (Nardil)
D. flooding
E. counterphobic attitudes

18.20 First-line medication treatments of anxiety disorders may generally include all of the following *except*

A. fluoxetine (Prozac)
B. fluvoxamine (Luvox)
C. venlafaxine (Effexor)
D. diazepam (Valium)
E. nefazodone (Serzone)

18.21 Induction of panic attacks in patients with panic disorder can occur with

A. yohimbine
B. carbon dioxide
C. doxapram

D. cholecystokinin
E. all of the above

Directions

Each set of lettered headings below is followed by a list of numbered words or phrases. For each numbered word or phrase, select

A. if the item is associated with A only
B. if the item is associated with B only
C. if the item is associated with both A and B
D. if the item is associated with neither A nor B

Questions 18.22–18.25

A. Panic disorder
B. Agoraphobia

18.22 Higher rates for women than for men
18.23 Lifetime prevalence of 3 to 5.6 percent
18.24 Lifetime prevalence of 0.6 to 6 percent
18.25 Relatives have higher rates of this disorder than relatives of controls

Questions 18.26–18.30

A. Generalized anxiety disorder
B. Panic disorder

18.26 Response rates between 60 and 80 percent have been reported to buspirone
18.27 Patients with the disorder may still be responsive to buspirone after being exposed to benzodiazepine
18.28 Buspirone's use is limited to potentiating the effects of other antidepressants and counteracting the adverse sexual effects of selective serotonin reuptake inhibitors (SSRIs)
18.29 Relapse rates are generally high after discontinuation of medication
18.30 Tricyclic drugs have been reported to worsen anxiety symptoms in patients where first symptoms were precipitated by cocaine use

Questions 18.31–18.34

A. Cognitive-behavioral therapy
B. Psychodynamic therapy

18.31 Produces 80 to 90 percent panic-free status in panic disorder within at least 6 months of treatment
18.32 May be nearly twice as effective in the treatment of social phobia as a more educational-supportive approach
18.33 Goals are more ambitious and require more time to achieve
18.34 Combining treatment with medication may be superior to either treatment alone

Directions

Each set of lettered headings below is followed by a list of numbered words or statements. For each numbered word or statement, select the *one* lettered heading most closely associated with it. Each lettered heading may be selected once, more than once, or not at all.

Questions 18.35–18.39

A. Acrophobia
B. Cynophobia
C. Mysophobia
D. Xenophobia
E. Ailurophobia

18.35 Fear of dirt and germs
18.36 Fear of heights
18.37 Fear of strangers
18.38 Fear of dogs
18.39 Fear of cats

Questions 18.40–18.42

A. Norepinephrine
B. Serotonin
C. γ-Aminobutyric acid (GABA)

18.40 The cell bodies of the neurotransmitter's neurons are confined primarily to the locus ceruleus
18.41 Benzodiazepines enhance the neurotransmitter's effects at its receptors
18.42 The cell bodies of the neurotransmitter's neurons are localized primarily within the raphe nuclei

Questions 18.43–18.46

A. In vivo exposure
B. Interoceptive exposure
C. Systematic desensitization
D. Imaginal exposure

18.43 A patient is presented with photographs of snakes while practicing various relaxation techniques to overcome fear; gradually he practices relaxation while in the presence of live snakes.
18.44 A patient with OCD attempts to use public telephones and doorknobs while intentionally refraining from washing her hands afterwards.
18.45 A patient is asked to imagine his wartime experiences as vividly as possible, in order to confront his memory of the traumatic events.
18.46 A patient breathes through a thin straw in order to produce the sensation of not getting enough air; this activity produces a similar sensation to the distressing feeling of getting on an airplane.

ANSWERS

18.1 The answer is C

According to current conceptualizations, PTSD is associated with objective measures of *physiological arousal*. This includes *elevated baselines heart rate, increased blood pressure and excessive sweating* that have been reported in the context of trauma cue reactivity studies. Further, evidence from studies of baseline cardiovascular activity revealed a positive association between heart rate and PTSD. The chronicity of PTSD was a moderator of this association. The most chronic patients showed the largest heart rate elevation, suggesting that increased heart rate is a response to repeated stress.

The finding of elevated baseline heart rate activity is consistent with the hypothesis of tonic sympathetic nervous system arousal in PTSD. *Disturbance in ANS activity in PTSD is characterized by increased sympathetic and decreased parasympathetic tone.* Preliminary evidence suggests that this autonomic imbalance can be normalized with SSRI treatment. *There is no change in blood level of thyroxine in PTSD.*

18.2 The answer is B

Both post-traumatic stress disorder and acute stress disorder are characterized by the onset of psychiatric symptoms immediately after exposure to a traumatic event. DSM-IV-TR explicitly notes that such a traumatic event involves either witnessing or experiencing threatened death or injury or witnessing or experiencing threat to physical integrity. Further, the response to the traumatic event must involve intense fear or horror. Such traumatic experiences might include being involved in or witnessing a violent accident or crime, military combat, assault, being kidnapped, being involved in natural disasters, being diagnosed with a life-threatening illness, or experiencing systematic physical or sexual abuse.

In PTSD, the individual develops symptoms in three domains: reexperiencing the trauma, avoiding stimuli associated with the trauma, and experiencing symptoms of increased autonomic arousal, such as an enhanced startle. Flashbacks, in which the individual may act and feel as if the trauma were recurring, represent the classic form of reexperiencing. Other forms of reexperiencing include distressing recollections or dreams and either physiological or psychological stress reactions when exposed to stimuli that are linked to the trauma. The diagnosis of acute stress disorder is applied to syndromes that resemble PTSD but *last less than 1 month after a trauma.* Acute stress disorder is characterized by reexperiencing, avoidance, and increased arousal, much like PTSD.

Generalized anxiety disorder is characterized by a pattern of frequent, persistent worry and anxiety that is out of proportion to the impact of the event. *Adjustment disorder* is characterized by an emotional response to a stressful event that begins within 3 months of the stressor and remits within 6 months of the stressor being removed. *Panic disorder* is characterized by recurrent panic attacks, which are periods of abrupt and intense fear accompanied by autonomic symptoms.

18.3 The answer is E (all)

The results of community studies reveal that *women have greater rates of almost all of the anxiety disorders.* Despite differences in the magnitude of the rates of specific anxiety disorders across studies, the gender ratio is strikingly similar. Women have an approximately twofold elevation in lifetime rates of panic, generalized anxiety disorder, agoraphobia, and simple phobia compared to men in nearly all of the studies. The only exception is the *nearly equal gender ratio in the rates of OCD and social phobia.*

Studies of youth report similar differences in the magnitude of anxiety disorders among girls and boys. Similar to the gender ratio for adults, girls tend to have more of all subtypes of anxiety disorders, irrespective of the age composition of the sample. However, it has also been reported that, despite the greater rates of anxiety in girls across all ages, there is *no significant difference between boys and girls in the average age at onset of anxiety.*

18.4 The answer is A

Community studies have consistently found that rates of anxiety disorders in general are *greater among those at lower levels of socioeconomic status and education level.* Anxiety disorders are negatively associated with income and education levels. For example, there is almost a twofold difference between rates of anxiety disorders in individuals in the highest income bracket and those in the lowest and between those who completed more than 16 years of school and those who completed less than 11 years of school. In addition, certain anxiety disorders seem to be elevated in specific occupations. *Anxiety disorders are higher in homemakers* and those who are unemployed or have a disability. Similarly, higher levels of generalized anxiety disorder and phobias are found in homemakers, students, and other unemployed persons. Several community studies have also yielded greater rates of anxiety disorders, particularly phobic disorders, among African Americans. The reasons for *ethnic and social class differences* have not yet been evaluated systematically; however, both methodological factors and differences in exposure to stressors have been advanced as possible explanations.

18.5 The answer is E (all)

The magnitude of comorbidity in adults and adolescents with anxiety suggests that investigation of the role of other disorders in enhancing the risk for the initial development and persistence of anxiety disorders over time may be fruitful. *Disorders that may enhance the risk for the development of anxiety disorders include eating disorders, depression, and substance use and abuse.* In contrast, anxiety disorders have been shown to elevate the risk of subsequent substance use disorders and may comprise a mediator of the link between depression and the subsequent development of substance use disorders in a clinical sample.

Several studies have also suggested that there is an association between anxiety disorders and allergies, high fever, immunological diseases and infections, epilepsy, and connective tissue diseases. Likewise, prospective studies have revealed that the anxiety disorders may comprise risk factors for the development of some cardiovascular and neurological diseases, such as ischemic heart disease and migraine.

18.6 The answer is C

Panic disorder *typically has its onset in late adolescence or early adulthood*, although cases of childhood-onset and late adulthood–onset disorder have been described. There are only tentative data on the natural course of panic disorder. The best evidence on the course of any disorder, including panic disorder, is derived from prospective epidemiological research, as both retrospective and clinically based studies are vulnerable to biases that preclude firm conclusions on course. Unfortunately, few such studies exist. Research from retrospective or clinical studies suggest that panic disorder tends to exhibit a *fluctuating course*, with varying levels of persistence over the life span. Approximately one-third to one-half of patients appear psychiatrically healthy at follow-up, with the *majority of these patients living relatively normal lives*, despite either fluctuating or recurrent symptoms. Typically, patients with chronic disorders exhibit a *pattern of exacerbation and remissions rather than chronic disability*.

18.7 The answer is C

Post-traumatic stress disorder is characterized by the onset of psychiatric symptoms immediately following exposure to a traumatic event. DSM-IV-TR specifies that the traumatic event involves either witnessing or experiencing threatened death or injury or witnessing or experiencing threat to physical integrity. Further, the response to the traumatic event must involve intense fear or horror. Such traumatic experiences might include *being involved in or witnessing an accident or crime*, military combat, assault, being kidnapped, *being involved in natural disasters, being diagnosed with a life-threatening illness*, or experiencing systematic physical or sexual abuse. *Manmade disasters or events are more likely to elicit PTSD symptoms than natural disasters or events; hence rape is a common cause of PTSD*. PTSD also requires characteristic symptoms following such trauma. There is evidence of a relationship between the degree of trauma and the likelihood of symptoms. The proximity to, and intensity of, the trauma bear on the probability of developing symptomatology.

18.8 The answer is B

The presentation of obsessions and compulsions in patients with OCD may overlap and change with time, but there remains four major symptom patterns. The *most common pattern in an obsession of contamination*, followed by washing or accompanied by compulsive avoidance of the presumably contaminated object. The feared object is often hard to avoid (e.g., feces, urine, dust, or germs). Patients may literally rub the skin off their hands by excessive hand washing or may be unable to leave their homes because of fear of germs. Patients with contamination obsessions usually believe that the contamination is spread from object to object or person to person by the slightest contact.

The second most common pattern is an *obsession of doubt*, followed by a compulsion of checking. In the third most common pattern, there are *intrusive obsessional thoughts* without a compulsion. Such obsessions are usually repetitious thoughts of a sexual or aggressive act that is reprehensible to the patient. The fourth most common pattern is the *need for symmetry* or precision, which can lead to a compulsion of slowness. Patients can literally take hours to eat a meal or shave their faces. Religious obsessions and *compulsive hoarding* are other common patterns in patients with OCD.

18.9 The answer is E

Obsessions and compulsions are the essential features of OCD. An individual must exhibit either obsessions or compulsions to meet DSM-IV-TR criteria. DSM-IV-TR recognizes obsessions as "persistent ideas, thoughts, impulses, or images that are experienced as intrusive and inappropriate," causing distress. Obsessions provoke anxiety, which accounts for the categorization of OCD as an anxiety disorder. However, they must be differentiated from excessive worries about real-life problems and associated with efforts to either ignore or suppress the obsessions. The DSM-IV-TR diagnostic criteria for OCD indicate *the obsessions must be acknowledged as excessive or unreasonable (with the exception that children need not acknowledge this fact), there must be attempts to suppress these intrusive thoughts, and that the obsessions or compulsions are time consuming to the point of requiring at least one hour a day*, among other diagnostic criteria. As part of the criteria however, is *not that the thoughts are a product of outside the person, as in thought insertion, but that the person recognizes that the thoughts are a product of his or her own mind.*

18.10 The answer is D

Structural brain imaging studies, such as MRI, in patients with panic disorder have implicated *pathological involvement in the temporal lobes*, particularly the hippocampus. One MRI study reported abnormalities, especially *cortical atrophy*, in the right temporal lobe of these patients. Functional brain imaging studies, such as PET, have implicated *dysregulation of cerebral blood flow*. Specifically, anxiety disorders and panic attacks are associated with *cerebral vasoconstriction*, which may result in central nervous system symptoms such as dizziness and in peripheral nervous system symptoms that may be induced by hyperventilation and hypocapnia. Most functional brain-imaging studies have used a specific panic-inducing substance (e.g., lactate, caffeine, or yohimbine) in combination with PET or single photon emisision computed tomography (SPECT) to assess the effects of the panic-inducing substance and the induced panic attack on cerebral blood flow. *Increased blood flow to the basal ganglia has not been noted in patients with panic disorder.*

18.11 The answer is A

Buspirone is a serotonin *receptor partial agonist and is most likely effective in 60 to 80 percent of patients with generalized anxiety disorder*. Data indicate that buspirone is more effective in reducing the cognitive symptoms of generalized anxiety disorder than in reducing the somatic symptoms. The major disadvantage of buspirone is that its effects take 2 to 3 weeks to become evident, in contrast to the almost immediate anxiolytic effects of the benzodiazepines.

18.12 The answer is A

Specific phobias are often treated with as-needed benzodiazepines, such as lorazepam. In the clinical case described, this is the most appropriate choice of treatment given their high safety margin (e.g., in overdose) and their overall excellent efficacy and rapid onset of action. *Beta-adrenergic receptor antagonists (not agonists)* may be useful in the treatment of specific phobia, especially when the phobia is associated with panic attacks. The most commonly used treatment for specific phobia is *exposure therapy*. In this method therapists desensitize patients by using a series of gradual, self-paced exposures to the phobic stimulus, and thus would not be appropriate when immediate relief is required. *Paroxetine, an SSRI, is not indicated for the immediate treatment of phobias.*

18.13 The answer is D

An interesting set of findings concerns the possible relationship between a subset of cases of OCD and certain types of motor tic syndromes (i.e., Tourette's disorder and chronic motor tics). Increased rates of OCD, Tourette's disorder, and chronic motor tics were found in the relatives of Tourette's disorder patients as compared to relatives of controls whether or not the patient had OCD. However, most family studies of probands with OCD have found elevated rates of Tourette's disorder and chronic motor tics only among the relatives of probands with OCD who also have some form of tic disorder. Taken together these data suggest that *there is a familial and perhaps genetic relationship between Tourette's disorder and chronic motor tics and some cases of OCD.* Cases of the latter in which the individual also manifests tics are the most likely to be related to Tourette's disorder and chronic motor tics. As there is considerable evidence of a genetic contribution to Tourette's disorder, this finding also supports a genetic role in a subset of cases of OCDs.

18.14 The answer is A

Unexpected panic attacks are required for the diagnosis of *panic disorder,* but panic attacks can occur in several anxiety disorders. The clinician must consider the context of the panic attack when making a diagnosis. Panic attacks can be divided into two types: (1) unexpected panic attacks, which are not associated with a situational trigger, and (2) situationally bound panic attacks, which occur immediately after exposure in a situational trigger or in anticipation of the situational trigger. Situationally bound panic attacks are most characteristic of *social phobia* and *specific phobia.* In *generalized anxiety disorder* the anxiety cannot be about having a panic attack.

18.15 The answer is C

Brain-imaging studies of OCD patients using PET have found *abnormalities in frontal lobes, cingulum, and basal ganglia.* PET scans have shown *higher levels of metabolism* and blood flows to those areas in OCD patients than in controls. Volumetric computed tomography (CT) scans have shown *decreased caudate volumes bilaterally in OCD patients* compared with normal controls. Morphometric magnetic resonance imaging (MMRI) has revealed that *OCD patients have significantly more gray matter and less white matter* than normal controls. MRI has also shown *longer mean T1 relaxation times in the frontal cortex in OCD patients* than is seen in normal controls.

18.16 The answer is D

Some differences between DSM-IV-TR and earlier versions in the diagnostic criteria of panic disorder are interesting. For example, no longer is a specific number of panic attacks necessary in a specific period of time to meet criteria for panic disorder. *Rather, the attacks must be recurrent and at least one attack must be followed by at least 1 month of anticipatory anxiety or phobic avoidance.* This recognizes for the first time that although the panic attack is obviously the seminal event for diagnosing panic disorder, the syndrome involves a number of disturbances that go beyond the attack itself. *Isolated panic attacks without functional disturbances are not diagnosed as panic disorder.* Furthermore, *isolated panic attacks without functional disturbance are not uncommon, occurring in approximately 15 percent of the population.*

18.17 The answer is A

Sigmund Freud viewed phobias as resulting from conflicts centered on an unresolved childhood oedipal situation. In the adult, because the sexual drive continues to have a strong incestuous coloring, its arousal tends to create anxiety that is characteristically a fear of castration. The anxiety then alerts the ego to exert *repression* to keep the drive away from conscious representation and discharge. Because repression is not entirely successful in its function, the ego must call on auxiliary defenses. In phobic patients, the defenses, arising genetically from an earlier phobic response during the initial childhood period of the oedipal conflict, involves primarily the use of *displacement*—that is, the sexual conflict is transposed or displaced from the person who evoked the conflict to a seemingly unimportant, irrelevant object or situation, which has the power to elicit the entire constellation of affects, including anxiety. The phobic object or situation selected has a direct associative connection with the primary source of the conflict and has thus come naturally to symbolize it. Furthermore, the situation or object is usually such that the patient is able to keep out of its way and by the additional defense mechanism of *avoidance,* to escape suffering from serious anxiety.

Regression is an unconscious defense mechanism in which a person undergoes a partial or total return to early patterns of adaptation. *Condensation* is a mental process in which one symbol stands for a number of components. *Projection* is an unconscious defense mechanism in which persons attribute to another person generally unconscious ideas, thoughts, feelings, and impulses that are undesirable or unacceptable in themselves. Projection protects persons from anxiety arising from an inner conflict. By externalizing whatever is unacceptable, persons deal with it as a situation apart from themselves. In psychoanalysis, *isolation* is a defense mechanism involving the separation of an idea or memory from its attached feeling tone. Unacceptable ideational content is thereby rendered free of its disturbing or unpleasant emotional charge. *Dissociation* is an unconscious defense mechanism involving the segregation of any group of mental or behavioral processes from the rest of the person's psychic activity. Table 18.1 describes a more current view of seven of the psychodynamic themes in phobias.

18.18 The answer is B

Clinical trials of drugs have supported the hypothesis that *dysregulation of serotonin is involved in the symptom formation* of obsessions and compulsions. Data show that *serotonergic drugs are an effective, not an ineffective treatment,* but it is unclear whether serotonin is involved in the cause of OCD.

Clinical studies have shown that *measures of platelet binding sites of imipramine* and of *serotonin metabolites in cerebrospinal*

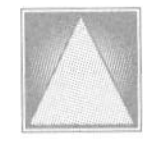

Table 18.1
Psychodynamic Themes in Phobias

Principal defense mechanisms include: displacement, projection, and avoidance.
Environmental stressors, including humiliation and criticism from an older sibling, parental fights, or loss and separation from parents, interact with a genetic constitutional diathesis.
A characteristic pattern of internal object relations is externalized in social situations in the case of social phobia.
Anticipation of humiliation, criticism, and ridicule is projected onto individuals in the environment.
Shame and embarrassment are the principal affect states.
Family members may encourage phobic behavior and serve as obstacles to any treatment plan.
Self exposure to the feared situation is a basic principle of all treatment.

fluid are variable, neither consistently abnormally low nor abnormally high.

18.19 The answer is E

A *counterphobic attitude* is not a therapy for phobias, although it may lead to counterphobic behavior. Many activities may mask phobic anxiety, which can be hidden behind attitudes and behavior patterns that represent a denial, either that the dreaded object or situation is dangerous or that one is afraid of it. Basic to this phenomenon is a reversal of the situation in which one is the passive victim of external circumstances to a position of attempting actively to confront and master what one fears. The counterphobic person seeks out situations of danger and rushes enthusiastically toward them. The devotee of dangerous sports, such as parachute jumping, rock climbing, bungee jumping, and parasailing, may be exhibiting counterphobic behavior. Such patterns may be secondary to phobic anxieties or may be used as a normal means of dealing with a realistically dangerous situation.

Both behavioral and pharmacological techniques have been used in treating phobias. The most common behavioral technique is *systematic desensitization,* in which the patient is exposed serially to a predetermined list of anxiety-provoking stimuli graded in a hierarchy from the least frightening to the most frightening. Patients are taught to self-induce a state of relaxation in the face of each anxiety-provoking stimulus. In *flooding,* patients are exposed to the phobic stimulus (actually [in vivo] or through imagery) for as long as they can tolerate the fear until they reach a point at which they can no longer feel it. The social phobia of stage fright in performers has been effectively treated with such β-adrenergic antagonists as *propranolol (Inderal),* which blocks the physiological signs of anxiety (for example, tachycardia). *Phenelzine (Nardil),* a monoamine oxidase inhibitor, is also useful in treating social phobia.

18.20 The answer is D

Antidepressant medication is increasingly seen as the medication treatment of choice for the anxiety disorders. More specifically, drugs with primary effects on the serotonin neurotransmission system have become first-line recommendations for panic disorder, social phobia, OCD, and PTSD. Evidence now exists that such medications are also effective for generalized anxiety disorder. Although they typically take longer to work than benzodiazepines, the selective serotonin reuptake inhibitors such as *fluoxetine (Prozac),* sertraline (Zoloft), paroxetine (Paxil), *fluvoxamine (Luvox),* and citalopram (Celexa), as well as *venlafaxine (Effexor) and nefazodone (Serzone) are probably more effective than benzodiazepines and easier to discontinue.* Increasingly, benzodiazepines such as *diazepam (Valium)* are used only for the temporary relief of extreme anxiety as clinician and patient wait for the effects of antidepressants to take hold. Longer-term administration of benzodiazepines is reserved for patients who do not respond to, or cannot tolerate, antidepressants.

Placebo-controlled trials leave little doubt that newer antidepressants are effective for anxiety disorders. Because they work fairly quickly and have fewer adverse effects than tricyclic drugs and monoamine oxidase inhibitors, a low threshold for prescribing them to anxious patients should be maintained. However, most clinicians believe that the best result for anxiety disorder patients comes with the combination of medication with one or more types of psychotherapy.

18.21 The answer is E (all)

Since the original finding that sodium lactate infusion can induce panic attacks in patients with panic disorder, many substances have shown similar panicogenic properties including the noradrenergic stimulant *yohimbine* (Yocon), *carbon dioxide, the respiratory stimulant doxapram* (Dopram), *and cholecystokinin.* Disordered serotonergic, noradrenergic, and respiratory systems are doubtless implicated in panic disorder, and the condition appears to be caused both by a genetic predisposition and some type of traumatic distress. More recently, neuroimaging studies revealed that patients with panic disorder have abnormally brisk cerebral vascular responses to stress, showing greater vasoconstriction during hypocapnic respiration than normal controls.

Answers 18.22–18.24

18.22 The answer is C

18.23 The answer is D

18.24 The answer is B

18.25 The answer is B

Analyses of relative risks show *higher rates of agoraphobia for women than for men, just as with panic disorder.*

Some individuals with panic disorder also develop agoraphobia while some do not and the reasons for this variation are not known. It is possible that panic disorder with agoraphobia is a more severe form of panic disorder. Alternatively, the development of agoraphobia may be related to separate inherited or environmental factors, or some mixture of these. Two studies have addressed these questions. Rates of panic disorder with and without agoraphobia in relatives of three groups of individuals: patients with panic disorder and no agoraphobia, patients with panic disorder and agoraphobia, and nonanxious controls were compared; results indicated *that relatives of the agoraphobia patients had higher rates of both panic disorder (7.0 versus 3.5) and agoraphobia (14.9 versus 3.5) than the relatives of the controls, although the difference reached the .05 level of significance only in the latter group.* In contrast, the relatives of the panic disorder patients had significantly higher rates of panic disorder (14.9 versus 3.5, $P<.005$) but no agoraphobia (1.7 versus 3.5, not significant) as compared to relatives of controls. These data may be interpreted as indicating that with respect to intergenerational transmission, agoraphobia (with panic attacks) is either a more severe form of panic disorder or possibly a different but partially overlapping illness. *The lifetime prevalence of panic attacks (not panic disorder) is 3 to 5.6 percent.* Panic disorder is 1.5 to 5 percent. *Lifetime prevalence of agoraphobia has been reported to range from as low as 0.6 percent to as high as 6 percent.*

Answers 18.26–18.30

18.26 The answer is A

18.27 The answer is A

18.28 The answer is B

18.29 The answer is C

18.30 The answer is B

Buspirone was promoted as a less sedating alternative to benzodiazepines in the treatment of panic disorder. Buspirone has lower potential for abuse and dependence than benzodiazepines and produces relatively few adverse effects and no withdrawal syndrome. Buspirone does not alter cognitive or psychomotor function, does not interact with alcohol, and is not a muscle relaxant or an anticonvulsant. However, the efficacy of buspirone in panic disorder is disappointing, and with its further handicap of delayed onset of action and the need for multiple dosings, its *use is limited to potentiating the efficacy of other antidepressants and counteracting the adverse sexual effects of SSRIs*. Also, *buspirone seems even less effective in patients previously exposed to benzodiazepines.*

Bupropion, maprotiline (Ludiomil), and trazodone have not been found efficacious for panic disorder in controlled studies, while the anticonvulsants divalproex (Depakote) and gabapentin (Neurontin), the polyol second-messenger precursor inositol, nefazodone, and the calcium-channel inhibitor verapamil (Calan, Isoptin) have shown promise as antipanic agents.

Although the short-term efficacy of antipanic medications has been established, the question of how long to treat a panic patient who responds to treatment remains open. The results of follow-up studies are mixed. *Several reports indicate that most panic patients relapse within 2 months to 2 years after the medication is discontinued.* A recent review concludes that following medication discontinuation, only about 30 to 45 percent of the patients remain well, and even remitted patients rarely revert back to significant phobic avoidance or serious vocational or social disability. Improvement may continue for years following a single course of medication treatment. This favorable outcome may be explained by the heterogeneity of panic disorder, spontaneous learning experience of patients in clinical trials, and concomitant self-monitoring. Given the uncertainty about the optimal duration of treatment, the current recommendation is to continue full-dosage medication for panic-free patients for at least 1 year. Medication taper should be slow, with careful monitoring of symptoms. Distinction should be made among return symptoms, withdrawal, and rebound anxiety.

Since longer duration of illness at baseline predicts poor long-term outcome, all efforts should be made to identify and treat panic patients as early as possible. More severe phobic avoidance and comorbid depression and social phobia at baseline also predict poor long-term outcome. Higher depression scores coincide with greater severity of avoidance and disability. The poorer overall outcome in panic disorder patients with comorbid recurrent depression is more likely due to the simultaneous presence of the two conditions. Comorbid depression usually improves in parallel with panic symptoms.

Atypical responses to medications have been reported in panic patients whose first panic attacks were precipitated by cocaine use. These patients respond preferentially to benzodiazepines and anticonvulsants, *while tricyclic drugs seem to worsen their anxiety symptoms.* This pattern of medication response suggests that cocaine-induced panic attacks may be related to a kindling-like phenomenon.

Patients with generalized anxiety disorder suffer from excessive and uncontrollable anxiety and worry for at least 6 months and experience a series of somatic symptoms such as restlessness, irritability, insomnia, and muscle tension. The illness is chronic, with periodic exacerbations and relative quiescence. The relative sparsity of biological data and pharmacotherapy research is due to a number of factors. First, because of their multiple somatic complaints, patients with generalized anxiety disorder are usually seen by generalists and medical specialists other than psychiatrists; generalized anxiety disorder is more likely to be diagnosed as a comorbid condition in psychiatric practices. Second, pharmacotherapy is considered less effective in generalized anxiety disorder than in some other anxiety disorders. Third, the diagnostic features are not clear-cut, and comorbid conditions make the diagnosis difficult.

The efficacy of benzodiazepines in the pharmacological treatment of generalized anxiety disorder gave rise to theories implicating the benzodiazepine γ-aminobutyric acid (GABA) receptor system in the pathophysiology of generalized anxiety disorder, but evidence exists for the involvement of the serotonergic and noradrenergic systems as well. Data do not support the advantage of any one benzodiazepine over others, and no correlation has been established between clinical response and dosage or plasma concentration. A daily equivalent of 15 to 25 mg of diazepam usually suffices to relieve most symptoms in up to 70 percent of generalized anxiety disorder patients. Both somatic and psychic anxiety symptoms respond within the first week of treatment. Tolerance to the sedative effects of benzodiazepines develops quickly, but the antianxiety effect of a given dosage is well maintained over time in generalized anxiety disorder. *However, the relapse rate upon discontinuation of benzodiazepines is high, as is the risk for dependency.*

Buspirone is a potential alternative to benzodiazepine treatment in generalized anxiety disorder. *Response rates between 60 and 80 percent have been reported at levels ranging from 30 to 60 mg a day in three divided doses.* While response rates seem comparable, more patients drop out of buspirone trials than benzodiazepine trials. The relative merits of buspirone and benzodiazepines are further detailed under panic disorder. One notable exception is that *generalized anxiety disorder patients exposed to benzodiazepines may still be responsive to buspirone, unlike panic patients.*

Answers 18.31–18.34

18.31 The answer is A

18.32 The answer is A

18.33 The answer is B

18.34 The answer is C

Some studies have shown that cognitive-behavioral treatment of panic disorder, or panic control therapy, produces 80 to 90 percent panic-free status within at least 6 months of treatment. Two-year follow-up indicates that more than 50 percent of those patients who originally responded to panic control therapy have occasional panic attacks and more than a quarter will seek additional treatment. Nonetheless, these treatment responders do tend to have a significant decline in panic-related symptoms and most maintain many of their treatment gains.

As with panic disorder, considerable progress in the psychological treatment of social anxiety or social phobia is linked to the application of cognitive-behavioral methods. Unlike more traditional psychotherapies, cognitive-behavioral approaches do not focus on the origins of social anxiety, but instead focus on the use of coping strategies that can be implemented in current fearful situations. The most thoroughly studied form of cognitive-behavioral therapy for social phobia is a group therapy consisting of several discrete entities including (1) presentation of a three-system (cognitive-behavioral-physiological) model of social anxiety; (2) training in identification and restructuring of irrational beliefs regarding social performance; (3) in-session exposure to feared social situations via group role-playing scenarios; and (4) homework assignments directing patients to utilize cognitive and exposure techniques in vivo. Groups are particularly amenable to the treatment of social phobia in that they provide natural opportunities for patients to practice feared behaviors in a supportive and informative context.

Outcome research is somewhat limited but one study showed that cognitive-behavioral group therapy was nearly twice as effective as standard educational-supportive group psychotherapy. Responders to cognitive-behavioral group therapy were also shown to maintain treatment gains to a considerable extent at 5-year follow-up. Questions remain as to the effective treatment component in these therapies that blend cognitive and exposure-based methods. For example, it is unclear whether exposure to feared situations alone, without cognitive therapy, would be just as effective as the combined treatment. Also, it is not known whether group therapies other than educational or supportive group therapy, such as interpersonal group therapy, may be effective in treating social phobia.

Psychodynamic psychotherapy is based on the concept that symptoms result from mental processes that may be outside of the patient's conscious awareness and that elucidating these processes can lead to remission of symptoms. Moreover, in order to lessen the patient's vulnerability to panic, the psychodynamic therapist considers it necessary to identify and alter core conflicts. *The goals of psychodynamic psychotherapy are more ambitious and require more time to achieve than those of a more symptom-focused treatment approach.* Thus, these therapies are inherently more difficult to study than more concrete, focused, manual-based therapies. There are some case reports of brief dynamic psychotherapies that took no longer than cognitive-behavioral therapy to achieve reasonable treatment goals for patients with panic disorder.

In psychodynamic psychotherapy, the successful emotional and cognitive understanding of the various elements of psychic conflict (impulses, conscience, internal standards that are often excessively harsh, psychological defense patterns, and realistic concerns) and reintegration of these elements in a more adaptive way may result in symptom resolution and fewer relapses. To achieve this insight and acceptance, the therapist places the symptoms in the context of the patient's life history and current realities and extensively uses the therapeutic relationship to focus on unconscious symptom determinants.

Investigators have examined use of the combination of medication and cognitive behavior therapy for patients with panic disorder and agoraphobia. *Several short-term treatment studies have shown that the combination* of the tricyclic medication imipramine (Tofranil) with one component of cognitive behavior therapy, behavioral exposure, *may be superior to either treatment alone.* Another study showed that selective serotonin reuptake inhibitors, such as paroxetine (Paxil), plus cognitive therapy worked significantly better for patients with panic disorder than cognitive therapy plus placebo. There has been one study of the combination of psychodynamic psychotherapy with medication. *This study suggested that psychodynamic psychotherapy may improve the long-term outcome of medication-treated patients.*

Answers 18.35–18.39

18.35 The answer is C

18.36 The answer is A

18.37 The answer is D

18.38 The answer is B

18.39 The answer is E

Specific phobia is divided into four subtypes (animal type, natural environment type, blood–injury type, and situational type) in addition to a residual category for phobias that do not clearly fall into any of these four categories. The key feature in each type of phobia is that the fear is circumscribed to a specific object, both temporally and with respect to other objects. Phobias have traditionally been classified according to the specific fear by means of Greek or Latin prefixes, as indicted by the examples below.

Acrophobia: fear of heights
Agoraphobia: fear of open places
Ailurophobia: fear of cats
Hydrophobia: fear of water
Claustrophobia: fear of closed spaces
Cynophobia: fear of dogs
Mysophobia: fear of dirt and germs
Pyrophobia: fear of fire
Xenophobia: fear of strangers
Zoophobia: fear of animals

Answers 18.40–18.42

18.40 The answer is A

18.41 The answer is C

18.42 The answer is B

The three major neurotransmitters associated with anxiety are norepinephrine, serotonin, and GABA. The general theory regarding the role of *norepinephrine* in anxiety disorders is that affected patients may have a poorly regulated noradrenergic system that has occasional bursts of activity. In that system *the cell bodies of the neurotransmitter's neurons are localized primarily to the locus ceruleus* in the rostral pons, and they project their axons to the cerebral cortex, the limbic system, the brainstem, and the spinal cord. Experiments in primates have shown that stimulation of the locus ceruleus produces a fear response.

The interest in *serotonin* was initially motivated by the observation that serotonergic antidepressants have therapeutic effects in some anxiety disorders—for example, clomipramine (Anafranil) in OCD. The effectiveness of buspirone (BuSpar), a serotonergic type 1A (5-HT_{1A}) receptor agonist, in the treatment of anxiety disorders also suggests the possibility of an association between serotonin and anxiety. *The cell bodies of most of the serotonergic neurons are in the raphe nuclei* in the rostral brainstem, especially the amygdala in the hippocampus, and the hypothalamus.

The role of *GABA* in anxiety disorders is most strongly supported by the undisputed efficacy of *benzodiazepines, which enhance the activity of GABA at the* $GABA_A$ *receptor in the treatment of some types of anxiety disorders.*

Answers 18.43–18.46

18.43 The answer is C

18.44 The answer is A

18.45 The answer is D

18.46 The answer is B

Exposure therapy involves intentionally confronting feared, but otherwise not dangerous, objects, situations, thoughts, memories, and physical sensations for the purpose of reducing fear reactions associated with the same or similar stimuli. Systematic desensitization was the first exposure therapy technique to undergo scientific investigation. Although an effective treatment for some anxiety disorders, it has generally fallen out of use among researchers and cognitive-behavioral therapists. The contemporary use of exposure therapy may be usefully divided into three classes of procedures: in vivo exposure, imaginal exposure, and interoceptive exposure.

In vivo exposure involves helping patients to directly confront feared objects, activities, and situations. It is usually conducted in a graduated fashion according to a mutually agreed-on (between patient and therapist) hierarchy. For example, a hierarchy for a specific animal phobia, such as a snake or spiders, may begin with looking at pictures and other representations of the feared animal, followed by looking at the actual animal kept in a cage, first at a distance and then gradually moving closer. In the case of OCD, in vivo exposure is explicitly combined with response prevention, in which the patient agrees to not engage in compulsions or rituals designed to reduce anxiety when exposed to an object that elicits obsessional fears or designed to control feared harmful consequences. For example, a person with fears of contamination may be asked to touch and use a variety of common objects such as door knobs, public phones, and public restrooms while intentionally refraining from washing or taking specific measures to limit the spread of contamination (e.g., using a tissue as a barrier between the skin and the contaminated object).

Imaginal exposure typically involves having the patient close his or her eyes and imagine feared stimuli as vividly as possible. The primary use of this type of exposure is to help patients confront feared thoughts, images, and memories. For example, individuals with OCD may experience obsessional thoughts and images about causing harm to people they love. In the case of PTSD, imaginal exposure is used to help the patient confront his or her memory of the traumatic event. For these conditions, imaginal exposure to these feared thoughts and consequences is used to promote habituation of emotional reactivity to the image and to help the patient distinguish between thoughts of the actual traumatic event and the current memory of the event, which, although distressing, is not harmful. A second use of imaginal exposure is in lieu of in vivo exposure when arranging direct contact with the feared situation is not safe or feasible or as a preparatory exercise to facilitate subsequent in vivo exposures.

Interoceptive exposure is the most recent form of exposure therapy to be introduced. This procedure is designed to induce feared physiological sensations under controlled circumstances. A number of specific exercises have been developed to induce specific panic-like sensations. For example, the step-up exercise, in which the patient repeatedly steps up and down on a single step as rapidly as possible, produces rapid heart rate and shortness of breath. Spinning in a chair or spinning in place produces dizziness and, in some people, mild nausea. Breathing through a thin straw produces the sensation of not getting enough air. The goal is to find an activity that produces similar sensations to the ones that patients find unduly distressing and attempt to avoid. Interoceptive exposure exercises are most commonly used in the treatment of panic disorder and certain specific phobias.

Systematic desensitization requires initial training in progressive muscle relaxation and the development of one or more carefully constructed hierarchies of feared stimuli. Treatment then involves the pairing of mental images of the lowest items on the hierarchy with relaxation until the image can be held in mind without it producing significant distress. This process is then repeated with each item on the hierarchy. Although systematic desensitization has been found to be effective in the treatment of specific phobias and social anxiety, it is generally no longer used among contemporary cognitive-behavioral therapists and researchers.

19 Somatoform Disorders

The term *somatoform* is derived from the Greek word *soma,* which means body. Somatoform disorders are a broad group of illnesses that have bodily signs and symptoms as a major component. These disorders encompass mind-body interactions in which the brain, in ways still not well understood, sends various signals that impinge on the patient's awareness, indicating a serious problem in the body. Additionally, minor or as yet undetectable changes in neurochemistry, neurophysiology, and neuroimmunology may result from unknown mental or brain mechanisms that cause illness.

The fourth revised edition of the *Diagnostic and Statistical Manual of Mental Disorders* (DSM-IV-TR) classifies them as somatization disorder, conversion disorder, hypochondriasis, body dysmorphic disorder, and pain disorder, as well as undifferentiated somatoform disorder not otherwise specified.

Before a somatoform disorder is diagnosed, the clinician must initiate a thorough medical evaluation to rule out the presence of actual medical pathology. A certain percentage of these patients will turn out to have real underlying medical pathology, but it does not usually account for the symptoms described by the patient. The disorders may be chronic or episodic, they may be associated with other mental disorders, and the symptoms described are always worsened by psychological stress.

Treatment is often very difficult, as the symptoms tend to have deeply rooted and unconscious psychological meanings for most patients, and these are patients who do not or cannot express their feelings verbally. Unconscious conflicts are expressed somatically and seem to have a particular tenaciousness and resistance to psychological treatment.

Treatment involves both biological and psychological strategies, including cognitive-behavioral treatments, psychodynamic therapies, and psychopharmacologic approaches. If other psychiatric disorders, such as depression or anxiety disorders, are also present, they must be treated concomitantly. Different medications are effective with the range of disorders and the student should be knowledgeable about this.

The student should study the questions and answers below for a useful review of these disorders.

HELPFUL HINTS

The student should be able to define the terms listed below.

- amobarbital (Amytal) interview
- anorexia nervosa
- antidepressants
- antisocial personality disorder
- astasia-abasia
- autonomic arousal disorder
- biofeedback
- body dysmorphic disorder
- Briquet's syndrome
- conversion disorder
- cytokines
- depression
- differential diagnosis
- dysmorphophobia
- endorphins
- generalized anxiety disorder
- hemianesthesia
- hypochondriasis
- hysteria
- identification
- instinctual impulse
- *la belle indifférence*
- major depressive disorder
- malingering
- pain disorder
- pimozide (Orap)
- primary gain and secondary gain
- pseudocyesis
- pseudoseizures
- secondary symptoms
- somatization disorder
- somatoform disorder not otherwise specified
- somatosensory input
- stocking-and-glove anesthesia
- symbolization and projection
- undifferentiated somatoform disorder
- undoing

QUESTIONS

Directions

Each of the statements or questions below is followed by five suggested responses or completions. Select the *one* that is *best* in each case.

19.1 Which of the following is *not* a recommended treatment strategy for a patient with somatization disorder?

A. Increasing the patient's awareness that psychological factors may be involved

B. Several different clinicians involved in caring for the patient

C. Avoiding additional laboratory and diagnostic procedures
D. Seeing patients during regularly scheduled visits at regular intervals
E. Listening to somatic complaints as emotional expressions rather than medical complaints

19.2 Which of the following is a theory for the etiology of hypochondriasis?

A. Symptoms are viewed as a request for admission to the sick role made by a person facing challenges in his or her life.
B. Persons with hypochondriasis have low thresholds for, and low tolerance of, physical discomfort.
C. Aggressive and hostile wishes toward others are transferred (through repression and displacement) into physical complaints.
D. Hypochondriasis is a variant form of other mental disorders, such as depressive or anxiety disorders.
E. All of the above

19.3 Body dysmorphic disorder is associated with

A. major depressive disorder
B. obsessive-compulsive disorder
C. social phobia
D. family history of substance abuse
E. all of the above

19.4 Pseudocyesis

A. involves abdominal enlargement, breast engorgement, and labor pains at the expected date of delivery
B. is listed as a specific somatoform disorder in the 10th edition of International Classification of Diseases (ICD-10)
C. can be explained by medical conditions involving endocrine changes
D. all of the above
E. none of the above

19.5 Conversion reactions

A. are always transient
B. are invariably sensorimotor as opposed to autonomic
C. conform to usual dermatomal distribution of underlying peripheral nerves
D. seem to change the psychic energy of acute conflict into a personally meaningful metaphor of bodily dysfunction
E. all of the above

19.6 Characteristic signs of conversion disorder include all of the following *except*

A. astasia-abasia
B. stocking-and-glove anesthesia
C. hemianesthesia of the body beginning precisely at the midline
D. normal reflexes
E. cogwheel rigidity

19.7 All of the following mental disorders are frequently seen in patients with somatization disorder (relative to the general population) *except*

A. schizophrenia
B. generalized anxiety disorder
C. obsessive-compulsive personality disorder
D. bipolar I disorder
E. major depressive disorder

19.8 Medical disorders to be considered in a differential diagnosis of somatization disorder include

A. multiple sclerosis
B. systemic lupus erythematosus
C. acute intermittent porphyria
D. hyperparathyroidism
E. all of the above

19.9 The most frequently occurring of the somatoform disorders is

A. conversion disorder
B. somatization disorder
C. hypochondriasis
D. pain disorder
E. body dysmorphic disorder

19.10 A patient with somatization disorder

A. presents the initial physical complaints after age 30
B. has had physical symptoms for 3 months
C. has complained of symptoms not explained by a known medical condition
D. usually experiences minimal impairment in social or occupational functioning
E. may have a false belief of being pregnant with objective signs of pregnancy, such as decreased menstrual flow or amenorrhea

19.11 Many patients with pseudoseizures have

A. interictal EEG abnormalities
B. neuropsychological impairment
C. abnormalities on MRI and CT scan
D. true convulsions or other true neurological conditions
E. all of the above

19.12 The most accurate statement regarding pain disorder is

A. Peak ages of onset are in the second and third decades.
B. First-degree relatives of patients have an increased likelihood of having the same disorder.
C. It is least common in persons with blue-collar occupations.
D. It is diagnosed equally among men and women.
E. Depressive disorders are no more common in patients with pain disorder than in the general public.

19.13 In body dysmorphic disorder

A. plastic surgery is usually beneficial.
B. a comorbid diagnosis is unusual.

C. anorexia nervosa may also be diagnosed.
D. some 50 percent of patients may attempt suicide.
E. serotonin-specific drugs are effective in reducing the symptoms.

19.14 True statements about hypochondriasis include all of the following *except*

A. Depression accounts for a major part of the total picture in hypochondriasis.
B. Hypochondriasis symptoms can be part of dysthymic disorders, generalized anxiety disorder, or adjustment disorder.
C. Hypochondriasis is a chronic and somewhat disabling disorder.
D. Recent estimates are that 4 to 6 percent of the general medical population meets the specific criteria for the disorder.
E. Significant numbers of patients with hypochondriasis report traumatic sexual contacts, physical violence, and major parental upheaval before the age of 17.

19.15 Historically, conversion disorders have been associated with

A. Pierre Briquet
B. Jean-Martin Charcot
C. Sigmund Freud
D. Pierre Janet
E. all of the above

19.16 Mrs. J, 30-year-old woman, is referred for psychiatric evaluation by her internist after her fourth request for mammography in 6 months. Two years ago a close friend died of breast cancer. Since that time, she has been preoccupied with the possibility that she also has the disease. She examines herself several times a day and when she finds something that seems unusual she goes to her doctor for medical evaluation. Initially, the doctor's reassurance was enough to convince her that her fears were exaggerated. However, over the past year she has required a mammogram to prove to herself that she does not have cancer. Each time when the mammography is reported to be normal, she is momentarily relieved but within several days starts to doubt the accuracy of the test and suspects that she does have undetected cancer. There are periods in which she is so convinced that she becomes despondent and is unable to do normal work around the house. She has started to neglect her 3-year-old son because of painful thoughts that he will be left motherless. She now spends several hours a day searching the internet for information on breast cancer or in breast cancer support chat rooms.

She is married to a successful architect, and by mutual agreement she quit her job as a financial analyst 3 years ago in order to spend full time at home with her son. She is friends with several of the mothers in her son's play group and occasionally sees colleagues from her former office. Despite her concerns, her health is good. Her most recent physical examination was unremarkable except for small bruises over both breasts that were the result of repeated self-examination. She drinks an occasional glass of wine with meals. She smoked marijuana in college but has not used any illicit drugs for 6 years.

After psychiatric examination, she appears mildly anxious. She describes herself as being at her wits' end, saying that the fear of cancer is ruining her life. She acknowledges that the fear is greatly exaggerated, but she feels powerless to control it. She denies ever having had hallucinations. She is alert, oriented, her memory is good, and concentration is mildly impaired.

Which of the following is the most likely diagnosis?

A. Obsessive-compulsive disorder
B. Major depressive disorder with psychotic features
C. Delusional disorder
D. Hypochondriasis
E. Body dysmorphic disorder

19.17 In the case above, which of the following is the most likely outcome without treatment?

A. Complete recovery
B. Chronic waxing and waning of symptoms
C. Development of cognitive impairment
D. Development of physical impairment
E. Development of psychotic symptoms

19.18 A 34-year-old woman presented with chronic and intermittent dizziness, paresthesias, pain in multiple areas of her body, and intermittent nausea and diarrhea. She reported that these symptoms had been present most of the time, although they had been undulating since she was approximately 24. In addition, she complained of mild depression, was disinterested in many things in life, including sexual activity, and had been to many doctors to try to find out what was wrong with her. Physical examination, including a neurological exam, was normal. There were no abnormalities on laboratory testing. Her doctor diagnoses somatization disorder. Which of the following about this disorder is true?

A. The symptoms typically begin in middle age.
B. These patients usually give a very thorough and complete report of their symptoms.
C. It occurs more commonly in men.
D. It is more common in urban populations.
E. These patients are no more likely to develop another medical illness than people without the disorder.

19.19 Hypochondriacs

A. are often thatophobic
B. seek treatment more than explanations
C. are usually women
D. do not respond to reassurance
E. in postmortem examinations have a greater degree of upper GI inflammation and congestion than normal controls

19.20 Conversion disorder

A. usually has a chronic onset
B. is commonly comorbid with a schizoid personality disorder
C. is associated with antisocial personality disorder
D. is associated with symptoms that conform to known anatomical pathways
E. responds well to a confrontation of the "false nature" of the symptoms

Directions

Each set of lettered headings below is followed by a list of numbered phrases. For each numbered phrase, select:

A. if the item is associated with A only
B. if the item is associated with B only
C. if the item is associated with both A and B
D. if the item is associated with neither A nor B

Questions 19.21–19.24

A. DSM-IV-TR
B. ICD-10

19.21 Categories of somatoform disorders include somatization, hypochondriasis, and pain disorder
19.22 Notes that when physical disorders are present, they cannot account for patients' symptoms or distress
19.23 Body dysmorphic disorder is considered a subcategory of hypochondriacal disorder
19.24 Includes the diagnosis neurasthenia, which has symptoms that overlap with anxiety and depression

Questions 19.25–19.26

A. Undifferentiated somatoform disorder
B. Somatization disorder

19.25 Estimated lifetime prevalence of between 4 and 11 percent
19.26 Course is generally chronic and relapsing

Questions 19.27–19.31

A. Somatization disorder
B. Pain disorder

19.27 Affects women more than men
19.28 Most often begins during a person's teens
19.29 Responds to antidepressants
19.30 May involve serotonin in its pathophysiology
19.31 Is commonly associated with anorexia nervosa

Questions 19.32–19.37

A. Somatization disorder
B. Conversion disorder

19.32 Prevalence is highest in rural areas and among the poorly educated.
19.33 Is associated with Pierre Briquet.
19.34 Comorbidity with an Axis II disorder is common.
19.35 Only one or two complaints.
19.36 Is chronic and relapsing, by definition.
19.37 Most symptoms remit spontaneously.

Questions 19.38–19.42

A. Undifferentiated somatoform disorder
B. Somatoform disorder not otherwise specified

19.38 A diagnostic category for patients with somatic symptoms not covered in other somatoform disorders
19.39 Patients have physical complaints not accounted for by another mental disorder
19.40 Examples are autonomic arousal disorder (involving the autonomic nervous system) and neurasthenia (involving sensations of fatigue)
19.41 Defined by unexplained physical effects lasting for at least 6 months that are below the threshold for diagnosing somatization disorder
19.42 A patient's somatic complaints may not have met the 6-month criterion of other somatoform disorders

Questions 19.43–19.47

A. Hypochondriasis
B. Body dysmorphic disorder

19.43 Beliefs and symptoms may reach delusional intensity
19.44 Has high rates of coexisting depressive and anxiety disorders
19.45 Patients actively seek out attention for their symptoms
19.46 Causes persistent distress or interference with personal functioning
19.47 May be related to the defense mechanisms of repression and displacement

ANSWERS

19.1 The answer is B

Somatization disorder is best treated *when the patient has a single identified physician as primary caretaker*. When more than one clinician is involved, patients have increased opportunities to express somatic complaints. Primary physicians should see patients *during regularly scheduled visits, usually at monthly intervals*. The visits should be relatively brief, although a partial physical examination should be conducted to respond to each new somatic complaint. *Additional laboratory and diagnostic procedures should generally be avoided*. Once somatization disorder has been diagnosed, the treating physician should *listen to the somatic complaints as emotional expressions rather than as medical complaints*. Nevertheless, patients with somatization disorder can also have bona fide physical illnesses; therefore, physicians must always use their judgment about what symptoms to work up and to what extent. A reasonable long-range strategy for a primary care physician who is treating a patient with somatization disorder is to *increase the patient's awareness of the possibility that psychological factors are involved in the symptoms* until the patient is willing to see a mental health clinician.

19.2 The answer is E (all)

A reasonable body of data indicates that persons with hypochondriasis augment and amplify their somatic sensations; *they have low thresholds for, and low tolerance of, physical discomfort.* They may focus on bodily sensations, misinterpret them, and become alarmed by them because of a faulty cognitive scheme. A second theory is that hypochondriasis is understandable in terms of a social learning model. *The symptoms of hypochondriasis are viewed as a request for admission to the sick role made by a person facing seemingly insurmountable and unsolvable problems.* The sick role offers an escape that allows a patient to avoid noxious obligations, to postpone unwelcome challenges, and to be excused from usual duties and obligations. A third theory suggests that hypochondriasis is *a variant form of other mental disorders, among which depressive disorders and anxiety disorders are most frequently included.* An estimated 80 percent of patients with hypochondriasis may have coexisting depressive or anxiety disorders. Patients who meet the diagnostic criteria for hypochondriasis may be somatizing subtypes of these other disorders. The psychodynamic school of thought has produced a fourth theory of hypochondriasis. According to this theory, *aggressive and hostile wishes toward others are transferred (through repression and displacement) into physical complaints.* The anger of patients with hypochondriasis originates in past disappointments, rejections, and losses. Hypochondriasis is also viewed as a defense against guilt, a sense of innate badness, and expression of low self-esteem, and a sign of excessive self-concern. Pain and somatic suffering thus become means of atonement and expiation (undoing) and can be experienced as deserved punishment for past wrongdoing (either real or imaginary) and for a person's sense of wickedness and sinfulness.

19.3 The answer is E

Body dysmorphic disorder is not uncommon as a comorbid condition in patients with major depressive disorder, obsessive-compulsive disorder, and social phobia. Indeed in one study of 30 patients, all met DSM-III-R criteria for at least one other psychiatric diagnosis at some point in their lives, and usually concurrently.

The cause of body dysmorphic disorder is unknown. The high comorbidity with depressive disorders, a higher-than-expected family history of mood disorders and obsessive-compulsive disorder, and the reported responsiveness to SSRIs indicates that, in at least some patients, the pathophysiology of the disorder may involve serotonin and may be related to other disorders. There may be significant cultural or social effects on patients with body dysmorphic disorder because of the emphasis on stereotyped concepts of beauty that may be emphasized in certain families and within the culture at large. In psychodynamic models, body dysmorphic disorder is seen as reflecting the displacement of a sexual or an emotional conflict onto a nonrelated body part; such a putative association occurs through the defense mechanisms of repression, dissociation, distortion, symbolization, and projection.

Family histories of substance abuse and mood disorder are common in documented cases. Also predisposing to the disorder may be certain types of personality characteristics, especially a mixture of obsessional and avoidant traits, but no single personality pattern predominates. Reportedly, the patients are shy, self-absorbed, and overly sensitive to their imagined defect as a focus of notice or criticism.

19.4 The answer is A

Pseudocyesis, or the false belief that one is pregnant, is an example of a somatoform disorder "not otherwise specified." This diagnostic category of somatoform disorders is a residual category for patients who have symptoms suggesting a somatoform disorder, but do not meet the specific diagnostic criteria for other somatoform disorders. *The ICD-10 does not list pseudocyesis as a specific somatoform disorder* (the main difference between the categorizations of somatoform disorders between the DSM-IV-TR and the ICD-10 is that the ICD-10 classifies body dysmorphic disorder as a subcategory of hypochondriasis). Pseudocyesis is associated with objective signs of pregnancy, which may include *abdominal enlargement* (although the umbilicus does not become everted), reduced menstrual flow, amenorrhea, subjective sensation of fetal movement, nausea, *breast engorgement* and secretions, and *labor pains at the expected date of delivery*. Endocrine changes may be present, but *the syndrome cannot be explained by a general medical condition that causes endocrine changes* (e.g., a hormone-secreting tumor).

19.5 The answer is D

Many conversion disorders simulate acute neurological pathology (e.g., strokes and disturbances of speech, hearing, or vision). However, conversion disorders are not associated with the usual pathological neurodiagnostic signs or the underlying somatic pathology. *Conversion symptoms* (e.g., anesthesias and paresthesias produced by a conversion disorder) *do not conform to usual dermatomal distribution of the underlying peripheral nerves*; rather, the signs and symptoms of a conversion disorder typically conform to the patient's concept of the medical condition.

Conversion disorders seem to change or convert the psychic energy of the turmoil of acute conflict into a personally meaningful metaphor of bodily dysfunction. Turbulence of the mind is transformed into a somatic statement, condensing and focusing concepts, role models, and communicative meanings into one or several physical signs or symptoms of dysfunction. These somatic representations often simulate an acute medical calamity; initiate urgent, sometimes expensive medical investigation; and produce disability. In primitive settings, however, certain conversion symptoms have been taken as tokens of religious faith and even as expressions of witchcraft.

Although most conversion reactions are transient (hours to days), some can persist. Chronic conversion disorders can actually produce permanent conversion complications, such as disuse contractures of a "paralyzed" limb that remains long after the psychic strife that prompted the conversion has been resolved. In many cases a chronic conversion disorder serves to help stabilize an otherwise dysfunctional family. *In addition to sensorimotor symptoms, marked autonomic disturbances such as protracted (psychogenic) vomiting, hyperemesis gravidarum, urinary retention, and pseudocyesis are also seen, although less commonly.* Conversion disorders challenge the diagnostic competence of internists, neurologists, otolaryngologists, ophthalmologists, and psychiatrists.

Like the other somatoform disorders, conversion disorders are not volitional. Rather, ego defense mechanisms of repression and dissociation act outside of the patient's awareness. Many patients with conversion disorders experience *la belle indifférence*, an emotional unconcern or even flatness in a setting of catastrophic illness; but some patients do experience considerable anguish over their new symptoms.

19.6 The answer is E

Cogwheel rigidity is an organic sign secondary to disorders of the basal ganglia and not a sign of conversion disorder. In conversion disorder, anesthesia and paresthesia, especially of the extremities, are common. All sensory modalities are involved, and the distribution of the disturbance is inconsistent with that of either central or peripheral neurological disease. Thus, one sees the characteristic *stocking-and-glove anesthesia* of the hands or feet or *hemianesthesia of the body beginning precisely at the midline*. Motor symptoms include abnormal movements and gait disturbance, which is often a wildly ataxic, staggering gait accompanied by gross, irregular, jerky truncal movements and thrashing and waving arms (also known as *astasia-abasia*). *Normal reflexes* are seen. The patient shows no fasciculations or muscle atrophy, and electromyography findings are normal.

19.7 The answer is D

Several studies have noted that somatization disorder commonly coexists with other mental disorders. About two thirds of all patients with somatization disorder have identifiable psychiatric symptoms, and up to half have other mental disorders. Commonly associated personality traits or personality disorders are those characterized by avoidant, paranoid, self-defeating, and *obsessive compulsive* features. Patients with *major depressive disorder, generalized anxiety disorder,* and *schizophrenia* may all have an initial complaint that focuses on somatic symptoms. In all these disorders, however, the symptoms of depression, anxiety, and psychosis eventually predominate over the somatic complaints. Two disorders that are *not* seen more commonly in patients with somatization disorder than in the general population are *bipolar I disorder* and substance abuse.

19.8 The answer is E (all)

The clinician must always rule out organic causes for the patient's symptoms. Medical disorders that present with nonspecific, transient abnormalities pose the greatest diagnostic difficulty in the differential diagnosis of somatization disorder. The disorders to be considered include *multiple sclerosis, systemic lupus erythematosus, acute intermittent porphyria*, and *hyperparathyroidism*. In addition, the onset of many somatic symptoms late in life must be presumed to be caused by a medical illness until testing rules it out. Table 19.1 lists a few of the disorders commonly confused with somatoform disorders, especially early in their courses.

19.9 The answer is A

Conversion disorders may be the most frequently occurring of the somatoform disorders. DSM-IV-TR gives a range from a low of 11 to a high of 500 cases per 100,000. Affected persons can range in age from early childhood into old age. The annual incidence of conversion disorders seen by psychiatrists in a New York county has been estimated to be 22 cases per 100,000. In a general hospital setting 5 to 16 percent of all psychiatric consultation

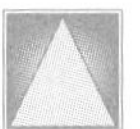

Table 19.1
Conditions Commonly Confused with Somatoform Disorder

Multiple sclerosis
Central nervous system syphilis
Brain tumor
Hyperparathyroidism
Acute intermittent porphyria
Lupus erythematosus
Hyperthyroidism
Myasthenia gravis

patients manifest some conversion symptoms. In a study of a rural Veterans Administration general hospital, 25 to 30 percent of all male patients had a conversion symptom at some time during their admission. By contrast, in a psychiatric emergency room or psychiatric clinic, the incidence of conversion disorder is far lower (1 percent of all psychiatric admissions), as different selection factors supervene. Lifetime figures for ever having any conversion symptoms, even if only on a transient basis, are far higher, with some studies reporting a 33 percent prevalence rate. Conversion disorder occurs mainly in women, with a ratio of 2 to 1 up to 5 to 1 in some studies. However, there does not seem to be an overrepresentation of conversion disorder in female children.

19.10 The answer is C

During the course of somatization disorder, the patient *has complained of* pain, gastrointestinal, sexual, and pseudoneurological symptoms that are *not explained by a known medical condition*. In addition, the patient *presents the initial physical complaints before, not after, age 30*. The patient *has had physical symptoms for at least several years, not just 3 months*. The patient has had interpersonal problems and tremendous psychological distress and *usually experiences significant, not minimal, impairment in social or occupational functioning*. A patient who has *a false belief of being pregnant* and objective signs of pregnancy, such as decreased menstrual flow or amenorrhea, does not have somatization disorder. Instead, the patient has pseudocyesis, a somatoform disorder not otherwise specified.

19.11 The answer is E (all)

Pseudoseizures are paroxysmal episodes of altered behavior resembling epileptic attacks but devoid of the characteristic clinical epileptic and electrographic features. Convulsive behaviors identified as a conversion disorder often take place when the clinician walks into the patient's room or when the family visits. Variously termed *psychogenic* or *hysterical seizures* in the past, these clinical episodes terminate without the patient having a period of sluggishness, sleepiness, or confusion (as might be seen following a true convulsion). Pseudoseizures, but not complex partial seizures, tend not to manifest extreme stereotypy in the overt motor sequence and lack a neurological indicator. These patients do not show evidence of an elevated serum prolactin level immediately following the clinical episode. The EEG of the pseudoseizure patient during the clinical episode does not show any of the correlates of an epileptic seizure, such as increasing frequency of spike discharges, sudden onset of focal or diffuse rhythmic activity, or postictal slow waves.

The induction of a seizure by suggestion, formerly considered a hallmark of hysterical seizures, is also seen in complex partial seizures when there is elevated electrical lability. Semipurposeful movements, thrashing, and pelvic thrusting, often considered to be the hallmarks of pseudoseizures, can be seen with direct stimulation of the cingulate region and are common correlates of complete partial seizures with frontotemporal foci. *Moreover, more than 70 percent of patients with pseudoseizures without documented bona fide seizures show interictal EEG abnormalities, neuropsychological impairment, or abnormalities on magnetic resonance imaging (MRI) and computed tomography (CT) scans.*

Although tongue-biting, urinary incontinence, injury during falls, and seeming loss of consciousness do not usually occur with a pseudoseizure, all of these can occur. However, the preservation of corneal, pupillary, and gag reflexes, plus the absence of extensor plantar responses and the preservation of normal color during the attack, all suggest a pseudoseizure.

The proportion of pseudoseizures in a given study typically reflects the nature of the referral source and their relationship with the evaluation. From a clinician's perspective, about *one-third of patients evaluated for a pseudoseizure do not have a convulsive disorder or pseudoseizures but rather have some other neurological condition; another third of patients have true convulsions as well as pseudoseizures; and another third have just pseudoseizures.*

19.12 The answer is B

The most accurate statement about pain disorder is that *first-degree relatives of pain disorder patients have an increased likelihood of having the same disorder*, thus indicating the possibility of genetic inheritance or behavioral mechanisms in the transmission of the disorder. Pain disorder is in fact *diagnosed twice as frequently in women as in men*. The *peak ages of onset are in the fourth and fifth decades*, when the tolerance for pain declines. Pain disorder is *most common in persons with blue-collar occupations*, perhaps because of increased job-related injuries. *Depressive disorders, anxiety disorders, and substance abuse are also more common in families of pain disorder patients* than in the general population.

19.13 The answer is E

Serotonin-specific drugs such as clomipramine (Anafranil) and fluoxetine (Prozac) *are effective in reducing the symptoms in at least 50 percent of patients with body dysmorphic disorder*. In any patient with a coexisting mental disorder or an anxiety disorder, the coexisting disorder should be treated with the appropriate pharmacotherapy and psychotherapy. How long treatment should be continued when the symptoms of body dysmorphic disorder have remitted is unknown. *Plastic surgery is not usually beneficial* in the treatment of patients with body dysmorphic disorder. In fact, surgical, dermatological, dental, and other medical procedures to address the alleged defects rarely satisfy the patient.

A comorbid diagnosis is not unusual. Body dysmorphic disorder commonly coexists with other mental disorders. One study found that more than 90 percent of body dysmorphic disorder patients had experienced a major depressive episode in their lifetimes, about 70 percent had had an anxiety disorder, and about 30 percent had a psychotic disorder. However, *anorexia nervosa should not be diagnosed* along with body dysmorphic disorder, since distortions of body image occur in anorexia nervosa, gender identity disorders, and some specific types of brain damage (for example, neglect syndromes).

The effects of body dysmorphic disorder on a person's life can be significant. Almost all affected patients avoid social and occupational exposure. As many as a third of the patients may be housebound by their concern about being ridiculed for their alleged deformities, and as many as *20 percent, not 50 percent, of patients attempt suicide.*

19.14 The answer is A

Hypochondriacal symptoms can be a part of another disorder such as major depressive disorder, dysthymic disorders, generalized anxiety disorder, or adjustment disorder. However, primary hypochondriasis or hypochondriacal disorder is a chronic and somewhat disabling disorder with hypochondriacal symptoms, not merely a part of another psychiatric condition.

Hypochondriasis was included as a diagnostic entity in DSM-I. The diagnostic criteria continued to be revised in DSM-II, DSM-III, and DSM-III-R; however, the changes have been primarily linguistic, not substantive. The only change between DSM-III-R and DSM-IV-TR is the addition of a specifier to note that the patient has poor insight during the current episode. The ICD-10 criteria for hypochondriasis are essentially the same as those of DSM-IV-TR.

Hypochondriasis is rather common in primary care settings. In various locales, the prevalence has varied from 3 to 14 percent. Recent work indicates that in a 6-month period of observation, *4 to 6 percent of the general medical population meets the specific criteria for this disorder.* The prevalence in either sex is comparable to that within the general medical population. There are no specific tendencies for overrepresentation based on social position, education, marital status, or other sociodemographic descriptors. There is a wide range of ages at onset. Although the disorder can begin at any age, onset is thought to be most common between 20 and 30 years of age. A preliminary family study of 19 cases and their 72 first-degree relatives demonstrated no increase in the rate of hypochondriasis among their relatives compared with a control group.

Comorbidity with other psychiatric disorders is common with hypochondriasis and must be treated accordingly. As an example, when case-matched controls and 42 hypochondriasis patients from a medical clinic were evaluated psychiatrically, the hypochondriasis patients had twice as many lifetime Axis I disorders and three times the number of personality disorders. Of the hypochondriasis patients in the study, 88 percent had one or more additional Axis I disorders, the overlap being greatest with depressive and anxiety disorders. *Depression only accounts for a minor part of the total picture in hypochondriasis, however, so it is a mistake to think that all hypochondriasis is the result of some other Axis I disorder.*

The developmental background of hypochondriacal patients is of interest in that significantly more of these patients than matched controls report traumatic sexual contacts, physical violence, and major parental upheaval before the age of 17.

19.15 The answer is E (all)

Until the middle of the 19th century, somatization disorder and conversion disorder (which often travel together) were considered to be one condition called *hysteria.* The term hysteria was derived from the Greek word *hystera*, meaning uterus.

Descriptions of conversion disorders appeared as far back as 1900 B.C. when multiple symptoms were attributed by Egyptian physicians to a wandering of the uterus within the body.

In the middle of the century, *Pierre Briquet originated the modern concept of conversion disorder.* He considered the disorder to result from a dysfunction of the central nervous system (CNS). He proposed that conversion symptoms occurred in those with a constitutional predisposition when a receptive part of the brain was affected by extreme stress. Later, Russell Reynolds described clinical cases in which the loss of function or the persistence of severe pain could be attributed to an idea that the patient had about the body.

Jean-Martin Charcot then expanded on the biological concepts of Briquet and the psychological constructs of Reynolds, adding heredity to factors that influence predisposition. Moreover, Charcot suggested that a traumatic event gave rise to the idea, which then led to the brain's dynamic dysfunction; Charcot also suggested that the idea could be produced in the brain by hypnosis.

The term conversion was first used by Sigmund Freud and his associate Josef Breuer. It was used to describe the clinical case of Anna O., whose undischarged psychic energy was bound in a somatic symptom. This symptom represented the unconscious conflict. That is, a repressed thought was converted to a somatic symptom. Freud then worked out his concept of talking therapy as a catharsis through which unconsciously repressed material might become conscious. With catharsis in psychotherapy and with hypnotic suggestion, somatic conversion symptoms were shown to diminish and even disappear.

In 1929, following from Charcot, *Pierre Janet observed that conversion disorders were preceded by a lowering of consciousness threshold and were associated with dissociation.* He recognized that a constitutional weakness in an individual might be accentuated by shock or fatigue, resulting in aspects of consciousness being split off. His concept of what is now considered to be conversion disorder did not, however, include the concept of repression; thus, he was not concerned with the significance of the dynamic unconscious as Freud was.

19.16 The answer is D

It is important early on in the assessment of any psychiatric patient to determine whether or not she has psychotic symptoms. This woman presents with the recurrent false belief that she has breast cancer; it is disrupting her life and causing considerable distress. The belief is *probably not delusional*, however, because she is able to be reassured, at least momentarily, and she recognizes that the fear is exaggerated. A delusion is, by definition, fixed and impervious to outside evidence that contradicts the belief. Accordingly, *it is most unlikely that she is suffering a delusional disorder or a major depressive disorder with psychotic symptoms. Obsessive-compulsive disorder* (OCD) is a serious consideration: She has obsessive, intrusive, and unwanted thoughts, and compulsive-like behavior in her self-examinations and time spent on the internet. However, DSM-IV-TR does not permit a diagnosis of OCD if the symptoms are limited to health concerns. Body dysmorphic disorder describes concerns about appearance, not underlying disease. *The appropriate diagnosis is hypochondriasis.* Intriguingly, some researchers are now speculating that hypochondriasis is part of an OCD spectrum of disorders. Although it has historically been regarded as difficult to treat, there are now data showing good response to selective serotonin reuptake inhibitors in doses similar to those used to treat OCD—typically higher than doses to treat depression alone.

19.17 The answer is B

The usual course of hypochondriasis is chronic, *with symptoms waxing and waning over the years*, often worsening during periods of stress. There are several features in Harriet's case to suggest the prognosis may be brighter. The onset of symptoms was acute, there is no clear secondary gain, and there is nothing in the case description to suggest that she suffers from a personality disorder, all of which are associated with a better prognosis. There is no specific psychotherapy for hypochondriasis. Cognitive-behavioral therapy is helpful to some individuals. It is worth noting that her cancer fears began not only in the context of a friend's illness and death, but also of a dramatic change in life circumstances. She left a job that required considerable training and skills, which provided constant interaction with other smart, educated adults, in order to stay home alone with the demands of a young baby. Consideration should be given to a psychotherapy that would help her explore her feelings, motivations, and reactions to this important decision.

19.18 The answer is E

Patients with somatization disorder consider themselves to be medically ill. Despite this, there is good evidence *that they are no more likely to develop another medical illness in the next twenty years than people without somatization disorder.* The *onset is before 25 years of age in 90 percent of people with the disorder*, but initial symptoms generally develop during adolescence. Partly because of the undulating nature of the disorder, *people with somatization are usually poor historians, and they seem to exaggerate various symptoms, each at different times. The female to male ratio ranges from 5 to 1 to 20 to 1. It is relatively more common in rural areas* and in people who are nonwhite, unmarried and have less education.

19.19 The answer is A

People with hypochondriasis are highly thanatophobic (fear of death), which is a central clinical feature of the disorder. They are *persistent seekers of explanations rather than of treatment*, are largely unsatisfied with their medical care, and often feel that physicians have not recognized their needs. The onset of the disorder is most commonly in the third and fourth decade of life, and it is *equally common in men and women.* Reassurance that is delivered confidently by a competent doctor using multiple modalities, including skillful examination, effective communication, and helpful education is the cornerstone of treatment of the hypochondriacal patient. Without successful reassurance, more specific treatments are not likely to be accepted or adhered to by the patient. There is no known somatic pathology specific to hypochondriasis. Investigators who conducted *postmortem examinations of hypochondriacs found no evidence of inflammation and congestion in the upper GI tract.*

19.20 The answer is C

There is an association between conversion disorder and antisocial personality disorder. The onset of the disorder is usually acute, and symptoms or deficits are usually of short duration. The *symptoms usually do not conform to known anatomical pathways* and physiological mechanisms, but instead follow the individual's conceptualization of his or her illness. *Confronting the patient about the so-called "false nature" of their symptoms is contraindicated.* In acute cases, reassurance and suggestion of recovery coupled with early rehabilitation are the treatments of choice. *Schizoid disorder is not comorbid in patients with conversion disorder.*

Answers 19.21–19.24

19.21 The answer is C

19.22 The answer is C

19.23 The answer is B

19.24 The answer is B

In the 10th revision of *International Statistical Classification of Diseases and Related Health Problems* (ICD-10), somatoform disorders are described as a "repeated presentation of physical symptoms, together with persistent requests for medical investigation," although patients have been reassured by their physicians that the symptoms have no physical basis. *If physical disorders are present, they cannot account for patients' symptoms or for their distress.* The *categories of somatoform disorders are similar in DSM-IV-TR and ICD-10 (including, for example, somatization disorder, pain disorder, and hypochondriasis/hypochondriacal disorder),* except that *in ICD-10, body dysmorphic disorder is a subcategory of hypochondriacal disorder.* ICD-10 also *includes the diagnosis of neurasthenia, which has many signs and symptoms that overlap with the DSM-IV-TR categories of anxiety, depression, and somatization.*

Answers 19.25–19.26

19.25 The answer is A

19.26 The answer is C

Many who work in the general medical setting find the diagnosis of undifferentiated somatoform disorder helpful. Research indicates the validity of distinguishing undifferentiated somatoform disorder from somatization disorder. There appears to be a dimensional or quantitative difference between undifferentiated somatoform disorder and somatization disorder rather than a qualitative difference between the two. However, the natural history of both disorders seems to be similar. The disorder was not included in DSM-I, DSM-II, and DSM-III; it was first introduced in DSM-III-R because somatization disorder was considered to be too restrictive by primary care providers to provide adequate coverage for many patients with significant somatoform complaints. Thus, the subsyndromal grouping was formalized to facilitate learning about the natural course of a large cluster of patients. The criteria for undifferentiated somatoform disorder in ICD-10 are similar to the diagnostic criteria in DSM-IV-TR.

Undifferentiated somatoform disorder is characterized by one or more unexplained physical complaints of at least 6 months' duration. These symptoms impair the patient in some domain and are temporally associated with a stressor. Psychological factors are assumed to be associated with the symptoms or complaints because of a contemporaneous relationship between the initiation or exacerbation of the symptoms and stressors, conflicts, or needs. The complaint must be unattributable to any other known psychiatric condition or pathophysiological mechanism or, when it is related to a nonpsychiatric condition, the physical complaints or resulting social and occupational impairments must be grossly in excess of what would ordinarily be expected from the findings.

The importance of undifferentiated somatoform disorder comes from the fact that it may be 30 to 100 times more prevalent than full-blown somatization disorder. *Undifferentiated somatoform disorder has an estimated lifetime prevalence in the general population of between 4 and 11 percent.* The estimated lifetime prevalence of somatization disorder is 0.2 to 2 percent in women and less in men.

The course of undifferentiated somatoform disorder is generally chronic and relapsing just as with somatization disorder; however, little systematic research on the disorder has been accomplished to date. It is likely that some cases of the disorder can resolve after a single episode.

Answers 19.27–19.31

19.27 The answer is C

19.28 The answer is A

19.29 The answer is C

19.30 The answer is C

19.31 The answer is D

Both somatization disorder and pain disorder affect *women more than men.* Somatization disorder has a 5 to 1 female-to-male ratio. The lifetime prevalence of somatization disorder among women in the general population may be 1 to 2 percent. Pain disorder is diagnosed twice as commonly in women as in men. Somatization disorder is defined as beginning before age 30, and it *most often begins during a person's teens.* As for pain disorder, the peak of onset is in the fourth and fifth decades, perhaps because the tolerance for pain decreases with age.

Antidepressants, such as fluoxetine (Prozac), sertraline (Zoloft), and clomipramine (Anafranil), *are effective* in the treatment of pain disorder and somatization disorder. *Serotonin may be involved in the pathophysiology of both disorders.* It is probably the main neurotransmitter in the descending inhibitory pathways. Endorphins also play a role in the central nervous system modulation of pain. *Anorexia nervosa is not commonly associated with either pain disorder or somatization disorder.* Anorexia nervosa is an eating disorder that presents a dramatic picture of self-starvation, peculiar attitudes toward food, weight loss (leading to the maintenance of the patient's body weight at least 15 percent below that expected), and an intense fear of weight gain.

Answers 19.32–19.37

19.32 The answer is C

19.33 The answer is C

19.34 The answer is C

19.35 The answer is B

19.36 The answer is A

19.37 The answer is B

The prevalence of conversion *is highest in rural areas and among the undereducated* and the lower socioeconomic classes. It is more prevalent in military populations, especially in those exposed to combat. It is also more common in underprivileged persons, in those of subnormal intelligence, and in industrial settings where compensation neurosis may become an issue. There may be a tendency for familial aggregation and for the patient to be the youngest sibling in the family. The incidence of the disorder may be on the decline.

Persons that meet the full criteria for somatization disorder are typically unmarried, nonwhite, *poorly educated, and from rural areas.*

In 1859 Pierre Briquet emphasized the multisymptomatic aspects of somatization and its protracted course. His report of the 430 cases observed at the Hospital de la Charité in Paris focused on polysymptomatic facets of the disorder. Briquet also recognized hysteria in men and attributed the disorder to emotional causes.

In the early 1960s two studies confirmed the original findings of a definable clinical syndrome, demonstrating diagnostic stability of the multisymptomatic concept of hysteria. In 1970 the eponym *Briquet's syndrome* was proposed to denote multisymptomatic hysteria. The disorder, characterized by at least 25 symptoms from ten symptom groups, was known as *Briquet's syndrome* until the publication of the DSM-III. Ironically, after the decision was made to incorporate Briquet's syndrome as part of the new diagnostic nomenclature, an unrelated decision was made to drop all eponyms. Hence a new name—*somatization disorder*—had to be created. *Pierre Briquet also originated the modern concept of conversion disorder.*

Axis II personality disorders frequently accompany a conversion disorder, especially the histrionic type (in 5 to 21 percent of cases), the passive-dependent type (9 to 40 percent of cases), and the passive-aggressive type of personality disorder. However, conversion disorders can occur in persons with no predisposing medical, neurological, or psychiatric disorder. Several recent studies using structured diagnostic interviews in patients from primary care settings found that 61 to 72 percent of *patients with somatization disorder also have co-occurring personality disorders*. This rate would seem to be 2.5 to 11.6 times more common in somatization disorder patients than in general medical patients. *Conversion disorder is characterized by focus on any one or two symptoms*, whereas somatization patients focus on complaints about multisystem symptoms that lead them to have an inordinately high number of surgical procedures and consume an excessive amount of health care.

By definition, somatization disorder is a chronic relapsing condition with no known cure. It usually begins in middle to late adolescence, but may start as late as the third decade of life. Most patients diagnosed with conversion disorder experience a quick symptomatic recovery. Rapid improvement is especially seen in cases where symptoms are of recent onset.

Most conversion symptoms remit spontaneously or after behavioral treatment, suggestion, and a supportive environment. Thus, for symptoms of very recent onset a variety of other therapies have also been utilized successfully. In practice, clinicians tend to choose therapies that reflect their training. Irrespective of the technique used, most approaches seem to work when symptoms are not reinforced and when the patient's psychosocial plight is the focus of attention.

A favorable prognosis of conversion disorder is associated with sudden onset; readily identifiable stressful events; good premorbid health with no comorbid psychiatric, medical, or neurological disease; and no ongoing compensation litigation.

Because the cause of somatization disorder is unknown and no curative or ameliorative treatment has been found, the clinician needs to focus on management rather than treatment, on coping rather than curing (care rather than cure).

Answers 19.38–19.42

19.38 The answer is B

19.39 The answer is C

19.40 The answer is A

19.41 The answer is A

19.42 The answer is B

According to the DSM-IV-TR, *undifferentiated somatoform disorder is defined as unexplained physical effects that last for at least 6 months and are below threshold for diagnosing somatization disorder*. This diagnosis is appropriate for patients with one or more physical complaints that cannot be explained by a known medical condition or that grossly exceed the expected complaints in a medical condition but do not meet the diagnostic criteria for a specific somatoform disorder. The disturbance is also *not better accounted for by another mental disorder* (e.g., another somatoform disorder, sexual dysfunction, mood disorder, anxiety disorder, sleep disorder, or psychotic disorder). Two types of symptom patterns may be seen in patients with undifferentiated somatoform disorder: *those involving the autonomic nervous system and those involving sensations of fatigue or weakness*. In what is sometimes referred to as *autonomic arousal disorder*, some patients are affected with somatoform disorder symptoms that are limited to bodily functions innervated by the autonomic nervous system. Such patients have complaints involving the cardiovascular, respiratory, gastrointestinal, urogenital, and dermatological systems. Other patients complain of mental and physical fatigue, physical weakness and exhaustion, and inability to perform many everyday activities because of their symptoms. Some clinicians believe this syndrome is *neurasthenia*, a diagnosis used primarily in Europe and Asia.

The DSM-IV-TR diagnostic category of somatoform disorder not otherwise specified is a residual category for patients who have symptoms suggesting a somatoform disorder but do not meet the specific diagnostic criteria for other somatoform disorders. *Such patients may have a symptom not covered in other somatoform disorders* or *may not have met the 6-month criterion of the other somatoform disorders*. Such disorders involve nonpsychotic hypochondriacal symptoms (of less than 6 months' duration) and involve unexplained *physical complaints that are not due to another mental disorder.*

Answers 19.43–19.47

19.43 The answer is D

19.44 The answer is C

19.45 The answer is A

19.46 The answer is C

19.47 The answer is C

Hypochondriasis and *body dysmorphic disorder* have several similarities in their proposed root causes and diagnostic criteria, which is perhaps why the ICD-10 includes body dysmorphic disorder as a subcategory of hypochondriacal disorder. In psychodynamic models of etiology, *both hypochondriasis and body dysmorphic disorder may be related to the defense mechanisms of repression and displacement.* In hypochondriasis, for example, aggressive and hostile wishes toward others are believed to be transferred through repression and displacement into physical complaints; body dysmorphic disorder, meanwhile, is seen as reflecting the *displacement* of a sexual or emotional conflict onto a nonrelated body part. Such association occurs through the defense mechanisms of *repression*, dissociation, distortion, symbolization, and projection. According to the DSM-IV-TR, the preoccupation with symptoms in both disorders cause *clinically significant distress or impairment in social, occupational, or other important areas of functioning.* In all the somatoform disorders, patients firmly believe that their physical complaints are real, but these convictions *do not reach delusional intensity*; if they do, the appropriate diagnosis is delusional disorder. Moreover, all of the somatoform disorders are related to high rates of comorbid mental disorders, such as depressive or anxiety disorders. Hypochondriasis, for example, is often accompanied by symptoms of depression and anxiety and *commonly coexists with a depressive or anxiety disorder.* Similarly, body dysmorphic disorder commonly coexists with other mental disorders: one study found that more than 90 percent of patients with body dysmorphic disorder had experienced a major depressive episode in their lifetimes, and about 70 percent had experienced an anxiety disorder. Although these two categories of somatoform disorders have some similarities, the DSM-IV-TR maintains them as separate entities because of fundamental differences in their presentation. For example, patients with body dysmorphic disorder wish to appear normal but believe that others notice that they are not, whereas those with hypochondriasis *seek out attention for their presumed diseases.*

20 Chronic Fatigue Syndrome and Neurasthenia

Chronic fatigue syndrome (referred to as myalgic encephalomyelitis in the United Kingdom and Canada) is characterized by 6 months or more of severe, debilitating fatigue, often accompanied by myalgia, headaches, pharyngitis, low-grade fever, cognitive complaints, gastrointestinal symptoms, and tender lymph nodes. The search for an infectious cause of chronic fatigue syndrome has been active because of the high percentage of patients who report abrupt onset after a severe flulike illness.

In 1988, the U.S. Centers for Disease Control and Prevention (CDC) defined specific diagnostic criteria for chronic fatigue syndrome. Since then, the disorder has captured the attention of both the medical profession and the general public. The problems associated with studying chronic fatigue syndrome are of great interest in the United States today. The disorder is classified in the 10th revision of International Statistical Classification of Diseases and Related Health Problems (ICD-10) as an ill-defined condition of unknown etiology under the heading "Malaise and Fatigue" and is subdivided into asthenia and unspecified disability.

The student should study the questions and answers below for a useful review of this syndrome.

HELPFUL HINTS

Students should know the terms listed here.

- anhedonia
- asthenia
- autonomic nervous system
- George Miller Beard
- CDC guidelines
- chronic fatigue syndrome
- chronic stress
- depletion hypothesis
- endocrine disorders
- environmental components
- epidemiology
- Epstein-Barr virus
- etiology
- flu-like illness
- growing pains
- ICD-10 classification
- immune abnormalities
- incidence and prevalence
- insight-oriented psychotherapy
- laboratory examination
- major depression
- malaise
- methylphenidate (Ritalin)
- nervous diathesis
- nervous exhaustion
- neurasthenia
- neuroendocrine dysregulations
- pathognomonic features
- pharmacotherapy
- premature diagnostic closure
- spontaneous recovery
- supportive treatment
- treatment options
- undifferentiated somatoform disorder
- unspecified disability

QUESTIONS

Directions

Each of the questions or incomplete statements below is followed by five lettered responses or completions. Select the *one* that is most appropriate in each case.

20.1 Chronic fatigue syndrome

A. is associated with antibodies to the Epstein-Barr virus
B. is observed primarily in the elderly
C. has no comorbidity with major depressive disorder
D. shows responsiveness to NSAIDS (non steroidal anti-inflammatory drugs)
E. is twice as likely to occur in women as in men

20.2 Which of the following about neurasthenia is *true*?

A. The term was coined by Sigmund Freud.
B. It is most commonly diagnosed in the central United States.
C. It is thought to be the result of unconscious psychological conflict.
D. It has a biphasic course, occurring most often in adolescence and middle age.
E. Bodily complaints dominate the clinical picture.

20.3 A highly accomplished energetic 40-year-old woman was referred for psychiatric consultation after her physicians were unable to offer a definitive physiological diagnosis despite extensive medical workup after the acute onset of profound fatigue occuring in the wake of a mild viral illness. This fatigue caused her to be totally incapacitated and bedridden for many months and left her feeling quite helpless and distraught. The fatigue slowly improved over many years.

Which of the following about chronic fatigue syndrome is *true*?

A. It is associated with neurally mediated hypotension.
B. It has minimal association with depressive syndromes.
C. The symptoms often respond to evening primrose oil.
D. It is associated with infection with Babesia microti.
E. It is more severe in patients who have a dysregulated immune system.

20.4 Chronic fatigue syndrome

A. is proved to be a viral or postviral syndrome
B. has not been linked with fibromyalgia
C. has been viewed as a vehicle for negotiation of change in interpersonal worlds
D. patients in magnetic resonance imaging studies (MRI) displayed a specific pattern of white matter abnormality
E. prevalence reports show that fewer than 10 percent of cases have antecedent psychiatric disorders

20.5 *True* statements about chronic fatigue syndrome include

A. Studies indicate that many chronic fatigue syndrome patients have somatization disorder.
B. The syndrome is most likely to be a heterogeneous condition with fatigue as a final common pathway.
C. Treatment is invariably physiologic.
D. Cognitive-behavioral therapy (CBT) has been shown to have little or no impact on the disability and symptoms of patients.
E. None of the above

20.6 The symptoms of neurasthenia include

A. paresthesia
B. tachycardia
C. headaches
D. physical aches and pains
E. all of the above

ANSWERS

20.1 The answer is E

Chronic fatigue syndrome *has a prevalence of 0.52 percent in women and 0.29 percent in men.* The cause is unknown, and while investigators have tried to implicate the Epstein-Barr herpesvirus (EBV) as the etiological agent, *the specific antibodies and atypical lymphocytosis which are noted in EBV infection, are absent in chronic fatigue syndrome.* In fact, chronic fatigue syndrome has *no pathognomonic features*, but up to 80 percent of patients with chronic fatigue syndrome meet the diagnostic criteria for major depression. *No effective medical treatment is known* either. Symptomatic treatment is the usual approach, like analgesics for arthralgias and muscular pains, *but nonsteroidal anti-inflammatory drugs (NSAIDS) are not effective.* A recent study found a specific gene associated with chronic fatigue syndrome; however, it required replication.

20.2 The answer is D

Neurasthenia *most often occurs during adolescence or middle age.* The *term was introduced in the 1860s by the American neuro-psychiatrist George Miller Beard, not Sigmund Freud.* The disorder is not considered a distinct diagnostic entity in the United States, and the fourth edition of the Diagnostic and Statistical Manual of Mental Disorders (DSM-IV-TR) categorizes neurasthenia as undifferentiated somatoform disorder. It is however, an accepted condition in Europe and Asia, and in many cultures in which people resist having a mental disorder, neurasthenia is a preferred diagnosis; *it is most commonly diagnosed in eastern Asia.* It *is thought to result from chronic stress, not from unconscious psychological conflicts*, with the idea that stress can cause structural change in an organ system. Hallmarks of neurasthenia are a patient's emphasis on fatigability and weakness and concern about lowered mental and physical efficiency, in contrast to the somatoform disorders, in which bodily complaints and *preoccupation with physical disease dominate the picture.*

20.3 The answer is A

Some patients with chronic fatigue syndrome-like symptoms *may have neurally mediated hypotension (NMH)*, a dysfunction of the autonomic nervous system. Medications effective for NMH may lead to relief from chronic fatigue syndrome. *There are high rates of depressive disorders among patients with chronic fatigue.* Controlled clinical trials, however, *do not support the use of antidepressants, corticosteroids or evening primrose oil.* Although certain organisms, such as *Babesia microti and B. burgdorferi, can result in a chronic fatigue-like picture, most cases of chronic fatigue syndrome are not linked to these agents.* Similarly, although evidence of *immune dysregulation has been reported among patients with chronic fatigue, the data are not consistent, and do not reflect illness severity.*

20.4 The answer is C

In the absence of a clear cause, chronic fatigue syndrome has been disparagingly called "the yuppie flu," neurasthenia, and masked depression. Viral or postviral etiologies have also been considered, with diagnoses such as myalgic encephalomyelitis and chronic Epstein-Barr virus disorder being in vogue for a while. *Studies of these viral etiologies have not seemed to be relevant to a large segment of those with chronic fatigue syndrome,* but recent research notes a persistent enterovirus or herpesvirus 6 in some cases. *An overlap with fibrositis or fibromyalgia has also been considered,* but this is not particularly illuminating because it only links a poorly understood rheumatic condition with another even less clearly defined, fatigue-centered condition of uncertain etiology.

Medical anthropologists have seen chronic fatigue syndrome as a vehicle for negotiation of change in interpersonal worlds. A physiologist recently suggested that there might be a nasal fatigue reflex, akin to the diving reflex (bradycardia in cold water). According to this hypothesis, the nasal fatigue reflex could produce the debilitating fatigue that would in turn give the afflicted individual the time to heal before having to face a hostile environment. Brain magnetic resonance imaging (MRI) studies of 43 patients with chronic fatigue syndrome, compared to controls, demonstrated that *no MRI pattern of white matter abnormalities is specific.*

Psychiatric factors have been strongly associated with the etiology of chronic fatigue syndrome. For example, certain clinical samples have reported that *almost half of their cases have had antecedent psychiatric disorders such as depression, phobias, or other anxiety disorders.* In a recent matched study of 214 subjects with chronic fatigue syndrome from a nonspecialist, nonreferral setting, most of the index subjects were at considerably greater risk of current psychiatric disorder than were control subjects. The likelihood of psychiatric disorder was six times greater in these chronic fatigue syndrome patients than in the matched controls when evaluated either by interview or by questionnaire. Other studies of subjects who have undergone neuropsychological testing indicate that at least a subset of patients with chronic fatigue syndrome experience significant impairments in learning and memory. However, a primary psychiatric etiology for chronic fatigue syndrome is, typically, stoutly denied by patients with this syndrome, especially by those who are members of the chronic fatigue syndrome national peer support groups.

20.5 The answer is B

Fatigue is one of the most common symptoms in all of medical practice. The nature of chronic fatigue syndrome, however, remains very controversial. This syndrome was defined by the CDC in 1988 as a disabling disorder with a combination of a certain number of nonspecific symptoms such as fluctuating levels of fatigue, various combinations of neuromuscular and neuropsychological symptoms, chronic pain, malaise, mild fevers, and anxiety. According to the latest CDC criteria, it is a condition that has been clinically evaluated and still remains an unexplained, persistent, or relapsing chronic fatigue that is of new or definite onset in a previously healthy person; is not the result of exertion; is not substantially alleviated by rest; and leads to substantial reduction in previous levels of occupational, educational, social, or personal activities (Table 20.1).

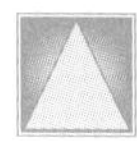

Table 20.1
CDC Criteria for Chronic Fatigue Syndrome

A. Severe unexplained fatigue for over 6 months that is:
   (1) of a new or definite onset
   (2) not due to continuing exertion
   (3) not resolved by rest
   (4) functionally impairing

B. The presence of four or more of the following new symptoms:
   (1) impaired memory or concentration
   (2) sore throat
   (3) tender lymph nodes
   (4) muscle pain
   (5) pain in several joints
   (6) new pattern of headaches
   (7) unrefreshing sleep
   (8) postexertional malaise lasting more than 24 hours

Table 20.2
Signs and Symptoms Reported by Patients with Neurasthenia

General fatigue	Sexual dysfunction, e.g., erectile disorder, anorgasmia
Exhaustion	Dysmenorrhea
General anxiety	Paresthesia
Difficulty concentrating	Insomnia
Physical aches and pains	Poor memory
Dizziness	Pessimism
Headache	Chronic worry
Intolerance of noise (hyperacusis) or bright lights	Fear of disease
Chills	Irritability
Indigestion	Feelings of hopelessness
Constipation or diarrhea	Dry mouth or hypersalivation
Flatulence	Arthralgias
Palpitations	Heat insensitivity
Extrasystole	Dysphagia
Tachycardia	Pruritus
Excess sweating	Tremors
Flushing of skin	Back pain

Chronic fatigue syndrome is most likely to be a heterogenous condition, with fatigue being only a final common pathway. At this phase of research on the condition, it is not possible to speak with certainty about its etiology.

Whether chronic fatigue syndrome should be considered as a special class of mood disorder with somatic symptoms (specifically fatigue), or a somatoform disorder not otherwise specified, or a combination of a psychiatric disorder with an unidentified infectious agent, or even some composite of these conditions, remains to be clarified. Using strict DSM-IV-TR criteria, one study demonstrates that *very few chronic fatigue syndrome patients have somatization disorder.*

Treatments for a presumably heterogenous condition with an unknown cause typically should involve a multidisciplinary approach involving psychological, physiological, and social factors. Possible concomitant psychiatric disorders could most likely benefit from a psychopharmacological trial. Many other types of treatments are being used for this debilitating illness, with even electric plum blossom needle therapy having its adherents in the literature. Two randomized controlled trials of cognitive-behavioral therapy (compared with relaxation therapy or routine practitioner care) indicate that *cognitive-behavioral therapy has substantial impact on the disability and symptoms of patients with this disorder.*

20.6 The answer is E (all)

All the listed choices—*paresthesia, tachycardia, headaches, and physical aches and pains*—are symptoms of neurasthenia. There are many more symptoms, such as difficulty in concentrating, dizziness, indigestion, constipation and diarrhea, palpitations, excess sweating, chills, noise or light intolerance, flushing, insomnia, and tremors (Table 20.2).

21 Factitious Disorders

According to the American Heritage Dictionary, the word *factitious* means "artificial; false," derived from the Latin word *facticius* which means "made by art." Those with factitious disorder simulate, induce, or aggravate illness, often inflicting painful, deforming, or even life-threatening injury on themselves or those under their care. Unlike malingerers who have material goals, such as monetary gain or avoidance of duties, factitious disorder patients undertake these tribulations primarily to gain the emotional care and attention that comes with playing the role of the patient. In doing so, they practice artifice and art, creating hospital drama that often causes frustration and dismay. Clinicians may thus dismiss, avoid, or refuse to treat factitious disorder patients. Strong countertransference of clinicians can be major obstacles toward the proper care of these patients who arguably are among the most psychiatrically disturbed.

The best known factitious disorder is perhaps factitious disorder with predominantly physical signs and symptoms, popularly known as Munchausen syndrome. This presentation involves persons who travel from hospital to hospital, gaining admission, receiving multiple diagnoses and treatments, until they are found out by staff, and then quickly move on to the next hospital to repeat the same rituals again. Common complaints or presenting symptoms include hematomas, abdominal pain, fever, and seizures. Patients have been known to do such bizarre things as inject themselves with feces to induce infections or to willingly undergo repeated unnecessary surgeries.

Despite potentially high stakes, relatively little empirical knowledge is available about the etiology, epidemiology, course and prognosis, and effective treatment of factitious disorders. Most knowledge comes from case reports, information that is frequently suspect, given the false, unreliable nature of the information these patients give. The DSM-IV-TR categories for the disorder include predominantly physical signs and symptoms, predominantly psychological signs and symptoms, both physical and psychological signs and symptoms, and factitious disorder not otherwise specified.

The student should study the questions and answers below for a useful review of these disorders.

HELPFUL HINTS

The student should be able to define each of these terms.

- approximate answers
- as-if personality
- borderline personality disorder
- Briquet's syndrome
- depressive-masochistic personality
- dissociative disorder not otherwise specified
- factitious disorder:
  - by proxy
  - not otherwise specified
  - with predominantly physical signs and symptoms
  - with predominantly psychological signs and symptoms
- Ganser's syndrome
- gridiron abdomen
- identification with the aggressor
- impostorship
- malingering
- Munchausen syndrome
- pseudologia fantastica
- pseudomalingering
- regression
- schizophrenia
- sick role
- somatoform disorders
- substance abuse
- symbolization
- unmasking ceremony

QUESTIONS

Directions

Each of the questions incomplete statements below is followed by five suggested responses completions. Select the *one* that is *best* in each case.

21.1 Factitious disorder

A. occurs more frequently in women than in men
B. is associated with a history of childhood abuse
C. is not associated with economic gain
D. may result in death due to needless medical interventions
E. all of the above

21.2 Ganser's syndrome

A. is a factitious disorder
B. is more common in women than in men

C. is associated with a severe personality disorder
D. has a chronic remitting and relapsing course
E. is motivated by involuntary phenomena

21.3 Which of the following occurs in factitious disorder by proxy?

A. The mother has had some medical education
B. The patient fails to respond to appropriate treatments
C. Maternal lying is observed
D. Unexplained illnesses have occurred in the mother
E. All of the above

21.4 Which of the following symptoms would a patient with Munchausen syndrome most likely present with?

A. Depression
B. Amnesia
C. Pain disorder
D. Hemoptysis
E. Psychosis

21.5 Factitious disorders are best treated by which of the following?

A. Immediate discharge from the hospital
B. Focusing on management rather than cure
C. Confrontation about the patient's deceit
D. Performing only minimally invasive procedures to satisfy the patient
E. Using low-dose neuroleptics to decrease the patient's physical distress

21.6 Which of the following is the gold standard for diagnosis of factitious disorder by proxy?

A. Discovery of illness-inducing agents in the caregiver's possession
B. Finding inconsistencies in the medical records
C. Confession by the child
D. Improvement when the child is removed from the caretaker
E. Direct observation of the caretaker doing harm

21.7 You are interviewing a patient to determine if a factitious disorder is present. You ask him to give you the sum of 2 plus 2. He replies, "5." Which of the following diagnoses is most likely?

A. Briquet's syndrome
B. Malingering
C. Ganser's syndrome
D. Munchausen syndrome
E. None of the above

21.8 You begin treatment of a new patient with a previously known history of factitious disorder. Within the first few sessions, you also become aware that this patient meets criteria for a diagnosis of antisocial personality disorder as well.

Which of the following statements regarding this patient is true?

A. Persons with both of these disorders do not usually volunteer for invasive procedures.
B. Persons with both of these disorders have repeated hospitalizations.
C. It is rare for persons with factitious disorder to also present with antisocial traits.
D. Factitious disorder symptoms almost always precede antisocial traits.
E. All of the above.

21.9 You are asked by the court to evaluate a 21-year-old man arrested in a robbery because his lawyer raised the issue of his competence to stand trial. He has no known psychiatric history, and no psychotic symptoms have been previously reported. During the interview the man appears calm and in control, sits slouched in the chair, and has good eye contact. His affect shows a good range. His thought processes are logical, sequential, and spontaneous even when he describes many difficulties with his thinking. He seems guarded in his answers, particularly to questions about his psychological symptoms.

He claims to have precognition on occasion, knowing, for instance, what is going to be served for lunch in the jail, and that he does not like narcotics because Jean Dixon doesn't like narcotics either, and she is in control of his thoughts. He states that he has seen a vision of General Lee in his cell as well as "little green men from Mars," and that his current incarceration is a mission in which he is attempting to be an undercover agent for the police, although none of the local police realize this. Despite the overtly psychotic nature of these thoughts as described, the patient does not seem to be really engaged in the ideas; he seems to be simply reciting a list of what appears to be crazy rather than recounting actual experiences and beliefs. When the interviewer expresses some skepticism about his described beliefs, he responds by saying that he has "many other crazy ideas" that he can share.

Which of the following is the most likely diagnosis?

A. malingering
B. schizophrenia, paranoid type
C. factitious disorder with predominantly psychological symptoms
D. delusional disorder
E. Capgras's syndrome

21.10 Factitious disorder patients with Munchausen syndrome are typically

A. middle-aged men
B. unmarried
C. unemployed
D. estranged from their families
E. all of the above

21.11 Patients with factitious disorders, either physical or psychological, most often demonstrate

A. a below-average IQ
B. a formal thought disorder
C. poor sexual adjustment

D. generally adequate frustration tolerance
E. all of the above

21.12 True statements about patients with factitious disorder with predominantly psychological signs and symptoms include

A. Virtually all patients with this type of factitious disorder have a personality disorder.
B. The rate of suicide is generally reported to be low in this population.
C. Prognosis is slightly better than for most other Axis I disorders.
D. Factitious psychosis, in particular, almost never represents the prodrome to an authentic psychosis.
E. None of the above

21.13 Clinical indicators of poor treatment responsiveness in patients with factitious disorders include

A. the coexistence of other Axis I disorders, such as mood, anxiety, or substance-related disorders
B. borderline or antisocial elements
C. religious affiliations
D. capacity to accept confrontation in therapy
E. all of the above

21.14 The differential diagnosis of a factitious disorder includes

A. somatization disorder
B. hypochondriasis
C. antisocial personality disorder
D. malingering
E. all of the above

21.15 Factitious disorders

A. usually begin in childhood
B. are best treated with psychoactive drugs
C. usually have a good prognosis
D. are synonymous with Ganser's syndrome
E. may occur by proxy

21.16 True statements about factitious disorder by proxy include all of the following *except*

A. The average length of time to establish a diagnosis after the initial presentation is about 2 months.
B. Often a sibling has died of undiagnosed causes before the disorder is recognized.
C. The disorder currently accounts for fewer than 1,000 of the almost 3 million cases of child abuse reported each year in the United States.
D. Prevalence of the disorder has been estimated to be approximately 5 percent in children presenting with allergies.
E. The prevalence of the disorder in life-threatening episodes treated with cardiopulmonary resuscitation has been estimated to be as high as 9 percent.

21.17 The perpetrators in factitious disorder by proxy

A. often suffer from psychotic or dissociative disorders
B. rarely have personal histories of factitious or somatoform disorders
C. most often suffered direct abuse in childhood themselves
D. are commonly unresponsive to their infants when their behavior is unwitnessed
E. all of the above

ANSWERS

21.1 The answer is E (all)

The prevalence of factitious disorder in the general population is unknown, but it *occurs more frequently in women than in men*, and the severe syndromes are more frequent in women. Anecdotal case reports indicate that many of the *patients suffered childhood abuse* or deprivation, resulting in frequent hospitalizations during early development. The motivation for the behavior is to assume the sick role, and external incentives, such as *economic gain*, avoiding legal responsibility, or improving physical well-being, as in malingering, are absent. The prognosis in most cases is poor, and although there are no adequate data about the ultimate outcome for the patients, a *few of them probably die as a result of needless medication, instrumentation, or surgery*.

21.2 The answer is C

Ganser's syndrome, the voluntary production of severe psychiatric symptoms, sometimes described as giving approximate answers or talking past the point, *is strongly associated with a severe personality disorder*. It *is more common in men than in women*, and it most typically associated with prison inmates. It was previously classified as a factitious disorder, but is commonly associated with dissociative phenomena such as amnesia, fugue, perceptual disturbances and conversion symptoms, and is *thus classified as a dissociative disorder. Recovery from the syndrome is sudden; patients claim amnesia for the events.*

21.3 The answer is E (all)

In factitious disorder by proxy, classified in DSM-IV-TR as a factitious disorder not otherwise specified, a person intentionally produces physical signs or symptoms in another person who is under the first person's care. The most common cases involve *mothers who deceive medical personnel* into believing that their child is ill. In this disorder, it has been noted that the symptoms and pattern of illness are extremely unusual. The mothers have often had some medical or nursing education, are observed to lie, and are the only witnesses to the onset of signs and symptoms. *Unexplained illnesses have occurred in the mother or her other children* and she often welcomes even invasive and painful tests. The ICD-10 classifies this condition under child abuse, not factitious disorders.

21.4 The answer is D

Munchausen syndrome is another name for factitious disorder with predominantly physical signs and symptoms. A primary feature of this disorder is a patient's ability to present physical symptoms such as *hemoptysis* so well that he or she gains admission to a hospital. A patient may feign symptoms of a severe disorder with which he or she is familiar and may also give a history good enough to deceive a skilled clinician. The patient usually demands surgery or other treatment and can become abusive when negative test results threaten to reveal the factitious behavior. The other choices listed, depression, amnesia, pain disorder, and psychosis, are common presentations of patients with factitious disorder with predominantly psychological signs and symptoms.

21.5 The answer is B

No specific psychiatric therapy has been effective in treating factitious disorders. It is a clinical paradox that patients with the disorders simulate serious illness and seek and submit to unnecessary treatment while they deny to themselves and others their true illness and this avoid possible treatment for it. *Treatment is thus best focused on management rather than cure*. Perhaps the single most important factor in successful management is a physician's early recognition of the disorder.

Physicians should try not to feel resentment when patients humiliate their diagnostic prowess, and they should *avoid any unmasking ceremony that sets up the patients as adversaries* and precipitates their flight from the hospital. The staff *should not perform unnecessary procedures or discharge patients abruptly*, both of which are manifestations of anger. Pharmacotherapy for factitious disorders is of limited use. Comorbid Axis I disorder (e.g. schizophrenia) will respond to antipsychotic medication, but in all cases medication should be administered carefully because of the potential for abuse.

21.6 The answer is E

Factitious disorder by proxy should not be considered a diagnosis of exclusion. Confirmatory evidence should be actively pursued, so as to lessen risk to the child. Safety of the child should be ensured at the same time. *The gold standard for confirming factitious disorder by proxy is direct observation of a parent causing harm to a child.* Covert video has also shown cases in which mothers, who appear concerned in the presence of staff, behave indifferently toward their children when they are not aware of being watched. Covert video should only be undertaken after consultation with legal counsel. A court order may need to be obtained, and a bioethics consultation may be helpful to weigh the potential benefits to the child versus compromises of privacy for the parent.

Other means of confirming factitious disorder by proxy include searching the mother's belongings for illness-inducing agents, reviewing collateral information and past medical records for inconsistencies, gathering information on siblings, recording temporal associations between parental visits and the child's signs and symptoms, observing the child's well-being when removed from the parent's care for extended periods, and analyzing specimens taken in the presence of the parent compared to those taken in the parent's absence.

21.7 The answer is C

Ganser's syndrome, a controversial condition most typically associated with prison inmates, is characterized by the use of approximate answers. Persons with the syndrome respond to simple questions with astonishingly incorrect answers. For example, when asked about the color of a blue car, the person answers "red" or answers "2 plus 2 equals 5." Ganser's syndrome may be a variant of malingering, in that the patients' avoid punishment or responsibility for their actions. Ganser's syndrome is classified in DSM-IV-TR as a dissociative disorder not otherwise specified and in ICD-10 under other dissociative or conversion disorders. However, patients with factitious disorder with predominantly psychological signs and symptoms may intentionally give approximate answers.

In *Briquet's syndrome*, another name for somatization disorder, the symptoms are not produced voluntarily, hospitalization is not frequent, and patients do not seek to undergo numerous mutilating procedures. *Malingering* is the voluntary production of false or exaggerated physical or psychological symptoms for secondary gain. *Munchausen syndrome* is another name for factitious disorder with predominantly physical signs and symptoms.

21.8 The answer is A

Because of their pathological lying, lack of close relationships with others, hostile and manipulative behavior, and associated substance abuse and criminal history, factitious disorder patients are often classified as having antisocial personality disorder. Antisocial persons, however, *do not usually volunteer for invasive procedures or resort to a way of life marked by repeated or long-term hospitalization.* There is no evidence that factitious disorder symptoms precede the development of antisocial personality traits or vice versa.

Because of attention seeking and an occasional flair for the dramatic, patients with factitious disorder may be classified as having histrionic personality disorder. Consideration of the patient's chaotic lifestyle, past history of disturbed interpersonal relationships, identity crisis, substance abuse, self-damaging acts, and manipulative tactics may lead to the diagnosis of borderline personality disorder.

21.9 The answer is A

Malingering is the most likely diagnosis based on the clinical presentation. Until his arrest, there was no previous psychiatric history or previously reported psychiatric symptoms. The man's mental status examination is apparently normal; there are no disorganized thoughts or loosening of associations. The patient claims a variety of unrelated bizarre beliefs, presenting responses in a manner that is inconsistent with the disorganization of psychological functioning that would be expected if the symptoms were genuine. In this case the "psychotic" symptoms are under voluntary control, and since there is external incentive (avoiding prosecution) and no evidence of an intrapsychic need to maintain a sick role, the diagnosis of *factitious disorder with predominantly psychotic features* is ruled out. The patient expresses no paranoid feelings, as would be seen in *schizophrenia, paranoid type.* His delusions lack conviction and are therefore not indicative of the unshakable beliefs in a *delusional disorder. Capgras's syndrome,* the delusion that familiar people have been replaced by identical impostors, is not seen here.

21.10 The answer is E (all)

Overall, demographic analyses of factitious disorders in the literature have distinguished two general patterns. Factitious disorder patients with Munchausen syndrome are *typically middle-aged men who are unmarried, unemployed, and estranged from their families*; the remaining patients are generally women aged 20 to 40 years. A number of reports suggest that those in the second group are commonly employed in or intimately familiar with health care occupations such as nursing and physical therapy. In a 10-year retrospective study of hospitalized patients, 28 of 41 patients with factitious disorder identified worked in medically related fields, 15 as nurses.

21.11 The answer is C

Patients with factitious disorders, whether physical or psychological, most often demonstrate *an average or above-average intelligence quotient (IQ), absence of a formal thought disorder,* a poor sense of identity, *poor sexual adjustment, poor frustration tolerance,* strong dependency needs, and narcissism.

21.12 The answer is A

The literature on factitious disorder with predominantly psychological signs and symptoms is notable for the magnitude of the psychological dysfunction present in patients. *Almost all have serious personality disorders,* often associated with substance abuse. Several authors have reported that *there is a high rate of suicide in this population* and that factitious psychological disorders *have a worse prognosis than most other Axis I disorders.*

The patient's simulation of a mental disorder *may actually represent the prodrome to an authentic mental disorder* with a serious outcome. In particular, clinicians *should be cautious in diagnosing factitious psychosis because in two small studies a majority of these patients eventually manifested clear-cut psychotic disorders such as schizophrenia.* In other cases, an ostensibly feigned condition such as depression has responded to psychotropic medications, validating at least some element of the presentation. Because virtually all patients with this type of factitious disorder have a personality disorder (usually borderline, histrionic, or antisocial), caregivers must also recognize that the simulated mental disorder coexists with an authentic one. Comorbidity with substance-related disorders and somatoform disorders has been reported as well, and dissociative disorders may result in alterations of memory and the patient's providing inconsistent factual information.

21.13 The answer is B

Overall, several clinical indicators of *enhanced* treatment responsiveness in patients with factitious disorders have been elucidated. They include: (1) *underlying psychiatric syndromes, such as mood, anxiety, substance-related,* or conversion disorders; (2) *personality traits without borderline or antisocial elements;* (3) psychosocial supports, such as ongoing relationships with significant others, employment or employability, or *religious affiliations;* and (4) ability to establish a therapeutic alliance as characterized by the capacity to establish and maintain rapport, *accept confrontation,* and comply with treatment recommendations.

21.14 The answer is E (all)

A factitious disorder is differentiated from *somatization disorder* (Briquet's syndrome) by the voluntary production of factitious symptoms, the extreme course of multiple hospitalizations, and the patient's seeming willingness to undergo an extraordinary number of painful, even mutilating, procedures.

Hypochondriasis differs from factitious disorder in that the hypochondriacal patient does not voluntarily initiate the production of symptoms, and hypochondriasis typically has a later age of onset. As is the case with somatization disorder, patients with hypochondriasis do not usually submit to potentially mutilating procedures.

Because of their pathological lying, lack of close relationships with others, hostile and manipulative manner, and associated substance and criminal history, factitious disorder patients are often classified as having *antisocial personality disorder.* However, persons with antisocial personality disorder do not usually volunteer for invasive procedures or resort to a way of life marked by repeated or long-term hospitalizations.

Factitious disorder must be distinguished from *malingering.* Malingerers have an obvious, recognizable environmental goal in producing signs and symptoms of illness. They may seek hospitalization to secure financial compensation, evade the police, avoid work, or merely obtain free bed and board for the night; yet they always have some apparent end for their behavior.

21.15 The answer is E

Factitious disorders *may occur by proxy*; such disorders are dually classified as factitious disorder by proxy and factitious disorder not otherwise specified.

Factitious disorders *usually begin in early adult life*, although they may appear during childhood or adolescence. The onset of the disorder or of discrete episodes of treatment-seeking may follow a real illness, loss, rejection, or abandonment. Usually, the patient or a close relative had a hospitalization in childhood or early adolescence for a genuine physical illness. Thereafter, a long pattern of successive hospitalizations unfolds, beginning insidiously.

Factitious disorders *are not best treated with psychoactive drugs.* Pharmacotherapy is of limited use. No specific psychiatric therapy has been effective in treating factitious disorders. Although no adequate data are available about the ultimate outcome for patients, a number of them probably die as a result of needless medication, instrumentation, or surgery. They *usually have a poor prognosis.*

Factitious disorders *are not synonymous with Ganser's syndrome,* a controversial condition that is characterized by the use of approximate answers. Ganser's syndrome may be a variant of malingering, in that patients avoid punishment or responsibility for their actions. Ganser's syndrome is classified as a dissociative disorder not otherwise specified.

21.16 The answer is A

Factitious disorder by proxy currently accounts for *fewer than 1,000 of the almost 3 million cases of child abuse reported each year in the United States,* but this number may rise as mass media and professional attention increase recognition of these cases. Authors have attempted to elucidate the prevalence of factitious disorder by proxy within particular populations, such as children presenting with apnea (0.27 percent), *allergy (5 percent)*, asthma (1 percent), apparent life-threatening episodes (1.5 percent), and *life-threatening episodes treated with cardiopulmonary resuscitation (over 9 percent* among children in whom final diagnoses were established). *The average length of time to establish a diagnosis of factitious disorder by proxy after the initial presentation is 15 months,* and *often a sibling has died of undiagnosed causes before the disorder is recognized.* Table 21.1 summarizes the most common presentations of the disorder.

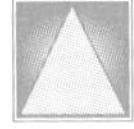

Table 21.1
Ranking of the Most Common Bibliographic References to Signs and Symptoms of Factitious Disorder by Proxy

Poisoning (includes Munchausen syndrome by proxy and intentional poisoning)
Seizures or vomiting
Apnea
Diarrhea
Unconsciousness
Fevers
Lethargy
Dehydration or hematemesis
Ataxia or hematuria

Adapted from Schreier HA, Libow JA. *Hunting for Love: Munchausen by Proxy Syndrome.* New York: Guilford Press; 1993; and Rosenberg DA. Web of deceit: a literature review of Munchausen syndrome by proxy. *Child Abuse Negl.* 1987;11:533.

21.17 The answer is D

By definition, factitious disorder by proxy requires that any external gains for the victim's fabricated or induced illnesses, such as disability payments or respite from child-rearing responsibilities during hospitalization, are incidental to the pursuit of the vicarious sick role. Several analyses have referred to a disorder of empathy among perpetrating mothers fueled by depression and isolation. With their spouses typically unavailable or uninvolved, they vitiate these painful feelings by mobilizing attention and nurturance through this disorder. A related hypothesis involves projective identification. Through this defense mechanism, the mother projects onto her child her own unconscious longings for nurturance, then ensures—through her own indefatigable attention as well as that of healthcare providers and others—that the child receives the attention she herself so desperately craves. Others have referred to factitious disorder by proxy as an epiphenomenon of the parent's narcissism and sociopathy with glee arising from the capacity to dupe highly educated professionals. The perpetrator may also be displacing onto the child sadistic impulses toward herself or others. A recent theory suggests that an unsatisfactory relationship with a desired but unavailable father contributes to a perverse relationship with physicians and hospital staff members, surrogate parents whom the abusing mother simultaneously pursues and punishes. In this context the mother perceives her child as an object to be used to manipulate an intensely ambivalent relationship with the medical establishment. Concrete evidence for this last observation has been provided through covert videotapes. In contrast to the devoted, even symbiotic, parenting style they reveal in public, these mothers *are commonly unresponsive to their infants* when their behavior is unwitnessed. Despite the perversity of their behavior, they *rarely suffer from psychotic or dissociative disorders,* although they *often have personal histories of factitious or somatoform disorders.* Although they may have been neglected or undervalued, most perpetrators *did not suffer direct abuse in childhood.* Table 21.2 lists the clinical indicators that may suggest factitious disorder by proxy.

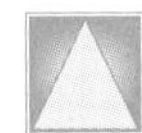

Table 21.2
Clinical Indicators That May Suggest Factitious Disorder by Proxy

The symptoms and pattern of illness are extremely unusual, or inexplicable physiologically.
Repeated hospitalizations and workups by numerous caregivers fail to reveal a conclusive diagnosis or cause.
Physiological parameters are consistent with induced illness; e.g., apnea monitor tracings disclose massive muscle artifact prior to respiratory arrest, suggesting that the child has been struggling against an obstruction to the airways.
The patient fails to respond to appropriate treatments.
The vitality of the patient is inconsistent with the laboratory findings.
The signs and symptoms abate when the mother has not had access to the child.
The mother is the only witness to the onset of signs and symptoms.
Unexplained illnesses have occurred in the mother or her other children.
The mother has had medical or nursing education, or exposure to models of the illnesses afflicting the child (e.g., a parent with sleep apnea).
The mother welcomes even invasive and painful tests.
The mother grows anxious if the child improves.
Maternal lying is proved.
Medical observations yield information that is inconsistent with parental reports.

Adapted from Feldman MD, Eisendrath SJ. *The Spectrum of Factitious Disorders.* Washington, DC: American Psychiatric Press; 1996.

22 Dissociative Disorders

Most persons see themselves as human beings with one basic personality; they experience a unitary sense of self. Persons with dissociative disorders, however, have lost the sense of having one consciousness. They feel as though they have no identity, they are confused about who they are, or they experience multiple identities. Everything that usually gives persons their unique personalities—their integrated thoughts, feelings, and actions—is abnormal in persons with dissociative disorders. The revised fourth edition of the *Diagnostic and Statistical Manual of Mental Disorders* (DSM-IV-TR) classifies dissociative disorders as dissociative amnesia, dissociative fugue, dissociative identity disorder (or more popularly, multiple personality disorder), depersonalization disorder, and dissociative disorder not otherwise specified.

Normal people can experience feelings of dissociation or depersonalization under a variety of circumstances, such as fatigue, isolation, or hypnosis. These feelings tend to be temporary, and, while perhaps briefly uncomfortable, are not experienced as overly distressful. Dissociative disorders are much more severe and disabling. Pathological dissociative states are associated with histories of childhood physical, emotional, and sexual abuse, or may be seen in people who have undergone traumatic wartime or disaster experiences. A careful and thorough medical evaluation is necessary to rule out any possible organic cause for the dissociative symptoms.

The student should study the questions and answers below for a useful review of these disorders.

HELPFUL HINTS

The terms below relate to dissociative disorders and should be defined.

- anterograde amnesia
- approximate answers
- automatic writing
- brainwashing
- coercive persuasion
- continuous amnesia
- crystal gazing
- denial
- depersonalization
- derealization disorder
- dissociation
- dissociative amnesia
- Dissociative Experience Scale
- dissociative fugue
- dissociative identity disorder
- dissociative trance
- dominant personality
- double orientation
- doubling
- epidemiology of dissociative disorders
- false memory syndrome
- Ganser's syndrome
- hemidepersonalization
- highway hypnosis
- hypnotizability
- Korsakoff's syndrome
- localized amnesia
- malingering
- multiple personality disorder
- paramnesia
- possession state
- reduplicative paramnesia
- repression
- retrograde amnesia
- secondary gain
- selective amnesia
- sleepwalking disorder
- temporal lobe functions
- transient global amnesia
- unitary sense of self
- wandering

QUESTIONS

Directions

Each of the questions or incomplete statements below is followed by five suggested responses or completions. Select the *one* that is *best* in each case.

22.1 *Reduplicative paramnesia* is a condition of which of the following disorders:

A. Dissociative identity disorder
B. Dissociative fugue
C. Depersonalization disorder
D. Dissociative amnesia
E. Déjà vu

22.2 Which of the following statements regarding transient global amnesia is *false*?

A. It is an acute retrograde amnesia
B. It affects recent memories more than remote memories
C. It usually lasts 6 to 24 hours
D. It complete recovery does not occur
E. It is most often caused by transient ischemic attacks

22.3 The mental status examination of a patient with dissociative identity disorder would most likely reveal which of the following?

A. Normal exam
B. Orientation difficulties

C. Impaired recent memory
D. Flat affect
E. Decreased concentration

22.4 The first stage in coercive processes such as brainwashing is

A. the emergence of a new pseudoidentity
B. inflicting pain
C. the idealization of captors
D. the development of dissociative state
E. traumatic infantilism

22.5 You begin therapy with a young woman who has a very limited memory of her childhood years but knows that she was removed from her parents due to abuse and neglect. She frequently cannot account for hours and even days of her life. Occasionally, she does not remember how or when she arrived at a particular location. She also finds clothes in her closet that she does not like and cannot remember buying. Her friends are puzzled because sometimes she acts in a childish, dependent way; other times she is uncharacteristically aggressive and hostile.

Which of the following is the most likely diagnosis?

A. Dissociative amnesia
B. Schizophrenia
C. Depersonalization disorder
D. Dissociative identity disorder
E. Somatization disorder

22.6 Dissociative fugue

A. has new identities that are more complete than in dissociative identity disorder
B. identities can alternate as in dissociative identity disorder
C. occurs more often during wartime and natural disasters
D. is caused by heavy alcohol use
E. all of the above

22.7 Patients with dissociative amnesia

A. do not retain the capacity to learn new information
B. commonly retain awareness of personal identity, but have amnesia for general information
C. present very similarly to patients with dementia
D. typically behave in a confused and disorganized way
E. none of the above

22.8 Dissociative amnesia is thought to be

A. the least common of the dissociative disorders
B. more common in women than men
C. more common in older adults than younger
D. decreased in times of war and natural disaster
E. none of the above

22.9 Organic amnesias are distinguished from dissociative amnesias by which of the following?

A. They do not normally involve recurrent identity alteration.
B. The amnesia is not selectively limited to personal information.
C. The memories do not focus on an emotionally traumatic event.
D. The amnesia is more often anterograde than retrograde.
E. All of the above

22.10 DSM-IV-TR includes dissociative symptoms in the criteria for all but which of the following mental disorders?

A. acute stress disorder
B. somatization disorder
C. posttraumatic stress disorder
D. obsessive-compulsive disorder
E. none of the above

22.11 Depersonalization disorder is characterized by

A. impaired reality testing
B. ego-dystonic symptoms
C. occurrence in the late decades of life
D. gradual onset
E. a brief course and a good prognosis

22.12 All of the following are true statements about dissociative fugue *except*

A. It is a rare type of dissociative disorder.
B. It is not characterized by behavior that appears extraordinary to others.
C. It is characterized by a lack of awareness of the loss of memory.
D. It is usually a long-lasting state.
E. Recovery is spontaneous and rapid.

22.13 The most common cause of organic fugue is probably

A. head trauma
B. hypoglycemia
C. epilepsy
D. brain tumors
E. migraines

22.14 Culture-bound syndromes in which dissociative fugue is a prominent feature include

A. *latah*
B. *amok*
C. *grisi siknis*
D. *piblokto*
E. all of the above

22.15 The mainstay of treatment of dissociative fugue is

A. psychodynamic psychotherapy
B. hypnosis
C. sodium amobarbital interviewing
D. antidepressant medication
E. none of the above

22.16 A patient normally without cognitive deficits, who seems out of touch with the environment and in a dream-like state for a brief period of time, and who has amnesia regarding the experience when it is ended is likely to have

A. dementia
B. dissociative fugue
C. localized amnesia
D. generalized amnesia
E. sleepwalking disorder

22.17 Patients predisposed to dissociative fugue include those with all of the following *except*

A. mood disorders
B. schizophrenia
C. histrionic personality disorders
D. heavy alcohol abuse
E. borderline personality disorders

22.18 Which of these statements regarding the prognosis of dissociative identity disorder is *incorrect*?

A. Recovery is generally complete.
B. The earlier the onset of dissociative identity disorder, the poorer the prognosis is.
C. The level of impairment is determined by the number and types of various personalities.
D. Individual personalities may have their own separate mental disorders.
E. One or more of the personalities may function relatively well.

Directions

These lettered headings are followed by a list of numbered phrases. For each numbered phrase, select

A. if the item is associated with A only
B. if the item is associated with B only
C. if the item is associated with both A and B
D. if the item is associated with neither A nor B

Questions 22.19–22.22

A. Dissociative amnesia
B. Amnesia secondary to organic etiology

22.19 More likely to involve interruption of the episodic-autobiographical memory
22.20 More likely to involve interruption of general cognitive functioning
22.21 More likely to involve interruption of language capacity
22.22 More likely to be localized

Directions

The lettered headings below are followed by a list of numbered statements. For each numbered statement, select the *one* lettered heading that is most closely associated with it. Each lettered heading may be selected once, more than once, or not at all.

Questions 22.23–22.26

A. Dissociative amnesia
B. Dissociative fugue
C. Dissociative identity disorder
D. Depersonalization disorder

22.23 A 25-year-old man comes to the emergency room and cannot remember his name
22.24 A 35-year-old man states that his body feels unreal, not attached to him
22.25 A 16-year-old girl is found in another city far from her home and does not recall how she got there
22.26 A 30-year-old woman suddenly has a new child-like voice in the interview

ANSWERS

22.1 The answer is C

An occasional phenomenon of *depersonalization disorder* is doubling; patients feel that the point of consciousness is outside their bodies, often a few feet overhead, and from there they observe themselves, as if they were totally separate persons. Sometimes, patients believe that they are in two places at the same time, a condition called *reduplicative paramnesia* or *double orientation*. Most patients are aware of their disturbed sense of reality; this awareness is considered one of the salient characteristics of the disorder. *Dissociation* is defined as an unconscious defense mechanism involving the segregation of any group of mental or behavioral processes from the rest of the person's psychic activity; may entail the separation of an idea from its accompanying emotional tone, as seen in dissociative and conversion disorders. *Déjà vu* is an illusions of visual recognition in which a new situation is incorrectly regarded as a repetition of a previous experience.

22.2 The answer is D

Transient global amnesia is an acute and *transient retrograde amnesia* that *affects recent, more than remote, memories*. Although patients are usually aware of the amnesia, they may still perform highly complex mental and physical acts during the *6 to 24 hours that transient global amnesia episodes usually last. Recovery from the disorder is usually complete.* Transient global amnesia is *most often caused by transient ischemic attacks* (TIAs) that affect limbic midline brain structures. It can also be associated with migraine headaches, seizures, and intoxication with sedative-hypnotic drugs.

22.3 The answer is A

On examination, *patients with dissociative identity disorder frequently show nothing unusual in their mental status*, other than a possible amnesia for periods of varying duration. Often, a clinician can detect the presence of multiple personalities only with prolonged interviews or many contacts with a patient with dissociative identity disorder. Sometimes, by having a patient keep a diary, the clinician finds the multiple personalities revealed in the diary entries. An estimated 60 percent of patients switch to alternate personalities only occasionally; another 20 percent of patients not only have rare episodes but also are adept at covering the switches.

22.4 The answer is B

The first stage in coercive processes has been likened to the *artificial creation of an identity crisis*, with the emergence of a *new pseudoidentity* that manifests characteristics of a dissociative state. Under circumstances of extreme and malignant dependency, overwhelming vulnerability, and danger to one's existence, individuals develop a state characterized by extreme idealization of their captors, with ensuing identification with the aggressor and externalization of their superego, regressive adaptation known as traumatic infantilism, paralysis of will, and a state of frozen fright. The coercive techniques that are typically used to induce such a state in the victim have been amply described and include isolation of the subject, degradation, control over all communications and basic daily functions, induction of fear and confusion, peer pressure, assignment of repetitive and monotonous routines, unpredictability of environmental supplies, renunciation of past relationships and values, and various deprivations. *Pain* is associated with torture, not brainwashing.

22.5 The answer is D

Losing time and memory gaps, including significant gaps in autobiographical memory, are typical symptoms of *dissociative identity disorder*. Patients also report fluctuations in their skills, well-learned abilities, and habits. The transition from one personality to another is often sudden and dramatic. During each personality state, patients generally are amnestic about other states and the events that took place when another personality was dominant. In classic cases, each personality has a fully integrated, highly complex set of associated memories and characteristic attitudes, personal relationships, and behavior patterns. Despite stories in the popular press about patients with more than 20 personalities, the median number of personalities in dissociative identity disorder is in the range of 5 to 10. *Dissociative amnesia* is the appropriate diagnosis when the dissociative phenomena are limited to amnesia. Its key symptom is the inability to recall information, usually about stressful or traumatic events in persons' lives.

22.6 The answer is C

The behavior of patients with dissociative fugue is unusual and dramatic. The term fugue is used to reflect the fact that patients physically travel away from their customary homes or work situations and fail to remember important aspects of their previous identities (name, family, occupation). Such patients often, but not always, take on an entirely new identity and occupation, although *the new identity is usually less complete than the alternate personalities in dissociative identity disorder*, and the *old and new identities do not alternate*, as they do in dissociate identity disorder. Dissociative fugue is rare and, like dissociative amnesia, *occurs most often during wartime, after natural disasters*, and as a result of personal crises with intense internal conflicts. According to DSM-IV-TR there is a prevalence rate of 0.2 percent in the general population. Although *heavy alcohol abuse may predispose persons to dissociative fugue, the cause of the disorder is thought to be basically psychological*. The essential motivating factor seems to be a desire to withdraw from emotionally painful experiences.

22.7 The answer is E (none)

The symptom of amnesia is common to dissociative amnesia, dissociative fugue, and dissociative identity disorder. Dissociative amnesia is the appropriate diagnosis when the dissociative phenomena are limited to amnesia. Its key symptom is the inability to recall information, usually about stressful or traumatic events in people's lives. This inability cannot be explained by ordinary forgetfulness, and there is no evidence of an underlying brain disorder. People retain the *capacity to learn new information.*

A common form of dissociative amnesia involves *amnesia for personal identity*, but *unimpaired memory of general information.* This *clinical picture is exactly the reverse of the one seen in dementia,* in which patients may remember their names but forget general information, such as what they had for lunch. Except for their amnesia, patients with dissociative amnesia appear completely intact and *function coherently.* By contrast, in most amnesias due to a general medical condition (such as postictal and toxic amnesias), patients may be confused and behave in a disorganized manner. Other types of amnesias (for example, transient global amnesia and post-concussion amnesia) are associated with an ongoing anterograde amnesia, which does not occur in patients with dissociative amnesia.

22.8 The answer is B

Amnesia is the most common dissociative symptom and occurs in almost all the dissociative disorders. Dissociative amnesia is thought to be the *most common of the dissociative disorders,* although epidemiological data for all the dissociative disorders are limited and uncertain. Dissociative amnesia is thought to occur *more often in women than in men* and *more often in young adults than in older adults.* Inasmuch as the disorder is usually associated with stressful and traumatic events, its incidence probably *increases during times of wars and natural disasters.* Cases of dissociative amnesia related to domestic settings—for example, spouse abuse and child abuse—are probably constant in number.

22.9 The answer is E (all)

Amnestic disorders are caused by a variety of organic conditions. Examples of organic causes of amnesia are epileptic seizure, head trauma, alcoholic blackouts, Korsakoff's syndrome, stroke, postoperative amnesia, postinfectious amnesia, post-ECT, surgery, infection and transient global amnesia. Less common causes are cerebrovascular disease, metabolic abnormalities, and toxic states.

Organic amnesias have several distinguishing features: they *do not normally involve recurrent identity alteration,* the amnesia is *not selectively limited to personal information,* the memories *do not focus on or result from an emotionally traumatic event,* and the amnesia *is more often anterograde* than retrograde. In cases of amnesia of organic etiology (excluding substance abuse, transient global amnesia, or metabolic abnormalities), the amnesia is usually permanent and does not lend itself to therapeutic technique. Whereas dissociative amnesia represents a displacement of the memory from awareness, organic amnesias represent the erasure or destruction of that memory through disturbance of the neuropsychological process.

22.10 The answer is D

DSM-IV-TR does not include dissociative symptoms in the criteria for *obsessive-compulsive disorder. Acute stress disorder, somatization disorder,* and *posttraumatic stress disorder* all include dissociative symptoms in their criteria as given in DSM-IV-TR. A diagnosis of dissociative disorder is not given if the symptoms occur exclusively during the course of one of these disorders. DSM-IV-TR notes that neurological or other medical conditions should be considered before diagnosing conversion disorder.

22.11 The answer is B

Depersonalization disorder is characterized by *ego-dystonic symptoms*—that is, symptoms distressing to the patient. However, the person maintains *intact (not impaired) reality testing;* he or she is aware of the disturbances. Depersonalization *rarely occurs in the late decades of life;* it most often starts between the ages of 15 and 30 years. In the large majority of patients, the symptoms first appear suddenly; only a few patients report a *gradual onset.* A few follow-up studies indicate that in more than half the cases, depersonalization disorder tends to have *a long-term (not brief) course and a poor (not good) prognosis.*

22.12 The answer is D

A dissociative fugue is *usually brief (not long-lasting)* (i.e., hours to days). Generally, *recovery is spontaneous and rapid,* and recurrences are rare. Dissociative fugue is considered *rare*, and like dissociative amnesia, it occurs most often during wartime, after natural disasters, and as a result of personal crises with intense conflict. Dissociative fugue is characterized by a *lack of awareness of the loss of memory* but *not by behavior that appears extraordinary* to others.

22.13 The answer is C

The differential diagnosis of fugue states is vast. Genuine dissociative fugue must be excluded as a diagnosis if dissociative identity disorder is present or if the fugue is caused by the direct physiological effects of drugs, medications, or alcohol; it cannot be diagnosed if it is due to a general medical condition such as epilepsy.

Probably the most common organic fugue is secondary to *epilepsy,* especially complex partial seizure disorder. During such seizures or postictally the individual may exhibit wandering behaviors. The clinical differentiation is usually fairly easily accomplished by a good clinical history regarding epileptic symptoms and electroencephalographic studies.

Several medical conditions besides epilepsy can cause organic fugue. These conditions include *brain tumor*, *head trauma*, *migraine*, cerebrovascular accidents, hypertensive neuropathy, limbic system dysfunction, *hypoglycemia*, uremia, dementia, and malaria.

Organic fugue states may be caused by a wide variety of medications including hallucinogenic drugs, steroids, barbiturates, phenothiazines, triazolam (Halcion), and L-asparaginase. The alcohol blackout can be easily confused with dissociative fugue, but this can be differentiated through a good clinical history and alcohol concentrations, if drawn during acute intoxication. The clinician should remember, however, that dissociative fugue and alcohol blackouts may coexist in the same individual.

22.14 The answer is E (all)

There are a number of culture-bound psychiatric syndromes in which fugue is a prominent feature. These syndromes include the "running" syndromes, which include *latah* and *amok*, that occur in several nations along the western Pacific rim; *grisi siknis,* occurring among the Miskito of Nicaragua and Honduras; and *piblokto* (Arctic hysteria), occurring among the Eskimos of northern Greenland. These syndromes are characterized by a high level of agitation, running about, trance-like states, and amnesia for the episode.

22.15 The answer is A

The mainstay of treatment of dissociative fugue is *psychodynamic psychotherapy.* A gently exploratory and expressive form is preferred in most cases, although a largely supportive form will usually suffice for those of low ego strength. The clinician should begin with a thorough clinical history and pay close attention to possible precipitating events. In many cases, encouraging persons with dissociative fugue to talk about what they already remember will bring the return of other memories; in some cases free association has proven helpful.

In situations where acute traumatic events have precipitated the dissociative fugue, a gentle abreaction of the trauma is indicated. However, the clinician should be very careful to not proceed with abreactive work until a stable therapeutic alliance has been established. In addition, abreactive work should be suspended, at least temporarily, if the patient's condition worsens (e.g., if the patient becomes depressed or suicidal).

If the individual with dissociative fugue continues to be densely amnesic for identity and autobiographical memory, the use of *hypnosis* or *sodium amobarbital interviewing* may be tried cautiously, keeping in mind that the dissociative fugue serves a defensive purpose, and that if the amnesia is suddenly lifted the individual may become depressed or even suicidal. Also, after the hypnotic session is completed, the amnesia may recur. Informed consent should be obtained whenever hypnosis or sodium amobarbital is used.

After the amnesia has been lifted, continued psychotherapy is indicated to help the individual cope with the underlying psychological conflicts that initially caused the dissociative fugue. Ideally, the patient should be helped to integrate the memories of the dissociative fugue state into a cohesive self and memory. *Antidepressant medication* may be helpful in the treatment of depressive symptoms that may accompany the fugue state.

22.16 The answer is E

Patients with *sleepwalking disorder*, classified in DSM-IV-TR as a type of sleep disorder, often behave like someone in a dissociative state. They appear out of touch with their environment and preoccupied with a private world; they may act emotionally upset and speak excitedly and incomprehensibly. When the episode has ended, patients have amnesia for it. By contrast, patients with *localized* or *generalized amnesia* do not seem out of touch with the environment and do not appear to be dreaming; to observers, they seem to act normally and are alert both before and after amnesia appears.

Dissociative fugue is similar to dissociative amnesia, but in dissociative fugue patients' behavior seems more integrated with their amnesia than it is for patients with dissociative amnesia.

Patients with dissociative fugue travel away from home or work and forget their name, occupation, and other aspects of their identity. Patients often take on a new identity and profession.

When patients with *dementia* have symptoms of amnesia, the dementia is often advanced, and the amnesia does not give way to a clear memory. Social awareness and ability to perform complex activities are also diminished, and personality is affected.

22.17 The answer is B

Schizophrenia does not predispose patients to dissociative fugue state. *Heavy alcohol abuse* may predispose a person to dissociative fugue, but the cause is thought to be basically psychological.

The essential motivating factor appears to be a desire to withdraw from emotionally painful experiences. Patients with *mood disorders* and certain personality disorders (for example, *borderline,* schizoid, and *histrionic personality disorders*) are predisposed to dissociative fugue.

22.18 The answer is A

In dissociative identity disorder, while *recovery is possible*, it is *generally incomplete.* This is considered the most severe and chronic of the dissociative disorders. The earlier the onset of dissociative identity disorder, *the poorer the prognosis is*. The *level of impairment* ranges from moderate to severe and is determined by variables such as the number, the type, and the chronicity of the various personalities.The *individual personalities* may have their own separate mental disorders; mood disorders, personality disorders, and other distinctive disorders are most common. One or more of the *personalities may function relatively well,* while others function marginally.

Answers 22.19–22.22

22.19 The answer is A

22.20 The answer is B

22.21 The answer is B

22.22 The answer is A

Dissociative amnesia is more likely to involve *interruption of the episodic-autobiographical memory* than the implicit-semantic memory. The memories unavailable for recall tend toward historical factual information (i.e., where was I; who was I with; and what did I do, think, and feel during the unaccountable period of time?) rather than *interruption of general cognitive functioning* or *language capacity.* This period of amnesia usually centers around a traumatic event or series of events and is *usually localized*, occurring during a specific period of time lasting anywhere from a few hours to several years. Occasionally the amnesia may be selective or systematized, whereby it is restricted to certain memories such as those involving a particular individual. Other forms of amnesia also occur (generalized amnesia, when the amnesia extends over the patient's entire life, and continuous amnesia, when the amnesia extends from a specific time up to the present), but are much more rare and are often associated with more severe dissociative disorders.

Dissociative amnesia is one of the most difficult disorders to assess because it cannot be observed directly except in cases of global amnesia; patients rarely complain about amnesia itself. Clinically, the patient may present symptoms of anxiety, depression, confusion, difficulty concentrating, and a history of blank spells or gaps in memory. Even once amnesia is confirmed, clinicians typically find it difficult to obtain from patients reliable estimates of the frequency and extent of their amnestic episodes.

Answers 22.23–22.26

22.23 The answer is A

22.24 The answer is D

22.25 The answer is B

22.26 The answer is C

Dissociative amnesia, as in the case of the man who *cannot remember his name*, is characterized by inability to remember information, usually related to a stressful or traumatic event, which cannot be explained by ordinary forgetfulness, the ingestion of substances, or a general medical condition. *Dissociative fugue*, as in the case of the girl who is *found in another city* far from her home, is characterized by sudden and unexpected travel away from home or work, associated with an inability to recall one's past, confusion about one's past, and confusion about one's personal identity or the adoption of a new identity. *Dissociative identity disorder*, as in the case of the woman who suddenly has *a new child-like voice* in the interview, is characterized by the presence of two or more distinct personalities within a single person; dissociative identity disorder is generally considered the most severe and chronic of the dissociative disorders. *Depersonalization disorder*, as in the case of the man who states that *his body feels unreal*, is characterized by recurrent or persistent feelings of detachment from one's body or mind.

23 Human Sexuality

Sexuality is determined by anatomy, physiology, psychology, the culture in which one lives, one's relationship with others, and developmental experiences throughout the life cycle. It includes the perception of being male or female and all those thoughts, feelings, and behaviors connected with sexual gratification and reproduction, including the attraction of one person to another.

Abnormal sexuality is defined as that which is destructive, compulsive, associated with overwhelming guilt and anxiety, unable to be directed toward a partner, and is generally pervasive, recurrent, and habitual. The revised fourth edition of the *Diagnostic and Statistical Manual of Mental Disorders* (DSM-IV-TR) broadly classifies sexual disorders as sexual dysfunctions, paraphilias, and sexual disorder not otherwise specified. There is also a classification for gender identity disorders, and this will be discussed in Chapter 24.

Sexual dysfunctions describe disturbed sexual desire and psychophysiologic changes in the sexual response cycle. Paraphilias are characterized by recurrent sexual urges or fantasies involving unusual objects, activities, or situations. Sexual disorder not otherwise specified describes sexual dysfunction not classifiable in any other category.

There are several terms related to human sexuality that are often misunderstood and misused. Sexual identity is a person's biological sexual characteristics, including genes, external and internal sexual organs, hormonal makeup, and secondary sex characteristics. Gender identity is a person's sense of being female or male. Sexual orientation describes the object of a person's sexual impulses: heterosexual, homosexual, or bisexual. Sexual behavior is the physiological experience triggered by psychological and physical stimuli.

Clinicians should be familiar with the sexual disorders as well as with the variety of treatments available to address these disorders. Students should study the following questions and answers related to the topic for a helpful review.

HELPFUL HINTS

The student should know the following terms and their definitions.

- anorgasmia
- autoerotic asphyxiation
- biogenic versus psychogenic
- bisexuality
- castration
- chronic pelvic pain
- clitoral versus vaginal orgasm
- coming out
- coprophilia
- cystometric examination
- desensitization therapy
- Don Juanism
- dual-sex therapy
- dyspareunia
- erection and ejaculation
- excitement
- exhibitionism
- female orgasmic disorder
- female sexual arousal disorder
- fetishism
- frotteurism
- FSH
- gender role
- heterosexuality
- HIV, AIDS
- homophobia
- homosexuality
- hymenectomy
- hypoactive sexual desire disorder
- hypoxyphilia
- incest
- infertility
- intersexual disorders
- intimacy
- Alfred Kinsey
- libido
- male erectile disorder
- male orgasmic disorder
- William Masters and Virginia Johnson
- masturbation
- moral masochism
- necrophilia
- nocturnal penile tumescence
- orgasm
- orgasm disorders
- orgasmic anhedonia
- paraphilias
- penile arteriography
- Peyronie's disease
- phases of sexual response
- postcoital dysphoria
- postcoital headache
- premature ejaculation
- prenatal androgens
- prosthetic devices
- psychosexual stages
- rape (male and female)
- refractory period
- resolution
- retarded ejaculation
- retrograde ejaculation
- satyriasis
- scatologia
- sensate focus
- sex addiction
- sexual arousal disorders
- sexual aversion disorder
- sexual desire disorders
- sexual dysfunction not otherwise specified
- sexual identity and gender identity
- sexual masochism and sexual sadism
- sexual orientation distress
- sexual pain disorders

- spectatoring
- spouse abuse
- squeeze technique
- statutory rape
- steal phenomenon
- sterilization
- stop–start technique
- sympathetic and parasympathetic nervous systems
- telephone scatologia
- transvestic fetishism
- tumescence and detumescence
- unconsummated marriage
- urophilia
- vagina dentata
- vaginismus
- vaginoplasty
- voyeurism
- zoophilia

QUESTIONS

Directions

Each of the questions or incomplete statements below is followed by five suggested responses or completions. Select the *one* that is *best* in each case.

23.1 Sexuality depends on which of the following psychosexual factors?

A. Sexual Identity
B. Gender Identity
C. Sexual orientation
D. Sexual behavior
E. All of the above

23.2 With regard to innervation of sex organs, all of the following are true *except*

A. Penile tumescence occurs through the synergistic activity of parasympathetic and sympathetic pathways.
B. Clitoral engorgement results from parasympathetic stimulation.
C. Vaginal lubrication results from sympathetic stimulation.
D. Sympathetic innervation is responsible for ejaculation.
E. Sympathetic innervation facilitates the smooth muscle contraction of the vagina, urethra, and uterus during orgasm.

23.3 *Primal scene* is a term used by Freud which described

A. a person's first coitus
B. genital self-stimulation in children under 24 months old
C. sexual learning adversely affected by abusive adults
D. a child seeing sex between their parents
E. None of the above

23.4 Among the following, the sexual dysfunction *not* correlated with phases of the sexual response cycle is

A. sexual aversion disorder
B. vaginismus
C. premature ejaculation
D. post-coital dysphoria
E. male erectile disorder

23.5 Paraphilias

A. are usually not distressing to the person with the disorder
B. are found equally among men and women
C. according to the classic psychoanalytic model, are due to a failure to complete the process of genital adjustment
D. with an early age of onset are associated with a good prognosis
E. such as pedophilia usually involve vaginal or anal penetration of the victim

23.6 When compared to children of heterosexual parents, children of gay and lesbian parents

A. have significantly different outcomes in gender identity
B. have significantly different outcomes in gender role
C. have significantly different outcomes in sexual orientation
D. may have to struggle with their difference from heterosexual families
E. all of the above

23.7 Mr. C a 35-year-old man, is referred from prison for a psychiatric evaluation because of exposing his genitals and masturbating in front of female corrections officers. He has been arrested for public masturbation and as a repeat offender is being held in jail prior to his first court hearing. He acknowledges the behavior and explains that he thought it would be sexually exciting to the officers and that they might want to have sex with him.

As an adolescent, Mr. C had numerous sexual encounters with other adolescents, with prepubertal children, and with adults of both sexes. He began going to pornographic movie theaters in his late teens, where he would always masturbate and, on occasion, have an anonymous sexual encounter with a stranger. During his 20s, he began masturbating in public with the belief that it would lead to sex with strangers. However, on those rare occasions when his exposure did lead to a proposition for sexual favors, he became frightened and ran away. He discovered that squeezing the urethra at the head of his penis would help delay orgasm, and he used the technique to prolong masturbation. When he learned (erroneously) that this would cause retrograde ejaculation into the bladder, he began to eat his own semen and drink his urine, variously describing the reasons for so doing as "saving sperm" or "as a perfect source of protein." He acknowledged that the practice does not literally save sperm and that most people would think it bizarre.

Mr. C had two psychiatric hospitalizations 8 and 12 years ago, each for hallucinations and paranoid delusions in the context of crack cocaine use. He insists that he has never had hallucinations when he was not using cocaine. He has used no illicit drugs for the past 5 years, but he drinks one or two beers each night and once or twice a month he will drink to the point of being unsteady on his feet and slurring his words. He has five prior arrests for public indecency but until now has never served time in jail. Mr. C has never married and denies ever having had a long-term romantic relationship. He graduated from high school and works the late-night shift at a local convenience store.

Which of the following is the most likely Axis I diagnosis?

A. Social phobia
B. Exhibitionism
C. Schizophrenia
D. Obsessive-compulsive disorder
E. Sexual aversion disorder

23.8 In the case described above, which of the following is the most likely Axis II diagnosis?

A. Antisocial personality disorder
B. Borderline personality disorder
C. Obsessive-compulsive personality disorder
D. Histrionic personality disorder
E. Schizotypal personality disorder

23.9 In the case described above, without treatment, which of the following is the most likely long-term course for Mr. C's Axis I condition?

A. Gradual decrease in symptomatic behavior
B. Progressive functional deterioration
C. Development of a recurrent psychotic disorder
D. Progression to pedophilia
E. Progressive cognitive deterioration

23.10 Which of the following statements about fetishism is *false*?

A. A fetish is an inanimate object that is used as the preferred or necessary adjunct to sexual arousal.
B. A fetish may be integrated into sexual activity with a human partner.
C. A fetish is a device that may function as a hedge against separation anxiety.
D. A fetish is a device that may function to ward off castration anxiety.
E. Fetishism is a disorder found equally in males and females.

23.11 Research has indicated that

A. a majority of married people are unfaithful to their spouses
B. the median number of sexual partners over a lifetime for men is six and for women two
C. vaginal intercourse is considered the most appealing type of sexual experience by a large majority of men and women
D. masturbation is more common among those 18 to 24 than among those 24 to 34 years old
E. the percentage of single women reporting "usually or always" having an orgasm during intercourse is greater than the percentage of married women reporting this

23.12 Measures used to help differentiate organically caused impotence from functional impotence include

A. monitoring of nocturnal penile tumescence
B. glucose tolerance tests
C. follicle-stimulating hormone (FSH) determinations
D. testosterone level tests
E. all of the above

23.13 Psychiatric interventions used to assist the paraphilia patient include

A. dynamic psychotherapy
B. external control
C. cognitive-behavioral therapy
D. treatment of comorbid conditions
E. all of the above

23.14 Which of the following substances has *not* been associated with sexual dysfunction?

A. cocaine
B. trazodone
C. amoxapine
D. antihistamines
E. all of the above

23.15 In the most severe forms of paraphilia

A. persons never experience any sexual behavior with partners
B. the specific paraphilia imagery or activity is absolutely necessary for any sexual function
C. the need for sexual behavior consumes so much money, time, concentration, and energy that the person describes self as out of control
D. orgasm does not produce satiety in the same way it typically does for age mates
E. all of the above

23.16 Which of the following conditions is classified as a psychological or behavioral disorder associated with sexual development or orientation?

A. fetishism
B. voyeurism
C. frotteurism
D. necrophilia
E. transsexualism

23.17 Premature ejaculation

A. is less common among college-educated men than among men with less education

B. is mediated via the sympathetic nervous system
C. is strongly influenced by the sex partner in an ongoing relationship
D. is defined within a specific time frame
E. all of the above

23.18 True statements about what research has shown about gay men and lesbians include

A. A majority of lesbians and gay men report being in a committed romantic relationship.
B. Lesbian couples tend more frequently to be sexually exclusive than male couples.
C. Gay men and lesbians, in comparison with heterosexual couples, generally have more equality in their relationships.
D. Gay men and lesbians report the same degree of global satisfaction in their relationships as heterosexual men and women.
E. All of the above

Directions

Each set of lettered headings below is followed by a list of numbered words or statements. For each numbered word or statement, select the *one* lettered heading most closely associated with it. Each lettered heading may be selected once, more than once, or not at all.

Questions 23.19–23.23

A. Vaginismus
B. Sexual aversion disorder
C. Anorgasmia
D. Hypoactive sexual desire disorder
E. Dyspareunia

23.19 Avoidance of genital sexual contact with a sexual partner
23.20 Patient has few or no sexual thoughts or fantasies
23.21 Recurrent and persistent inhibition of female orgasm
23.22 Recurrent pain during intercourse
23.23 Involuntary and persistent constrictions of the outer one-third of the vagina

Questions 23.24–23.26

A. Fetishism
B. Voyeurism
C. Frotteurism
D. Exhibitionism
E. Sexual masochism
F. Sexual sadism
G. Transvestic fetishism

23.24 Rubbing up against a fully clothed woman to achieve orgasm
23.25 Sexual urges by heterosexual men to dress in female clothes for purposes of arousal
23.26 Preoccupation with fantasies and acts that involve observing people who are naked or engaging in sexual activity.

Questions 23.27–23.29

A. Sensate focus exercises
B. Squeeze technique

23.27 Intercourse is interdicted initially
23.28 Raises the threshold of penile excitability
23.29 Attempts to decrease "spectatoring"

Questions 23.30–23.34

A. Desire phase
B. Excitement phase
C. Orgasm phase
D. Resolution phase

23.30 Vaginal lubrication
23.31 Orgasmic platform
23.32 Testes increase in size by 50 percent
23.33 Slight clouding of consciousness
23.34 Detumescence

Questions 23.35–23.39

A. Sexual identity
B. Gender identity
C. Sexual orientation
D. Sexual behavior

23.35 Sense of maleness or femaleness
23.36 The object of a person's sexual impulses
23.37 Chromosomes
23.38 Gonads and secondary sex characteristics
23.39 Desire and fantasies

Questions 23.40–23.46

A. Virilizing adrenal hyperplasia (adreno-genital syndrome)
B. Turner's syndrome
C. Klinefelter's syndrome
D. Androgen insensitivity syndrome (testicular-feminizing syndrome)
E. Enzymatic defects in XY genotype (e.g., 5-α-redyctase deficiency, 17-hydroxy-steroid deficiency)
F. Hermaphroditism
G. Pseudohermaphroditism

23.40 Interruption in production of testosterone
23.41 Genotype is XXY
23.42 Assigned as males or females, depending on morphology of genitals
23.43 Excess androgens in fetus with XX genotype
23.44 Absence of second female sex chromosome (XO)
23.45 Inability of tissues to respond to androgens
23.46 Both testes and ovaries

ANSWERS

23.1 The answer is E (all)

Sexuality depends on four interrelated psychosexual factors: sexual identity, gender identity, sexual orientation, and sexual behavior. These factors affect personality, development, and functioning.

Sexual identity is the pattern of a person's biological sexual characteristics: chromosomes, external and internal genitalia, hormonal composition, gonads, and secondary sex characteristics. In normal development, these characteristics form a cohesive pattern that leaves individuals in no doubt about their sex.

Gender identity is an individual's sense of maleness or femaleness. By the age of 2 or 3 years, almost everyone has a firm conviction that "I am a boy" or "I am a girl." Gender identity results from an almost infinite series of clues derived from experiences with family members, peers, and teachers, and from cultural phenomena. For instance, male infants tend to be handled more vigorously and female infants tend to be cuddled more. Fathers spend more time with their infant sons than with their daughters, and they also tend to be more aware of their sons' adolescent concerns than of their daughters' anxieties. Boys are more likely to be physically disciplined than girls are. A child's sex affects parental tolerance for aggression and reinforcement or extinction of activity and of intellectual, aesthetic, and athletic interests. Physical characteristics derived from a person's biological sex (e.g., physique, body shape, and physical dimensions) interrelate with an intricate system of stimuli, including rewards, punishment, and parental gender labels, to establish gender goals. Recent studies of children with intersex conditions have drawn attention to a physiological basis for gender identity. In particular, they have focused on the masculinization or feminization of the fetal brain.

Sexual orientation describes the object of a person's sexual impulses: heterosexual (opposite sex), homosexual (same sex), or bisexual (both sexes). The overwhelming majority of people have a heterosexual orientation. In the United States, 2.8 percent of men and 1.4 percent of women identify themselves as homosexual. These numbers are compatible with figures from Western European countries as well. However, a higher percentage of persons have had at least one same-sex experience in their lives. Additionally, homosexuals congregate in urban areas, so the incidence of homosexuality in some large cities is as high as 8 or 9 percent.

Sexual behavior includes desire, fantasies, pursuit of partners, autoeroticism, and all the activities engaged in to express and gratify sexual needs. It is an amalgam of psychological and physiological responses to internal and external stimuli.

23.2 The answer is C

Innervation of the sexual organs is mediated primarily through the autonomic nervous system (ANS). *Penile tumescence* occurs through the synergistic activity of two neurophysiologic pathways. A parasympathetic (cholinergic) component mediates reflexogenic erections via impulses that pass through the pelvic splanchnic nerves (S2, S3, and S4). A thoracolumbar, pathway transmits psychologically induced impulses. Both parasympathetic and sympathetic mechanisms are thought to play a part in relaxing the smooth muscles of the penile corpora cavernosa, which allow the penile arteries to dilate and cause the inflow of blood that results in penile erection. Relaxation of cavernosal smooth muscles is aided by the release of nitric oxide, an endothelium-derived relaxing factor. *Clitoral engorgement* and *vaginal lubrication* also result from parasympathetic stimulation that increases blood flow to genital tissue. Adrian Zorgniotti has compared the erection phenomenon that results from increased penile blood inflow and decreased blood outflow with the inflation of an automobile tire, which requires an inflow of air and an intact casing.

Evidence indicates that the sympathetic (adrenergic) system is responsible for *ejaculation*. Through its hypogastric plexus the adrenergic impulses innervate the urethral crest, the muscles of the epididymis, and the muscles of the vas deferens, seminal vesicles, and prostate. Stimulation of the plexus causes emission. In women, the sympathetic system facilitates the *smooth muscle contraction* of the vagina, urethra, and uterus that occurs during orgasm.

The ANS functions outside of voluntary control and is influenced by external events (e.g., stress, drugs) and internal events (hypothalamic, limbic, and cortical stimuli). It is not surprising, therefore, that erection and orgasm are so vulnerable to dysfunction.

23.3 The answer is D

Children who view the *primal scene*—the term Freud used to *describe a child seeing sex between their parents*—may be traumatized. This is particularly the case if they interpret coital sounds and movements as a physical aggression between the parents.

Genital self-stimulation is a normal activity of babies. It is particularly pronounced between the ages of 15 and 19 months, and it is part of the general interest of children in their bodies. The activity is reinforced by the pleasurable sensations it produces. As youngsters acquire playmates, curiosity about their own and others' genitalia motivates episodes of exhibitionism or genital exploration.

Sexual learning in childhood is *adversely affected by exploitative, abusive adults*. Incestuous activity, with or without penetration, or sexual abuse by other adults (babysitter, other older relatives, teachers, coaches, etc.) is damaging to the child. It may precipitate sexual dysfunction in adult life, as well as promiscuity and problems with intimacy. It may produce delinquent activities and behavioral problems in adolescence, as well as learning problems in school.

23.4 The answer is B

Seven major categories of sexual dysfunction are listed in DSM-IV-TR: (1) sexual desire disorders, (2) sexual arousal disorders, (3) orgasm disorders, (4) sexual pain disorders, (5) sexual dysfunction due to a general medical condition, (6) substance-induced sexual dysfunction, and (7) sexual dysfunction not otherwise specified.

In DSM-IV-TR sexual dysfunctions are categorized as Axis I disorders. All of the syndromes listed except *vaginismus*, including *sexual aversion disorder*, *premature ejaculation*, *post-coital dysphoria*, and *male erectile disorder*, are correlated with the sexual physiological response cycle, which is divided into four phases: desire, excitement, orgasm, and resolution. The essential feature of the sexual dysfunctions is inhibition in one or more of the phases, including disturbance in the subjective sense of pleasure or desire, or disturbance in the objective performance.

Either type of disturbance can occur alone or in combination. Sexual dysfunctions are diagnosed only when they are a major part of the clinical picture. They can be lifelong or acquired, generalized or situational, and can be due to psychological factors, physiological factors, or combined factors. If they are attributable entirely to a general medical condition, substance use, or adverse effects of medication, then sexual dysfunction due to a general medical condition or substance-induced sexual dysfunction is diagnosed.

Vaginismus is an involuntary muscle constriction of the outer third of the vagina that interferes with penile insertion and intercourse. It can also occur during a gynecological exam. It is not correlated with phases of the sexual response cycle.

23.5 The answer is C

Paraphilias, *according to the classic psychoanalytic model*, are due to a failure to complete the process of genital adjustment. However bizarre its manifestation, the paraphilia provides an outlet for the sexual and aggressive drives that would otherwise have been channeled into proper sexual behavior. Paraphilias are *usually distressing* to the person with the disorder. Paraphilias are *not found equally among men and women.* As usually defined, paraphilias seem to be largely male conditions. Paraphilias with an *early age of onset* are associated with a poor prognosis, as are paraphilias with a high frequency of the acts (Table 23.1), no guilt or shame about the acts, and substance abuse. Paraphilias such as *pedophilia* usually do not involve vaginal or anal penetration of the victim. The majority of child molestations involve genital fondling or oral sex.

23.6 The answer is D

Many lesbians and gay men have had children, historically most often within heterosexual marriages and more recently through other avenues as well, including adoption, artificial insemination, and co-parenting arrangements outside of marriage. Numerous studies since the late 1970s have demonstrated the characteristics of gay and lesbian families and the impact of having a gay or lesbian parent on children. A significant change in recent years has been the greater visibility of families with gay and lesbian parents and the increased viability for gay men and lesbians to be involved in childrearing.

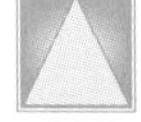

Table 23.1
Frequency of Paraphiliac Acts Committed by Paraphilia Patients Seeking Outpatient Treatment

Diagnostic Category	Paraphilia Patients Seeking Outpatient Treatment (%)	Paraphiliac Acts per Paraphilia Patient[a]
Pedophilia	45	5
Exhibitionism	25	50
Voyeurism	12	17
Frotteurism	6	30
Sexual masochism	3	36
Transvestic fetishism	3	25
Sexual sadism	3	3
Fetishism	2	3
Zoophilia	1	2

[a]Median number.
Courtesy of Gene G. Abel, M.D.

Research on gay and lesbian families was initially undertaken to disprove psychological and judicial assumptions about the harm that might be done to children raised by gay and lesbian parents. The findings resulting from such research have confirmed that lesbian and gay parents neither affect their children in a negative way psychologically nor produce *significantly different outcomes* in the *gender identity*, *gender role*, or *sexual orientation* of their children when compared with the children of heterosexual parents. Children with gay and lesbian parents *may have to struggle with their difference from heterosexual families* and may have difficulty overcoming the possible stigma associated with this situation. The first era of research into the effects of gay and lesbian parents on their children has now yielded to a period of greater emphasis on understanding the dynamics of and determining the potential differences between families with heterosexual, gay, and lesbian parents. Future studies may involve greater methodological precision, focusing more on family process than on structure alone and allowing for improved understanding of differences between gay and lesbian families, derived from religion, age, class, race, and other characteristics, as well as sex and sexual orientation.

The emergence of families with openly gay, lesbian, and bisexual parents and children since the 1970s represents one of the most significant shifts in the structure of the family during the latter part of the 20th century. The psychiatrist must recognize and validate the importance of this phenomenon in the lives of millions of men, women, and children and not confound the clinical evaluation and approach to treatment of patients from these families with negative portrayals derived from political, religious, or psychological biases.

23.7 The answer is B

At first glance the diagnosis for Mr. C seems fairly straightforward. He has a long history of public exposure and masturbation that has continued despite repeated arrests and, astoundingly, even while he was in jail. The absence of any long-term romantic relationships adds to the impression that exposing himself and publicly masturbating is his preferred method of sexual expression, all of which leads to a diagnosis of *exhibitionism*, one of the sexual paraphilias. An intriguing question, however, is whether Mr. C also has an underlying psychotic disorder. He has been hospitalized twice in the past with hallucinations and delusions, but he insists that they occurred only when he used crack cocaine. The behavior of eating his own semen and drinking his urine is, as he recognizes, profoundly bizarre. It does not, however, seem to be driven by any delusional belief, and without further information, it is difficult to conclude that it is not just bizarre but psychotic. Because of impaired judgment and disinhibition, people with *schizophrenia* or other cognitive or psychotic disorders may have isolated episodes of unusual sexual behavior. Mr. C, however, has a pattern of numerous, repeated episodes of public exposure over many years, despite a number of arrests.

23.8 The answer is E

Because personality disorder diagnoses are intended to describe deeply ingrained, maladaptive fixed habits over an individual's lifetime, it is always difficult to make an Axis II diagnosis based on a short case history. Nevertheless the features attributed to Mr. C are most consistent with a diagnosis of *schizotypal personality disorder*, most remarkably his social isolation and his strange beliefs and behavior, which fall short of being psychotic. *Antisocial personality disorder* describes a broader pattern of systematically violating the rights of others than just repeated public exposure. *Borderline personality disorder* implies intense, chaotic relationships, not the absence of relationships. Individuals with the diagnosis of *histrionic personality disorder* often have a quality of promiscuous flirtatiousness but without the extraordinary lack of judgment, violation of the law, and compulsiveness described here.

23.9 The answer is B

There is no evidence that exhibitionism progresses to another paraphilia or other Axis I disorder. However, a poor prognosis is associated with an earlier age of onset, a high frequency of acts, no guilt or shame, substance abuse, a lack of a history of coitus, and referral from a legal authority, all present in this case.

23.10 The answer is E

Fetishism is a disorder *found almost exclusively in males*. The essential feature of a fetish is a nonliving object that is used as the preferred or necessary *adjunct to sexual arousal*. Sexual activity may involve the fetish alone, or the fetish may be *integrated into sexual activities with a human partner.* In the absence of the fetish, the male may be impotent. According to psychoanalytic theory, the fetish may function as *a hedge against separation anxiety* from the love object and may be *used to ward off castration anxiety.*

23.11 The answer is C

A 1994 study, which was based on a representative United States population between the ages of 18 and 59, found the following:

1. Eighty-five percent of married women and 75 percent of married men are *faithful to their spouses*.
2. Forty-one percent of married couples have sex twice a week or more, compared with 23 percent of single persons.
3. Cohabiting single persons have the most sex of all, twice a week or more.
4. The median *number of sexual partners* over a lifetime for men is 12 (not six) and for women, six (not two).
5. A homosexual orientation was reported by 2.8 percent of men and 1.4 percent of women, with 9 percent of men and 5 percent of women reporting that they had at least one homosexual experience after puberty.
6. *Vaginal intercourse* is considered the most appealing type of sexual experience by the majority of both men and women.
7. Among married partners, 93 percent are of the same race, 82 percent are of similar educational level, 78 percent are within 5 years of each other's age, and 72 percent are of the same religion.
8. Both men and women who as children had been sexually abused by an adult were more likely as adults to have had more than ten sex partners, to engage in group sex, to report a homosexual or bisexual identification, and to be unhappy.
9. Fewer than 8 percent of the participants reported having sex more than four times a week; about two-thirds said they had sex a few times a month or less, and about three in ten have sex a few times a year or less.
10. About one man in four and one woman in ten masturbates at least once a week, and *masturbation* is less common (not more common) among those 18 to 24 years of age than among those 24 to 34 years old.
11. Three-quarters of the married women said "they usually or always" had an *orgasm during sexual intercourse,* compared with 62 percent of the single women. Among men, married or single, 95 percent said they usually or always had an orgasm.
12. More than half of the men said that they thought about sex every day or several times a day, compared with only 19 percent of the women.

23.12 The answer is E (all)

A variety of measures is used to differentiate organically caused impotence from psychologically caused impotence. The *monitoring of nocturnal penile tumescence* is a noninvasive procedure; normally, erections occur during sleep and are associated with rapid eye movement (REM) sleep periods. Tumescence may be determined with a simple strain gauge. In most cases in which organic factors account for the impotence, the man has minimal or no nocturnal erections. Conversely, in most cases of psychologically caused or psychogenic impotence, erections do occur during REM sleep.

Other diagnostic tests that delineate organic bases of impotence include *glucose tolerance tests, follicle stimulating hormone (FSH) determinations,* and *testosterone level tests.* The glucose tolerance curve measures the metabolism of glucose over a specific period and is useful in diagnosing diabetes, of which impotence may be a symptom. FSH is a hormone produced by the anterior pituitary that stimulates the secretion of estrogen from the ovarian follicle in the female; it is also responsible for the production of sperm from the testes in men. An abnormal finding suggests an organic cause for impotence. Testosterone is the male hormone produced by the interstitial cells of the testes. In the male, a low testosterone level produces a lack of desire as the chief complaint, which may be associated with impotence. If the measure of nocturnal penile tumescence is abnormal, indicating the possibility of organic impotence, a measure of plasma testosterone is indicated.

23.13 The answer is E (all)

Five types of psychiatric interventions are used to assist the paraphilia patient to rebalance internal control mechanisms, cease victimization of others, and enhance the capacities to relate to others: *external control*, reduction of sexual drives, *treatment of comorbid conditions*, *cognitive-behavioral therapy*, and *dynamic psychotherapy*. The art of therapy is to select and modify these various elements for the individual patient.

When sexual victimization of others has occurred, new external controls should be instituted. Prison is an external control for sexual crimes that usually does not contain a treatment element. All relevant persons in the environment need to know what the person has done and is capable of doing again under opportune conditions. For intrafamilial abuse of children, for instance, the adults and other children in the family are informed of the abuse. The children in the family are not permitted to be alone with the offender again as long as they are unable to adequately protect themselves. With such controls implemented, those who victimize girls in their own home have recidivism rates of less than 5 percent. The more socially, economically, and psychologically disruptive alternative is to remove the offender from the home. When professionals who have sexually offended return to their work settings, external controls take the form of restricting access to potential victims and monitoring by administration, coworkers, and sometimes by patients with the use of exit questionnaires. Perpetrators and their professional colleagues can be educated about boundary crossings. When a therapist agrees to keep the knowledge of the patient's victimizing sexual patterns from family members, administrators, or colleagues on the basis of confidentiality, the single most effective psychiatric intervention is removed from the treatment plan. The therapist will probably be the last to know of the resumption of victimizing behaviors.

Psychiatrists need to consider the role of inadequately treated comorbid states when planning to treat sexual compulsivity or impulsivity. Alcohol and substance abuse, major depressive disorder, grief, psychotic disorder, attention-deficit/hyperactivity disorder, bipolar II disorder, and others may be the cofactor that enables a compensated sexual pattern to deteriorate and come to clinical attention.

It is frequently observed that sex offenders lack the social skills necessary to live effectively and create nonproblematic sexual relationships. Correcting some of these deficits is a goal of most cognitive-behavioral treatment programs for sexually offending paraphiliac individuals. Each intervention is an aspect of a therapy approach that assumes that a paraphiliac lifestyle is learned and can be significantly modified. The specific techniques can be implemented in individual or group settings.

The nonviolent paraphilias and the paraphilia-related disorders are often treated with traditional individual or group therapies using a combination of supportive, growth-promoting tactics. Such therapies aim at creating an evolving hypothesis about the unique developmental origin of the patient's eroticism. The defensive function of the impulse to act out (the anxiety reduction function) is defined so that the person can deal directly with the unpleasant feelings that trigger the impulses. Hypotheses get more complex as more developmental details emerge. The vast majority of patients need many therapeutic opportunities to work through the paraphiliac defense so that they can simply feel and cope with their particular life issue. Dynamic psychotherapy approaches emphasize the importance of the trusting relationship with the therapist to enable the work to occur. Therapists often face a delicate situation because most paraphilia embodies the capacity to transform the pain of childhood misery—for instance, "Mother didn't love me" into the pleasure of sexual arousal—"I'll exhibit myself to a teenager." Although the patient may no longer want to act out sexually, his desire to avoid reexperiencing his painful past may be greater. When the therapist decides to assist the patient in working through some of his distressing memories, a great deal of support may be needed. Generally speaking, the more globally impaired the paraphiliac is, the less likely it is that he (or she) can be treated in a dynamic psychotherapy.

23.14 The answer is E (all)

Intoxication with *cocaine* and alcohol, among other substances, produces sexual dysfunction. Medications such as *antihistamines,* antidepressants, and antiepileptics, among others, can cause arousal and orgasmic disorders as well as decreased sexual interest. *Trazodone* is one of the substances associated with priapism, and *amoxapine* is associated with painful orgasm. Still other substances implicated in sexual dysfunction include antihypertensives, antiparkinsonian agents, anxiolytics, hypnotics, sedatives, amphetamines, and anabolic steroids.

23.15 The answer is E (all)

DSM-IV-TR recognizes the paraphilias as consisting of recurrent, intensely sexually arousing fantasies, sexual urges, or sexual behaviors that involve nonhuman objects, the suffering of the self or partner, or children, or nonconsenting persons. To qualify as a diagnosis, however, these patterns must have existed for at least 6 months and they have to cause clinically significant distress or impairment in social, occupational, or some other important area, such as sexual function.

DSM-IV-TR specifies nine paraphiliac diagnoses: exhibitionism or genital exposure; voyeurism or clandestine observation of another person's undressing, toileting, or sexual behavior; sadism or causing suffering during sexual behavior; masochism or being humiliated during sexual behavior; pedophilia or sexual behavior with prepubescent or peripubertal children; fetishism or use of nonliving objects for sexual behavior; frotteurism or rubbing against or touching a nonconsenting person; transvestic fetishism or use of clothing of the opposite sex for arousal; and paraphilia not otherwise specified for other observed atypical sexual patterns such as dressing in diapers, requiring a partner who has an amputated limb, and others.

All paraphilia behaviors are rehearsed repeatedly in fantasy; often these unusual fantasies have been present since childhood or puberty. Some persons with paraphilias *never experience any sexual behavior with partners.* The shame of the paraphilia interest and the fear of negative consequences may contribute to a lifelong avoidance of intimate contact. Sexual behaviors consist entirely of masturbation, often with magazine or Internet pictures and bulletin boards, videotapes, reading material, clothing, or mechanical props. People in this category are the most psychologically unprepared for sexual expression within an ordinary relationship.

In the most severe forms of paraphilia, the *specific paraphiliac imagery or activity is absolutely necessary* for any sexual function. Without it, the person is always sexually apathetic—there is no desire for sexual behavior with the partner, no sustainable arousal, or no orgasmic attainment. When embarrassment prevents the paraphiliac from sharing the secret, the relationship may never be consummated and the partner is either baffled or settles on a wrong explanation. If the paraphiliac is able to integrate the paraphiliac requirements into the lovemaking, either by engaging in the behavior or imagining it, sexual functioning may even be normal.

The final parameter of severity is the degree of drive to masturbate or act out the fantasy with a partner.

The most severe form of compulsivity is the loss of autonomy. The loss of autonomy has three characteristics: (1) the *need for sexual behavior* consumes so much money, time, concentration, and energy that the patient describes himself as out of control; (2) intrusive, unwanted paraphiliac thoughts prevent concentration on other life demands and are the source of anxiety; and (3) *orgasm does not produce satiety* in the way it typically does for age mates. Thus, a man may masturbate six times a day, visit a prostitute twice in a day, or spend hundreds of dollars on phone sex. Although such drivenness may exist for long periods of time and is presented to the clinician as uncontrollable, a careful history often reveals that both the thoughts and the behaviors can be interrupted by other life demands.

23.16 The answer is E

Transsexualism is described as a gender identity disorder that is characterized by a desire to live and be accepted as a member of the opposite sex, rather than a disorder of sexual preference. In transsexualism, a person feels uncomfortable about his or her own anatomic sex and often wishes to undergo treatments to change the body to the preferred sex.

The other choices refer to disorders of sexual preferences. *Fetishism* is a reliance on a nonliving object as a stimulus for sexual arousal and gratification. Many fetishes are extensions of the human body, such as shoes or articles of clothing; others have a particular texture, such as leather or plastic. When fetishes are used, they need not always be primary but may simply enhance sexual excitement.

In *voyeurism*, a person feels impelled to look at people engaging in sexual activity or other intimate behavior, such as undressing. *Frotteurism* is a desire to seek sexual stimulation by rubbing against people in crowded places, such as on a subway. *Necrophilia* refers to a desire to be near dead bodies or to have an impulse to have sex with a dead body.

23.17 The answer is C

In premature ejaculation, the man recurrently achieves orgasm and ejaculates before he wishes to do so. *There is no definite time frame within which to define the dysfunction.* The diagnosis is made when the man regularly ejaculates before or immediately after entering the vagina or following minimal sexual stimulation. The clinician should consider factors that affect duration of the excitement phase, such as age, novelty of the sexual partner, and the frequency and duration of coitus. Masters and Johnson conceptualized the disorder in terms of the couple and consider a man a premature ejaculator if he cannot control ejaculation long enough during intravaginal containment to satisfy his partner in at least half of their episodes of coitus. That definition assumes that the female partner is capable of an orgasmic response. As with other dysfunctions, the disturbance is diagnosed only if it is not caused exclusively by medical factors or is not symptomatic of any other Axis I syndrome.

Premature ejaculation is *more common (not less common) today among college-educated men* than among men with less education and is thought to be related to their concern for partner satisfaction. It is estimated that about 35 to 40 percent of men treated for sexual disorders have premature ejaculation as the chief complaint.

Difficulty in ejaculatory control may be associated with anxiety regarding the sex act. Ejaculation is *mediated by the parasympathetic (not the sympathetic) nervous system.* Other psychological factors that have been noted include sexual guilt, a history of parent–child conflict, interpersonal hypersensitivity, and perfectionism or unrealistic expectations about sexual performance.

Current research also suggests that a subgroup of premature ejaculators (particularly those with a lifelong history of the dysfunction) may be biologically predisposed to this problem. Some researchers believe that certain males are constitutionally more vulnerable to sympathetic stimulation, hence they ejaculate rapidly. Other workers have found a shorter bulbocavernosus reflex nerve latency time in men with lifelong premature ejaculation than in men who had acquired the dysfunction.

Premature ejaculation also may result from negative cultural conditioning. The man who has most of his early sexual contacts with prostitutes who demand that the sex act proceed quickly or in situations in which discovery would be embarrassing, such as in an apartment shared with roommates or in the parental home, may become conditioned to achieving orgasm rapidly. *In ongoing relationships* the partner has been found to have great influence on the premature ejaculator. A stressful marriage exacerbates the disorder.

23.18 The answer is E (all)

The majority of gay men and lesbians report *being in a committed romantic relationship*, with some surveys indicating that 45 to 80 percent of lesbians and 40 to 60 percent of gay men are currently in such relationships. From 8 to 14 percent of lesbian couples and from 18 to 25 percent of gay male couples report that they have lived together for more than 10 years. Although same-sex marriage is still legally prohibited in most states, many same-sex couples live in relationships that are as enduring and emotionally significant as any heterosexual relationship, in spite of discrimination against these relationships, the absence of rituals and laws that support them, and the denial of equal protection and benefits to these couples.

Findings from the limited but growing research on gay and lesbian couples reveal that *lesbian couples tend more frequently to be sexually exclusive* than male couples. In addition, *gay male and, particularly, lesbian couples*, in comparison with heterosexual couples, generally have *more equality in their relationships* and do not differentiate household functions according to gender-based categories of work. Gay men and lesbians report the *same degree of global satisfaction in their relationships* as heterosexual men and women. However, undoubtedly as a result of gender socialization, women tend to appraise the value of and rewards from their relationships more highly than men, but gay and heterosexual men and lesbian and heterosexual women describe similar levels of valuing and rewards.

Empirical research by David McWhirter and Andrew Mattison led to the description of six stages in the development of male–male relationships: blending, nesting, maintaining, building, releasing, and renewing. Each stage is marked by specific characteristics and a time span, although the stages may overlap and occur in a different sequence for some couples and the characteristics may appear in more than one stage. The relevance of this stage model for lesbians has not been determined, but some variation from the gay male experience should be expected.

Answers 23.19–23.23

23.19 The answer is B

23.20 The answer is D

23.21 The answer is C

23.22 The answer is E

23.23 The answer is A

Sexual aversion disorder is defined in DSM-IV-TR as a "persistent or recurrent and extreme aversion to, and avoidance of, all or almost all, genital sexual contact with a sexual partner." Some researchers consider the line between hypoactive desire disorder and sexual aversion disorder blurred, and, in some cases, both diagnoses are appropriate. Low frequency of sexual interaction is a symptom common to both disorders. The clinician should think of the words "repugnance" and "phobia" in relation to the patient with sexual aversion disorder.

Hypoactive sexual desire disorder is experienced by both men and women; however, they may not be hampered by any dysfunction once they are involved in the sex act. Conversely, hypoactive desire may be used to mask another sexual dysfunction. Lack of desire may be expressed by decreased frequency of coitus, perception of the partner as unattractive, or overt complaints of lack of desire. Upon questioning, the patient is found to have few or no sexual thoughts or fantasies, a lack of awareness of sexual cues, and little interest in initiating sexual experiences.

Female orgasmic disorder (also known as inhibited female orgasm or *anorgasmia*) is defined as the recurrent and persistent inhibition of the female orgasm, manifested by the absence or delay of orgasm after a normal sexual excitement phase that the clinician judges to be adequate in focus, intensity, and duration. Women who can achieve orgasm with noncoital clitoral stimulation but cannot experience it during coitus in the absence of manual stimulation are not necessarily categorized as anorgasmic.

Dyspareunia refers to recurrent and persistent pain during intercourse in either a man or a woman. In women, the dysfunction is related to and often coincides with vaginismus. Repeated episodes of vaginismus may lead to dyspareunia and vice versa, but, in either case, somatic causes must be ruled out. Dyspareunia should not be diagnosed as such when a medical basis for the pain is found or when (in a woman) it is associated with vaginismus or with lack of lubrication.

Vaginismus is an involuntary and persistent constriction of the outer one-third of the vagina that prevents penile insertion and intercourse. The response may be demonstrated during a gynecological examination when involuntary vaginal constriction prevents introduction of the speculum into the vagina, although some women only have vaginismus during coitus.

Answers 23.24–23.26

23.24 The answer is C

23.25 The answer is G

23.26 The answer is B

In fetishism the sexual focus is on objects (such as shoes, gloves, pantyhose, and stockings) that are intimately associated with the human body. The particular fetish may be linked to someone involved closely with the patient during childhood, and has some quality associated with that loved, needed, or even traumatizing person. *Voyeurism* is the recurrent preoccupation with fantasies and *acts that involve observing people who are naked or engaging in sexual activity*. It is also known as scopophilia. Masturbation to orgasm usually occurs during or after the event.

Frotteurism is usually characterized by the male's *rubbing up against a fully clothed woman to achieve orgasm*. The acts usually occur in crowded places, particularly subways and buses. Exhibitionism is the recurrent urge to expose one's genitals to a stranger or an unsuspecting person. Sexual excitement occurs in anticipation of the exposure, and orgasm is brought about by masturbation during or after the event.

Persons with sexual masochism have a recurrent preoccupation with sexual urges and fantasies involving the act of being humiliated, beaten, bound, or otherwise made to suffer. Persons with sexual sadism have fantasies involving harm to others. According to psychoanalytic theory, sexual sadism is a defense against fears of castration—the persons with sexual sadism do to others what they fear will happen to them. Pleasure is derived from expressing the aggressive instinct.

Transvestic fetishism is marked by *fantasies and sexual urges by heterosexual men to dress in female clothes for purposes of arousal* and as an adjunct to masturbation or coitus. Transvestic fetishism begins typically in childhood or early adolescence. As years pass, some men with transvestic fetishism want to dress and live permanently as women. Such persons are classified as persons with transvestic fetishism, with gender dysphoria.

Answers 23.27–23.29

23.27 The answer is A

23.28 The answer is B

23.29 The answer is A

Treatment of sexual dysfunction tends to be short term and behaviorally oriented. Specific exercises are prescribed to help the couple with their particular problem. Sexual dysfunction often involves a fear of inadequate performance. Thus, couples are specifically prohibited from any sexual play other than that prescribed by the therapist. Initially, *intercourse is interdicted*, and couples learn to give and receive bodily pleasure without the pressure of performance. Beginning exercises usually focus on heightening sensory awareness to touch, sight, sound, and smell.

During those exercises, called *sensate focus exercises,* the couple is given much reinforcement to lessen anxiety. They are urged to use fantasies to distract them from obsessive concerns about performance, which is termed *spectatoring*. The needs of both the dysfunctional partner and the nondysfunctional partner are considered. If either partner becomes sexually excited by the exercises, the other is encouraged to bring him or her to orgasm by manual or oral means. That procedure is important to keep the nondysfunctional partner from sabotaging the treatment. Open communication between the partners is urged, and the expression of mutual needs is encouraged. Resistances, such as claims of fatigue or not enough time to complete the exercises, are common and must be dealt with by the therapist. Genital stimulation is eventually added to general body stimulation. The couple is taught sequentially to try various positions for intercourse without necessarily completing the act, and to use varieties of stimulating techniques before they are permitted to proceed with intercourse.

The specific exercises vary with differing presenting complaints, and special techniques are used to treat the various dysfunctions. In cases of vaginismus, for instance, the woman is advised to dilate her vaginal opening with her fingers or with size-graduated vaginal dilators as part of the therapy. In cases of premature ejaculation, an exercise known as the *squeeze technique* is used *to raise the threshold of penile excitability.* In that exercise the man or the woman stimulates the erect penis until the earliest sensations of impending orgasm and ejaculation are felt. Penile stimulation is then stopped abruptly, and the coronal ridge of the penis is squeezed forcibly for several seconds. The technique is repeated several times. A variation is the stop–start technique in which stimulation is interrupted for several seconds but no squeeze is applied. Masturbation to the point of imminent orgasm raises the threshold of excitability to a more tolerant stimulation level. The man is encouraged to focus on sensations of excitement rather than distract himself from them. This makes him more familiar with his excitement pattern and lets him feel in control rather than overwhelmed by sensations of arousal. Communication between the partners is improved, because the man must let his partner know his level of sexual excitement so that she can squeeze his penis before the ejaculatory process has started. Sex therapy has been successful with some premature ejaculators; however, a subgroup of dysfunctional men may need pharmacotherapy as well.

A man with sexual desire disorder or erectile disorder is sometimes told to masturbate to demonstrate that full erection and ejaculation are possible. A woman with lifelong female orgasmic disorder is directed to masturbate, sometimes using a vibrator. Kegel's exercises may be introduced to strengthen the pubococcygeal muscles; that is, the woman is encouraged to contract her abdominal and perineal muscles at various times, including during masturbation and coitus. When a man has erectile disorder, the woman may be instructed to stimulate or tease his penis. The same technique is used with men who suffer from retarded ejaculation, with stimulation sometimes involving a vibrator. Retarded ejaculation is managed by extravaginal ejaculation initially, and gradual vaginal entry after stimulation to the point of near ejaculation.

Answers 23.30–23.34

23.30 The answer is B

23.31 The answer is B

23.32 The answer is B

23.33 The answer is C

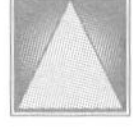

Table 23.2
Male Sexual Response Cycle[a]

Organ	Excitement Phase	Orgasmic Phase	Resolution Phase
Skin	Just before orgasm: sexual flush inconsistently appears; maculopapular rash originates on abdomen and spreads to anterior chest wall, face, and neck and can include shoulders and forearms	Well-developed flush	Flush disappears in reverse order of appearance; inconsistently appearing film of perspiration on soles of feet and palms of hands
Penis	Erection in 10 to 30 secs caused by vasocongestion of erectile bodies of corpus cavernosa of shaft; loss of erection may occur with introduction of asexual stimulus, loud noise; with heightened excitement, size of glans and diameter of penile shaft increase further	Ejaculation; emission phase marked by three to four 0.8-sec contractions of vas, seminal vesicles, prostate; ejaculation proper marked by 0.8-sec contractions of urethra and ejaculatory spurt of 12 to 20 inches at age 18, decreasing with age to seepage at 70	Erection: partial involution in 5 to 10 secs with variable refractory period; full detumescence in 5 to 30 mins
Scrotum and testes	Tightening and lifting of scrotal sac and elevation of testes; with heightened excitement, 50 percent increase in size of testes over unstimulated state and flattening against perineum, signaling impending ejaculation	No change	Decrease to baseline size because of loss of vasocongestion; testicular and scrotal descent within 5 to 30 mins after orgasm; involution may take several hours if no orgasmic release takes place
Cowper's glands	2 to 3 drops of mucoid fluid that contain viable sperm are secreted during heightened excitement	No change	No change
Other	Breasts: inconsistent nipple erection with heightened excitement before orgasm Myotonia: semispastic contractions of facial, abdominal, and intercostal muscles Tachycardia: up to 175 beats a min Blood pressure: rise in systolic 20 to 80 mm; in diastolic 10 to 40 mm Respiration: increased	Loss of voluntary muscular control Rectum: rhythmical contractions of sphincter Heart rate: up to 180 beats a minute Blood pressure: up to 40 to 100 mm systolic; 20 to 50 mm diastolic Respiration: up to 40 respirations a minute	Return to baseline state in 5 to 10 mins

[a]A desire phase consisting of sex fantasies and desire to have sex precedes excitement phase.

23.34 The answer is D

The fourth revised edition of *Diagnostic and Statistical Manual of Mental Disorders* (DSM-IV-TR) defines a four-phase sexual response cycle: phase 1, desire; phase 2, excitement; phase 3, orgasm; phase 4, resolution.

The *desire phase* is distinct from any phase identified solely through physiology, and it reflects the psychiatrist's fundamental interest in motivations, drives, and personality. It is characterized by sexual fantasies and the desire to have sexual activity. The *excitement phase* is brought on by psychological stimulation (fantasy or the presence of a love object) or physiological stimulation (stroking or kissing) or a combination of the two. It consists of a subjective sense of pleasure. The excitement phase is characterized by penile tumescence leading to erection in the man and by *vaginal lubrication* in the woman. Initial excitement may last several minutes to several hours. With continued stimulation, the woman's vaginal barrel shows a characteristic constriction along the outer third, known as the *orgasmic platform*, and the man's *testes increase in size 50 percent* and elevate.

The *orgasm phase* consists of a peaking of sexual pleasure, with the release of sexual tension and the rhythmic contraction of the perineal muscles and the pelvic reproductive organs. A subjective sense of ejaculatory inevitability triggers the man's orgasm. The forceful emission of semen follows. The male orgasm is also associated with four to five rhythmic spasms of the prostate, seminal vesicles, vas, and urethra. In the woman, orgasm is characterized by three to 15 involuntary contractions of the lower third of the vagina and by strong sustained contractions of the uterus, flowing from the fundus downward to the cervix. Blood pressure rises 20 to 40 mm (both systolic and diastolic), and the heart rate increases up to 160 beats a minute. Orgasm lasts 3 to 25 seconds and is associated with a *slight clouding of consciousness.*

The *resolution phase* consists of the disgorgement of blood from the genitalia *(detumescence)*, and that detumescence brings the body back to its resting state. If orgasm occurs, resolution is rapid; if it does not occur, resolution may take 2 to 6 hours and may be associated with irritability and discomfort.

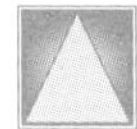

Table 23.3
Female Sexual Response Cycle[a]

Organ	Excitement Phase	Orgasmic Phase	Resolution Phase
Skin	Just before orgasm: sexual flush inconsistently appears; maculopapular rash originates on abdomen and spreads to anterior chest wall, face, and neck; can include shoulders and forearms	Well-developed flush	Flush disappears in reverse order of appearance; inconsistently appearing film of perspiration on soles of feet and palms of hands
Breasts	Nipple erection in two-thirds of women, venous congestion and areolar enlargement; size increases to one fourth over normal	Breasts may become tremulous	Return to normal in about $\frac{1}{2}$ hr
Clitoris	Enlargement in diameter of glans and shaft; just before orgasm, shaft retracts into prepuce	No change	Shaft returns to normal position in 5 to 10 secs; detumescence in 5 to 30 mins; if no orgasm, detumescence takes several hours
Labia majora	Nullipara: elevate and flatten against perineum Multipara: congestion and edema	No change	Nullipara: increase to normal size in 1 to 2 mins Multipara: decrease to normal size in 10 to 15 mins
Labia minora	Size increased 2 to 3 times over normal; change to pink, red, deep red before orgasm	Contractions of proximal labia minora	Return to normal within 5 mins
Vagina	Color change to dark purple; vaginal transudate appears 10 to 30 secs after arousal; elongation and ballooning of vagina; lower third of vagina constricts before orgasm	3 to 15 contractions of lower third of vagina at intervals of 0.8 sec	Ejaculate forms seminal pool in upper two thirds of vagina; congestion disappears in seconds or, if no orgasm, in 20 to 30 mins
Uterus	Ascends into false pelvis; labor-like contractions begin in heightened excitement just before orgasm	Contractions throughout orgasm	Contractions cease, and uterus descends to normal position
Other	Myotonia A few drops of mucoid secretion from Bartholin's glands during heightened excitement Cervix swells slightly and is passively elevated with uterus	Loss of voluntary muscular control Rectum: rhythmical contractions of sphincter Hyperventilation and tachycardia	Return to baseline status in seconds to minutes Cervix color and size retum to normal, and cervix descends into seminal pool

[a]A desire phase consisting of sex fantasies and desire to have sex precedes excitement phase.

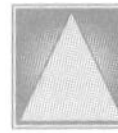

Table 23.4
Classification of Intersexual Disorders[a]

Syndrome	Description
Virilizing adrenal hyperplasia (adrenogenital syndrome)	Results from excess androgens in fetus with XX genotype; most common female intersex disorder; associated with enlarged clitoris, fused labia, hirsutism in adolescence
Turner's syndrome	Results from absence of second female sex chromosome (XO); associated with web neck, dwarfism, cubitus valgus; no sex hormones produced; infertile; usually assigned as females because of female-looking genitals
Klinefelter's syndrome	Genotype is XXY; male habitus present with small penis and rudimentary testes because of low androgen production; weak libido; usually assigned as male
Androgen insensitivity syndrome (testicular-feminizing syndrome)	Congenital X-linked recessive disorder that results in inability of tissues to respond to androgens; external genitals look female and cryptorchid testes present; assigned as females, even though they have XY genotype; in extreme form patient has breasts, normal external genitals, short blind vagina, and absence of pubic and axillary hair
Enzymatic defects in XY genotype (e.g., 5-α-reductase deficiency, 17-hydroxysteroid deficiency)	Congenital interruption in production of testosterone that produces ambiguous genitals and female habitus; usually assigned as female because of female-looking genitalia
Hermaphroditism	True hermaphrodite is rare and characterized by both testes and ovaries in same person (may be 46 XX or 46 XY)
Pseudohermaphroditism	Usually the result of endocrine or enzymatic defect (e.g., adrenal hyperplasia) in persons with normal chromosomes; female pseudohermaphrodites have masculine-looking genitals but are XX; male pseudohermaphrodites have rudimentary testes and external genitals and are XY; assigned as males or females, depending on morphology of genitals

[a]Intersexual disorders include a variety of syndromes that produce persons with gross anatomical or physiological aspects of the opposite sex.

Tables 23.2 and 23.3 describe the male and female sexual response cycles.

Answers 23.35–23.39

23.35 The answer is B

23.36 The answer is C

23.37 The answer is A

23.38 The answer is A

23.39 The answer is D

Sexual identity is the pattern of a person's biological sexual characteristics: *chromosomes*, external and internal genitalia, hormonal composition, *gonads, and secondary sex characteristics.* In normal development, these characteristics form a cohesive pattern that leaves persons in no doubt about their sex.

Gender identity is a person's *sense of maleness or femaleness.* By the age of 2 or 3 years, almost everyone has a firm conviction that "I am male" or "I am female." Gender identity results from an almost infinite series of clues derived from experiences with family members, peers, and teachers and from cultural phenomena. For instance, male infants tend to be handled more vigorously and female infants to be cuddled more. Fathers spend more time with their infant sons than with their daughters, and they also tend to be more aware of their sons' adolescent concerns than of their daughters' anxieties. Boys are more likely than girls to be physically disciplined. A child's sex affects parental tolerance for aggression and reinforcement or extinction of activity and of intellectual, aesthetic, and athletic interests. Physical characteristics derived from a person's biological sex (e.g., physique, body shape, and physical dimensions) interrelate with an intricate system of stimuli, including rewards, punishment, and parental gender labels, to establish gender goals.

Sexual orientation describes the *object of a person's sexual impulses:* heterosexual (opposite sex), homosexual (same sex), or bisexual (both sexes). In the United States, research indicates that 2.8 percent of men and 1.4 percent of women identify themselves as homosexual. These numbers are compatible with figures from Western European countries as well. However, a higher percentage of persons have had at least one same-sex experience in their lives. Additionally, gay people more typically settle in urban areas, so the incidence of homosexuality in some large cities is as high as 9 or 10 percent.

Sexual behavior includes *desire, fantasies*, pursuit of partners, autoeroticism, and all the activities engaged in to express and gratify sexual needs. It is an amalgam of psychological and physiological responses to internal and external stimuli.

Answers 23.40–23.46

23.40 The answer is E

23.41 The answer is C

23.42 The answer is G

23.43 The answer is A

23.44 The answer is B

23.45 The answer is D

23.46 The answer is F

See Table 23.4 for classification of intersexual disorders.

24 Gender Identity Disorders

Gender identity refers to the sense one has of being male or being female which corresponds, normally, to the person's anatomical sex. The revised fourth edition of the *Diagnostic and Statistical Manual of Mental Disorders* (DSM-IV-TR) define *gender identity disorders* (GID) as a group whose common feature is a strong, persistent preference for living as a person of the other sex. The affective component of gender identity disorders is gender dysphoria, discontent with one's designated birth sex and a desire to have the body of the other sex, and to be regarded socially as a person of the other sex. Gender identity disorder in adults was referred to in early versions of the DSM as *transsexualism*.

In DSM-IV-TR, no distinction is made for the overriding diagnostic term *gender identity disorder* as a function of age. In children, it may be manifested as statements of wanting to be the other sex and as a broad range of sex-typed behaviors conventionally shown by children of the other sex. Gender identity crystallizes in most persons by age 2 or 4 years.

The student should study the questions and answers below for a useful review of these disorders.

HELPFUL HINTS

The student should know the gender identity syndromes and terms listed below.

- adrenogenital syndrome
- agenesis
- ambiguous genitals
- androgen insensitivity syndrome
- asexual
- assigned sex
- Barr chromatin body
- bisexuality
- buccal smear
- cross-dressing
- cross-gender
- cryptorchid testis
- dysgenesis
- effeminate boys and masculine girls
- gender confusion
- gender identity
- disorder not otherwise specified
- gender role
- genotype
- hermaphroditism
- heterosexual orientation
- homosexual orientation
- hormonal treatment
- intersex conditions
- Klinefelter's syndrome
- male habitus
- phenotype
- prenatal androgens
- pseudohermaphroditism
- rough-and-tumble play
- sex of rearing
- sex-reassignment surgery
- sex steroids
- sexual object choice
- testicular feminization syndrome
- transsexualism
- transvestic fetishism
- Turner's syndrome
- virilized genitals
- X-linked

QUESTIONS

Directions

Each of the questions or incomplete statements below is followed by five suggested responses or completions. Select the *one* that is *best* in each case.

24.1 In gender identity disorders

A. there is no distinction made for age
B. there is discontent with one's designated birth sex
C. there is a desire to have the body of the other sex
D. there is a wish to be regarded socially as a person of the other sex
E. all of the above

24.2 Which of the following is true?

A. girls with congenital virilizing adrenal hyperplasia are less interested in dolls
B. polycystic ovaries has not been considered as associated with transexualism
C. mothers, more than fathers, give negative responses to boys playing with dolls
D. boys with GID are more likely to be right-handed than control boys
E. boys with GID generally tend to have more sisters than brothers

24.3 Sex reassignment

A. is often the best solution in treating gender dysphoria
B. usually involves a full-time social transition to living in the desired gender before hormonal treatment
C. includes daily doses of oral estrogen in persons born male
D. may involve sex reassignment surgery
E. all of the above

24.4 Gender constancy

A. is a task of separation-individuation
B. has no age-related stage-like sequence because it is inherent
C. includes a sense of "gender stability"
D. cannot be tested in the clinical situation
E. none of the above

24.5 In patients born with ambiguous genitalia, which of the following is the predominant factor by which assigned sex is determined?

A. Wishes of the parents
B. Genetic phenotype and potential for reproduction
C. Extent of virilization
D. Surgical team capabilities
E. Wishes of the patient at time of puberty

24.6 A boy with gender identity disorder

A. usually begins to display signs of the disorder after age 9
B. experiences sexual excitement when he cross-dresses
C. has boys as his preferred playmates
D. is treated with testosterone
E. may say that his penis or testes are disgusting

24.7 Girls with gender identity disorder in childhood

A. regularly have male companions
B. may refuse to urinate in a sitting position
C. may assert that they have or will grow a penis
D. may give up masculine behavior by adolescence
E. all of the above

24.8 Which of the following statements does *not* apply to the treatment of gender identity disorder?

A. Adult patients generally enter psychotherapy to learn how to deal with their disorder, not to alter it.
B. Before sex-reassignment surgery, patients must go through a trial of cross-gender living for at least 3 months.
C. A one-to-one play relationship is used with boys in which adults role-model masculine behavior.
D. Hormonal therapy is not required as a preceding event in sex-reassignment surgery.
E. During hormonal treatments, both males and females need to be watched for hepatic dysfunction and thromboembolic phenomena.

24.9 In biological men undertaking estrogen hormone treatment, all of the following side effects are common *except*

A. Testicular atrophy
B. Change in pitch of voice
C. Diminished erectile capacity
D. Breast enlargement
E. Decrease in density of body hair

24.10 True statements about the epidemiology of gender identity disorders include

A. As many as five boys are referred for each girl referred.
B. Among a sample of 4- to 5-year-old boys referred for a range of clinical problems, the reported desire to be the opposite sex was 15 percent.
C. Most parents of children with gender identity disorder report that cross-gender behaviors were apparent before age 3.
D. The prevalence rate of transsexualism is estimated to be about 1 case per 10,000 males.
E. All of the above

24.11 In biological women undertaking testosterone hormone treatment, all of the following side effects are common *except*

A. Temporary deepening of vocal pitch
B. Enlargement of clitoris
C. Increased libido
D. Male hair pattern
E. Increased muscle mass

24.12 In a patient with Turner's Syndrome, all of the following are common findings *except*

A. Atypical female sex identification
B. Gonadal dysgenesis
C. Female genitalia
D. Small uterus
E. Dyspareunia

Directions

The lettered heading below are followed by a list of numbered statements. For each numbered statement, select the *one* lettered heading that is most closely associated with it. Each lettered heading may be selected once, more than once, or not at all.

Questions 24.13–24.17

A. Klinefelter's syndrome
B. Turner's syndrome
C. Congenital virilizing adrenal hyperplasia
D. True hermaphroditism
E. Androgen insensitivity syndrome

24.13 A 17-year-old girl presented to a clinic with primary amenorrhea and no development of secondary sex characteristics. She was short in stature and had a webbed neck.

24.14 A baby was born with ambiguous external genitalia. Further evaluation revealed that both ovaries and testes were present.

24.15 A baby was born with ambiguous external genitalia. Further evaluation revealed that ovaries, a vagina, and a uterus, were normal and intact.

24.16 A buccal smear from a phenotypically female patient revealed that the patient was XY. A further workup revealed undescended testes.

24.17 A tall, thin man presented for infertility problems was found to be XXY.

ANSWERS

24.1 The answer is E (all)

In the current diagnostic system *no distinction is made for the definition of gender identity disorders as a function of age*. They are defined in DSM-IV-TR as a group whose common feature is a strong, persistent preference for living as a person of the other sex. *The affective component is gender dysphoria, discontent with one's designated birth sex* and *a desire to have the body of the other sex*, and to be *regarded socially as a person of the other sex*.

24.2 The answer is A

Evidence for hormonal influence in gender identity disorder derives from several sources. *Girls with congenital virilizing adrenal hyperplasia overproduce adrenal androgen in utero, and, as girls, are less interested in dolls*, and more likely to be considered tomboys than girls who do not have the disorder. Reports describe *polycystic ovaries as more common in female-to-male transsexuals than in the typical female population*. In social learning theories that focus on the differential reinforcement of sex-typed behavior by parents, starting shortly after birth, *it has been noted that fathers, more than mothers, give negative responses to boys playing with dolls*. Handedness may relate to prenatal sex steroid levels, and *boys with GID are significantly more likely to be non-right handed than control boys*. Similarly, *boys with GID have been reported to have significantly more brothers than sisters*.

24.3 The answer is E (all)

No drug treatment has been shown to be effective in reducing cross-gender desire, and when *gender dysphoria is severe and intractable, sex reassignment may be the best solution*. This involves an extensive set of clinical management guidelines, and many clinicians *require that the patient begin the Real Life Test or Real Life Experience before hormonal treatment*. The Real Life Test is typically 1 to 2 years of full-time cross-gender living, including at least one year of employment in the desired gender role and one year on high doses of cross-sex hormones. *For born males, this includes high doses of oral estrogens*; biological women are treated with monthly or three weekly injections of testosterone. Sex reassignment surgery is often the last stage in the reassignment process.

24.4 The answer is C

Gender constancy is a *piagetian construct of the constancy of gender and its possibility to change by altering superficial characteristics*. It is *not described by Mahler in separation-individuation*. It *involves an age-related stage-like sequence*, in which children first self-categorize the gender of self and others, "gender identity," then appreciate its invariance over time, "gender stability." Finally, it involves understanding that invariance in the face of superficial transformations of gender, such as changing sex-typed clothing or hair length. Although no psychological test is diagnostic of gender identity disorder in children, *the It-Scale for Children and the Draw-A-Person test have been used to assess GID in the clinical situation*.

24.5 The answer is B

In patients born with ambiguous genitalia, *the determination of genetic phenotype and considerations for reproduction generally dominates other factors in the designation of assigned sex*. Decision making in this area of pediatric urology is multi-factorial, requiring biological, surgical and social factors to be evaluated. Controversy surrounds pediatric sex assignment because decisions are most often made without patient input, and challenges to traditional factors such a "phallic adequacy" and *surgical capability* have been made in response to reassignment by patients at later dates. Some in the lay community advocate *waiting until puberty before making an assignment*, to allow the patient to made the determination. Surgeons tend to support earlier intervention, generally before 5 years of age.

A 2006 survey by the American Academy of Pediatrics produced consensus data around two standard cases. In the case of a genetic female (XX) who had been exposed to excess androgen and had virilized genitalia, (i.e., Prader V 46XX with congenital adrenal hyperplasia), 99 percent of the pediatric urologists agreed that female assignment would be preferred. The foremost reason being the potential for reproduction. The lack of exogenous steroids and overall better outcomes with female assignment were also cited. If required, surgery was advised to take place between 3 and 18 months of age.

In the case of a genetic male (XY) cloacal exstrophy with rudimentary phallic structures, 70 percent of pediatric urologists concurred that a male assignment would be optimal. The effect of androgens on the development of the male nervous system was cited as the foremost reason. The desire not to remove both gonads and fertility were also prominent. Physicians who designated female assignment cited difficulty with creating a functional phallus as a reason. Of note, one study found over 50 percent of these patients assigned female sex with gonadectomy desired reassignment to male at a later date, therefore calling into question the validity of surgical capability as a dominant criteria in this case.

24.6 The answer is E

A boy with gender identity disorder *may say that his penis or testes are disgusting* and that he would be better off without them. Persons with this disorder *usually begin to display signs of the disorder before age 4 (not after age 9)*, although it may present at any age. Cross-dressing may be part of the disorder, but boys *do not experience sexual excitement when they cross-dress*. A boy with a gender identity disorder is generally preoccupied with female stereotypical activities and usually *has girls (not boys) as his preferred playmates*. Gender identity disorder *is not treated with testosterone*.

24.7 The answer is E (all)

Girls with gender identity disorder in childhood *regularly have male companions* and an avid interest in sports and rough-and-tumble play; they show no interest in dolls and playing house. In a few cases, a girl with this disorder *may refuse to urinate in a sitting position, may assert that she has or will grow a penis*, does not want to grow breasts or menstruate, and says that she will grow up to become a man. Girls with gender identity disorder in childhood *may give up masculine behavior by adolescence*.

24.8 The answer is D

Hormone treatment is required and must be received by patients for about a year prior to sex-reassignment surgery, with estradiol and progesterone in male-to-female changes and testosterone in female-to-male changes. Many transsexuals like the changes in their bodies that occur as a result of that treatment, and some stop at that point, not progressing on to surgery. Another requirement before sex-reassignment surgery is that patients *must go through a trial of cross-gender living for at least 3 months* and in many cases up to 1 year. *Adult patients* generally *enter psychotherapy to learn how to deal with their condition, not to alter it*. In boys with gender identity disorder, a one-to-one play relationship is used, in which *adults or peers role-model masculine behavior. During hormonal treatments*, both males and females need to be watched for hepatic dysfunction and thromboembolic phenomena.

24.9 The answer is B

The pitch of the male voice is determined primarily by the resonance and volume of the chest and not affected by estrogen treatment. Speech therapy can be undertaken to achieve a more feminine pitch and laryngeal surgery is an option, although the range may be decreased by the procedure. Biological men undergoing hormonal treatment with daily doses of estrogen can expect the *enlargement of breast tissue, testicular atrophy*, decreased libido, *diminished erectile tissue, and decreased body hair*. Facial hair most often requires electrolysis. Maximal breast tissue development is generally achieved within 2 years of hormonal treatment and surgical augmentation may be required to achieve aesthetic goals. In addition to estrogen, a variety of anti-androgenic compounds (cytoproterone acetate, flutamide, spironolactone) and gonadectomy can be used to counter the effects of testosterone.

24.10 The answer is E (all)

The prevalence of the gender identity disorder of childhood can only be estimated because no epidemiological studies have been published. A rough estimate can be obtained from two items on Thomas Achenbach's Child Behavior Checklist that are consistent with components of the diagnosis: behaves like opposite sex and wishes to be of opposite sex. In one study, among *a sample of 4- to 5-year-old boys* referred for a range of clinical problems, the reported desire to be of the opposite sex was 15 percent. Among 4- to 5-year-old boys not referred for behavioral problems, it was only 1 percent. For ages 6 to 7, the rates were 2.7 and 0 percent; for ages 8 to 9, 5.1 and 0 percent; and for ages 10 to 11, 1.1 and 2.3 percent. For clinically referred girls, there was more uniformity across the ages, with the highest being 8 percent at age 9 and the lowest being 4 percent for other ages. For nonreferred girls, the highest rate was 5 percent at ages 4 to 5 and less than 3 percent for other ages.

As many as five boys are referred for each girl referred, for which several explanations are possible. First, there is greater parental concern with sissiness than with tomboyishness and greater peer group stigma attaches to substantial cross-gender behavior in boys. Thus, there may be an equal prevalence of gender identity disorder in boys and girls but a differential referral rate. Another possibility is that a genuine disparity results from the male's more perilous developmental course. The fundamental mammalian state is female. No sex hormones are required for prenatal female anatomical development (XO children with gonadal dysgenesis [Turner's syndrome] appear female at birth). Sex hormones are required at critical developmental times for male anatomical differentiation. If the mechanisms of behavioral development track anatomical development, the masculine behavioral system requires adequate levels of hormones at the appropriate time for normative expression. Finally, the psychodynamic developmental model explaining the disparate referral rates views both boys and girls as initially identifying with the female parent, with only boys needing to make the developmental shift for later normative male identification.

Most children with a gender identity disorder are referred for clinical evaluation in early grade school. Parents typically report that *cross-gender behaviors were apparent before age 3.*

There is no basis for estimating the proportion of adults who would qualify for a DSM-IV-TR diagnosis of gender identity disorder. The only relevant data are for transsexuals, who comprise only a subgroup of gender-dysphoric adults, and even those figures may be underestimates. The available data (from the United Kingdom, the Netherlands, Sweden, and Australia) place *the prevalence rate of transsexualism* at about 1 case per 10,000 males and 1 in 30,000 females.

24.11 The answer is A

Deepening of the voice due to testosterone hormonal treatment is irreversible. Results are typically seen within 6 to 10 weeks. The standard regimen is 200 mg of intra-muscular testosterone ester given biweekly. *Testosterone will enlarge the clitoris by two to three times the pretreatment size* and approximately 5 percent of post-treatment patients are capable of vaginal intercourse. *Increases in libido are reported, lean muscle mass is increased,* and acne is a common side effect of testosterone. Breast tissue glandular activity is reduced although overall size in not affected by testosterone treatment.

24.12 The answer is A

Patients with Turner's syndrome have typical female identification (Fig. 24.1). The majority report heterosexual identification though they tend to have fewer sexual relationships. During adolescence, many patients have difficulties reading social cues, and experience social isolation and anxiety. Most patients with Turner's Syndrome have *gonadal dysgenesis* and require

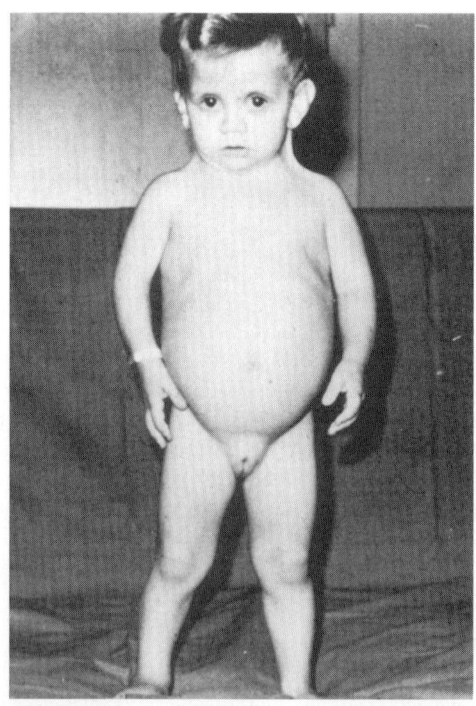

FIGURE 24.1

Photograph of patient with Turner's syndrome. The main characteristics are webbed neck, short stature, broad chest, and absence of sexual maturation. (Reprinted with permission from Sadler T. *Langman's Medical Embryology*. 5th ed. Baltimore: Williams & Wilkins; 1985:121.)

exogenous estrogen to complete growth and develop secondary sex characteristics. However, in patients with 45,X0/46,XX mosaicism, spontaneous menarche is common (40 percent) and in rare cases, pregnancy is possible. These patients typically experience ovarian failure at a later date. *Turner's Syndrome patients have female genitalia. The uterus may be small* but structural abnormalities are not typical. *The lack of estrogen may shorten the vagina and contribute to dyspareunia.*

Answers 24.13–24.17

24.13 The answer is B

24.14 The answer is D

24.15 The answer is C

24.16 The answer is E

24.17 The answer is A

In *Turner's syndrome* (Fig. 24.1), one sex chromosome is missing (XO). The result is an absence (agenesis) or minimal development (dysgenesis) of the gonads; no significant sex hormones, male or female, are produced in fetal life or postnatally. The sexual tissues remain in a female resting state. Because the second X chromosome, which seems to be responsible for full femaleness, is missing, the girls have an incomplete sexual anatomy and, lacking adequate estrogens, have *amenorrhea and* develop *no secondary sex characteristics* without treatment. They often have other stigmata, such as a webbed neck, low posterior hairline margin, short stature, and cubitus valgus. The infant is born with normal-appearing female external genitals and so is unequivocally assigned to the female sex and is so reared. All the children develop as unremarkably feminine, heterosexually oriented girls.

True hermaphroditism is characterized by the presence of both ovaries and testes in the same person. The genitals' appearance at birth determines the sex assignment, and the core gender identity is male, female, or hermaphroditic, depending on the family's conviction about the child's sex. Usually, a panel of experts determines the sex of rearing; they base their decision on buccal smears, chromosome studies, and parental wishes.

Congenital virilizing adrenal hyperplasia results from an excess of androgen acting on the fetus. When the condition occurs in girls, excessive fetal androgens from the adrenal gland cause *ambiguous external genitals, ranging from mild clitoral enlargement to* external genitals that look like *a normal scrotal sac, testes, and a penis*; but they also have *ovaries, a vagina, and a uterus* (Fig. 24.2).

Androgen insensitivity syndrome, a congenital X-linked recessive-trait disorder, results from an inability of the target tissues to respond to androgens. Unable to respond, the fetal tissues remain in their female resting state, and the central nervous system is not organized as masculine. The infant at birth *appears to be female*, although she is later found to have *undescended testes*, which produce the testosterone to which the tissues do not respond, and minimal or absent internal sexual organs. Secondary sex characteristics at puberty are female because of the small but sufficient amounts of estrogens typically produced by the testes. The patients invariably sense themselves to be female and are feminine. They are clinically considered to be female. Intersex conditions, such as androgen insensitivity syndrome and congenital adrenal hyperplasia, are diagnosed as gender identity disorders not otherwise specified.

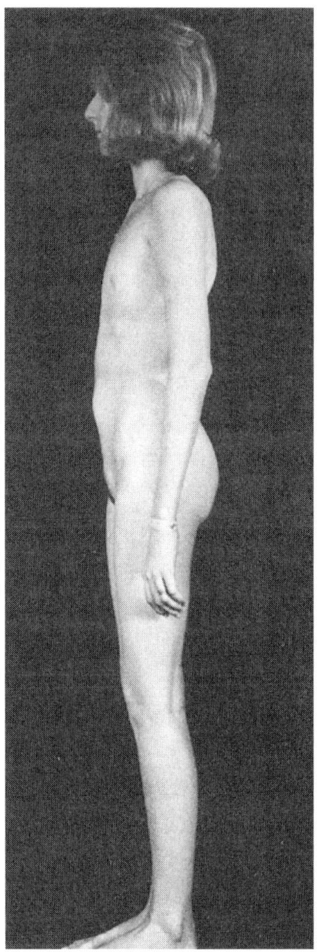

FIGURE 24.2

A phenotypic female with XY karyotype. The vaginal canal was normal without clitoral enlargement. At laparotomy, dysgenetic gonads and a uterus with Fallopian tubes were present. On cyclic estrogen-progestogen therapy, menses were induced at regular intervals and good breast development resulted.

In *Klinefelter's syndrome* the person (usually *XXY*) has a male habitus, under the influence of the Y chromosome, but the effect is weakened by the second X chromosome. Although the patient is born with a penis and testes, the testes are small and *infertile*, and the penis may also be small. Beginning in adolescence, some patients develop gynecomastia and other feminine-appearing contours. Their sexual desire is usually weak. Sex assignment and rearing should lead to a clear sense of maleness, but the patients often have gender disturbances, ranging from transsexualism to an intermittent desire to put on women's clothes. As a result of lessened androgen production, the fetal hypogonadal state in some patients seems to have interfered with the completion of the central nervous system organization that should underlie masculine behavior. In fact, patients may have any of a wide variety of neuro- and psychopathologies, ranging from emotional instability to mental retardation.

25 Eating Disorders

Despite their often innocuous, culturally syntonic origins, eating disorders have undoubtedly been present in various forms for thousands of years, but their prevalence has increased substantially since the 1950s. They now present as common and serious clinical syndromes. Eating disorders have some of the highest rates of premature mortality in psychiatry—up to 19 percent within 20 years of onset among those initially requiring hospitalization. For this reason, eating disorders, defined as severe disturbances in eating behavior in the revised 4th edition of the *Diagnostic and Statistical Manual of Mental Disorders* (DSM-IV-TR), remain an important focus for the psychiatrist, with the goal of engraving on the public consciousness the presence and seriousness of the disorders.

Anorexia nervosa is defined as occurring at onset in a person, usually an adolescent girl, who refuses to maintain a minimally normal body weight, fears gaining weight, and has a disturbed perception of body shape and size. Bulimia nervosa is characterized by a person engaging in binge eating and using inappropriate and dangerous compensatory methods, such as induced vomiting or use of laxatives, to prevent weight gain. Besides those who clearly fit diagnostic criteria for these disorders, there are many others who may exhibit various aspects and degrees of them. Bulimia nervosa is more common than anorexia nervosa.

Eating disorder patients tend to be high achievers and perfectionistic and come from families with similar characteristics. Psychological struggles center around issues of autonomy and control, as well as on conflicts surrounding sexual maturation. There is often a family history of depression. Biological treatments for both disorders may involve the use of antidepressants, with serotonin and norepinephrine neurotransmitters being particularly implicated.

Anorexia nervosa and bulimia nervosa are strikingly similar in some regards but differ dramatically in others. The student needs to be aware of these differences as well as of the various treatments available. Family therapy has traditionally been considered a mainstay of treatment, especially with younger anorexic patients. Treatment in some severe cases of both disorders is ineffective, and death can result.

The student should study the questions and answers below for a useful review of these disorders.

HELPFUL HINTS

These terms relate to impulse-control disorders and should be defined by the student.

- alopecia
- anticonvulsants
- attention-deficit/hyperactivity disorder
- behavior therapy
- benzodiazepines
- biofeedback
- desperate stage
- enuresis
- epileptoid personality
- 5-HIAA
- hydroxyzine hydrochloride
- hypnotherapy
- impulse-control disorder
- impulse-control disorder not otherwise specified
- intermittent explosive disorder
- kleptomania
- limbic system
- lithium
- lust angst
- multidetermined
- oniomania
- parental factors
- pathological gambling
- pleasure principle, reality principle
- progressive-loss stage
- psychodynamics
- pyromania
- social gambling
- SSRIs
- testosterone
- trichophagy
- trichotillomania
- winning phase

QUESTIONS

Directions

Each of the incomplete statements below is followed by five suggested completions. Select the *one* that is *best* in each case.

25.1 Which of the following is the most common comorbid disorder associated with anorexia nervosa?

A. Depression
B. Social phobia
C. Obsessive-compulsive disorder
D. Bulimia
E. Body dysmorphic disorder

25.2 Which of the following is *not* an endocrine or structural change noted as a result of starvation?

A. Hypercortisolemia
B. Thyroid suppression
C. Enlarged ventricles
D. Increased total brain volume
E. Gonadotropin-releasing hormone suppression

25.3 Which of the following percentages below expected weight does an anorexic patient generally fall before being recommended for inpatient hospitalization?

A. 20 percent
B. 40 percent
C. 60 percent
D. 80 percent
E. None of the above

25.4 Pickwickian syndrome is

A. when persons eat excessively after they have had their evening meal
B. binge eating without the inappropriate compensatory behaviors
C. when a person is 100 percent over desirable weight with cardiorespiratory pathology
D. when obese persons feel their bodies are grotesque and loathsome
E. sudden, compulsive ingestion of very large amounts of food in a short time

25.5 Which of the following statements regarding anorexia and bulimia is *false*?

A. Bulimia patients find the disorder more ego-dystonic than do anorexic patients.
B. Both anorexia and bulimia have increased incidences of familial depression.
C. Anorexic patients are generally more angry and impulsive than bulimic patients.
D. Bulimia nervosa is more prevalent than anorexia nervosa.
E. Bulimia nervosa often has a later age of onset than anorexia nervosa.

25.6 Which of the following professionals is most likely to develop anorexia nervosa?

A. Executive chef working exclusively in food preparation
B. Female stock broker with stressful job demands
C. Male advertising executive with a history of depression
D. Ballet dancer vying for the lead role in her next production
E. Actress from upper economic class background

25.7 Treatments that have shown some success in ameliorating anorexia nervosa include

A. cyproheptadine
B. electroconvulsive therapy (ECT)
C. chlorpromazine
D. fluoxetine
E. all of the above

25.8 Ms. L was a gaunt 15-year-old high-school student evaluated at the insistence of her parents, who were concerned about her weight loss. She was 5 feet 3 inches tall and had reached her greatest weight, 100 pounds, a year earlier. Shortly thereafter she decided to lose weight to be more attractive. She felt "chubby" and thought she would be more appealing if she were thinner. First she eliminated all carbohydrate-rich foods, and gradually intensified her dieting until she was eating only a few vegetables a day. She also started a vigorous exercise program. Within 6 months, she was down to 80 pounds. She then became preoccupied with food and started collecting recipes from magazines in order to prepare gourmet meals for her family. She had difficulty sleeping and was irritable and depressed, having several crying spells every day. Her menses started the previous year, but she had only a few normal periods.

Ms. L had always had high grades in school and had spent a great deal of time studying. She had never been active socially and had never dated. She was conscientious and perfectionistic in everything she undertook. She had never been away from home longer than a week. Her father was a business manager. Her mother was a housewife who for the past 2 years had a problem with hypoglycemia and was on a low-carbohydrate diet.

During the interview, Ms. L said she felt fat, even though she weighed 80 pounds, and she described a fear of losing control and eating so much food that she would become obese. She did not feel she was ill and thought that hospitalization was unnecessary.

The diagnosis of anorexia nervosa can be made on the basis of Ms. L's

A. 20-pound weight loss
B. feeling fat at a weight of 80 pounds and a height of 5 feet 3 inches
C. having had only a few normal periods
D. fear of becoming obese
E. all of the above

25.9 Features associated with anorexia nervosa include

A. normal hair structure and distribution
B. the fact that 7 to 9 percent of those affected are male
C. onset between the ages of 10 and 30
D. mortality rates of 20 to 25 percent
E. all of the above

25.10 The binge-eating/purging type of anorexia nervosa when compared to the restricting type is more often associated with

A. suicide attempts
B. drug abuse
C. premorbid obesity
D. familial obesity
E. all of the above

25.11 Studies suggest that

A. The overall incidence of anorexia nervosa has decreased in the last 50 years.

B. The overall incidence of bulimia nervosa has increased in the last 50 years.
C. The incidence rate of anorexia nervosa in industrialized countries is approximately 20 per 100,000 population per year.
D. The lifetime prevalence rate of anorexia nervosa in the United States has been estimated to be 5 percent.
E. Bulimia nervosa has a prevalence rate of about 10 percent in adolescents and young adult women.

25.12 Medical complications of eating disorders related to weight loss include all of the following *except*

A. erosion of dental enamel with corresponding decay
B. bradycardia
C. constipation and delayed gastric emptying
D. abnormal taste sensation
E. osteoporosis

25.13 Ipecac intoxication is associated with

A. pericardial pain and cardiac failure
B. dyspnea
C. generalized muscle weakness
D. hypotension
E. all of the above

25.14 Characteristic laboratory test results in anorexia nervosa include

A. ST-segment and T-wave changes on electrocardiogram
B. decreased serum cholesterol levels
C. increased fasting serum glucose concentrations
D. decreased serum salivary amylase concentrations
E. all of the above

25.15 Biological complications of eating disorders may include

A. salivary gland and pancreatic inflammation
B. gastric or esophageal tearing or rupture
C. cardiac arrhythmias, loss of cardiac muscle, and cardiomyopathy
D. leukopenia
E. all of the above

25.16 Which of the following features can be associated with bulimia nervosa?

A. undeveloped breasts
B. abnormal insulin secretion
C. widespread endocrine disorder
D. a previous episode of anorexia nervosa
E. body weight at least 15 percent below normal

25.17 Anorexia nervosa has a mortality rate of up to approximately

A. 1 percent
B. 18 percent
C. 30 percent
D. 42 percent
E. 50 percent

Directions

The questions below consist of lettered headings followed by a list of numbered phrases. For each numbered phrase, select

A. if the item is associated with A only
B. if the item is associated with B only
C. if the item is associated with both A and B
D. if the item is associated with neither A nor B

Questions 25.18–25.25

A. Anorexia nervosa
B. Bulimia nervosa

25.18 Severe weight loss and amenorrhea
25.19 Visual agnosia, compulsive licking and biting, hypersexuality
25.20 After 5 to 10 years, at least 50 percent will be markedly improved
25.21 Higher fatality rate
25.22 Family therapy is not widely used
25.23 Cognitive-behavioral therapy is the benchmark, first-line treatment
25.24 Decreased appetite only occurs in the most severe stages
25.25 Body weight of less than 85 percent of the patient's expected weight

ANSWERS

25.1 The answer is A

The diagnostic challenges of eating disorders are only partly addressed when a specific eating disorder is identified, because, in the large majority of cases, comorbid psychiatric disorders accompany the eating disorder, with two to four separate additional diagnoses on Axis I or II of DSM-IV-TR commonly seen. *Anorexia nervosa is associated with depression in 65 percent of cases, social phobia in 34 percent of cases, and obsessive-compulsive disorder in 26 percent of cases.* There is also a high comorbidity of anorexia nervosa with *body dysmorphic disorder*—estimated at 20 percent—in which patients additionally have obsessional preoccupations regarding specific body parts not related to weight or shape in particular.

In addition to identifying Axis I mood, anxiety, obsessive-compulsive, and substance abuse disorders and Axis II personality vulnerabilities and disorders, the temporal relationship of these disorders to the eating disorder should be noted. Mood disorders that precede eating disorders differ significantly from those that first occur after the eating disorder is initiated. Mood disorders starting before eating disorders usually require separate and specific treatment, whereas those starting in the wake of an eating disorder often improve on their own during recovery from the eating disorder.

25.2 The answer is D

Endogenous opiates may contribute to the denial of hunger in patients with anorexia nervosa. Preliminary studies show dramatic weight gains in some patients given opiate antagonists. Starvation results in many biochemical changes, some of which are also present in depression, such as *hypercortisolemia* and nonsuppression by dexamethasone. *Thyroid function is suppressed as well.* These abnormalities are corrected by realimentation. Starvation produces amenorrhea, which reflects *lowered hormonal levels (luteinizing, follicle-stimulating, and gonadotropin-releasing hormones).* Some anorexia nervosa patients, however, become amenorrheic before significant weight loss. Several computed tomography (CT) studies reveal *enlarged CSF spaces (enlarged sulci and ventricles)* in anorectic patients during starvation, a finding that is reversed by weight gain. While *decreases in total brain volume* and increases in brain ventricular size are usually seen, normal brain structural studies may also be seen in some very malnourished patients.

25.3 The answer is A

The first consideration in the treatment of anorexia nervosa is to restore patients' nutritional state: dehydration, starvation, and electrolyte imbalances can seriously compromise health and, in some cases, lead to death. The decision to hospitalize a patient is based on the patient's medical condition and the amount of structure needed to ensure patient cooperation. In general, *anorexia nervosa patients who are 20 percent below the expected weight for their height are recommended for inpatient programs*, and patients who are 30 percent below their expected weight require psychiatric hospitalization for 2 to 6 months.

25.4 The answer is C

Pickwickian syndrome is said to exist when a person is *100 percent over desirable weight* and has associated respiratory and cardiovascular pathology. The *night-eating syndrome* is one in which persons eat excessively after they have had their evening meal, and seems to be precipitated by stressful life circumstances. *Binge-eating disorder* is recurrent episodes of binge eating in the absence of the inappropriate compensatory behaviors characteristic of bulimia nervosa; these patients are not fixated on body shape and weight. *Body dysmorphic disorder* is when some obese persons feel that their bodies are grotesque and loathsome and that others view them with hostility and contempt. The *binge-eating syndrome* (bulimia) is characterized by sudden, compulsive ingestion of very large amounts of food in a short time.

25.5 The answer is C

Patients with bulimia nervosa, like those with anorexia nervosa, have difficulties with adolescent demands, but *bulimia nervosa patients are more outgoing, angry, and impulsive than anorexia nervosa patients.* These patients generally *experience their uncontrolled eating as more ego-dystonic than do anorexia nervosa patients* and so seek help more readily.

Bulimia nervosa is more prevalent than anorexia nervosa. Estimates of bulimia nervosa range from 1 to 3 percent of young women. Like anorexia nervosa, bulimia nervosa is significantly more common in women than in men, but its *onset is often later in adolescence than that of anorexia nervosa.* Patients with bulimia nervosa, like those with anorexia nervosa tend to be high achievers and to respond to societal pressures to be slender. *As with anorexia nervosa, many patients with bulimia are depressed and have increased familial depression*, but the families of patients with bulimia nervosa are generally less close and more conflictual than the families of anorexia nervosa patients.

25.6 The answer is D

Anorexia nervosa is seen with the greatest frequency among *young women in professions that require thinness*, such as modeling and ballet. Anorexia nervosa occurs 10 to 20 times more often in females than males, and occurs in about 0.5 percent of adolescent girls. Although the disorder was initially reported predominantly in the upper economic classes, recent epidemiological surveys do not show that distribution. Although the other professions listed may result in increased stress and involve food preparation, these professions are not most likely to develop anorexia.

25.7 The answer is E (all)

Medications can be useful adjuncts in the treatment of anorexia nervosa. The first drug used in treating anorectic patients was *chlorpromazine.* This medication is particularly helpful for severely ill patients who are overwhelmed with constant thoughts of losing weight and behavioral rituals for losing weight. There are few double-blind controlled studies to definitively prove this drug's effectiveness for calming such patients and inducing needed weight gain. *Cyproheptadine (Periactin)* in high dosages (up to 28 mg a day) can facilitate weight gain in anorectic restrictors and also has an antidepressant effect. Some recent studies indicate that *fluoxetine* may be effective in preventing relapse in patients with anorexia nervosa.

Amitriptyline (Elavil) has been reported to have some benefit in patients with anorexia nervosa, as have imipramine (Tofranil) and desipramine (Norpramin). There is some evidence that *electroconvulsive therapy (ECT)* is beneficial in certain cases of anorexia nervosa associated with major depressive disorder.

25.8 The answer is E (all)

The diagnosis of anorexia nervosa can be made on the basis of Ms. L's *20-pound weight loss*, her *feeling fat* at a weight of 80 pounds and a height of 5 feet 3 inches, her having had *only a few normal periods*, and her *fear of becoming obese.*

25.9 The answer is C

Features associated with anorexia nervosa include *onset between the ages of 10 and 30; lanugo* (neonatal-like body hair), not normal hair structure and distribution; *mortality rates of 5 to 18 percent (not 20 to 25 percent); and the fact that 4 to 6 percent (not 7 to 9 percent) of those affected are male.*

25.10 The answer is E (all)

DSM-IV-TR divides anorexia nervosa into two subtypes: the restricting type and the binge-eating/purging type. There are significant differences between anorexia nervosa patients who engage in bulimic or purging behaviors and those who consistently restrict their dietary intake. Impulsive behaviors such as stealing, *drug abuse, suicide attempts*, and self-mutilations are significantly more prevalent in the binge-eating/purging type compared with the restricting type. The bulimic group of anorexia nervosa patients also has a higher prevalence of *premorbid obesity, familial obesity*, mood lability, and debilitating personality characteristics; the latter are often in the context of a Cluster B (impulsive) personality disorder cluster. The binge-eating/purging type of patients is similar to persons with bulimia nervosa in behaviors and characteristics. They are not classified as having bulimia nervosa because they have lost large amounts of weight and meet the criteria for anorexia nervosa. The specific mechanisms by which the binge-eating/purging type patients are able to obtain and maintain large weight losses are still unknown to researchers and are being investigated.

25.11 The answer is B

One of the major problems in studying the epidemiology of eating disorders over time is the change in criteria for these syndromes since the late 1960s. Despite this problem, studies suggest that *the overall incidence of both anorexia nervosa and bulimia nervosa has increased in the past 50 years.* There was a consistent increase in the registered incidence of anorexia nervosa from 1931 to 1986 in cases presenting to the health care system in several industrialized countries. A study in northeastern Scotland showed that between 1965 and 1991 there was almost a sixfold increase in the incidence of anorexia nervosa—from 3/100,000 to 17/100,000. A study conducted in southwest London between July 1991 and June 1992 showed an incidence of anorexia nervosa to be 2.7 cases per 100,000 total population. In females aged 15 to 29 years, the incidence was 19.2 cases per 100,000. In Rochester, Minnesota, a recent study found an overall adjusted incidence for females of 14.6 per 100,000; for men, the corresponding figure was 1.8. When estimates are based on the population at large, *the incidence rate of anorexia nervosa in industrialized countries is estimated at 8.1 (not 20.1) per 100,000 population per year.* A recent prevalence study of anorexia nervosa was found to be 20.2 cases per 100,000 population (0.02 percent total population) in the United Kingdom. In a recent study conducted *in the United States, lifetime prevalence rates for anorexia nervosa were found to be 0.51 percent (narrowly defined) and 3.7 percent (not 5 percent) (broadly defined).* A summary of numerous prevalence studies across European countries reported an average prevalence of anorexia nervosa, using strict diagnostic criteria, of 0.28 percent of young females.

There are very few studies of the incidence of bulimia nervosa. A large representative sample of the Dutch population in Holland showed an incidence of bulimia nervosa at 11.4 per 100,000 population per year during the period from 1985 through 1989.

A review of over 50 prevalence studies of bulimia nervosa conducted from 1981 through 1989 in Europe and the United States showed a remarkable consistency in finding that *bulimia nervosa* had *a prevalence rate of about 3 percent (not 10 percent) in adolescents and young adult women.* Partial or subthreshold eating disorders occur at a far greater frequency in the general community—in about 5 to 10 percent of young women. In a recent Canadian study, the lifetime prevalence rate for bulimia nervosa was 1.1 percent for females and 0.1 percent for males. In industrialized countries, the prevalence is about 1 percent for bulimia nervosa.

25.12 The answer is A

Erosion of dental enamel with corresponding decay is associated with the purging behavior of eating disorders, not to the weight loss of eating disorders. Table 25.1 lists medical complications related to weight loss and purging in eating disorders. Among these complications are *bradycardia, delayed gastric emptying,* disturbed *taste sensation,* and *osteoporosis.*

25.13 The answer is E (all)

Bulimia nervosa patients who engage in self-induced vomiting and who abuse purgative or diuretic medications are susceptible to the same complications as anorexia nervosa patients involved in this behavior. Exposure to gastric juices through vomiting can cause severe erosion of the teeth, pathological pulp exposures, diminished masticatory ability, and an unaesthetic facial appearance. Parotid gland enlargement is associated with elevated serum amylase concentrations and is commonly observed in patients who binge and vomit. Acute dilatation of the stomach is a rare emergency condition for patients who binge eat, and esophageal tears can occur in the process of self-induced vomiting. Severe abdominal pain in the bulimia nervosa patient should alert the physician to a diagnosis of gastric dilatation and the need for nasal gastric suction, X-rays, and surgical consultation. Cardiac failure caused by cardiomyopathy from ipecac toxication is a medical emergency that usually results in death. Symptoms of *pericardial pain, dyspnea,* and *generalized muscle weakness* associated with *hypotension,* tachycardia, and electrocardiogram (ECG) abnormalities should alert medical personnel to possible ipecac intoxication.

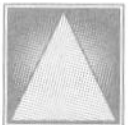

Table 25.1
Medical and Biological Complications of Eating Disorders

Related to weight loss

Cachexia: Loss of fat, muscle mass, reduced thyroid metabolism (low T_3 syndrome), cold intolerance, difficulty in maintaining core body temperature

Cardiac: Loss of cardiac muscle; small heart; cardiac arrhythmias, including atrial and ventricular premature contractions, prolonged His bundle transmission (prolonged QT interval), bardycardia, ventricular tachycardia; sudden death

Digestive-gastrointestinal: Delayed gastric emptying, bloating, constipation, abdominal pain

Reproductive: Amenorrhea, low levels of leutenizing hormone a (LH) and follicle-stimulating hormone (FSH)

Dermatological: Lanugo (fine baby-like hair over body), edema

Hematological: Leukopenia

Neuropsychiatric: Abnormal taste sensation (?zinc deficiency), apathetic depression, mild cognitive disorder

Skeletal: Osteoporosis

Related to purging (vomiting and laxative abuse)

Metabolic: Electrolyte abnormalities, particularly hypokalemic, hypochloremic alkalosis; hypomagnesemia

Digestive-gastrointestinal: Salivary gland and pancreatic inflammation and enlargement with increase in serum amylase, esophageal and gastric erosion, dysfunctional bowel with haustral dilation

Dental: Erosion of dental enamel, particularly of front teeth, with corresponding decay

Neuropsychiatric: Seizures (related to large fluid shifts and electrolyte disturbances), mild neuropathies, fatigue and weakness, mild cognitive disorder

(From Yager I. Eating disorders. In: Stoudemire A, ed. *Clinical Psychiatry for Medical Students.* Philadelphia: JB Lippincott; 1990:324, with permission.)

25.14 The answer is A

There are no laboratory tests that can provide a diagnosis of anorexia nervosa. The medical phenomena present in this disorder result from the starvation or purging behaviors. There are several relevant laboratory tests that should be obtained in these patients. A complete blood count will often reveal a leukopenia with a relative lymphocytosis in emaciated anorexia nervosa patients. If binge eating and purging are present, serum electrolytes will reveal a hypokalemic alkalosis. *Fasting serum glucose concentrations are often low (not increased)* during the emaciated phase, and *serum salivary amylase concentrations are often elevated (not decreased)* if the patient is vomiting. An *electrocardiogram may show ST-segment and T-wave changes,* which are usually secondary to electrolyte disturbances; emaciated patients will have hypotension and bradycardia. Adolescents may have an *elevated (not decreased) serum cholesterol level.* All these values revert to normal with nutritional rehabilitation and cessation of purging behaviors. Endocrine changes that occur, such as amenorrhea, mild hypothyroidism, and hypersecretion of corticotrophin-releasing hormone, are due to the underweight condition and revert to normal with weight gain.

25.15 The answer is E (all)

Most of the physiological and metabolic changes in anorexia nervosa are secondary to the starvation state or purging behaviors. These changes usually revert to normal with nutritional rehabilitation or cessation of the purging behavior (Table 25.1).

25.16 The answer is D

A previous episode of anorexia nervosa is often associated with bulimia nervosa. This episode may have been fully or only moderately expressed.

Undeveloped and underdeveloped breasts, *abnormal insulin secretion*, widespread *endocrine disorder*, and *body weight at least 15 percent below normal* are all associated with anorexia nervosa, not bulimia nervosa.

25.17 The answer is B

Most studies show that anorexia nervosa has a range of mortality rates from 5 percent to *18 percent.*

Answers 25.18–25.25

25.18 The answer is A

25.19 The answer is D

25.20 The answer is C

25.21 The answer is A

25.22 The answer is B

25.23 The answer is B

25.24 The answer is A

25.25 The answer is A

If binging and purging behaviors are occurring in a person who meets diagnostic criteria for anorexia nervosa, bulimia nervosa cannot be the diagnosis. *Severe weight loss and amenorrhea* are two features differentially distinguishing anorexia nervosa from bulimia nervosa.

On rare occasions a central nervous system tumor may be associated with bulimic behaviors. Overeating episodes also occur in the Klüver-Bucy syndrome, which consists of *visual agnosia, compulsive licking and biting,* inability to ignore any stimulus, *and hypersexuality*. Another uncommon syndrome associated with hyperphagia is the Kleine-Levin syndrome, which is characterized by periodic hypersomnia lasting for several weeks.

Ten-year outcome studies in the United States have shown that about one-fourth of anorexic patients recover completely and another *one-half are markedly improved* and functioning fairly well. The other one-fourth includes an overall 7 percent mortality rate and those who are functioning poorly with a chronic underweight condition. Swedish and English studies over a 20- and 30-year period have a mortality rate of 18 percent. Good prognostic indicators across studies include an earlier age of onset (under age 18), no previous hospitalization for the illness, and no purging behaviors. Some factors such as parental conflict, degree of denial, immaturity, and self-esteem have been related to outcome in some studies but not others. Importantly, about half of anorexia nervosa patients will eventually have the symptoms of bulimia, usually within the first year after the onset of anorexia nervosa, which has a higher *fatality rate.*

After between 5 and 10 years about 50 percent of bulimic patients will be fully recovered; 20 percent will continue to meet diagnostic criteria for bulimia nervosa. About one-third of recovered bulimic patients will relapse within 4 years of presentation. Patients with personality disorders marked by problems with impulse control generally have a worse prognosis compared with bulimia nervosa patients with no personality disorder problems.

The severity of illness will determine the intensity of treatment required for the anorexia nervosa patient. Treatment levels can range from an inpatient specialized and multimodal eating disorder unit, to a partial hospitalization or day program, to outpatient care depending on the weight, medical status, and other psychiatric comorbidity of the patient. Decisions about particular treatment modalities and strategies must be based on the needs of the individual patients as well as the capabilities of the treatment setting. Understandably, it has been extremely difficult to subject severely medically ill patients with anorexia nervosa to controlled treatment studies during the emaciated state of the illness. Since patients with anorexia nervosa are resistant to, uninterested in, and fearful of treatment, there are very few (outpatient) controlled treatment studies. Open studies have indicated that a multifaceted treatment approach is the most effective, which includes medical management, psychoeducation, and one-to-one therapy utilizing cognitive and behavior therapy principles. Controlled studies have shown that youth under the age of 18 do better if they participate in family therapy.

In contrast to the relatively *few outpatient treatment studies of anorexia nervosa,* treatment outcome studies of bulimia nervosa have proliferated since the late 1980s.

Family therapy is not widely used in the treatment of bulimia nervosa, as it is for anorexia nervosa, because most patients with bulimia nervosa are in their 20s or older and live away from their family of origin. There is a consensus that families of younger patients should be involved with their treatment; however, controlled studies are needed to prove this.

A family analysis should be done on all anorexia nervosa patients who are living with their families. On the basis of this analysis, a clinical judgment can be made as to what type of family therapy or counseling is advisable. In some cases, family therapy is not possible. However, in those cases, issues of family relationships can be addressed in individual therapy. In some cases, brief counseling sessions with immediate family members may be the extent of family therapy required.

Cognitive-behavioral therapy should be considered the benchmark, first-line treatment for bulimia nervosa. It has been found to be the most effective treatment in over 35 controlled psychosocial studies. About 40 to 50 percent of patients are abstinent from both binge eating and purging at the end of treatment (16 to 20 weeks). Altogether, improvement by a reduction in binge eating and purging occurred in a range from 70 to 95 percent of patients. Additionally, another 30 percent of those who did not show improvement immediately post-treatment nevertheless showed improvement to full recovery 1 year after treatment. In patients with a depressive disorder and bulimia nervosa, cognitive-behavioral therapy was also found to decrease depression.

Cognitive and behavior therapy principles can be applied in both inpatient and outpatient settings in anorexia nervosa, but there are no large-sample-size controlled studies of formal cognitive-behavioral therapy with anorexia nervosa patients.

Generally, a patient with a depressive disorder has a decreased appetite, whereas an anorexia nervosa patient may deny the existence of, yet still have, an appetite. It is *only in the most severe stages of anorexia nervosa that the patient actually has a decreased appetite.*

The diagnostic criteria of anorexia nervosa include a persistent refusal to maintain body weight at or above a minimum expected weight (for example, loss of weight leading to a *body weight of less than 85 percent of the patient's expected weight*) or a failure to gain the expected weight during a period of growth, leading to a body weight less than 85 percent of the expected weight.

26

Normal Sleep and Sleep Disorders

Sleep is absolutely essential for normal, healthy function. The importance to the psychiatrist lies in the fact that sleep disorders are very common, with insomnia being the most frequently reported. The revised 4th edition of the *Diagnostic and Statistical Manual of Mental Disorders* (DSM-IV-TR) organizes the disorders first as primary ones (dyssomnias and parasomnias), then as those related to another mental disorder (such as anxiety, depression, or mania), as due to a general medical condition (the physiological effects of the condition of the sleep-wake cycle), and as substance-induced, due to either intoxication or withdrawal, and from either recreational drugs or medications.

To understand sleep disorders, one must first have a solid understanding of the processes involved in normal sleep. Normal sleep has two essential phases: nonrapid eye movement sleep (NREM) and rapid eye movement sleep (REM). NREM sleep is composed of stages 1 through 4, and is characterized as the phase of sleep associated with a strong reduction in physiological functioning. REM sleep, on the other hand, is characterized by a highly active brain with physiological levels similar to the awake state.

REM sleep is associated with dreaming and is characterized by low-voltage random fast activity with sawtooth waves. The four stages of NREM sleep are qualitatively different, with such differences being displayed in electroencephalogram (EEG) voltages and wave forms. NREM sleep normally changes over to the first REM episode about 90 minutes after a person falls asleep. In disorders such as depression and narcolepsy, this latency is markedly shortened, and REM sleep begins much sooner. Many antidepressants act to suppress REM sleep, thus effectively increasing this latency period back toward normal.

The necessary amount of sleep can vary greatly from person to person. Many factors interfere with sleep, from emotional or physical stress, to multiple substances and medications. Sleep deprivation can lead to ego disorganization, hallucinations, and delusions, and has been shown to lead to death in animals. Students should be aware of how biological rhythms can affect sleep, and how the 24-hour clock affects the natural body clock of 25 hours. Dyssomnias are disturbances in the amount, quality, or timing of sleep, and parasomnias are abnormal or physiological events that occur in connection with various sleep stages or during the sleep-wake transition. To effectively treat sleep disorders, the clinician must have a firm understanding of normal sleep and the factors that interfere with it.

The student should study the questions and answers below for a useful review of these disorders.

HELPFUL HINTS

The student should know and be able to define each of these terms.

- acetylcholine
- advanced sleep phase syndrome
- alveolar hypoventilation syndrome
- circadian rhythm sleep disorder
- delayed sleep phase syndrome
- dysesthesia
- dyssomnias
- EEG
- familial sleep paralysis
- hypersomnia
- idiopathic CNS hypersomnolence
- insomnia:
  - nonorganic
  - organic
  - persistent
  - primary
  - secondary
  - transient
- jactatio capitis nocturna
- K complexes
- Kleine-Levin syndrome
- melatonin
- microsleeps
- narcolepsy
- nightmare disorder
- nightmares
- normal sleep
- paradoxical sleep
- parasomnias
- paroxysmal nocturnal hemoglobinuria
- *pavor nocturnus, incubus*
- poikilothermic
- REM, NREM
- REM latency
- sleep apnea
- sleep deprivation, REM-deprived
- sleep drunkenness
- sleep paralysis, sleep attacks
- sleep patterns
- sleep-related abnormal swallowing syndrome
- sleep-related asthma
- sleep-related bruxism
- sleep-related cardiovascular symptoms
- sleep-related cluster headaches and chronic paroxysmal hemicrania
- sleep-related epileptic seizures
- sleep-related gastroesophageal reflux
- sleep-related (nocturnal) myoclonus syndrome
- sleep spindles
- sleep terror disorder
- sleepwalking disorder
- slow-wave sleep (SWS)
- somniloquy
- somnolence
- L-Tryptophan
- variable sleepers

QUESTIONS

Directions

Each of the questions or incomplete statements below is followed by five suggested responses or completions. Select the *one* that is *best* in each case.

26.1 Sleep is best described as the integrated product of the following two factors

A. transition from day to night (dusk) and night to day (dawn)
B. Melatonin peak and temperature nadir
C. age and health
D. sleep homeostat and the circadian clock
E. seasonality and photoperiods

26.2 Which of the following is the treatment of choice for patients with obstructive sleep apnea?

A. Benzodiazepines
B. Nasal continuous positive airway pressure
C. Weight loss
D. Uvulopalatoplasty
E. Theophylline

26.3 Which of the following is a component of good sleep hygiene?

A. Take daytime naps as needed
B. Establish physical fitness with exercise in the evening
C. Eat larger meals near bedtime
D. Arise at the same time daily
E. All of the above

26.4 Sleep latency is defined as

A. Period of time from the onset of sleep until the first REM period of the night
B. Period of time from turning out the lights until the appearance of stage 2 sleep
C. Time of being continuously awake from the last stage of sleep until the end of the sleep record
D. Period of time from the onset of sleep until the first sleep spindle
E. None of the above

26.5 You begin treating a blind woman who presents with difficulty sleeping. This patient is most likely to be experiencing which of the following circadian disturbances?

A. Delayed sleep phase syndrome
B. Advanced sleep phase syndrome
C. Non–24-hour sleep-wake cycle
D. Irregular sleep-wake rhythm
E. No disturbances

26.6 All of the following statements regarding nightmares are true *except*

A. Massive autonomic signs often accompany nightmares in children
B. REM-suppressing drugs can bring about nightmares
C. Creative people have been shown to have nightmares more frequently
D. Children who have nightmares do not awaken confused
E. Nightmares occur in as much as 50 percent of children aged 3 to 6

26.7 An experiment is performed in which sleeping patients are awakened at the beginning of REM cycles. They are then allowed to sleep with repeated interruption. Which of the following will be the result of this experiment?

A. Decrease in the length of REM periods
B. Increase in the number of REM periods
C. More frequent nighttime awakenings
D. Increase in REM latency
E. No change in sleep patterns

26.8 True statements about circadian processes include all of the following *except*

A. It is easier to shift sleep-wake rhythms to earlier rather than later.
B. Circadian rhythms are endogenously regulated.
C. Slow-wave activity is driven mainly through homeostatic processes, whereas REM sleep is driven by the circadian system.
D. A circadian clock may be located in the retina.
E. Exposure to bright light in the evening and darkness in the morning may help with jet lag when traveling westward.

26.9 Antidepressant effects have been linked to

A. total sleep deprivation
B. selective REM sleep deprivation
C. sleep deprivation in the last half of the night
D. all of the above
E. none of the above

26.10 The characteristic 4-stage pattern of EEG changes from a wakeful state to sleep are

A. regular activity, delta waves at three to seven cycles a second, sleep spindles and K complexes
B. regular activity at three to seven cycles a second, delta waves, sleep spindles, and K complexes
C. regular activity, sleep spindles and K complexes, delta waves at three to seven cycles a second
D. regular activity, delta waves, sleep spindles and K complexes at three to seven cycles a second
E. regular activity at three to seven cycles a second, sleep spindles and K complexes, delta waves

26.11 An 11-year-old girl asked her mother to take her to a psychiatrist because she feared she was going crazy. Several times during the past 2 months she had awakened confused about where she was until she realized that she was on the living room couch or in her little sister's bed, even though she went to bed in her own room. When she woke up in her older brother's bedroom, she became concerned and felt guilty about it. Her younger sister said that she had seen the patient walking during the night, looking like "a zombie," that she did not answer when called, and that she had walked at night several times but usually went back to her bed. The patient feared she had amnesia because she had no memory of anything happening during the night.

Which of the following statements about the patient's disorder is *false*?

A. Usually the disorder begins between the ages of 4 and 8 and peaks at age 12.
B. Patients often have vivid hallucinatory recollections of an emotionally traumatic event with no memory upon awakening.
C. There is no impairment in consciousness several minutes after awakening.
D. The disorder is more commonly seen in girls than in boys.
E. There is a tendency for the disorder to run in families.

26.12 In REM sleep

A. there is infrequent genital tumescence
B. cardiac output is decreased
C. cerebral glucose metabolism is decreased
D. respiratory rate is decreased
E. brain temperature is decreased

26.13 Anatomical sites implicated in the generation of NREM sleep include

A. basal forebrain area
B. thalamus and hypothalamus
C. dorsal raphe nucleus
D. medulla
E. all of the above

26.14 Figure 26.1 illustrates the stages of a patient's sleep pattern. Which of the following statements regarding this sleep pattern is true?

A. The sleep pattern is abnormal because of the shortened latency of REM sleep.
B. The sleep pattern represents human sleep between the ages of newborn and young adult.
C. The sleep pattern is consistent with that found in a patient with depression.
D. The sleep pattern is consistent with that found in a patient with narcolepsy.
E. The sleep pattern is normal.

26.15 During REM sleep

A. the pulse rate is typically five to ten beats below the level of restful waking
B. a poikilothermic condition is present
C. frequent involuntary body movements are seen
D. dreams are typically lucid and purposeful
E. sleepwalking may occur

26.16 The symptoms of narcolepsy include all of the following *except*

A. catalepsy
B. daytime sleepiness
C. hallucinations
D. sleep paralysis
E. cataplexy

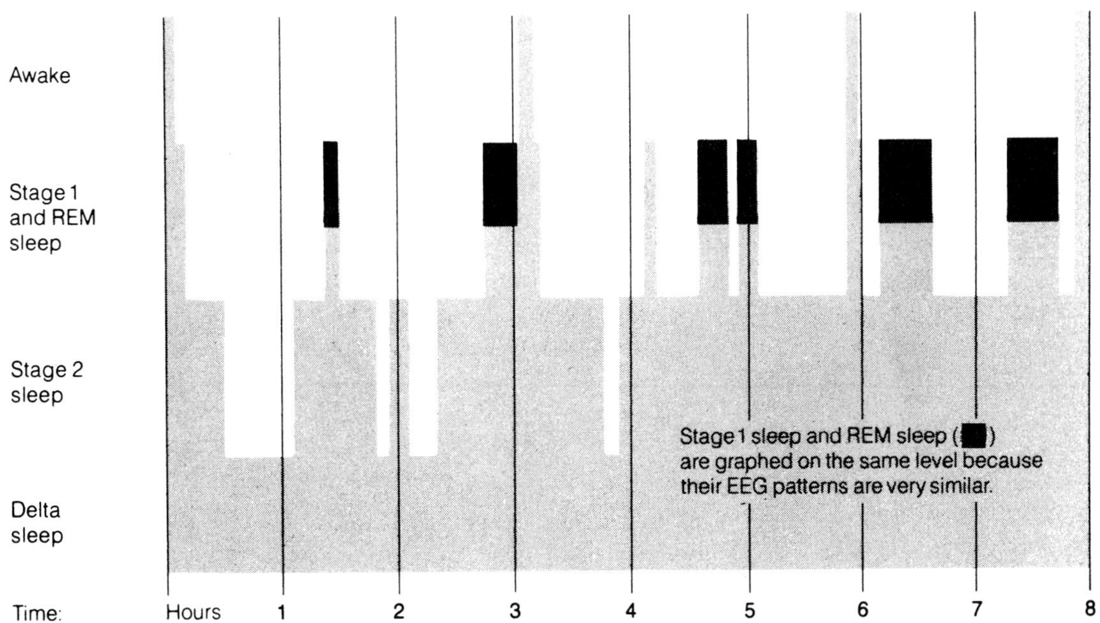

FIGURE 26.1

Reproduced with permission from Hauri P. *The Sleep Disorders.* Current Concepts. Kalamazoo, MI: Upjohn; 1982:82.

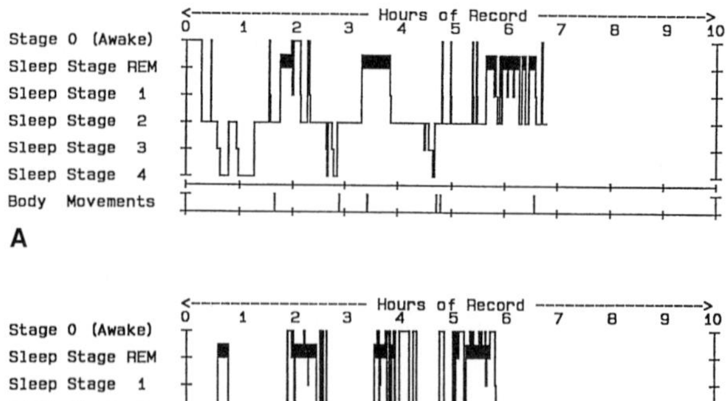

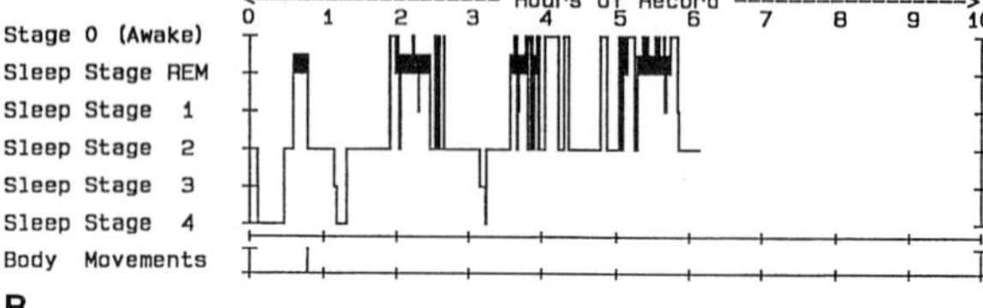

FIGURE 26.2

Reproduced with permission from Hauri P. *The Sleep Disorders.* Current Concepts. Kalamazoo, MI: Upjohn; 1982:82.

26.17 Which of the following statements about the sleep stage histograms shown in Figure 26.2 is true?

A. *A* is characteristic of obstructive sleep apnea syndrome.
B. *A* is characteristic of anxiety disorder.
C. *B* is characteristic of major depressive disorder.
D. *A* is characterized by an abnormal latency to REM sleep.
E. Both are within normal limits.

26.18 True statements about sleep in the elderly include all of the following *except*

A. After the age of 65, one-third of women and one-fifth of men report that they take over 30 minutes to fall asleep.
B. The incidence of nocturnal myoclonus increases with age.
C. Average daily total sleep time decreases after the age of 65.
D. Death rates are higher in the elderly both in people who sleep more than 9 hours and those who sleep fewer than 5 hours.
E. Individuals with periodic limb movements sleep about an hour less per night than controls.

26.19 Many benzodiazepine hypnotic medications cause

A. profound hypersomnia during withdrawal
B. increases in slow wave sleep
C. reductions in REM sleep
D. abnormally decreased EEG beta and sleep spindle activity
E. all of the above

26.20 Which of the following features is *not* typical of REM sleep?

A. Dreams are typically concrete and realistic.
B. Polygraph measures show irregular patterns.
C. The resting muscle potential is lower in REM sleep than in a waking state.
D. Near-total paralysis of the postural muscles is present.
E. A condition of temperature regulation similar to that in reptiles occurs.

26.21 Which of the following statements does *not* correctly describe sleep regulation?

A. Melatonin secretion helps regulate the sleep-wake cycle.
B. Destruction of the dorsal raphe nucleus of the brainstem reduces sleep.
C. L-Tryptophan deficiency is associated with less time spent in NREM sleep.
D. REM sleep can be reduced by increased firing of noradrenergic neurons.
E. Disrupted REM sleep patterns in patients with depression show shortened REM latency.

Directions

Each group of questions below consists of lettered headings followed by a list of numbered words or phrases. For each numbered word or phrase, select the *one* lettered heading that is most closely associated with it. Each lettered heading may be selected once, more than once, or not at all.

Questions 26.22–26.31

A. REM sleep
B. NREM sleep

26.22 Sleepwalking
26.23 Bed-wetting (enuresis)
26.24 Paroxysmal hemicrania
26.25 Erections
26.26 D sleep
26.27 Paradoxical sleep
26.28 Slow wave sleep (SWS)
26.29 EEG synchronized sleep
26.30 Most occurs in the last half of the night
26.31 Autonomic functioning is usually slow and steady

Questions 26.32–26.36

A. Sleep terror disorder
B. Nocturnal myoclonus
C. Jactatio capitis nocturnus
D. Sleep-related hemolysis
E. Sleep-related bruxism

26.32 Urge to move the legs
26.33 Brownish-red morning urine
26.34 Patient wakes up screaming
26.35 Head banging
26.36 Damage to the teeth

ANSWERS

26.1 The answer is D

Sleep is the integrated product of two oscillatory processes. The first process, frequently referred to as the *sleep homeostat*, is an oscillation that stems from the accumulation and dissipation of sleep debt. The biological substrates encoding sleep debt are not known, although adenosine is emerging as a primary candidate neuromodulator of the sleep homeostat. The second oscillatory process is governed by *the circadian clock* and controls a daily rhythm in sleep propensity or, conversely, arousal.

The circadian cycle in arousal (wakefulness) steadily increases throughout the day, reaching a maximum immediately before the circadian *increase in plasma melatonin*. Arousal subsequently decreases to coincide with the circadian trough in *core body temperature*. Experiments imposing forced sleep schedules throughout the circadian day have shown that an uninterrupted 8-hour bout of sleep can only be obtained if sleep is initiated approximately 6 hours before the *temperature nadir*. This nadir typically occurs at approximately 5:00 AM to 6:00 AM. In healthy individuals, initiating sleep between 11:00 PM and 12:00 AM affords the highest probability of getting 8 solid hours of sleep.

Whether humans are truly seasonal is still a point of considerable debate. Several lines of evidence exist that suggest the presence of a residual tendency toward seasonality. A peak in the rate of suicide occurs in the summer; this peak is cross-cultural. Birth rates also tend to show a seasonal variation; a small but distinguishable peak in the rate of births occurs in spring and summer. This pattern, however, is itself variable and is heavily influenced by unknown cultural and geographical factors. Interestingly, the amplitude of the spring-summer birth rate peak has diminished as societies have become industrialized.

Age is one contribution to the sleep homeostat. Sleep deprivation studies have shown that the homeostat component of sleep is remarkably similar among individuals of similar age. There is a well-established age-dependent decline in sleep need.

Biological evidence exists for an adaptive system that allows humans to track the transition from *day to night (dusk)* and *night to day (dawn)*. This system could function to maintain proper sleep patterns during changing *photoperiods* (changing day length associated with seasonality). Ill health, emotional or physical can disrupt normal sleep physiology.

26.2 The answer is B

Nasal continuous positive airway pressure (nCPAP) is the treatment of choice for obstructive sleep apnea. Other procedures include *weight loss*, nasal surgery, tracheostomy, and *uvulopalatoplasty*. Some medications may normalize sleep in patients with apnea. SSRIs and heterocyclic antidepressant drugs sometimes help treat sleep apnea by decreasing the amount of time spent in REM sleep, the stage of sleep in which apneic episodes occur most often. In addition, *theophylline* has been shown to decrease the number of episodes of apnea; however, it may interfere with the overall quality of sleep, limiting its general utility. When apnea is established or suspected, patients must *avoid the use of sedative medication*, including alcohol, because it can considerably exacerbate the condition, which may then become life threatening.

26.3 The answer is D

A common finding is that a patient's lifestyle leads to sleep disturbance. This is usually phrased as *inadequate sleep hygiene*, referring to a problem in following generally accepted practices to aid sleep. These include, for instance, *keeping regular hours of bedtime and arousal*, avoiding excessive caffeine, *not eating heavy meals before bedtime*, and getting adequate exercise (exercise during the day, *not in the evening* as this may disturb sleep). In general, *napping is discouraged*, except in elderly and debilitated patients. Two caveats are in order when helping to educate a patient about sleep hygiene. The first is that these are general principles and are not applicable to all patients. The second is that when trying to modify a patient's behavior, it is usually better to focus on one or two changes at a time, rather than assaulting him or her with a panoply of desired changes, which can come across as overwhelming.

26.4 The answer is B

Common polysomnographic measures are used to diagnose and describe sleep disorders. *Sleep latency* is the period of time from turning out the lights until the appearance of stage 2 sleep. The period of time from the onset of sleep until the first REM period is known as *REM latency*. *Early morning awakening* is defined as a time of being continuously awake from the last stage of the sleep until the end of the sleep record (usually at 7 AM). There has been no defined measure of the period of time from the onset of sleep until the appearance of the first sleep spindle.

26.5 The answer is C

In a *non–24-hour sleep-wake cycle*, a patient may report intermittent insomnia that periodically recurs. It is usually found in blind individuals and results from a complete failure of the resetting mechanism of the pacemaker. The patient then begins to live with a propensity to have a sleep-wake rhythm with the inherent and uncorrected period of the internal pacemaker, approximately 24.15 hours. In a world in which day and night follow a 24.0-hour cycle, this means that the patient's propensity for sleep is constantly shifting forward relative to what would be appropriate to his or her surroundings. The result is that he or she experiences insomnia, which is periodically exacerbated when his or her internal rhythm is most out of phase with the environment and which improves as he or she moves more in phase with his surroundings. Melatonin administration has been demonstrated to be useful in regulating sleep in these individuals.

Delayed sleep phase syndrome is a persistent pattern of late sleep onset and late awakening times, with an inability to fall asleep and awaken at a desired earlier time. *Advanced sleep phase syndrome*, in contrast, early sleep onset and early awakening, with an inability to fall asleep and awaken at a desired later time. *Irregular sleep-wake rhythm* is characterized by constantly shifting hours of sleepiness and wakefulness. It is generally an affliction of disco aficionados and others who maintain a highly irregular schedule, although it is sometimes seen in persons who have had tumors or other pathology of the hypothalamus. Treatment is organized around altering behavior, encouraging the patient to keep regular hours of bedtime and arising and to avoid napping.

26.6 The answer is A

Nightmares are vivid dreams that become progressively more anxiety producing, ultimately resulting in an awakening. They can *occur occasionally in as much as one-half of children in the range of 3 to 6 years of age*. In contrast to night terrors, the *child is not confused, does not exhibit the massive autonomic signs*, and describes having had a scary dream. Nightmares in children are not associated with psychiatric illness; in contrast, approximately one-half of the roughly 1 percent of adults who experience frequent nightmares are found to have disorders, including borderline personality and schizophrenia. *Nightmares are sometimes brought out by REM-suppressing drugs*, in which case, the treatment is to gradually discontinue the medication, if possible. Some workers suggest that nightmares occur more frequently in persons with certain personality traits, including those with thin boundaries and *more creative individuals*. There is no widely accepted medical intervention.

26.7 The answer is B

Prolonged periods of sleep deprivation sometimes lead to ego disorganization, hallucinations, and delusions. Depriving persons of REM sleep by awakening them at the beginning of REM cycles *increases the number of REM periods and the amount of REM sleep* (rebound increase) when they are allowed to sleep without interruption. Studies have also shown that REM deprivation leads to a *shortening of REM latency (not an increase)*. There has been no evidence of increased frequency of nighttime awakenings in studies of REM deprivation.

REM-deprived patients may exhibit irritability and lethargy. In studies with rats, sleep deprivation produces a syndrome that includes a debilitated appearance, skin lesions, increased food intake, weight loss, increased energy expenditure, decreased body temperature, and death. The neuroendocrine changes include increased plasma norepinephrine and decreased plasma thyroxine levels.

26.8 The answer is A

The daily sleep-wake cycle is an example of a circadian rhythm (from the Latin *circa*, meaning "about," and *dies*, meaning "day"). *Circadian rhythms are endogenously regulated* by a biological clock located in the suprachiasmatic nuclei of the anterior hypothalamus, which in turn is synchronized with the environment by visual or other, nonphotic time clues (*Zeitgebers,* meaning "time givers"). For example, if humans and animals are kept in an environment devoid of time clues, the period length of the sleep-wake cycle and other biological rhythms, such as core body temperature or cortisol, increases from about 24 hours to about 24.2 hours; this condition is called free-running. If, however, a 24-hour light-dark cycle of sufficient amplitude is imposed on this environment, subjects revert to a 24-hour sleep-wake cycle, that is, the subjects and their rhythms are entrained to the 24-hour day.

Sleep and wakefulness are influenced strongly by two separate processes: (1) an endogenous biological clock, which drives the circadian rhythm of the propensity for sleep and the characteristics of sleep across the 24-hour day; and (2) a homeostatic process that increases sleep propensity the longer the period of wakefulness prior to sleep.

Studies have supported the hypothesis that *slow-wave activity is driven mainly through homeostatic processes* whereas REM sleep as well as sleep spindles are driven by the circadian system. Humans appear to have two peaks of daytime sleepiness. The first, and obvious, one is at night in the normally entrained individual; the second is in midafternoon ("siesta hour"). Not surprisingly, automobile accidents, in which the driver falls asleep at the wheel, peak during the last half of the night and in the midafternoon. If the circadian temperature curve is used to index the phase position of the circadian pacemaker, it is seen that the major period of sleepiness occurs near the nadir of temperature, that is, at about 3:00 to 5:00 AM in normal circumstances. Both the duration of sleep and the type of sleep are influenced strongly by the phase position of sleep onset. People tend to awaken on the rising limb of the temperature curve; thus, sleep tends to be longest when it starts near the peak of the temperature curve. Furthermore, REM sleep is most likely to occur near the temperature nadir; thus, REM latency is shorter and REM time higher during morning naps compared with afternoon or evening naps.

The 24-hour sleep-wake rhythm is driven by the suprachiasmatic nuclei synchronized to the environmental light–dark cycle by *Zeitgebers*. Lesions of the suprachiasmatic nuclei in animals result in arrhythmic rest-activity patterns, which no longer follow a circadian rhythm but are distributed in numerous short bouts of sleep and wakefulness during the 24-hour period. Despite the dramatic alteration of the temporal organization of sleep and wakefulness the total amount of sleep and wakefulness in 24 hours remains fairly constant in the suprachiasmatic nuclei-lesioned animal. Indeed, a suprachiasmatic nuclei-lesioned animal deprived of sleep shows the normal compensatory increase in sleep during the recovery period, thereby demonstrating that the homeostatic and circadian processes can be separated. Although the major circadian pacemaker in mammals is the suprachiasmatic nuclei, a second *circadian clock may be located in the retina.*

Because the endogenous period in humans is slightly longer than 24 hours, *it is easier to shift sleep-wake rhythms to later rather than earlier*. For example, most individuals cope with jet lag more easily when traveling west than when traveling east. It usually takes about 1 day to accommodate for each time zone traveled when moving in an easterly direction, somewhat faster in a westerly direction. In addition, shift workers seem to feel better and perform better when going from a day to an evening to a night shift (forward shifting) than from a day to a night to an evening shift (backward shifting). Appropriate administration of bright light and darkness may ameliorate jet lag and shift-work problems by hastening the resynchronization of the endogenous clock modulating sleep-wakefulness and controlling temperature and other psychobiological rhythms. For example, *exposure to bright light in the evening and darkness in the morning* may help with jet lag when traveling westward or shifting from an evening to a night schedule of work. In addition, the administration of exogenous melatonin may shift the phase position of the clock and offers hope for treating jet lag, shift work, and other circadian sleep-wake disorders in which rapid resynchronization of the internal clock with the sleep-wake cycle is required. At this time, however, neither the efficacy nor the safety of melatonin administration for more than very short-term use has been demonstrated.

26.9 The answer is D (all)

Although the morbidity associated with sleep deprivation has been emphasized, the paradoxical finding that *total sleep deprivation*, partial *sleep deprivation* (especially in the last half of the night), and *selective REM sleep deprivation* have antidepressant effects in depressed patients must not be overlooked; unfortunately, the beneficial effect of total and partial sleep deprivation only lasts until the next sleep period, after which the patient typically awakens depressed again. Hence, sleep may be depressogenic in some patients. There is some evidence suggesting that selective REM sleep deprivation repeated over about 2 weeks, or a continued sleep-phase advance protocol after total sleep deprivation, might result in a sustained antidepressant effect. However, so far the latter treatment modes have scientific rather than practical implications because these protocols are extremely costly and time-consuming.

Many of the following observations suggest that some depressed patients are overaroused, at least in some areas of the brain: the antidepressant effects of sleep deprivation, loss of delta sleep and sleep continuity, and increased core body temperature during sleep. Moreover, a preliminary PET study showed that cerebral glucose metabolism during the first NREM period was significantly elevated in depressed patients compared with normal controls and that depressed patients had some of the abnormalities during sleep that had previously been reported in other patients while awake, such as decreased relative metabolic activity in the anterior cingulate and ventral-medial prefrontal cortex. Consistent with the overarousal hypothesis, depressed patients who responded to sleep deprivation showed significantly elevated metabolic rates within the anterior cingulate gyrus before sleep deprivation as compared with nonresponders and normal controls. After clinical improvement, metabolic activity normalized in responders, but did not change in the two other groups.

26.10 The answer is E

The characteristic sequential pattern of electroencephalographic (EEG) changes from a wakeful state to sleep are *regular activity at 3 to 7 cycles a second, sleep spindles and K complexes, and delta waves*—not *regular activity*, *delta waves*, and *sleep spindles and K complexes* in other configurations.The waking EEG is characterized by alpha waves of 8 to 12 cycles a second and low-voltage activity of mixed frequency. As the person falls asleep, alpha activity begins to disappear. Stage 1, considered the lightest stage of sleep, is characterized by low-voltage regular activity at three to seven cycles a second. After a few seconds or minutes, that stage gives way to stage 2, a pattern showing frequent spindle-shaped tracings at 12 to 14 cycles a second (sleep spindles) and slow triphasic waves known as K complexes. Soon thereafter, delta waves—high-voltage activity at 0.5 to 2.5 cycles a second—make their appearance and occupy less than 50 percent of the tracing (stage 3). Eventually, in stage 4, delta waves occupy more than 50 percent of the record. It is common practice to describe stages 3 and 4 as delta sleep or slow-wave sleep because of their characteristic appearance on the EEG record.

26.11 The answer is D

The patient's diagnosis is sleepwalking disorder. This disorder is *more commonly seen in boys than in girls*. Patients often have *vivid hallucinatory recollections* of emotionally traumatic events with *no memory upon awakening*. Sleepwalking disorder consists of a sequence of complex behaviors initiated in the first third of the night during deep nonrapid eye movement (NREM) sleep (stages 3 and 4). It consists of arising from bed during sleep and walking about, appearing unresponsive during the episode, amnestic for the sleepwalking on awakening, and with *no impairment in consciousness several minutes after awakening*. Sleepwalking usually begins *between ages 6 and 12* and *tends to run in families*.

26.12 The answer is B

In REM sleep, there may be genital tumescence, *cardiac output is decreased*, cerebral glucose metabolism is unchanged or increased (not decreased), respiratory rate is variable (not decreased), and brain temperature is increased (not decreased).

26.13 The answer is E (all)

At least five anatomical sites have been implicated in the generation of NREM sleep: the *basal forebrain area, thalamus, hypothalamus, dorsal raphe nucleus, and* nucleus tractus solitarius of the *medulla*. For example, lesions of the preoptic basal forebrain area produce hyposomnia lasting 4 to 6 weeks in rats and cats, whereas electrical stimulation and local warming of this region elicit both EEG and behavioral signs of sleep. In addition, some noncholinergic neurons in the basal forebrain discharge selectively during NREM sleep. The thalamus in general and the reticular nucleus of the thalamus in particular appear to play an important role in the generation of cortical sleep spindles (12 to 14 Hz) and delta waves (0.5 to 3 Hz, 75 mV or greater in humans) during NREM sleep. Recently, Mircea Steriade and colleagues hypothesized that thalamocortical cells are hyperpolarized by corticothalamic cells and are depolarized by cholinergic input from basal forebrain and the lateral dorsal tegmental and pedunculopontine tegmental, as well as through noradrenergic, serotonergic, and excitatory amino-acid input. The thalamocortical cells, which drive and synchronize the ensembles of cortical cells to produce the major EEG rhythms, change their rhythms from spindle frequencies to delta frequencies as they hyperpolarize. This theory also explains why immediately prior to and during REM sleep, when cholinergic activity in the lateral dorsal tegmental and pedunculopontine tegmental is high, the EEG becomes gradually desynchronized. While histaminergic cells in the posterior hypothalamus maintain arousal, ventrolateral preoptic neurons in the anterior hypothalamus may be involved in the induction of slow-wave sleep. The dorsal tegmental, the origin of the serotonergic projections of the brain, may be involved in the induction of sleep, at least insofar as either selective lesions or depletion of serotonin induce a dramatic insomnia lasting several days. Finally, the nucleus tractus solitarius was implicated by experiments in which medullary anesthesia or cooling of the fourth ventricular floor caused EEG activation. Low-frequency stimulation of this region produced EEG synchronization and behavioral sleep while cells in this region increase their discharge rate during NREM sleep. These regions appear to facilitate sleep; however, none have been found to be essential.

26.14 The answer is E

Figure 26.1 represents a *normal sleep pattern* of a young human adult. The periods of REM sleep shown are consistent with that found in a normal young adult, occurring every 90 to 100 minutes during the night, with most REM sleep occurring in the last third of the night.

Depressed patients, in contrast, experience *shortened REM latency* (60 minutes or less), an increased percentage of REM sleep (over the normal 25 percent), and a shift in REM distribution from most occurring in the last half (normal) to most occurring in the first half of the night (abnormal).

Narcolepsy is characterized by abnormal manifestations of REM sleep, including the appearance of REM sleep within 10 minutes of sleep onset (sleep-onset REM periods), as well as hypnagogic and hypnopompic hallucinations, cataplexy, and sleep paralysis.

Sleep patterns change over the life span. In the neonatal period, REM sleep occurs during more than 50 percent of total sleep time, whereas in *young adulthood*, REM sleep occurs during 25 percent of total sleep time. In addition, the EEG pattern of *newborns* goes from the alert state directly to the REM state without going through stages 1 through 4.

26.15 The answer is B

During REM sleep *a poikilothermic condition is present.* Poikilothermia is a state in which body temperature varies with the temperature of the surrounding medium. In contrast, a homeothermic condition is present during wakefulness and NREM sleep; in that condition the body temperature remains constant regardless of the temperature of the surrounding medium.

In REM sleep *the pulse rate is not typically five to ten beats below the level of restful waking;* that is characteristic of NREM sleep. In fact, pulse, respiration, and blood pressure in humans are all high during REM sleep—much higher than during NREM sleep and often higher than during waking. Because of motor inhibition, *body movement is absent (not frequent)* during REM sleep. *Dreams* during REM sleep *are typically abstract and unreal (not lucid and purposeful).* Dreaming does occur during NREM sleep, but is typically more realistic. *Sleepwalking does not occur* in REM sleep but does occur during stages 3 and 4 of NREM sleep.

26.16 The answer is A

Catalepsy is a condition in which a person maintains the body position in which it is placed. It is a symptom observed in severe cases of catatonic schizophrenia. Excessive *daytime sleepiness,* naps, and the accessory symptoms of *cataplexy, sleep paralysis,* and hypnagogic *hallucinations* are the classically recognized symptoms of narcolepsy. Patients generally report the onset of daytime sleepiness before the accessory symptoms are noted.

The sleepiness may persist throughout the day, but more often it is periodic and may be relieved by a sleep attack or by a nap from which the patient characteristically awakens refreshed. Thus, there are often refractory periods of 2 or 3 hours of almost normal alertness. The sleep attacks are usually associated with characteristic times of the day, such as after meals, when some degree of sleepiness is quite normal. The attacks are typically irresistible and may even occur while eating, riding a bicycle, or actively conversing and also during sexual relations.

Cataplexy, which occurs in 67 to 95 percent of the cases, is paralysis of the antigravity muscles in the awake state. A cataplectic attack often begins during expressions of emotion, such as laughter, anger, and exhilaration. The attacks vary in intensity and frequency; they can consist of a weakening of the knees, a jaw drop, a head drop, or a sudden paralysis of all of the muscles of the body—except for the eyes and the diaphragm—leading to a complete collapse.

Sleep paralysis is a neurological phenomenon that is most likely due to a temporary dysfunction of the reticular activating system. It consists of brief episodes of an inability to move or speak when awake or asleep.

Hypnagogic hallucinations are vivid perceptual, dream-like experiences occurring at sleep onset. They occur in about 50 percent of patients. The accompanying affect is usually fear or dread. The hallucinatory imagery is remembered best after a brief narcoleptic sleep attack, when it is often described as a dream.

26.17 The answer is C

The sleep stage histograms demonstrate *normal sleep* in *A* and that found in a patient with *major depressive disorder* in *B*. As shown in histogram A, *REM sleep normally has a latency (time between sleep onset and first REM episode) of about 90 minutes.* In contrast, REM latency is shortened to 60 minutes or less in major depressive disorder, as shown in histogram B. Other findings in *B* consistent with major depressive disorder include disruption of sleep continuity and early morning awakenings.

Obstructive sleep apnea syndrome is characterized by repetitive episodes of upper airway obstruction that occur during sleep, usually associated with a reduction in blood oxygen saturation. Sleep is disturbed by frequent awakenings, while REM and slow-wave (stages 3 and 4) sleep are nearly absent.

26.18 The answer is C

After the age of 65, about one-third of women and one-fifth of men report that they take *over 30 minutes to fall asleep.* Wake time after sleep onset (WASO) tends to increase with age, perhaps because of the greater incidence of sleep-related breathing disorders (i.e., mild apnea) and *nocturnal myoclonus.* In general, the severity of apnea in older persons is mild compared with that seen in patients with clinical sleep apnea. *Periodic limb movements* during sleep are also common in the elderly, with prevalence rates ranging from 25 to 60 percent in various studies of the healthy elderly. Individuals with periodic limb movements are reported to sleep about an hour less per night than controls without periodic limb movements. Perhaps as a result, napping also increases with age, although it rarely accounts for a large proportion of total sleep time in healthy individuals.

Average daily total sleep time actually increases slightly (rather than decreases) after the age of about 65. Greater numbers of elderly individuals fall into either long-sleeping (>9 hours) or short-sleeping (<5 hours) subgroups. It is noteworthy that *death rates are higher both in long-sleeping and excessively short-sleeping individuals.* The reasons for that are still unknown, although there has been speculation that sleep apnea might contribute to increased mortality in the long-sleeping group.

Although the incidence of insomnia and certain other sleep-wake disorders tends to increase with age, clinicians should not assume that age explains these complaints. Rather, the clinician must search for underlying conditions that can be treated, such as medical, neurological, psychiatric, situational, pharmacological, or circadian factors.

26.19 The answer is C

Alcohol, anxiolytics, opioids, and sedative-hypnotics all promote sleep by sedation. However, the resulting sleep, while apparently of greater quantity, is of poorer quality. Many benzodiazepine hypnotic medications alter the basic architecture of sleep. Most *reduce (rather than increase) slow-wave sleep,* and *some reduce REM sleep. Abnormally increased (not decreased) EEG beta and sleep spindle activity* result from ingesting some hypnotic drugs. Alcohol may relax a tense person and thereby decrease latency to sleep; however, sleep later in the night is fragmented by arousals. As tolerance develops to chronic drug and alcohol use, increased dosage is needed to sustain effects; lower dosage produces an abstinence syndrome, and sleep regresses to its initial abnormal pattern. Furthermore, during withdrawal of hypnotic medication or after tolerance has developed, the sleep disturbance can rebound to a more severe level than the initial problem leading to insomnia.

By contrast, psychostimulant use poses a different problem. Cocaine, amphetamine and related stimulants, caffeine, and theobromine all produce CNS arousal that may persist into the sleep period and produce insomnia. Especially in cases of stimulant abuse, an individual usually becomes severely sleep deprived. Over time a massive sleep debt accumulates, and upon substance discontinuation, *profound hypersomnia* results. This compensatory sleep, or sleep rebound, continues for an extended time (several weeks or more in some instances).

26.20 The answer is A

In REM sleep, *dreams are typically abstract and surreal, not concrete and realistic.* People report dreaming 60 to 90 percent of the time during REM sleep. Dreaming also occurs during NREM sleep, but these dreams are lucid and purposeful.

During REM sleep, *polygraph measures show irregular patterns*, sometimes close to waking patterns. Aside from measures of muscle tone, physiological measures during REM periods could be inferred as those of a person in a waking state. Pulse, respiration, and blood pressure are all high during REM sleep, higher than during NREM sleep, and sometimes higher than during waking.

The *resting muscle potential is lower in REM sleep* than in a waking state. *Near-total paralysis of the postural muscles* is present during REM sleep, so that the body cannot move. This motor inhibition is sometimes thought to be associated with dreams of being unable to move. Also during REM sleep, a condition of *temperature regulation* similar to that in reptiles occurs; in this condition (poikilothermia) body temperature varies with the temperature of the environment.

26.21 The answer is C

L-Tryptophan deficiency is associated with less time spent in REM sleep, not in NREM sleep. Ingestion of large amounts of L-tryptophan reduces sleep latency and nocturnal awakening.

Melatonin secretion helps regulate the sleep-wake cycle; melatonin secretion is inhibited by bright light, so that the lowest concentrations occur during the day. A circadian pacemaker in the hypothalamus may regulate melatonin secretion. *Destruction of the dorsal raphe nucleus of the brainstem* reduces sleep, as nearly all of the brain's serotonergic cell bodies are located there. Reduced REM sleep can also be caused by *increased firing of noradrenergic neurons.*

Disrupted REM sleep patterns in patients with depression show shortened REM latency. As compared with normal sleep patterns, those of people with depression also show an increased percentage of REM sleep and a shift of REM sleep from the last to the first half of the night.

Answers 26.22–26.31

26.22 The answer is B

26.23 The answer is B

26.24 The answer is A

26.25 The answer is A

26.26 The answer is A

26.27 The answer is A

26.28 The answer is B

26.29 The answer is B

26.30 The answer is A

26.31 The answer is B

Sleepwalking occurs during the first third of the night during NREM sleep, stages 3 and 4. Bed-wetting *(enuresis)*, a repetitive and inappropriate passage of urine during sleep, is usually associated with NREM sleep, stages 3 and 4, but may occur during any stage of sleep. *Paroxysmal hemicrania* is a type of unilateral vascular headache that is exacerbated during sleep and that occurs only in association with REM sleep. Erections are associated with REM sleep. Almost every REM period is accompanied by a partial or full penile *erection* or clitoral erection in women.

Most mammals have two major phases of sleep: rapid eye movement (REM) sleep and nonrapid eye movement (NREM) sleep. REM sleep is sometimes called *dreaming or D sleep* insofar as it is associated with dreaming, or *paradoxical sleep*, because the electroencephalogram (EEG) becomes activated during this state of sleep. NREM sleep, on the other hand, conforms to traditional concepts of sleep as a time of decreased physiological and psychological activity; it is therefore sometimes called orthodox sleep or *slow wave sleep (SWS), EEG synchronized sleep*, or S sleep.

NREM sleep is further divided into four sleep stages on the basis of visually scored EEG patterns.

Sleep normally begins with stage 1, a brief transitional phase, before progressing successively into stages 2 through 4. Stage 2 sleep is defined by the presence of sleep spindles and K-complexes in the EEG. Stage 3 and stage 4 sleep, or delta sleep, are defined by the presence of delta waves in the EEG, a moderate (20 to 50 percent) and large (>50 percent) proportion of an epoch (usually 30 seconds long) of sleep, respectively.

REM sleep is characterized by an activated EEG, loss of tone in the major antigravity muscles, and periodic bursts of rapid eye movements. The REM latency is usually about 70 to 100 minutes in normal subjects but may be shortened significantly in some patients with depressive disorder, eating disorders, borderline personality disorder, schizophrenia, alcohol use disorder, or other psychiatric disorders. Thereafter, NREM and REM sleep oscillate with a cycle length of roughly 90 to 100 minutes. When it does occur, delta sleep is highest in the first NREM period of the night and declines with each successive NREM period. Most of the delta sleep occurs in the first half of the night and *most of the REM sleep occurs in the last half of the night.*

REM sleep and NREM sleep differ from each other in many psychological and physiological domains. On a psychological level, REM sleep is associated with dreaming mentation, while NREM sleep is more likely to be associated with abstract thinking. *Autonomic functioning* is often highly variable during REM sleep; it is usually slow and steady in NREM sleep.

Answers 26.32–26.36

26.32 The answer is B

26.33 The answer is D

26.34 The answer is A

26.35 The answer is C

26.36 The answer is E

Nocturnal myoclonus consists of highly stereotyped contractions of certain leg muscles during sleep. Though rarely painful, the syndrome causes an almost irresistible *urge to move the legs*, thus interfering with sleep. *Sleep-related hemolysis* (paroxysmal nocturnal hemoglobinuria) is a rare acquired chronic hemolytic anemia in which intravascular hemolysis results in hemoglobinemia and hemoglobinuria. Accelerated during sleep, the hemolysis and consequent hemoglobinuria color the *morning urine a brownish red.* Sleep-related hemolysis is diagnosed as sleep disorder due to a general medical condition.

In *sleep terror disorder* the patient typically sits up in bed with a frightened expression and *wakes up screaming*, often with a feeling of intense terror; patients are often amnestic for the episode. Sleep-related *head banging (jactatio capitis nocturnus)* consists chiefly of rhythmic to-and-fro head rocking, and less commonly of total body rocking, occurring just before or during sleep, rarely persisting into or occurring in deep non-rapid eye movement (NREM) sleep. According to dentists, 5 to 10 percent of the population suffers from *sleep-related bruxism* (tooth grinding) severe enough to produce noticeable *damage to the teeth.* Although the condition often goes unnoticed by the sleeper, except for an occasional feeling of jaw ache in the morning, the bed partner and roommates are acutely cognizant of the situation, as they are awakened repeatedly by the sound.

27 Impulse-Control Disorders Not Elsewhere Classified

Impulsive behavior can be quite common in the personalities of normal individuals. However, the hallmark of impulse-control disorders is the individual's inability to stop impulses that may cause harm to themselves or others. The revised 4th edition of the *Diagnostic and Statistical Manual of Mental Disorders* (DSM-IV-TR) lists several impulse-control disorders that are not classified under any other diagnostic heading in DSM-IV-TR, but are nonetheless serious enough to be highlighted. These are intermittent explosive disorder, kleptomania, pyromania, pathological gambling, trichotillomania, and impulse-control disorder not otherwise specified. These disorders are all quite different in their epidemiology, etiology, psychodynamic formulation, course, prognosis, and treatment, but share other characteristics. Affected individuals often feel anxiety or tension in considering these behaviors, and this anxiety or tension is relieved or diminished once the impulse is acted on.

Intermittent Explosive Disorder is evidenced by episodes of acting out aggression and causing bodily harm and/or property destruction. Kleptomania is evidenced by acting out the impulse to steal objects without the motive of monetary gain. Pyromania is evidenced by the uncontrollable urge to set fires. Pathological Gambling is evidenced by habitual, self-destructive gambling. Trichotillomania is evidenced by recurrent hair pulling resulting in significant hair loss, often to the point of baldness or to removing eyebrows and lashes.

As with most psychiatric disorders, both biological and psychological components contributing to the etiology of these disorders have been studied and identified. Biological investigations have been particularly relevant to the understanding of violent impulse-control disorders. Studies include investigations of the limbic system of the brain, the effects of testosterone, histories of head trauma and childhood abuse, childhood histories of attention deficit/hyperactivity disorder, and CSF levels of 5-hydroxyindolacetic acid (5-HIAA), a metabolite of serotonin. Alcohol abuse has been associated with some of the more violent impulse-control disorders and can act as a facilitator to losing control. Unfulfilled narcissistic, dependency, and self-object needs have also been implicated, as are exposure to parental impulse-control problems during development.

The student should study the questions and answers below for a useful review of these disorders.

HELPFUL HINTS

These terms relate to impulse-control disorders and should be defined by the student.

- alopecia
- anticonvulsants
- attention-deficit/hyperactivity disorder
- behavior therapy
- benzodiazepines
- biofeedback
- desperate stage
- enuresis
- epileptoid personality
- 5-HIAA
- hydroxyzine hydrochloride
- hypnotherapy
- impulse-control disorder
- impulse-control disorder not otherwise specified
- intermittent explosive disorder
- kleptomania
- limbic system
- lithium
- lust angst
- multidetermined
- oniomania
- parental factors
- pathological gambling
- pleasure principle, reality principle
- progressive-loss stage
- psychodynamics
- pyromania
- social gambling
- SSRIs
- testosterone
- trichophagy
- trichotillomania
- winning phase

QUESTIONS

Directions

Each of the questions or incomplete statements below is followed by five suggested responses or completions. Select the *one* that is *best* in each case.

27.1 Which of the following is a component of kleptomania?

A. Persons often do not have the means to pay for items they steal
B. Stealing occurs in order to meet personal needs
C. Stealing is often planned and carefully carried out

D. Persons never feel guilt or remorse following the theft
E. It is characterized by mounting tension before the act

27.2 Which of the following is *not* one of the phases typically seen in pathological gamblers?

A. Winning phase
B. Progressive-loss phase
C. Risk-taking phase
D. Desperate phase
E. Hopeless phase

27.3 All of the following have been noted to have an association with pyromania *except*?

A. Mild retardation
B. Delinquency
C. Cruelty to animals
D. Obsession with firefighters
E. Alcohol use disorders

27.4 The term *epileptoid personality* has been used in reference to patients with which of the following?

A. Seizure disorder
B. Intermittent explosive disorder
C. Pyromania
D. Kleptomania
E. Trichotillomania

27.5 A 28-year-old man had been repeatedly brutalized by his alcoholic mother throughout childhood and early adolescence. He felt particularly humiliated when she would slap his face during frequent bouts of uncontrollable anger. One evening, while they were drinking at a local tavern, a friend playfully slapped his cheek. The patient suddenly "saw red," broke a beer bottle over the man's head, and then mauled him severely. Which of the following defense mechanisms is this patient with intermittent explosive disorder exhibiting?

A. Identification with the aggressor
B. Passive-aggressive behavior
C. Regression
D. Controlling
E. Reaction formation

27.6 Which of the following is *not* a neuroendocrine change noted in patients with abnormal aggression?

A. Deranged serotonin neurotransmission
B. Low CSF levels of 5-hydroxyindolacetic acid (5-HIAA)
C. Decreased platelet serotonin reuptake
D. Elevated CSF testosterone
E. Increased glucose metabolism

27.7 True statements about pathological gambling include

A. Rates of pathological gambling are lower in locations where gambling is legal.
B. Rates of pathological gambling are lower among the poor and minorities.
C. Rates of pathological gambling have been shown to be lower in high school students than in the general population.
D. The natural history of the illness has been divided into four phases: winning, losing, desperation, and hopelessness.
E. All of the above

27.8 Which of the following drugs has been found to cause a paradoxical reaction of dyscontrol in some cases of impulse-control disorder?

A. lithium
B. phenytoin
C. carbamazepine
D. trazodone
E. benzodiazepines

27.9 All of the following have been identified as predisposing factors for the development of pathological gambling *except*

A. loss of a parent before the child is 15 years old
B. childhood enuresis
C. attention-deficit/hyperactivity disorder
D. inappropriate parental discipline
E. family emphasis on material symbols

27.10 People with trichotillomania

A. often have family histories of tics
B. often respond preferentially to serotonergic agents
C. have an increased prevalence of mood and anxiety disorders
D. often require a biopsy to confirm the diagnosis
E. all of the above

27.11 Intermittent explosive disorder

A. is relatively common
B. is characterized by discrete periods of aggressive episodes
C. is associated with lower than expected rates of depressive disorders in first-degree relatives of patients
D. is typically seen in small men with avoidant personality features
E. none of the above

27.12 Which of the following selections is *not* associated with intermittent explosive disorder?

A. Patients may feel helpless before an episode.
B. The disorder usually grows less severe with age.
C. A predisposing factor in childhood is encephalitis.
D. Dopaminergic neurons mediate behavioral inhibition.
E. Neurological examination can show left-right ambivalence.

Directions

Each set of lettered headings below is followed by a list of numbered words or phrases. For each numbered word or phrase, select

A. if the item is associated with A only
B. if the item is associated with B only
C. if the item is associated with both A and B
D. if the item is associated with neither A nor B

Questions 27.13–27.17

A. Compulsive buying
B. Kleptomania

27.13 Chronic condition
27.14 Recognized as a discrete disease entity by DSM-IV-TR
27.15 Preponderance in women
27.16 Increased lifetime rate of major mood disorders
27.17 Treatment has included both psychological and pharmacological modalities

Questions 27.18–27.23

A. Trichotillomania
B. Pyromania

27.18 More common in females than in males
27.19 Onset generally in childhood
27.20 Sense of gratification or release during the behavior
27.21 Treated with lithium
27.22 Associated with truancy
27.23 May be a response to an auditory hallucination

ANSWERS

27.1 The answer is E

The essential feature of kleptomania is a recurrent failure to resist impulses to steal *objects not needed for personal use or monetary value*. The objects are often given away, returned surreptitiously, or kept and hidden. Persons with kleptomania *usually have the money to pay for the objects they impulsively steal*. Like other impulse control disorders, kleptomania is characterized by mounting tension before the act, followed by gratification and lessening of tension with or without guilt, remorse, or depression after the act. The *stealing is not planned* and does not involve others. Although the thefts do not occur when immediate arrest is probable, persons with kleptomania do not always consider their chances of being apprehended, even though repeated arrests lead to pain and humiliation. These *persons may feel guilt and anxiety after the theft*, but they do not feel anger or vengeance. Furthermore, when the object stolen is the goal, the diagnosis is not kleptomania; in kleptomania the act of stealing is itself the goal.

27.2 The answer is C

Pathological gambling usually begins in adolescence for men and late in life for women. The disorder waxes and wanes and tends to be chronic. Four phases are seen in pathological gambling:

1. The *winning phase*, ending with a big win, equal to about a year's salary, which hooks patients. Women usually do not have a big win, but use gambling as an escape from problems.
2. *Progressive-loss phase*, in which patients structure their lives around gambling and then move from being excellent gamblers to stupid ones who take considerable risks, cash in securities, borrow money, miss work, and lose jobs.
3. The *desperate phase*, with patients frenziedly gambling with large amounts of money, not paying debts, becoming involved with loan sharks, writing bad checks, and possibly embezzling.
4. The *hopeless stage* of accepting that losses can never be made up, but the gambling continues because of the associated arousal or excitement. The disorder may take up to 15 years to reach the last phase, but then, within a year or two, patients have deteriorated totally.

27.3 The answer is D

Persons who set fires are more likely to be *mildly retarded* than are those in the general population. Some studies have noted an increased incidence of *alcohol use disorders* in persons who set fires. Fire setters also tend to have a history of antisocial traits, such as truancy, running away from home, and *delinquency*. Enuresis has been considered a common finding in the history of fire setters, although controlled studies have failed to confirm this. Studies have, however, found an association between *cruelty to animals* and fire setting. Childhood and adolescent fire setting is often associated with attention-deficit/hyperactivity disorder or adjustment disorders. There has been *no evidence of an association between obsession with firefighters and pyromania*.

27.4 The answer is B

Intermittent explosive disorder manifests as discrete episodes of losing control or aggressive impulses; these episodes can result in serious assault or the destruction of property. The symptoms, which patients may describe as spells or attacks, appear within minutes or hours and, regardless of duration, remit spontaneously and quickly. The term *epileptoid personality* has been used to convey the seizure-like quality of these characteristic outbursts. The outbursts are not typical of the patient's usual behavior, and the term also conveys the suspicion of an organic disease process, for example, damage to the central nervous system. Several associated features suggest the possibility of an epileptoid state: the presence of auras; postictallike changes in sensorium, including partial or spotty amnesia; and hypersensitivity to photic, aural, or auditory stimuli. *Trichotillomania* is the pulling of hair; *kleptomania* is compulsive stealing; and *pyromania* is the setting of fires.

27.5 The answer is A

Although research has been limited, it is generally assumed that intermittent explosive disorder—like other impulse-control disturbances—is caused by a varying confluence of psychosocial and neurobiological factors. Patients regularly describe chaotic family backgrounds, rife with explosive behavior and verbal and physical abuse, often in the context of acute alcohol intoxication. *Identification with the aggressor* is a common defense mechanism, in which the explosive violence of a parent or close relative is internalized. This sinister coping strategy replicates the acts of stormy violence to which patients have been exposed during their formative years. Situations that realistically or symbolically evoke memories of early oppression and trauma may spark explosive episodes. Typically, an acute sense of narcissistic injury, a lowered self-esteem, and profound feelings of shame and humiliation are evoked.

Passive-aggressive behavior is aggression toward an object expressed indirectly and ineffectively through passivity, masochism, and turning against the self. *Regression* is a return to a previous stage of development or functioning to avoid the anxieties involved in later stages. *Controlling* is the excessive attempt to manage events or objects in the environment in the interest of minimizing anxiety and solving internal conflicts. *Reaction formation* is the management of unacceptable impulses by permitting expression of the impulse in an antithetical form.

27.6 The answer is E

Modest neurobiological studies point to possible *deranged serotonin neurotransmission* in patients identified with intermittent explosive disorder; *low cerebrospinal fluid (CSF) levels of 5-hydroxyindoleacetic acid* (5-HIAA) in some impulsive, temper-prone individuals; and *lowered levels of platelet serotonin reuptake* in patients with episodic rage. A connection has also been inferred between *elevated CSF testosterone levels* and aggressive or openly violent behavior. An element of genetic loading is also suggested by the fact that blood relatives are more likely to have characteristic outbursts of explosive behavior compared to adoptive relatives. *Increased glucose metabolism* has not been implicated in patients with abnormal aggression.

27.7 The answer is D

Up to 3 percent of adults in the general population may be classified with probable pathological gambling. Based on treatment samples, the typical pathological gambler is an upper-middle-class or middle-class white man between the ages of 40 and 50. However, pathological gamblers in treatment may differ significantly from those in the general population. Surveys demonstrate that *rates of pathological gambling are higher (not lower) among the poor and minorities* and that these individuals are underserved by current treatment resources. Although male pathological gamblers outnumber women, the previous ratio of 2 to 1 may be high. Individuals under the age of 30 are probably underrepresented in treatment centers, and data suggest that the prevalence of pathological gambling among adolescents is increasing. Some surveys have shown *higher (not lower) rates of pathological gambling among high school students* than in the general population. Pathological gamblers tend to have had an alcohol- or other substance-abusing parent, and approximately 25 percent had a parent who was probably a pathological gambler. Surveys also demonstrate that *rates of pathological gambling are considerably higher (not lower) in locations where gambling is legal.*

The course of pathological gambling is insidious, and conversion to pathological gambling probably is precipitated either by increased exposure to gambling or by the occurrence of a psychological stressor or significant loss. In males, the onset of pathological gambling begins in adolescence; in females the onset occurs later in life.

The *natural history of the illness has been divided into four phases*. In the *first (winning)* phase, a big win stimulates feelings of omnipotence. Women do not generally experience a big win initially. They may see gambling as a means of escaping overwhelming problems in their environment or in their past. Thus, there are apparently two possible motivators for ongoing gambling activity: action seeking (characterized by the big win) or escape seeking. In the *second (losing)* phase, the person either has a string of bad luck or begins to find losing intolerable. Gamblers then alter their strategy in an attempt to win back everything at once (chasing). Debts accrue, and there is a sense of urgency and an attempt to cover up both the behavior and the losses by lies. Relationships suffer as the gambler becomes irritable and secretive. In the *third (desperation)* phase gamblers engage in uncharacteristic, often illegal behaviors. Bad checks are written, funds are embezzled, and they desperately seek ways to obtain money to continue gambling, both to recoup losses and to regain the feeling of arousal characteristic of the initial phase. Relationships deteriorate further. Symptoms of depression appear, including neurovegetative signs, suicidal ideation, and suicide attempts. The fourth and *final phase (hopelessness)* involves an acceptance that losses can never be made good. Nevertheless, gambling continues, with the main motivator being the attainment of arousal or excitement.

Although a few gamblers seek help while in the winning phase, most seek help much later, generally because their relationships are threatened or they have committed illegal acts.

The course of the disorder is accelerated by the use of alcohol or drugs, the death or loss (possibly through divorce) of a significant other, the birth of a child, physical illness, a job or career disappointment, or increasing interpersonal difficulties. Job promotion or success may also hasten the course of the disorder.

27.8 The answer is E

Anticonvulsants have long been used in treating explosive patients, with mixed results. *Phenothiazines* and antidepressants have been effective in some cases. *Benzodiazepines have been reported to produce a paradoxical reaction of dyscontrol* in some cases. *Lithium (Eskalith)* has been reported to be useful in generally lessening aggressive behavior, as have *carbamazepine (Tegretol)* and *phenytoin (Dilantin)*. Propranolol (Inderal), buspirone (BuSpar), and *trazodone (Desyrel)* have also been effective in some cases. Reports increasingly indicate that fluoxetine (Prozac) and other serotonin-specific reuptake inhibitors are useful in reducing impulsivity and aggression.

27.9 The answer is B

Childhood enuresis is the involuntary loss of urine (sometimes the condition is seen as voluntary). It is not a predisposing factor for the development of pathological gambling. *Loss of a parent* by death, separation, divorce, or desertion before the child is 15 years old may be a predisposing factor. Other possible factors include *attention-deficit/hyperactivity disorder, inappropriate parental discipline, family emphasis on material symbols,* and a lack of family emphasis on saving, planning, and budgeting.

27.10 The answer is E (all)

The cause of trichotillomania remains unclear and both psychological and biological mechanisms have been proposed.

Psychodynamic explanations suggest that the disorder is a response to loss or separation in childhood. Mothers of patients are often characterized as critical, and fathers are frequently passive or emotionally weak. Alternatively, behaviorists point out that the disorder is common in children and adolescents, and when it persists, it takes on the characteristics of a habit that remits with behavioral techniques. Biochemical explanations stem from the finding that patients have *an increased prevalence of both mood and anxiety disorders* and some symptoms of obsessive-compulsive disorder. The *family history* of patients with trichotillomania often *includes tics*, habits, and obsessive-compulsive symptoms. This disorder *responds preferentially to serotonergic agents*, which lends credence to a biochemical relation to either mood or anxiety disorders. However, since serotonergic agents are not always effective, the disorder most likely has more than one cause. Another biochemical theory points to the potential role of the opiate system, largely on the basis of the response of dogs with canine acral lick dermatitis to opioid antagonists. It was proposed that patients with trichotillomania have a general hypoalgesia that allows them to continue plucking hair without the perception of pain, but a recent study found no difference in pain perception thresholds.

Trichotillomania can be quite difficult to diagnose for a number of reasons. Although this disorder disrupts most patients' lives, they tend to deny the illness and frequently disguise it successfully for decades. Most often, people with this disorder pull hair from the scalp, most commonly the vertex, though people also pull frequently from the temporoparietal, occipital, and frontal regions. Generally, hair plucking involves multiple sites on the scalp or other body regions such as the eyebrows, eyelashes, facial hair, and the pubic area. The average dermatologist sees three to seven cases of trichotillomania a year. The affected site usually shows a mixture of short and long hairs in a linear or circular pattern. *A biopsy is often necessary* to confirm the diagnosis and distinguish it from alopecia areata or tinea capitis.

27.11 The answer is B

The notion that explosive violence may be linked to a discrete diagnosable condition is controversial. In DSM-IV-TR intermittent explosive disorder is characterized by aggressive impulses out of proportion to any precipitating psychosocial stressor. In the intervals between episodes there is no sign of impulsiveness or aggressiveness.

The existence of intermittent explosive disorder as a unique entity remains controversial. Many have difficulty with the idea of *a normal baseline with superimposed periods of aggressive episodes.* In addition, anger outbursts are a part of many other disease entities.

Intermittent explosive disorder is thought to be rare (not common) and occurs more frequently in males. High rates of firesetting behavior in persons with the disorder have been reported. Recent studies suggest higher than normal rates of intermittent explosive disorder in families of patients with the diagnosis. *First-degree relatives of patients with the disorder appear to have higher (not lower) than expected rates of depressive disorders* and alcohol and substance abuse.

Hypotheses about the cause of impulsive aggression derive from both psychological and biological perspectives. Psychoanalytic reports suggest that such outbursts occur in response to narcissistic injurious events. Rage outbursts serve as defenses that regulate interpersonal distance and protect against further narcissistic wounding. *Typical patients appear to be large (not small) men with dependent (not avoidant) personality features* who respond to feelings of uselessness or impotence with violent outbursts.

27.12 The answer is D

Serotonergic neurons (not dopaminergic neurons) mediate behavioral inhibition. Decreases in serotonergic transmission can reduce the effect of punishment as a deterrent of behavior, and the restoration of serotonin activity restores the behavioral effect of punishment. Researchers have suggested a connection between low levels of CSF 5-HIAA and impulsive behavior. Patients with intermittent explosive disorder are typically large, dependent men with a poor sense of masculine identity. *Patients may feel helpless* before an episode. A predisposing factor in childhood is *encephalitis,* as are perinatal trauma, minimal brain dysfunction, and hyperactivity. A patient's childhood was often violent and traumatic. Neurological examination can show *left-right ambivalence* and perceptual reversal. The disorder *usually grows less severe with age,* but heightened organic impairment can lead to frequent and severe episodes.

Answers 27.13–27.17

27.13 The answer is C

27.14 The answer is B

27.15 The answer is C

27.16 The answer is C

27.17 The answer is C

Kleptomania is a chronic illness, generally beginning in late adolescence and continuing over many years. The spontaneous remission rate and long-term prognosis are unknown.

Compulsive buying is a chronic condition that can have devastating financial, marital, and vocational consequences. Though individuals frequently attempt to stop the behavior on their own, they are usually unsuccessful. Limiting access to shopping, including credit cards, home catalogs, the Internet, and the home shopping network, has met with some success for this disorder.

Kleptomania has been recognized as a discrete disease entity by DSM-III, DSM-III-R, DSM-IV, and DSM-IV-TR. The disorder was excluded from the second edition of DSM (DSM-II) and was mentioned in the first edition of DSM (DSM-I) as an accessory term only. Features include a recurrent impulse to steal objects that are not needed for personal use or monetary value. DSM-IV-TR diagnostic criteria stipulate that the stealing is not an expression of anger or revenge, is not associated with a delusion or hallucination, and is not due to a conduct disorder, manic episode, or antisocial personality disorder.

Compulsive buying is not recognized by DSM-IV-TR as a unique subcategory, but some attempts have been made recently to develop a more formal definition of diagnostic criteria. Table 27.1 lists some proposed diagnostic criteria for compulsive buying.

Current estimates of the prevalence of compulsive buying range from 1.1 to 5.9 percent of the general population.

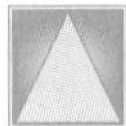

Table 27.1
Diagnostic Criteria for Compulsive Buying

A. Maladaptive preoccupation with buying or shopping, or maladaptive buying or shopping impulses or behavior, as indicated by at least one of the following:
   1. Frequent preoccupation with buying or impulses to buy that are experienced as irresistible, intrusive, and/or senseless.
   2. Frequent buying of more than can be afforded, frequent buying of items that are not needed, or shopping for longer periods of time than intended.

B. The buying preoccupations, impulses, or behaviors cause marked distress, are time consuming, significantly interfere with social or occupational functioning, or result in financial problems (e.g., indebtedness or bankruptcy).

C. The excessive buying or shopping behavior does not occur exclusively during periods of hypomania or mania.

Reprinted with permission from McElroy SL, Keck PE Jr, Pope HG Jr, Smith JM, Strakowski SM. Compulsive buying: a report of 20 cases. *J Clin Psychiatry,* 1994;55:242.

General population surveys of people meeting criteria for compulsive buying have shown that 80 to 92 percent are women. The onset of the disorder appears to be approximately 18 years of age, though frequently a decade passes before the buying pattern is recognized as a problem. Information from case reports points to a *preponderance of kleptomania in women,* although women are more likely to present for psychiatric evaluation than men.

Patients with kleptomania have an increased lifetime rate of major mood disorders, anxiety disorders, and eating disorders. They frequently have a history of sexual dysfunction. Persons with kleptomania do not meet the criteria for antisocial personality disorder. Those with a psychiatric disorder in addition to kleptomania generally state that of all their difficulties, stealing causes them the greatest grief.

Compulsive buying must be distinguished from spending that occurs exclusively during a hypomanic or manic period. Compulsive shoppers demonstrate a more enduring pattern of behavior that is not limited to episodes in which other symptoms of mania can be observed.

These individuals show a high comorbidity with other Axis I conditions. In one study of 20 patients, all met criteria for two or more Axis I conditions, and 13 met criteria for four or more conditions. *All of these patients met criteria for some form of mood disorder*, most commonly bipolar I or bipolar II disorder. Symptoms seemed to increase when individuals felt more dysphoric and to decrease when patients were hypomanic. Many of these individuals stated that buying relieved their depressive symptoms.

Other disorders comorbid with compulsive buying include anxiety disorders such as obsessive-compulsive disorder, panic disorder, and phobias. Substance abuse and dependence, eating disorders, and other impulse-control disorders are frequently seen in these patients.

Information regarding treatment of compulsive buying is based on case reports; no formal, rigorously controlled treatment studies exist for compulsive shopping. *Treatment of compulsive buying has included both psychological and pharmacological modalities,* though information is based upon case reports rather than clinical trials. Some patients receiving cognitive-behavioral, supportive, or insight-oriented therapy report gaining some control over their buying compulsions. Others have been helped by supportive self-help groups like Debtors Anonymous. Pharmacological data are limited, with mixed results. In one series, 9 of 20 patients receiving pharmacological interventions had complete or partial remission of symptoms. Medications that were at least somewhat effective included antidepressants, mood-stabilizing agents, anxiolytics, and antipsychotics that were used alone or in conjunction with other agents. Some individuals who did not improve had discontinued pharmacotherapy early in treatment because of adverse effects or induction of hypomania.

Other methods include the use of psychodynamic psychotherapy, behavioral techniques, and somatic interventions in the treatment of kleptomania, with variable outcomes. However, there are no controlled studies in the treatment of kleptomania. The use of long-term, insight-oriented psychotherapy is of questionable value to this patient population. Behavioral techniques have met with some success. Effective pharmacological interventions have been described in case reports, including the use of fluvoxamine (Luvox), amitriptyline (Elavil), imipramine (Tofranil), nortriptyline (Pamelor), trazodone (Desyrel), fluoxetine (Prozac), lithium (Eskalith), and valproate (Depakote). The use of electroconvulsive therapy (ECT) has also met with some success in case reports.

Answers 27.18–27.23

27.18 The answer is A

27.19 The answer is C

27.20 The answer is C

27.21 The answer is D

27.22 The answer is B

27.23 The answer is D

Both pyromania and trichotillomania have their *onset in childhood* and are characterized by a *sense of gratification or release during the act. Trichotillomania* is apparently *more common in females than in males. Pyromania* is associated with antisocial traits, such as *truancy*, running away from home, and delinquency. *Neither disorder is treated with lithium (Eskalith), and according to the DSM-IV-TR diagnostic criteria, neither can be a response to an auditory hallucination.*

28 Adjustment Disorders

Adjustment disorders are short-term maladaptive reactions to what a layperson would call a personal calamity but in psychiatric terms would be referred to as a psychosocial stressor. An adjustment disorder is expected to remit soon after the stressor ceases or, if it persists, a new level of adaptation is achieved.

According to the text revision of the 4th edition of *Diagnostic and Statistical Manual of Mental Disorders* (DSM-IV-TR), symptoms must appear within 3 months of a stressor's onset. The nature and severity of the stressors are not specified. However, the stressors are more often everyday events that are ubiquitous (e.g., loss of a loved one, change of employment or financial situation) rather than rare, catastrophic events (e.g., natural disasters, violent crimes). The disturbance must not fulfill the criteria for another major psychiatric disorder or bereavement (not considered a mental disorder, although it may be a focus of clinical attention). The symptoms of the disorder usually resolve within 6 months, although they may last longer if produced by a chronic stressor or one with long-lasting consequences.

The student should study the questions and answers below for a useful review of these disorders.

HELPFUL HINTS

The student should know these terms and types (including case examples) of adjustment.

- acute stress reaction
- adjustment disorder:
  - with anxiety
  - with depressed mood
  - with disturbance of conduct
  - with mixed anxiety and depressed mood
  - with mixed disturbance of emotions and conduct
- adolescent onset
- bereavement
- crisis intervention
- good-enough mother
- maladaptive reaction
- mass catastrophes
- posttraumatic stress disorder
- psychodynamic factors
- psychosocial stressor
- recovery rate
- resilience
- secondary gain
- severity of stress scale
- vulnerability
- Donald Winnicott

QUESTIONS

Directions

Each of the statements or questions below is followed by five suggested responses or completions. Select the *one* that is *best* in each case.

28.1 Which of the following is *not* a classification of adjustment disorder in DSM-IV-TR?

A. With disturbance of conduct
B. With depressed mood
C. With psychotic features
D. With mixed disturbance of emotions and conduct
E. With anxiety

28.2 Which of the following stressors most often leads to psychological impairment that could be diagnosed as an adjustment disorder?

A. rape
B. loss of a job
C. a plane crash
D. all of the above
E. none of the above

28.3 Adjustment disorders

A. must remit within 6 months following the cessation of the stressor
B. are in response, most often, to everyday events rather than rare, catastrophic events
C. have subtypes indicating that almost any subthreshold condition associated with a psychosocial stressor may meet criteria for the disorder
D. as a diagnosis may be used excessively and incorrectly by clinicians
E. all of the above

28.4 Adjustment disorder

A. correlates with the severity of the stressor
B. occurs more often in males than in females
C. is a type of bereavement

D. usually requires years of treatment
E. occurs in all age groups

28.5 Factors affecting the relationship of stress to the development of psychopathology include

A. preexisting mood symptomatology
B. preexisting adaptive skills
C. genetic influence
D. the nature of the preexisting event
E. all of the above

28.6 The rate of reliability in the diagnosis of adjustment disorders is

A. considered good
B. improved by the variability produced by cultural expectations regarding reactions to and management of stressful events
C. increased by the absence of any impairment criteria in the diagnostic algorithm that defines maladaption to stress
D. consistent with the fact that measurement of psychosocial stress on Axis IV has been found to be questionable
E. none of the above

28.7 The symptomatic profile and level of impairment in adjustment disorders with depressed mood has been found to be quite similar to

A. dysthymic disorder
B. major depressive disorder
C. bipolar I disorder
D. all of the above
E. none of the above

Directions

Each set of lettered headings below is followed by a list of numbered phrases. For each numbered phrase, select:

A. if the item is associated with A only
B. if the item is associated with B only
C. if the item is associated with both A and B
D. if the item is associated with neither A nor B

Questions 28.8–28.12

A. DSM-IV-TR
B. ICD-10

28.8 Places adjustment disorders in the same category as reactions to severe stress
28.9 Notes that once a stressor (or its consequences) has ceased, an adjustment disorder may not persist for more than 6 more months
28.10 Stipulates that onset of symptoms of an adjustment disorder must occur within 1 month of exposure to a psychosocial stressor
28.11 Notes that the criteria of another disorder (e.g., antisocial personality disorder) may be fulfilled in an adjustment disorder
28.12 Includes adjustment disorders with depressed mood, anxiety, and disturbance of conduct

Questions 28.13–28.17

A. Adolescents
B. Adults

28.13 Often require a longer recovery time from an adjustment disorder
28.14 Common precipitating stressor for an adjustment disorder may be divorce
28.15 Males and females equally diagnosed with adjustment disorders
28.16 The age group in which adjustment disorders are most frequently diagnosed
28.17 Females are diagnosed with adjustment disorders twice as often as males

ANSWERS

28.1 The answer is C

The clinical presentations of adjustment disorder can vary widely. The *DSM-IV-TR* lists six adjustment disorders: *adjustment disorder with depressed mood*; *adjustment disorder with anxiety*; adjustment disorder with mixed anxiety and depressed mood; *adjustment disorder with disturbance of conduct*; *adjustment disorder with mixed disturbance of emotions and conduct*; and adjustment disorder unspecified. In adjustment disorder with depressed mood, the predominant manifestations are depressed mood, tearfulness, and hopelessness, and it must be distinguished from major depressive disorder and uncomplicated bereavement. Symptoms of anxiety, such as palpitations, jitteriness, and agitation, are present in adjustment disorder with anxiety, which must be differentiated from anxiety disorders. In adjustment disorder with mixed anxiety and depressed mood, patients exhibit features of both anxiety and depression that do not meet the criteria for an already established anxiety or depressive disorder. In adjustment disorder with disturbance of conduct, the predominant manifestation involves conduct in which the rights of others are violated or age-appropriate societal norms and rules are disregarded. Examples of behavior in this category are truancy, vandalism, reckless driving, and fighting, and it must be differentiated from conduct disorder and antisocial personality disorder. A combination of disturbances of emotions and conduct sometimes occurs. Clinicians are encouraged to try to make one or the other diagnosis in the interest of clarity. Adjustment disorder unspecified is a residual category for atypical maladaptive reactions to stress. Examples include inappropriate responses to the diagnosis of physical illness, such as massive denial, severe noncompliance with treatment, and social withdrawal, without significant depressed or anxious mood. Maladjustment with some sub-threshold psychotic features would most likely fall into the adjustment disorder unspecified category, as *adjustment disorder with psychotic features* is not an adjustment disorder classification specified by the DSM-IV-TR.

28.2 The answer is B

By definition, an adjustment disorder is precipitated by one or more stressors. The severity of the stressor or stressors does not always predict the severity of the disorder; the stressor severity is a complex function of degree, quantity, duration, reversibility, environment, and personal context. The nature and severity of stressors that may lead to an adjustment disorder are not specified by the DSM-IV-TR. Stressors may be single, such as a divorce or the *loss of a job*, or multiple, such as the death of a person important to a patient, which coincides with the patient's own physical illness and loss of a job. Specific developmental stages, such as beginning school, leaving home, getting married, becoming a parent, failing to achieve occupational goals, having the last child leave home, and retiring, are often associated with adjustment disorders.

In adjustment disorders, a precipitating stress need not be severe or unusual in order to lead to impairment; however, in acute stress disorder or posttraumatic stress disorder (PTSD), symptoms develop following a traumatic event or events that are "outside the range of normal human experience." In other words, the stressors producing PTSD are expected to cause a psychological reaction in the average person, whereas those persons who develop adjustment disorders are responding maladaptively to a relatively common event. Stressors that can lead to PTSD often contain a psychological component and frequently a concomitant physical component that may directly damage persons' nervous systems. Persons may experience these stressors alone, as in *rape* or assault, or in groups, as in military combat or death camps. Mass catastrophes—such as hurricanes, floods, *airplane crashes*, and atomic bombings—are also identified stressors that can lead to PTSD or acute stress disorder.

28.3 The answer is E (all)

One of the most problematic diagnostic categories in DSM-IV-TR is adjustment disorders. The fact that the relationship between stress and psychiatric disorder is both complex and uncertain has caused many to question the theoretical basis of adjustment disorders. In addition, the absence of operationalized, symptom-based criteria and a threshold level of symptomatology required for diagnosis have resulted in the use of this category for patients who might otherwise fulfill criteria for another, more specific mental disorder. Because incorrect diagnosis may result in inadequate treatment, inappropriately conceptualizing a patient's problem as constituting an adjustment disorder may result in delays or errors in treatment planning. Misdiagnosis of other, more specific disorders when an adjustment disorder should be diagnosed is also a problem. For example, in one study, medical residents frequently diagnosed major depressive disorder when adjustment disorder with depressed mood was considered the correct diagnosis by an attending psychiatrist.

Problems with the use of the adjustment disorders category among child and adolescent psychiatrists were highlighted in a survey conducted as a means of informing the DSM-IV-TR work groups about the use of psychiatric disorders in clinical practice. Of those who responded to the survey, 55 percent indicated that they used adjustment disorders to avoid stigmatization of patients. Many of those who favored the use of this category were not trained formally in the revised third edition of DSM (DSM-III-R) and were not inclined to use not otherwise specified categories. Over half of these psychiatrists did not consider the temporal-onset criterion for adjustment disorders or the relevant exclusionary criteria in applying this diagnosis. *The survey results indicate that adjustment disorders diagnoses may be used excessively and incorrectly by some clinicians.*

Adjustment disorders are characterized in DSM-IV-TR by the development of emotional or behavioral symptoms in the context of one or more identified psychosocial stressors. The resultant symptomatology is deemed to be clinically significant by virtue of either impairment in social, occupational, or educational function or the subjective experience of distress in excess of what would normally be expected for the given stressors. The nature and severity of the stressors are not specified. *However, the stressors are more often everyday events that are ubiquitous* (e.g., loss of a loved one, change of employment or financial situation) *rather than rare, catastrophic events,* such as natural disasters or lethal crimes. The symptomatology must, by definition, occur within 3 months of the occurrence of the stressor and *must remit within 6 months following the cessation of the stressor.* Finally, the disturbance must not fulfill the criteria for another major psychiatric disorder or bereavement (not considered a mental disorder, although it may be a focus of clinical attention). A variety of symptomatic presentation subtypes of adjustment disorders are identified. The scope of symptomatology covered by these subtypes indicates that *virtually any subthreshold condition deemed to be associated with a psychosocial stressor may potentially meet the criteria for adjustment disorders.*

28.4 The answer is E

Adjustment disorder *occurs in all age groups*. It *does not always correlate with the severity of the stressor* and *appears to occur more often in females than in males.* Adjustment disorder *is not a type of bereavement.* The overall prognosis for a person with adjustment disorder is generally favorable with appropriate treatment. Most patients return to their previous level of functioning within 3 months and *do not require years of therapy.*

28.5 The answer is E (all)

The results of studies that have examined the relationship of stress to the development of psychopathology provide additional information to be considered in evaluating the model of stress–disease interaction in adjustment disorders. Several studies have found that individuals with and without preexisting symptoms respond differently to the presence of stressful events. This has been observed both in samples with adjustment disorders and in other conditions. *Preexisting mood symptomatology* was the only factor that predicted a prolonged course of adjustment disorders following cardiac surgery. In Israeli children who suffered the loss of their fathers in war, preexisting conduct symptoms were correlated highly with poor adjustment (although not necessarily adjustment disorders).

Other studies have focused on those factors that protect individuals from developing stress-related symptoms. For example, *preexisting adaptive skills* decrease the likelihood of symptoms developing in the face of stress. In child and adolescent populations, a warm and supportive relationship with the primary caregiver, easy and adaptable child temperament, and healthier adjustment of the family to stress all predict a more positive response to stress within the child. Finally, *the nature of preexisting life events* has important implications for the level of adjustment. Control over life events has generally been associated with improved adjustment even though it may increase stress. Similarly, pleasurable events are on the whole linked to psychological well-being, even though they may be stressful. In contrast, life events of a more dependent nature, which are undesirable and outside the control of the affected individual, are more likely to produce psychiatric symptoms.

The relationship of family, environmental, and genetic factors to adverse life events must also be considered. Findings from a study of over 2,000 twin pairs indicate that life events are correlated modestly in twin pairs, with monozygotes showing greater concordance than dizygotes. Family-environmental and genetic factors each accounted for approximately 20 percent of the variance in that study. Another twin study that examined *genetic contributions* to the development of symptoms of posttraumatic stress disorder (not necessarily at the level of full disorder and therefore relevant to adjustment disorders) similarly concluded that the likelihood of developing symptoms in the context of traumatic life events is partially under genetic control. The findings of these studies suggest that the occurrence of adverse life events and their consequences are not necessarily random. Certain individuals appear to be at increased risk both for the occurrence of these events and for the development of pathology once they occur.

28.6 The answer is D

The few extant *studies of reliability in adjustment disorders have produced unimpressive results.* One study determined the interrater agreement (κ) for adjustment disorders to be 0.05 (P = not significant) in a survey of psychiatrists and psychologists using 27 case histories of child and adolescent cases. The κ for the DSM-II category transient situational disorder was somewhat higher in this study ($\kappa = 0.28$; $P < 0.05$). The results of the United Kingdom World Health Organization (UK-WHO) study of reliability of the ninth revision of *International Statistical Classification of Disease* (ICD-9) categories in children and adolescents were consistent with these findings. The κ for adjustment disorders was 0.23, which was considerably lower than for many other categories. Reclassification using a glossary improved reliability to 0.33, suggesting that structured assessment can at least partially ameliorate the limited reliability of adjustment disorders.

There are many potential sources of poor reliability, although the lack of an operationalized symptom checklist and a threshold level of symptoms that demarcate entrance into the diagnosis seem paramount. *Other sources of poor (not improved) reliability include* (1) difficulties in determining when subjective distress or observable symptomatology exceeds what would normally be expected for a given stressor in an "average" individual; (2) *the absence of any impairment* criterion in the diagnostic algorithm that defines maladaptation to stress; and (3) *the variability produced by cultural expectations* regarding the reaction to and management of stressful events. The low reliability of adjustment disorders is consistent with the fact that *measurement of psychosocial stress on Axis IV* has repeatedly been found to be *questionable.*

28.7 The answer is A

Adjustment disorders has been described as a transitional diagnostic category because the level of symptomatology and impairment in adjustment disorders was found to be intermediate between that observed in comparison groups who only had a DSM-IV-TR problem-level diagnosis and patients with specific, above-threshold diagnoses. The symptomatic profile and level of impairment in patients with adjustment disorders with depressed mood was quite *similar to that found in dysthymic disorder* and atypical (minor) depression, although it was *distinct from major depressive disorder* and *bipolar I disorder,* suggesting poor discriminate validity of adjustment disorders with depressed mood with respect to minor depressive disorders. Adjustment disorders have also been described as an admission diagnosis or initial diagnosis for many adolescent and adult psychiatric inpatients. In one study, a large number (40 percent) of patients given this preliminary diagnosis were assigned a different diagnosis at the time of discharge. An even smaller number (18 percent) of those who were subsequently readmitted to the hospital were again diagnosed as having adjustment disorders.

Answers 28.8–28.12

28.8 The answer is B

28.9 The answer is C

28.10 The answer is B

28.11 The answer is D

28.12 The answer is C

The text revision of the fourth edition of the DSM-IV-TR and the 10th revision of the *International Statistical Classification of Diseases and Related Health Problems* (ICD-10) both include adjustment disorders, which are classified into categories such as adjustment disorder *with depressed mood, with anxiety,* and *with disturbance of conduct.* Like the DSM-IV-TR, the ICD-10 notes that the symptoms of an adjustment disorder must *not meet or fulfill the criteria for any other disorder.* The ICD-10 time pattern for adjustment disorders differs from that of DSM-IV-TR, with an *onset usually within a month of the stressful event or life change,* instead of the 3-month window prescribed by the DSM-IV-TR. However, like the DSM-IV-TR, the ICD-10 notes that *symptoms of an adjustment disorder may not persist for more than six months after a stressor or its consequences have ceased.* The ICD-10 *places adjustment disorders in the same category as reactions to severe stress,* and includes acute stress reaction and posttraumatic stress disorder in this category.

Answers 28.13–28.17

28.13 The answer is A

28.14 The answer is C

28.15 The answer is A

28.16 The answer is A

28.17 The answer is B

According to DSM-IV-TR, *women are diagnosed with adjustment disorders twice as often as men,* and single women are generally overly represented as most at risk. In children and *adolescents, boys and girls are equally diagnosed with adjustment disorders*. The disorders may occur at any age but *are most frequently diagnosed in adolescents*. Among adolescents of either sex, common precipitating stresses are school problems, parental rejection and *divorce*, and substance abuse. Among *adults*, common precipitating stresses are marital problems, *divorce*, moving to a new environment, and financial problems.

With appropriate treatment, the overall prognosis of an adjustment disorder is generally favorable. Most patients return to their previous level of functioning within 3 months. Some persons (particularly adolescents) who receive a diagnosis of an adjustment disorder later have mood disorders or substance-related disorders. *Adolescents usually require a longer time to recover than adults*.

29 Personality Disorders

Personality disorders are common and chronic. Approximately 10 to 20 percent of the population suffers from them; at least one in every five to ten people in a community has a personality disorder. These patients have chronic impairment in their ability to work and love. They consume a large portion of community service, social welfare benefits, and public health resources. About fifty percent of all psychiatric patients have personality disorders, which in and of themselves are predisposing factors for other psychiatric disorders.

According to *Diagnostic and Statistical Manual of Mental Disorders* (DSM-IV-TR) the critical criterion for distinguishing deviant personality traits is the prevalence or existence of long-term maladaptation and inflexibility that are manifested as subjective distress or socio-occupational functional impairment, or both. Personality disorders are classified into three clusters, each sharing clinical features. Cluster A includes three disorders with odd, aloof features, such as paranoid, schizoid, and schizotypal. Cluster B includes four disorders with dramatic, impulsive, and erratic features, such as borderline, antisocial, narcissistic, and histrionic. Cluster C includes three disorders sharing anxious and fearful features, such as avoidant, dependent, and obsessive-compulsive.

Patients with personality disorders typically blame other people for unfavorable circumstances for their own problems. Most of these patients perceive their own deviant behaviors as appropriate and adequate. In light of this, patients with personality disorders try to change others, not themselves, and most people with these disorders seldom seek or accept treatment. Typically, they seek help when their maladaptive behaviors culminate in severe marital, family, and career problems or for comorbid anxiety, depression, substance abuse, or eating disorders.

It is hard to find a psychotherapeutic method that has not been tried to treat personality disorders. Each school of psychotherapy provides a specific understanding of behavior and a particular method of intervention. In practice, many of these schools overlap or complement each other.

A growing body of evidence demonstrates that pharmacotherapy is at least equally important to psychotherapy in the overall treatment of these disorders. Pharmacotherapy is aimed at correcting neurobiological dispositions to underlying deviant traits or at correcting target symptoms of these disorders.

The terms personality, temperament, motivation, character and psyche are often used interchangeably. This is misleading, and the student is encouraged to review and distinguish these terms with more clarity. Students should also familiarize themselves with the complicated questions surrounding these disorders: are they clinical or social diagnoses, what is the categorical versus dimensional approach to these disorders, how are they measured?

The student should study the questions and answers below for a useful review of all these disorders.

HELPFUL HINTS

The student should be able to define the terms that follow.

- acting out
- alloplastic
- ambulatory schizophrenia
- anankastic
- antisocial
- as-if personality
- autoplastic
- avoidant
- borderline
- Briquet's syndrome
- castration anxiety
- chaotic sexuality
- character armor
- Stella Chess, Alexander Thomas
- clusters A, B, and C
- counterprojection
- denied affect
- dependent
- depressive
- dissociation
- ego-dystonic
- ego-syntonic
- emotionally unstable personality
- endorphins
- Erik Erikson
- extroversion
- fantasy
- free association
- genetic factors
- goodness of fit
- histrionic
- hypochondriasis
- idealization/devaluation
- ideas of reference
- identity diffusion
- inferiority complex
- internal object relations
- introversion
- isolation
- Carl Gustav Jung
- Heinz Kohut
- *la belle indifférence*
- macropsia
- magical thinking
- mask of sanity
- micropsychotic episodes
- narcissistic
- object choices
- obsessive-compulsive
- oral character
- organic personality disorder

- panambivalence
- pananxiety
- panphobia
- paranoid
- passive-aggressive
- personality
- platelet MAO
- projection
- projective identification
- psychotic character
- Wilhelm Reich
- repression
- saccadic movements
- Leopold von Sacher-Masoch
- Marquis de Sade
- sadistic personality
- sadomasochistic personality
- schizoid
- schizotypal
- secondary gain
- self-defeating personality
- self-mutilation
- splitting
- three Ps
- timid temperament
- turning anger against the self

QUESTIONS

Directions

Each of the questions or incomplete statements below is followed by five suggested responses or completions. Select the *one* that is *best* in each case.

29.1 Traits that have been identified as forming the stylistic components of behavior known as *temperament* include all of the following *except*

A. harm avoidance
B. novelty seeking
C. shyness
D. persistence
E. reward dependence

29.2 True statements about diagnosing specific personality disorders include

A. Diagnosis may not be made in children.
B. Antisocial personality disorder may be diagnosed in individuals under 18.
C. There is a potential sex bias in diagnosing personality disorders.
D. Real gender differences do not exist in the prevalence of personality disorders.
E. None of the above

29.3 Which of the following biological factors pertaining to personality disorders is *true*?

A. Compulsive traits are associated with high levels of testosterone
B. Low platelet monoamine oxidase levels have been noted in some patients with histrionic personality disorder
C. Antisocial personalities may have fast wave activity on EEG
D. Smooth pursuit eye movements are saccadic in persons who are introverted
E. 5-HIAA levels have been found to be high in suicide attempters

29.4 Antisocial personality disorder is associated with an increased risk for

A. major depressive disorder
B. anxiety disorders
C. somatization disorder
D. borderline personality disorder
E. all of the above

29.5 Persons with narcissistic personality disorders

A. may benefit from a psycho-analytic treatment approach
B. are usually immune to criticism
C. are easy to treat
D. handle aging well
E. are unlikely to feel depressed

29.6 The etiology of borderline personality disorder involves

A. childhood trauma
B. vulnerable temperament
C. biological vulnerabilities
D. familial aggregation
E. all of the above

29.7 Basic rules with regard to the treatment of patients with personality disorders include all of the following *except*

A. a passive therapist
B. use of pharmacotherapy
C. supervision and a support network for therapists
D. rare use of pure supportive psychotherapy
E. frequent sessions

29.8 Defense mechanisms

A. are unconscious processes
B. are implemented to abolish anxiety and depression
C. are employed to resolve internal conflicts
D. in personality disorder patients are often rigid and intractable
E. all of the above

29.9 Spectrum disorders

A. aggregate in the same family
B. co-occur in the same person
C. sometimes reflect differential expression of the same liability
D. may be phenotypically distinguishable
E. all of the above

29.10 Otto Kernberg's borderline level of personality organization involves

A. a lack of anxiety tolerance

B. a blurring of boundaries between the self and other
C. is centered around splitting
D. alternating perceptions of the self and other as all-good or all-bad
E. all of the above

29.11 Schizotypal personalities

A. are usually socially gregarious
B. occur more commonly in women with fragile X syndrome
C. demonstrate a full affective range
D. commonly suffer from mania
E. are not any more prevalent with schizophrenia than any other personality disorders

29.12 True statements about the aspects of personality called *temperament* include all of the following *except*

A. They are heritable.
B. They are observable early in childhood.
C. They are relatively stable in time.
D. They are inconsistent in different cultures.
E. They are predictive of adolescent and adult behavior.

29.13 Individuals high in novelty seeking are most likely

A. impulsive
B. disorderly
C. easily bored
D. extravagant
E. all of the above

29.14 True statements about paranoid personality disorder include

A. Patients are at decreased risk for major depression.
B. It may be a prepsychotic antecedent of delusional disorders, paranoid type.
C. Impairment is frequently severe.
D. The disorder is not complicated by brief psychotic disorder.
E. All of the above

29.15 Borderline personality disorder is associated with

A. decreased risk for psychotic symptoms
B. increased risk for premature death
C. decreased risk for other coexisting personality disorders
D. decreased risk for bulimia
E. decreased risk for posttraumatic stress disorder

29.16 Which of the following statements about borderline personality disorder is *false*?

A. Patients with borderline personality disorder have more relatives with mood disorders than do control groups.
B. Borderline personality disorder and mood disorders often coexist.
C. First-degree relatives of persons with borderline personality disorder show an increased prevalence of alcohol dependence.
D. Smooth-pursuit eye movements are abnormal in borderline personality disorder.
E. Monoamine oxidase inhibitors are used in the treatment of borderline personality disorder patients.

29.17 The defense mechanism most often associated with paranoid personality disorder is

A. hypochondriasis
B. splitting
C. isolation
D. projection
E. dissociation

29.18 A pervasive pattern of grandiosity, lack of empathy, and need for admiration suggests the diagnosis of which of the following personality disorders?

A. schizotypal
B. passive-aggressive
C. borderline
D. narcissistic
E. paranoid

29.19 Mr. S was a 45-year-old postal service employee who was evaluated at a clinic specializing in the treatment of depression. He claimed to have felt constantly depressed since the first grade, without a period of normal mood for more than a few days at a time. His depression was accompanied by lethargy, little or no interest or pleasure in anything, trouble in concentrating, and feelings of inadequacy, pessimism, and resentfulness. His only periods of normal mood occurred when he was home alone, listening to music or watching TV. On further questioning, Mr. S revealed that he could never remember feeling comfortable socially. Even before kindergarten, if he was asked to speak in front of a group of family friends, his mind would go blank. He felt overwhelming anxiety at children's social functions, such as birthday parties, which he either avoided or attended in total silence. He could answer questions in class only if he wrote down the answers in advance; even then, he frequently mumbled and could not get the answer out. He met new children with his eyes lowered, fearing their scrutiny, expecting to feel humiliated and embarrassed. He was convinced that everyone around him thought he was "dumb or a jerk."

During the past several years, he had tried several therapies to help him get over his shyness and depression. Mr. S had never experienced sudden anxiety or a panic attack in social situations or at other times. Rather, his anxiety built gradually to a constant level in anticipation of social situations. He had never experienced any psychotic symptoms.

The *best* diagnosis in the patient above is

A. avoidant personality disorder
B. schizoid personality disorder

C. schizotypal personality disorder
D. social phobia
E. adjustment disorder with anxiety

Directions

Each group of questions consists of lettered headings followed by a list of numbered statements. For each numbered phrase or statement, select the *one* lettered heading that is most closely associated with it. Each lettered heading may be selected once, more than once, or not at all.

Questions 29.20–29.27

A. Cluster A
B. Cluster B
C. Cluster C

29.20 Borderline personality disorder
29.21 Avoidant personality disorder
29.22 Narcissistic personality disorder
29.23 Obsessive-compulsive personality disorder
29.24 Paranoid personality disorder
29.25 Reward dependence
29.26 Novelty seeking
29.27 Harm avoidance

Questions 29.28–29.32

A. Schizoid personality disorder
B. Schizotypal personality disorder

29.28 Strikingly odd or eccentric behavior
29.29 Magical thinking
29.30 Ideas of reverence
29.31 Formerly called latent schizophrenia
29.32 Suspiciousness or paranoid ideation

Questions 29.33–29.36

A. ictal aggression
B. affective aggression
C. predatory aggression
D. organic-like aggression
E. None of the above

29.33 Aggression as a result of feeling threatened
29.34 Aggression seen often in patients with frontal lobe lesions
29.35 Aggression with intact impulse control
29.36 Unprovoked aggression associated with cerebral instability

Questions 29.37–29.40

A. character
B. temperament
C. personality
D. psyche
E. All of the above

29.37 Involves rational concepts about oneself and one's relationships
29.38 Involves basic emotions
29.39 Involves intuitive self-awareness
29.40 A dynamic system that is constantly evolving

ANSWERS

29.1 The answer is C

Temperament traits of *harm avoidance, novelty seeking, reward dependence, and persistence* are defined as heritable differences underlying one's automatic response to danger, novelty, and various typed of reward, respectively. These four temperament traits are closely associated with the four basic emotions of fear (harm avoidance), anger (novelty seeking), attachment (reward dependence), and ambition (persistence).

Individual differences in temperament and basic emotions modify the processing of sensory information and shape early learning characteristics, especially associative conditioning of unconscious behavior responses. Temperament is conceptualized as heritable biases in emotionality and learning that underlie the acquisition of emotion-based, automatic, behavioral traits and habits that are observable early in life and are relatively stable over one's life span.

The four temperament traits are understood to be genetically independent dimensions that occur in all factorial combinations, rather than mutually exclusive categories.

Persons who are harm avoidant are often shy, but *shyness* is only one variant of many that contributes to a harm avoidant temperament.

29.2 The answer is C

Diagnosis of specific personality disorders may be made in children or adolescents when observed maladaptive personality traits are pervasive, persistent, and unlikely to be limited to a particular developmental stage or an episode of an Axis I disorder. Diagnosis of a personality disorder in an individual under 18 years of age requires that the features be present for more than 1 year. The only exception to this *is antisocial personality disorder, which cannot be diagnosed in individuals under 18 years of age.*

Clinical experience points to *a potential sex bias in diagnosing personality disorders.* Certain personality disorders are diagnosed more frequently in men (e.g., antisocial and schizoid), whereas some disorders are diagnosed more frequently in women (e.g., borderline, histrionic, and dependent). Even though *real gender differences likely exist* in the prevalence of these disorders, clinicians are cautioned not to overdiagnose or underdiagnose certain personality disorders in males and females because of social stereotypes about typical gender roles and behaviors.

29.3 The answer is D

Smooth pursuit eye movements are often noted to be saccadic, or jumpy in persons who are introverted, have low self esteem, tend to withdraw, and who have schizotypal personality disorder. Persons with *impulsive, not compulsive traits,* often show high levels of testosterone, 17-estradiol, and estrone. *Low platelet monoamine oxidase* (MAO) levels have been associated in schizotypal disorders, not histrionic personalities. Changes in electrical conductance on EEG occur in some patients with personality disorders, most commonly antisocial and borderline types; these changes appear as *slow-wave activity on EEG. Levels of 5-hydroxyindoleacetic acid* (5-HIAA), a metabolite of serotonin, are low in persons who attempt suicide and in patients who are impulsive and aggressive.

29.4 The answer is E (all)

Antisocial patients are at increased risk for impulse control disorders, *major depression,* substance abuse or dependence, pathological gambling, *anxiety disorders*, and *somatization disorder.* The most common co-occurring personality disorders are narcissistic, *borderline*, and histrionic.

29.5 The answer is A

Heinz Kohut advocated using a *psychoanalytic approach* to effect change in the treatment of patients with narcissistic personality disorder. This said, because patients must renounce their narcissism to progress, the *treatment of these patients is difficult*. Their sense of entitlement is striking, and they are particularly *vulnerable to feeling criticized*, even if they appear immune to it. They handle criticism poorly and become enraged when criticized. They are constantly dealing with blows to their senses of self, *and age is handled poorly*; they often value beauty, strength and youthful attributes, to which they cling inappropriately. Because of their fragile self esteem, *they are prone to depression*.

29.6 The answer is E (all)

Numerous studies have pointed to *early traumatic experiences* as a cause of this personality disorder. Recently, a tripartite etiological model, including childhood trauma, *vulnerable temperament,* and a series of triggering events has been formulated. Dynamic and biological psychiatry agree that a combination of early traumatic events and *certain biological vulnerabilities* (mostly in the emotional domain) represent primary etiological factors. Physical and sexual abuse, neglect, hostile conflict, and early parental loss or separation are common in childhood histories of patients with this disorder. *Familial aggregation* of borderline personality disorder has been demonstrated repeatedly. Borderline personality disorder is five times more common among relatives of probands with this disorder than in the general population. The disorder is also associated with increased familial risk for antisocial personality disorder, substance abuse, and mood disorders.

29.7 The answer is A

As a rule, combinations of various orientations and formats along with emphasis on teamwork are optimal in the psychotherapy of personality disorders. Some basic guidelines and values are, nevertheless, strictly observed. Probably most crucial is having a stable therapeutic framework with consistent and reliable care. Next, behavior and feelings are used as the principal mode of communication. *The therapist is active, not passive*, and uses high-energy confrontation and care (so-called therapeutic pressing). The central message is "do something with the patient, not something to the patient." This way, patients feel more in control, which might keep them in treatment. Reflecting their splitting mechanism, these patients alternately feel inferior and omnipotent, angry at others and self-destructive, sensitive to rejection but usually provoking it. Flexibility in therapeutic approach but firmness in core values, with creativity and readiness to step away from the rules to get beyond "no way out" situations, is essential. Many of these patients cannot tolerate feeling better, as this means, at least in part, that the therapist is successful. These and similar frustrating situations cause countertransference problems, with a potential loss of professional objectivity; constant supervision and a *support network* are therefore necessary for the therapist treating borderline patients. Remember, these patients are almost never as good as they look when they are doing well, and almost never as bad as they look when they are not doing well.

Pure supportive psychotherapy is rarely used for personality disorders. Pure support, aimed at strengthening existing coping styles (which are, by definition, maladaptive in personality disorders), often reinforces the problems of these patients.

The psychobiological approach incorporates these psychodynamic strategies into a comprehensive treatment plan aimed at stimulating character development, primarily self-directedness and cooperativeness. The main focus is to change internalized conceptual representations of the self and the external objects (i.e., concepts about self, society, and the world as a whole). This is attempted either with cognitive methods (aimed at revising these concepts), with dynamic methods (aimed at generating maturation of internalized object relations), or, most frequently, with a combination of the two. Cognitive methods use emotions as the royal road to cognition. Also, object relations are a special kind of internalized concept about self and others associated with either positive or negative affects, depending on the nature of the relation. In other words, both cognitive and psychodynamic methods address emotional and conceptual aspects of deviant behaviors. Dynamic and cognitive methods are complemented by behavioral and experiential techniques, which are efficient in transforming concepts and insights into everyday life.

During therapy, as character matures and new concepts and their associated secondary emotions develop, they neutralize extreme temperament traits and their related basic emotions of fear and anger. Behaviors change accordingly, from being primarily reactive (i.e., steered by basic emotions and automatic responses regulated by temperament) to being primarily proactive (i.e., steered predominantly by secondary emotions and active symbolic constructs regulated by character traits).

Psychotherapy of personality disorders is a strategy rather than a strictly defined method because the therapy takes place constantly (during any contact with the patient), not only during the psychotherapy sessions proper. In fact, what is happening between sessions may be critical for the outcome of the treatment as a whole. With these patients, psychotherapy essentially means reparenting, which, although sometimes demanding, leaves space for various types of interventions, such as education, help with real-life problems, and encouragement. Frequent sessions (at least once a week) are needed to develop reasonably complex interactions in the relationship, for diagnostic and (especially) treatment purposes.

Increasing evidence shows pharmacotherapy to be at least as important as psychotherapy in the overall treatment of personality disorders. Pharmacotherapy is either (1) causal, aimed at correcting neurobiological dispositions underlying deviant traits; or (2) symptomatic, aimed at correcting target behaviors and symptoms of personality disorders. The third approach, based on the expectation that the treatment of diagnosable comorbid Axis I disorders might improve personality symptoms indirectly, receives least support in the literature.

29.8 The answer is E (all)

Defense mechanisms are *unconscious processes* used to resolve the conflicts of our inner lives. When they are most effective, especially in those with personality disorders, they can *abolish anxiety and depression*. Thus, abandoning a defense increases conscious anxiety and depression. Patients with personality disorders may be characterized by their defenses which are most *rigid and intractable*.

29.9 The answer is E (all)

Spectrum disorders *aggregate in the same family* and tend to *co-occur in the same person. Phenotypically distinguishable* disorders are referred to as spectrum disorders if they meet the two conditions previously mentioned. Spectrum disorders sometimes *reflect differential expression* of the same liability. They may also reflect a less deviant form of the other on a liability scale. Narcissistic, antisocial, and histrionic personality disorders are examples of spectrum-disorders.

29.10 The answer is E (all)

As defined by Otto Kernberg, the borderline level of personality organization is characterized by nonspecific manifestations of ego weakness, such as a lack of impulse control, and a *lack of anxiety tolerance*. There are specific ego defects, like partially *blurred boundaries* between the self and other. Object relations often *alternate between all-good and all-bad perceptions* of the self and external object. The defense mechanisms are primitive and *center on splitting* and identity disturbance.

29.11 The answer is B

While the sex ratio of schizotypal personality disorder is unknown, it is frequently diagnosed in *women with fragile X syndrome*. It is characterized by social and interpersonal deficits as indicated by pervasive discomfort with reduced capacity for close relationships. *Their affect is frequently constricted* or inappropriate. More than half of these patients have had at least one episode of *major depression, not mania*, and 30 to 50 percent have major depression concurrent with this personality disorder. There is an *increased prevalence* of the disorder among first degree relatives of probands with *schizophrenia*, and there is an increased prevalence of schizophrenia in the relatives of probands with schizotypal personality disorder.

29.12 The answer is D

Pioneering work by Alexander Thomas, M.D. and Stella Chess, M.D. conceptualized temperament as the stylistic component (how) of behavior, as differentiated from motivation (why) and content (what) of behavior. Modern concepts of temperament, however, emphasize its emotional, motivational, and adaptive aspects. Specifically, four major temperament traits have been identified: harm avoidance, novelty seeking, reward dependence, and persistence.

Temperament traits of harm avoidance, novelty seeking, reward dependence, and persistence are defined as *heritable differences* underlying one's automatic response to danger, novelty, and various types of reward, respectively. These four temperament traits are associated closely with the four basic emotions of fear (harm avoidance), anger (novelty seeking), attachment (reward dependence), and mastery (persistence). Individual differences in temperament and basic emotions modify the processing of sensory information and critically shape early learning characteristics, especially associative conditioning of unconscious behavior responses. In other words, temperament is conceptualized as heritable biases in emotionality and learning that underlie the acquisition of emotion-based, automatic behavior traits and habits *observable early in life and that are relatively stable over one's life span*.

Each of the four major dimensions is a normally distributed quantitative trait. The four dimensions were shown to be genetically homogeneous and independently inherited from one another in large, independent twin studies in the United States and Australia. Temperamental differences, which are not very stable initially, tend to stabilize during the second and third years of life. Accordingly, ratings of these four temperament traits at age 10 years predicted personality traits at ages 15, 18, and 27 years in a large sample of Swedish children. The four dimensions have been shown repeatedly to be *universal across different cultures*, ethnic groups, and political systems on five continents. In summary, these aspects of personality are called "temperament" because they are heritable, observable early in childhood, relatively stable in time, *moderately predictive of adolescent and adult behavior*, and consistent in different cultures.

29.13 The answer is E (all)

Novelty seeking reflects a heritable bias in the initiation or activation of appetitive approach in response to novelty, signals of reward, avoidance of conditioned signals of punishment, and skilled escape from unconditioned punishment. All four of these behaviors are hypothesized to co-vary as part of one heritable system of learning. They are observed as exploratory activity in response to novelty, impulsiveness, extravagance in approach to cues of reward, and active avoidance of frustration. Individuals high in novelty seeking are quick-tempered, curious, *easily bored, impulsive, extravagant*, and *disorderly*. Adaptive advantages of high novelty seeking are enthusiastic explorations of new and unfamiliar stimuli, leading potentially to originality, discoveries, and reward. The disadvantages include frequent and easy boredom, excessive impulsivity and angry outbursts, potential fickleness in relationships, and impressionism in efforts. Persons low in novelty seeking are slow tempered, stoic, reflective, frugal, reserved, and orderly. Their reflectiveness, stoic resilience, systematic efforts, and meticulous approach are clearly advantageous when these features are needed adaptively. The disadvantages include an uninquiring attitude, lack of enthusiasm, and tolerance of monotony, potentially leading to prosaic routinization of activities.

Mesolimbic and mesofrontal dopaminergic projections have a crucial role in incentive activation of each aspect of novelty seeking in animals. For example, dopamine-depleting lesions in the nucleus accumbens or the ventral tegmentum lead to neglect of novel environmental stimuli and reduce both spontaneous activity and investigative behavior. Behavioral activation by dopaminergic agonists depends on integrity of the nucleus accumbens but not the caudate nucleus. In human studies, individuals at risk for Parkinson's disease have low premorbid scores in novelty seeking but not other dimensions of personality, supporting the importance of dopamine in incentive activation of pleasurable behavior. The initiation and frequency of hyperactivity, binge eating, sexual hedonism, drinking, smoking, and other substance abuse (especially stimulants) are each associated with high scores in novelty seeking.

29.14 The answer is B

The hallmarks of paranoid personality disorder are excessive suspiciousness and distrust of others expressed as a pervasive tendency to interpret actions of others as deliberately demeaning, malevolent, threatening, exploiting, or deceiving. *Frequently, impairment is mild, not severe,* but the disorder typically includes occupational and social difficulties.

These patients are at *increased (not decreased) risk for major depressive disorder*, obsessive-compulsive disorder, agoraphobia, and substance abuse or dependence. The most common co-occurring personality disorders are schizotypal, schizoid, narcissistic, avoidant, and borderline personality disorders. The disorder *may be complicated by brief psychotic disorder*, particularly in response to stress. Paranoid personality disorder has been *postulated to be a prepsychotic antecedent of delusional disorder, paranoid type.*

29.15 The answer is B

The hallmarks of borderline personality disorder are pervasive and excessive instability of affects, self-image, and interpersonal relationships as well as marked impulsivity.

The disorder may be complicated by *psychotic-like symptoms* (hallucinations, body image distortions, hypnagogic phenomena, ideas of reference) in response to stress, and an increased risk for *premature death* (or physical handicap) from suicide and suicidal gestures, failed suicide, and self-injurious behavior. Frequent and severe impairment may lead to job losses, interrupted education, and broken marriages.

These patients are at *increased (not decreased) risk* for major depression, substance abuse or dependence, *eating disorders (notably bulimia), posttraumatic stress disorder*, and attention-deficit/hyperactivity disorder. Borderline personality disorder *co-occurs with most other personality disorders.*

29.16 The answer is D

Smooth pursuit eye movements are normal (not abnormal) in borderline personality disorder. They are abnormal in schizophrenic patients and patients with schizotypal personality disorder.

Patients with borderline personality disorders have *more relatives with mood disorders* than do members of control groups, and *borderline personality disorder and mood disorders often coexist.* First-degree relatives of persons with borderline personality disorder show an *increased prevalence of alcohol dependence* and substance abuse. *Monoamine oxidase inhibitors* (MAOIs) are used in the treatment of borderline personality disorder patients and have been effective in modulating affective instability and impulsivity in a number of patients. However, due to the high incidence of impulsivity, substance abuse, and eating disorders in borderline patients, MAOIs must only be used in selective patients, and even then with great restraint.

29.17 The answer is D

The defense mechanism most often associated with paranoid personality disorder is *projection*. The patients externalize their own emotions and attribute to others impulses and thoughts that they are unable to accept in themselves. Excessive fault finding, sensitivity to criticism, prejudice, and hypervigilance to injustice can all be understood as examples of projecting unacceptable impulses and thoughts onto others.

Hypochondriasis is a defense mechanism in some personality disorders, particularly in borderline, dependent, and passive-aggressive personality disorders. Hypochondriasis disguises reproach; that is, the hypochondriac complaint that others do not provide help often conceals bereavement, loneliness, or unacceptable aggressive impulses. The mechanism of hypochondriasis permits covert punishment of others with the patient's own pain and discomfort.

Splitting is used by patients with borderline personality disorder in particular. With splitting, the patient divides ambivalently regarded people, both past and present, into all-good or all-bad, rather than synthesizing and assimilating less-than-perfect caretakers.

Isolation is the defense mechanism characteristic of the orderly controlled person, often labeled an obsessive-compulsive personality. Isolation allows the person to face painful situations without painful affect or emotion and thus to remain always in control.

Dissociation consists of a separation of consciousness from unpleasant affects. It is most often seen in patients with histrionic or borderline personality disorder.

29.18 The answer is D

A pervasive pattern of grandiosity (in fantasy or behavior), lack of empathy, and need for admiration suggests the diagnosis of *narcissistic* personality disorder. The fantasies of narcissistic patients are of unlimited success, power, brilliance, beauty, and ideal love; their demands are for constant attention and admiration. Narcissistic personality disorder patients are indifferent to criticism or respond to it with feelings of rage or humiliation. Other common characteristics are a sense of entitlement, surprise and anger that people do not do what the patient wants, and interpersonal exploitiveness.

Schizotypal personality disorder is characterized by various eccentricities in communication or behavior coupled with defects in the capacity to form social relationships. The term emphasizes a possible relation with schizophrenia. The manifestation of aggressive behavior in passive ways—such as obstructionism, pouting, stubbornness, and intentional inefficiency—typify *passive-aggressive* personality disorder. *Borderline* personality disorder is marked by instability of mood, interpersonal relationships, and self-image. *Paranoid* personality disorder is characterized by rigidity, hypersensitivity, unwarranted suspicion, jealousy, envy, an exaggerated sense of self-importance, and a tendency to blame and ascribe evil motives to others.

29.19 The answer is A

The best diagnosis is *avoidant personality disorder.* Although feeling constantly depressed caused Mr. S to seek treatment, the pervasive pattern of social avoidance, fear of criticism, and lack of close peer relationships was of equal importance. Persons with avoidant personality show an extreme sensitivity to rejection, which may lead to social withdrawal. They are not asocial but are shy and show a great desire for companionship; they need unusually strong guarantees of uncritical acceptance. In the case presented, the patient exhibited a longstanding pattern of difficulty in relating to others. Persons with *schizoid personality disorder* do not evince the same strong desire for affection and acceptance; they want to be alone. *Schizotypal personality disorder* is characterized by strikingly odd or strange behavior, magical thinking, peculiar ideas, ideas of reference, illusions, and derealization. The patient described did not exhibit those characteristics. *Social phobia* is an irrational fear of social or performance situations such as public speaking and eating in public. A social phobia is anxiety concerning socially identified situations, not relationships in general.

A person with a personality disorder can have a superimposed adjustment disorder, but only if the current episode includes new clinical features not characteristic of the individual's personality. No evidence in the case described indicated that the anxiety was qualitatively different from what the patient always experienced in social situations. Thus, an additional diagnosis of *adjustment disorder with anxiety* is not made.

Answers 29.20–29.27

29.20 The answer is B

29.21 The answer is C

29.22 The answer is B

29.23 The answer is C

29.24 The answer is A

29.25 The answer is A

29.26 The answer is B

29.27 The answer is C

DSM-IV-TR arranges categorical personality disorders into three clusters, each sharing some clinical features: *Cluster A* includes three disorders with odd, aloof, and eccentric features (*paranoid*, schizoid, and schizotypal); *Cluster B* includes four disorders with dramatic, impulsive, and erratic features (*borderline*, antisocial, *narcissistic*, and histrionic); and *Cluster C* includes three disorders sharing anxious and fearful features (*avoidant*, dependent, and *obsessive-compulsive*). Several studies have supported the construct validity of these clusters except that the symptoms for compulsive disorder sometimes tend to form a fourth cluster. Note that the three dimensions underlying Clusters A, B, and C (i.e., detachment, impulsivity, and fearfulness) correspond closely to normal temperament traits (*reward dependence, novelty seeking, and harm avoidance,* respectively), suggesting that variation in these temperament traits might be significant in distinguishing among the three clusters of disorders.

Patients with *obsessive-compulsive personality disorder* are preoccupied with orderliness and perfectionism and are rigid and stubborn. In ICD-10 it is called anankastic personality disorder. Patients with *avoidant personality disorder* are unwilling to be involved with people unless certain of being liked. In ICD-10 this is called anxious personality disorder. *Borderline personality disorder* is characterized by identity disturbance, impulsivity, and recurrent suicidal behavior. In ICD-10 the disorder is called emotionally unstable personality disorder. Patients with *paranoid personality disorder* read hidden demeaning or threatening meanings into benign events and comments.

Answers 29.28–29.32

29.28 The answer is B

29.29 The answer is B

29.30 The answer is B

29.31 The answer is B

29.32 The answer is B

Unlike schizoid personality disorder, *schizotypal personality disorder* manifests with *strikingly odd or eccentric behavior. Magical thinking, ideas of reference*, illusions, and derealization are common; their presence formerly led to defining this disorder as borderline *or latent schizophrenia. Suspiciousness or paranoid ideation* occurs in schizotypal personality disorder, not schizoid personality disorder.

Answers 29.33–29.36

29.33 The answer is B

29.34 The answer is D

29.35 The answer is C

29.36 The answer is A

It is useful to distinguish different types of aggression. The most common form of aggression occurs when a quick-tempered person is provoked by *frustration or threats*. This is called *affective aggression*, and is frequent in impulsive-aggressive individuals. *Unprovoked aggression* can occur in patients with *cerebral instability* documented by an abnormal EEG, so-called ictal aggression, regardless of any associated personality traits. *Predatory aggression* or cruelty involves hostile revengefulness and taking pleasure in the victimization of others, often with *intact impulse control. Organic-like aggression* is often accompanied by poor social judgment and is often seen in patients with *frontal lobe lesions*.

Answers 29.37–29.40

29.37 The answer is A

29.38 The answer is B

29.39 The answer is D

29.40 The answer is C

Personality is complex and unique. It is the dynamic organization within the individual of those "psychosocial systems that determine his or her unique adjustment to his or her environment." It is a system that is constantly evolving and changing. *Temperament* involves basic emotions and refers to the body's biases in the modulation of conditioned behavioral responses to prescriptive physical stimuli. *Character* involves rational concepts about the self and interpersonal relationships. It refers to the mind, and is the conceptual core of personality. The *psyche* involves intuitive self-awareness and intelligence. It refers to a person's consciousness, self-awareness or spirit.

30

Psychosomatic Medicine and Consultation-Liaison Psychiatry

It is likely that no real "interface" existed between psychiatry and medicine until the early 20th century. Undoubtedly there was interest in applying psychiatry to patients with medical problems, but pursuit of this interest was usually quite personal and not formalized. Today, psychosomatic medicine has been a specific area of study within the field of psychiatry for more than 75 years. It is informed by two basic assumptions: There is a unity of mind and body (reflected in the term mind-body medicine); and psychological factors must be taken into account when considering all disease states.

The revised 4th edition of the *Diagnostic and Statistical Manual of Mental Disorders* (DSM-IV-TR) includes a classification specifically for psychological factors affecting medical conditions, and characterizes the factors as having to have a significant effect on the course or outcome of the condition, or place the patient at significantly higher risk for an adverse outcome. The nature of the various psychological factors are delineated in DSM-IV-TR and include mental disorder, psychological symptoms, personality traits or coping styles, maladaptive health behaviors, and unspecified psychological factors. DSM-IV-TR does not stipulate that these factors must directly cause the medical condition, but it does specify that there must be a close temporal relationship between the factors and the condition.

Consultation-liaison (C-L) psychiatry is the study, practice, and teaching of the relation between medical and psychiatric disorders. In C-L psychiatry, psychiatrists serve as consultants to medical colleagues (either another psychiatrist or, more commonly, a non-psychiatric physician) or to other mental health professionals (psychologist, social worker, or psychiatric nurse). C-L psychiatry is associated with all the diagnostic, therapeutic, research, and teaching services that psychiatrists perform in the general hospital and serves as a bridge between psychiatry and other specialties. Virtually every major system of the body has been investigated with regard to the relationship between psychological factors and disease. Psychological factors affecting the cardiovascular, respiratory, immune, endocrine, gastrointestinal, and dermatologic systems are well known. Even the apparently simple act of correctly following a medication regimen can be complicated, and perhaps undermined, by unaddressed or unrecognized psychological factors.

Psychosomatic concepts have contributed greatly to many approaches to medical care. Concepts derived from the field of psychosomatic medicine influenced the emergence of complementary and alternative medicine (CAM) which relies heavily on examining psychological factors in the maintenance of health and also influenced the field of holistic medicine with its emphasis on examining and treating the whole patient, not just his or her disease or disorder. The concepts of psychosomatic medicine also influenced the field of behavioral medicine, which integrates the behavioral sciences and the biomedical approach to the prevention, diagnosis, and treatment of disease.

The student should study the questions and answers below for a useful review of these factors.

HELPFUL HINTS

These terms relating to psychophysiological medicine should be defined.

- AIDS
- Franz Alexander
- alexithymia
- allergic disorders
- analgesia
- atopic
- autoimmune diseases
- behavioral medicine
- behavior modification deconditioning program
- biofeedback
- bronchial asthma
- bulimia nervosa and anorexia nervosa
- C-L psychiatry
- cardiac arrhythmias
- cell-mediated immunity
- chronic pain
- climacteric
- command hallucination
- compulsive personality traits
- congestive heart failure
- conversion disorder
- coronary artery disease
- crisis intervention
- Jacob DaCosta
- diabetes mellitus
- dialysis dementia
- Flanders Dunbar
- dysmenorrhea
- dysthymic disorder
- essential hypertension
- fibromyalgia
- Meyer Friedman and Roy Rosenman
- general adaptation syndrome
- giving up–given up concept

- gun-barrel vision
- hay fever
- hemodialysis units
- Thomas Holmes and Richard Rahe
- humoral immunity
- hyperhidrosis
- hyperthyroidism
- hyperventilation syndrome
- hypochondriasis
- ICUs
- idiopathic amenorrhea
- IgM and IgA
- immediate and delayed hypersensitivity
- immune disorders
- immune response
- life-change units
- low back pain
- menopausal distress
- migraine
- myxedema madness
- neurocirculatory asthenia
- obesity
- obsessional personalities
- oral-aggressive feelings
- organ transplantation
- pain clinics
- pain threshold and perception
- pancreatic carcinoma
- Papez circuit
- peptic ulcer
- personality types
- pheochromocytoma
- PMS
- postcardiotomy delirium
- premenstrual dysphoric disorder
- propranolol (Inderal)
- pruritus
- psyche and soma
- psychogenic cardiac nondisease
- psychophysiological
- psychosomatic
- Raynaud's phenomenon
- relaxation therapy
- rheumatoid arthritis
- Hans Selye
- skin disorders
- social readjustment rating scale
- somatization disorder
- specific versus nonspecific stress
- specificity hypothesis
- surgical patients
- systemic lupus erythematosus
- tension headaches
- tension myositis syndrome (TMS)
- thyrotoxicosis
- type A and type B personalities
- ulcerative colitis
- undermedication
- vasomotor syncope
- vasovagal attack
- Wilson's disease

QUESTIONS

Directions

Each of the questions or incomplete statements below is followed by five responses or completions. Select the *one* that is *best* in each case.

30.1 Antidepressants should be used cautiously in cardiac patients due to increased risk of which of the following?

A. Hypertension
B. Suicide
C. Conduction side effects
D. Noncompliance
E. All of the above

30.2 Which of the following is *not* a medical cause of hallucinations?

A. Alcohol use
B. Alcohol withdrawal
C. Cocaine use
D. Hyperthyroidism
E. None of the above

30.3 Which of the following statements regarding the Social Readjustment Rating Scale is *not* true?

A. It is based on the work of Thomas Holmes and Richard Rahe.
B. It suggests marriage is a more stressful event than divorce.
C. The life event incurring the most life change units is death of a spouse.
D. It helps correlates life stress with subsequent illness.
E. Accumulating 200 or more life change units increases the risk for illness.

30.4 Which of the following is the most common reason for a consultation-liaison psychiatrist to be consulted?

A. Anxiety
B. Depression
C. Disorientation
D. Treatment problems
E. Sleep disorders

30.5 You are the C-L psychiatrist called to consult on a patient who is scheduled for a liver transplant. You learn the patient now needs a transplant after he was infected with hepatitis C due to promiscuous sexual activity. Which of the following is this patient at increased risk for?

A. Medication noncompliance
B. Major depression
C. Organ rejection
D. Adjustment disorder
E. Suicide

30.6 Which of the following statements regarding tension headaches is *true*?

A. Competitive personalities are prone to tension headaches.
B. Antianxiety agents have been shown effective in treatment.
C. Psychotherapy is effective for treatment of chronic tension headaches.
D. Antidepressants can be helpful in some cases of tension headaches.
E. All of the above.

30.7 Which of the following is *not* a physiological response of the GI system to acute stress?

A. Increased resting tone of the upper esophageal sphincter
B. Decreased contraction amplitude in the distal esophagus
C. Decreased antral motor activity in the stomach

D. Reduced migrating motor function in the small intestine
E. Increased myoelectrical motility in the large intestine

30.8 Which of the following statements regarding psychiatric disorders and asthma is *true*?

A. Type B personalities have been associated with an increased prevalence of asthma.
B. Approximately one-third of persons with asthma also have panic disorder.
C. Patients with asthma have excessive dependency needs.
D. Fear may directly trigger asthma attacks.
E. All of the above

30.9 Which of the following statements regarding psychogenic excoriations is true?

A. Scratching does not occur in response to an itch.
B. Lesions are typically found in hard to reach areas.
C. The behavior never becomes ritualistic.
D. Freud believed the skin is susceptible to unconscious sexual urges.
E. All of the above

30.10 Dialysis dementia

A. Can occur after a patient's first dialysis treatment
B. Is a common occurrence
C. Can cause seizures and dystonias
D. Rarely leads to depression and suicide
E. All of the above

30.11 A review of the impact of biobehavioral factors on adult cancer pain concluded that

A. there was a consistent role of personality factors
B. the relationship to affective states was major
C. environmental influences were strong
D. all of the above
E. none of the above

30.12 A major advance in DSM-IV-TR in regard to the diagnostic criteria for psychological factors affecting medical condition is that it allows for emphasis on

A. environmental stimuli
B. psychological stimuli
C. somatoform disorders
D. conversion disorder
E. all of the above

30.13 A decrease in T lymphocytes has been reported in all of the following *except*

A. bereavement
B. caretakers of patients with dementia of the Alzheimer's type
C. women who are having extramarital affairs
D. nonpsychotic inpatients
E. medical students during final examinations

30.14 True statements about the effects of psychosocial interventions in cancer outcomes and prognosis include

A. There is no evidence that psychotherapy influences the outcome of metastatic breast cancer.
B. The mortality rates and recurrence rates in patients with malignant melanoma have been shown to be greater in patients who did not receive a structured group intervention than in those who did.
C. Group behavioral intervention in patients with breast cancer does not appear to have any effect on lymphocyte mitogen responses.
D. A lack of social support and depression has not been shown to be linked to diminished immune responses in women with breast cancer.
E. Hypothalamic-pituitary-adrenal axis hypoactivity induced by exposure of rats to stress is associated with increased tumor growth.

30.15 Exposure of rats to stress reliably

A. decreases plasma concentrations of ACTH
B. decreases plasma concentrations of corticosterone
C. increases secretion of growth hormone
D. increases secretion of CRF in locus ceruleus
E. all of the above

30.16 The most frequent functional gastrointestinal disorder is

A. functional abdominal bloating
B. functional chest pain
C. functional heartburn
D. irritable bowel syndrome
E. globus

30.17 True statements about research in psychocardiology include

A. The most consistent psychological correlates of hypertension are inhibited anger expression and excessive anger expression.
B. Stress leads to excess secretion of epinephrine, which raises cardiac contractility and conduction velocity.
C. Cardiac surgery patients at greatest risk for complications are depressed and in denial about their anxiety.
D. Mental stress leads to diminished cardiac perfusion.
E. All of the above

30.18 True statements about type A behavior include

A. Once coronary artery disease is present, global type A behavior appears to increase the risk of subsequent cardiac morbidity.
B. Of all the elements of the syndrome, hostility has been found to be the most toxic element.
C. Global type A behavior consistently predicts risk of coronary artery disease.
D. Expressive hostility and antagonistic interactions appear to be least strongly related to the risk of coronary artery disease in women.
E. Lifestyle modification has little effect on revascularization.

30.19 True statements about obesity include

A. The number of obese Americans is less than that of nonobese Americans.
B. The prevalence of obesity in America has doubled since the early 1900s.
C. Higher rates of obesity are linked with lower socioeconomic and educational levels and type of diet.
D. Its prevalence in children appears to be stabilized and even decreasing.
E. All of the above

30.20 A 53-year-old male patient is found to have an occipital lobe tumor. He would be *least likely* to exhibit which of the following symptoms and complaints?

A. Paranoid delusions
B. Visual hallucinations
C. Headache
D. Papilledema
E. Homonymous hemianopsia

30.21 In evaluating patients with complaints of chronic pain of whatever cause, the physician must be alert to

A. use of over-the-counter medications
B. alcohol dependence
C. withdrawal symptoms during the evaluation
D. an underlying medical illness
E. all of the above

30.22 A highly emetogenic anticancer agent is

A. cisplatin
B. doxorubicin
C. vincristine
D. vinblastine
E. bleomycin

30.23 Psoriasis has been shown to be

A. unaffected by such psychosocial interventions as meditation or relaxation
B. associated with lower levels of anxiety and depression than in the general population
C. triggered by external factors such as cold weather and physical trauma
D. rarely associated with personality disorders
E. none of the above

30.24 Antidepressants have been shown to be helpful in the treatment of

A. idiopathic pruritus
B. urticaria
C. vulvodynia
D. glossodynia
E. all of the above

30.25 Which of the following statements about psychoneuroimmunology is *true*?

A. Immunological reactivity is not affected by hypnosis.
B. Lymphocytes cannot produce neurotransmitters.
C. The immune system is affected by conditioning.
D. Growth hormone does not affect immunity.
E. Marijuana does not affect the immune system.

30.26 Phantom limb occurs after leg amputation in what percentage of patients?

A. 98 percent
B. 90 percent
C. 80 percent
D. 50 percent
E. 10 percent

30.27 In the psychotherapeutic treatment of patients with psychosomatic disorders, the most difficult problem is patients'

A. resistance to entering psychotherapy
B. erotic transference to the psychotherapist
C. positive response to the interpretation of the physiological meaning of their symptoms
D. overemphasis of the psychological component of their physiological symptoms
E. none of the above

Directions

The questions below consist of five lettered headings followed by a list of numbered phrases. For each numbered item, select the *one* lettered heading that is most closely associated with it. Each lettered heading may be selected once, more than once, or not at all.

Questions 30.28–30.32

A. Wilson's disease
B. Pheochromocytoma
C. Systemic lupus erythematosus
D. Acquired immune deficiency syndrome (AIDS)
E. Pancreatic cancer

30.28 Dementia syndrome with global impairment and seropositivity
30.29 Resemblance to steroid psychosis
30.30 Explosive anger and labile mood
30.31 Symptoms of a classic panic attack
30.32 Sense of imminent doom

ANSWERS

30.1 The answer is C

Consultation-liaison psychiatrists must make a careful assessment of drug-drug interactions prior to prescribing medications, and this should be undertaken in collaboration with the patient's primary physician. Antidepressants should be used cautiously in cardiac patients because of *conduction side effects and orthostatic hypotension* (not hypertension). It is typically depressed patients who may be at increased risk for *suicide* once started on antidepressants, not cardiac patients. *Noncompliance*, while an issue with all patients for various reasons, is not specifically troublesome with cardiac patients.

30.2 The answer is A

The most common cause of hallucinations is *delirium tremens,* a component of *alcohol withdrawal*, which usually begins 3 to 4 days after hospitalization. Also of concern are patients in intensive care units who experience sensory isolation and who may respond with hallucinatory activity. Conditions such as brief psychotic disorder, schizophrenia, and cognitive disorders are associated with hallucinations that respond rapidly to antipsychotic medication. Formication in which the patient believes they have bugs crawling over the skin is often associated with *cocainism.* Patients with severe cases of *thyrotoxicosis* may exhibit visual hallucinations, paranoid ideation, and delirium.

30.3 The answer is B

A major area of psychosomatic research involving social stress is based on the work of *Thomas Holmes and Richard Rahe*, using the Schedule of Recent Experience (SRE) and Social Readjustment Rating Scale. Recent life events (e.g. the death of a close relative, a job change, or a divorce) are assigned life change units. An expanded and revised version of the SRE, the Recent Life Change Questionnaire, also asks subjects to score recent life changes on the degree of perceived adjustment. Both instruments are designed to measure recent life stress and to *correlate the degree of life stress with subsequent illness*. The basic hypothesis is that stressful life occurrences are risk factors for the development of physical illness. Holmes and Rahe hypothesized that the *accumulation of 200 or more life change units in a single year increases the risk of developing a psychosomatic disorder in that year*. Numerous studies demonstrate a relation between stressful life events and one's chances of having a physical illness. Epidemiological research involving other types of stressful life events (e.g., natural disasters, social disruption, social changes, poor social support, and work-related stress) has shown similar trends toward an increased probability of physical illness and relatively poor medical outcome. Current models of psychosomatic research integrate the interaction of psychological variables, stressful social situations, and biological vulnerability with latent physical disease. Table 30.1 provides the Social Readjustment Rating Scale, which shows the life event *incurring the most life change units is death of a spouse*, and that *divorce incurs more life change units than marriage* (not marriage more than divorce).

30.4 The answer is D

C-L psychiatrists must deal with a broad range of psychiatric disorders. The most common reason for consultation being *treatment problems,* which account for 50 percent of the consultation requests made of psychiatrists. Other common symptoms are *anxiety, depression, and disorientation*. While sleep disorders are common complaints among hospitalized patients, treatment problems clearly surpass these disorders as a reason for consultation.

30.5 The answer is A

Transplantation programs have expanded over the past decade, and C-L psychiatrists play an important role in helping patients and their families deal with the many psychosocial issues

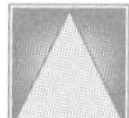

Table 30.1
Social Readjustment Rating Scale

Life Event	Mean Value
1. Death of spouse	100
2. Divorce	73
3. Marital separation from mate	65
4. Detention in jail or other institution	63
5. Death of a close family member	63
6. Major personal injury or illness	53
7. Marriage	50
8. Being fired at work	47
9. Marital reconciliation with mate	45
10. Retirement from work	45
11. Major change in the health or behavior of a family member	44
12. Pregnancy	40
13. Sexual difficulties	39
14. Gaining a new family member (through birth, adoption, elder moving in, etc.)	39
15. Major business readjustment (merger, reorganization, bankruptcy, etc.)	39
16. Major change in financial state (a lot worse off or a lot better off than usual)	38
17. Death of a close friend	37
18. Changing to a different line of work	36
19. Major change in the number of arguments with spouse (either a lot more or a lot less than usual regarding child rearing, personal habits, etc.)	35
20. Taking on a mortgage greater than $10,000 (purchasing a home, business, etc.)[a]	31
21. Foreclosure on a mortgage or loan	30
22. Major change in responsibilitities at work (promotion, demotion, lateral transfer)	29
23. Son or daughter leaving home (marriage, attending college, etc.)	29
24. In-law troubles	29
25. Outstanding personal achievement	28
26. Wife beginning or ceasing work outside the home	26
27. Beginning or ceasing formal schooling	26
28. Major change in living conditions (building a new home, remodeling, deterioration of home or neighborhood)	25
29. Revision of personal habits (dress, manners, associations, etc.)	24
30. Troubles with the boss	23
31. Major change in working hours or conditions	20
32. Change in residence	20
33. Changing to a new school	20
34. Major change in usual type or amount of recreation	19
35. Major change in church activities (a lot more or a lot less than usual)	19
36. Major change in social activities (clubs, dancing, movies, visiting, etc.)	18
37. Taking on a mortgage or loan less than $10,000 (purchasing a car, TV, freezer, etc.)	17
38. Major change in sleeping habits (a lot more or a lot less sleep or change in part of day when asleep)	16
39. Major change in number of family get-togethers (a lot more or a lot less than usual)	15
40. Major change in eating habits (a lot more or a lot less food intake or very different meal hours or surroundings)	15
41. Vacation	15
42. Christmas	12
43. Minor violations of the law (traffic tickets, jaywalking, disturbing the peace, etc.)	11

[a]This figure no longer has any relevance in the light of inflation; what is significant is the total amount of debt from all sources.

Reprinted with permission from Holmes T. Life situations, emotions, and disease. *Psychosom Med.* 1978;9:747.

involved: (1) which and when patients on a waiting list will receive organs, (2) anxiety about the procedure, (3) fear of death, (4) organ rejection, and (5) adaptation to life after successful transplantation. Posttransplant patients require complex aftercare, and achieving *compliance with medication* may be difficult without supportive psychotherapy. This is particularly relevant to patients who have received liver transplants as a result of hepatitis C brought on by promiscuous sexual behavior and to drug addicts who use contaminated needles.

While all the remaining choices are of concern for any transplant patient, they are not particularly relevant in this patient, as the primary concern should be his medication compliance. Within 1 year of transplant, almost 20 percent of patients experience a *major depression* or an *adjustment disorder* with depressed mood. In such cases evaluation for *suicidal ideation* and risk is important. In addition to depression, another 10 percent of patients experience signs of posttraumatic stress disorder, with nightmares and anxiety attacks related to the procedure.

30.6 The answer is E (all)

Tension headaches are frequently associated with anxiety and depression and occur to some degree in about 80 percent of persons during periods of emotional stress. Tense, high-strung, *competitive personalities are especially prone* to the disorder. In the initial stage persons may be treated with *antianxiety agents*, muscle relaxants, and massage or heat application to the head and the neck; *antidepressants may be prescribed when an underlying depression is present. Psychotherapy is an effective treatment for persons chronically afflicted* by tension headaches. Learning to avoid or cope better with tension is the most effective long-term management approach. Biofeedback using electromyogram (EMG) feedback from the frontal or temporal muscles may help some patients. Relaxation exercises and meditation also benefit some patients.

30.7 The answer is B

Acute stress can induce physiological responses in several GI target organs. In the esophagus, acute stress *increases resting tone of the upper esophageal sphincter* and increases *(not decreases)* contraction amplitude in the distal esophagus. Such physiological responses may result in symptoms that are consistent with globus or esophageal spasm syndrome. In the stomach, acute stress induces *decreased antral motor activity*, potentially producing functional nausea and vomiting. In the small intestine, *reduced migrating motor function* can occur, whereas in the large intestine, there can be *increased myoelectrical and motility activity* under acute stress. These effects in the small and large intestine may be responsible for bowel symptoms associated with irritable bowel syndrome (IBS).

30.8 The answer is E (all)

Asthma is a chronic, episodic illness characterized by extensive narrowing of the tracheobronchial tree. Symptoms include coughing, wheezing, chest tightness, and dyspnea. Nocturnal symptoms and exacerbations are common. Although patients with asthma are *characterized as having excessive dependency needs, no specific personality type has been identified*; however, *up to 30 percent of persons with asthma meet the criteria for panic disorder or agoraphobia*. The *fear of dyspnea may directly trigger asthma attacks*, and high levels of anxiety are associated with increased rates of hospitalization and asthma-associated mortality. Certain personality traits in asthma patients are associated with greater use of corticosteroids and bronchodilators and longer hospitalizations than would be predicted from pulmonary function alone. These traits include intense fear, emotional lability, sensitivity to rejection, and lack of persistence in difficult situations.

30.9 The answer is D

Psychocutaneous disorders encompass a wide variety of dermatological diseases that may be affected by the presence of psychiatric symptoms or stress and psychiatric illnesses in which the skin is the target of disordered thinking, behavior, or perception.

Psychogenic excoriations (also called psychogenic pruritus) are lesions caused by scratching or picking *in response to an itch or other skin sensation* or because of an urge to remove an irregularity on the skin from preexisting dermatoses such as acne. Lesions are typically found in *areas that the patient can easily reach* (e.g., the face, upper back, and the upper and lower extremities) and are a few millimeters in diameter and weeping, crusted, or scarred, with occasional postinflammatory hypopigmentation or hyperpigmentation. The behavior in psychogenic excoriation sometimes resembles obsessive-compulsive disorder in that it is *repetitive, ritualistic, and tension reducing*, and patients attempt (often unsuccessfully) to resist excoriating. The skin is an important erogenous zone, and *Freud believed it susceptible to unconscious sexual impulses*.

30.10 The answer is C

Dialysis patients are coping with lifelong, debilitating, and limiting disease; they are totally dependent on a multiplex group of caretakers for access to a machine controlling their well-being. Dialysis dementia is a *rare condition* characterized by loss of memory, disorientation, *dystonias, and seizures*. The dementia occurs in patients who have been receiving *dialysis treatment for many years*. The cause is unknown. Other complications of dialysis treatment can include psychiatric problems such as *depression*, and *suicide is not rare*. Sexual problems can be neurogenic, psychogenic, or related to gonadal dysfunction and testicular atrophy.

30.11 The answer is E (none)

Patients with pain have a significantly higher incidence of depression and anxiety. It has been suggested that chronic pain may be a depressive equivalent, that pain may cause psychiatric syndromes, and that pain may coexist with psychopathology in vulnerable subjects. In cancer patients, the evidence suggests that these emotional reactions both result from and contribute to the experience of pain, and that treatment of one improves the other. However, *a review of the impact of biobehavioral factors on adult cancer pain concluded that the role of personality factors was inconsistent (not consistent), the relationship to affective states minimal (not major), the environmental influences were weak (not strong)*, and the role of cognitive factors was unexplored. Hence, the psychiatric consultant is wise to avoid diagnostic inferences that minimize the patient's complaints. Patients with significant psychopathology are indeed more difficult to evaluate, so the consultant must help the staff make the same aggressive efforts at symptom relief for these patients as for other patients. The incidence of psychiatric complications is

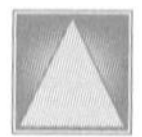

Table 30.2
Behavioral States Associated with In Vitro Immune Suppression

Disturbed sleep function
Examination stress
Loneliness
Unemployment
Marital discord
Divorce
Alzheimer's disease—caregivers' stress
Bereaved spouses (including anticipatory bereavement)
Clinical anxiety
Major depressive disorder

particularly high when pain is underestimated and undermedicated by caretakers, an event that recurs with a regularity that cries out for explanations.

30.12 The answer is B

A major advance in DSM-IV-TR from the third edition (DSM-III-R) is that DSM-IV-TR allows clinicians to specify the *psychological stimuli* that affect the patient's medical condition. In DSM-III-R, psychologically meaningful *environmental stimuli* were temporally related to the physical disorder. Excluded in DSM-III-R were *somatoform disorders*, such as *conversion disorder*, in which the physical symptoms are not based on organic pathology. The DSM-IV-TR emphasis on psychological factors permits a wide range of psychological stimuli to be noted (for example, personality traits, maladaptive health behaviors).

30.13 The answer is C

There are no studies on the T cells of *women who are having extramarital affairs.* Investigators have found a decrease in lymphocytic response in *bereavement* (conjugal and anticipatory), the *caretakers of patients with dementia of the Alzheimer's type,* in *nonpsychotic inpatients*, in resident physicians, in *medical students during final examinations*, in women who were separated or divorced, in the elderly with no social support, and in the unemployed. Table 30.2 lists some of the common behavioral states associated with in vitro immune suppression.

30.14 The answer is B

The growing interface between the social sciences and oncology between the 1930s and 1950s was the foundation for the emergence of the subspecialty called psychosocial oncology or psycho-oncology. This area, which has become a major contender in psychosomatic medicine research, seeks to study both the impact of cancer on psychological functioning and the role that psychological and behavioral variables may play in cancer risk and survival. A hallmark of psycho-oncology research has been intervention studies that attempt to influence the course of illness in patients with cancer. While most psychosocial interventions are aimed at providing psychological support rather than direct treatment of comorbid conditions such as major depressive disorder, important clinical observations have emerged that focus on such variables as cancer outcome and psychoneuroimmunology. For example, one landmark study demonstrated that *women with metastatic breast cancer* who received weekly group psychotherapy survived an average of 18 months longer than control patients randomly assigned to routine care. In their study of *patients with malignant melanoma*, one group of investigators found that control patients who did not receive a structured group intervention had a statistically significant recurrence of cancer and a greater mortality rate than patients who did receive such therapy. The malignant melanoma patients who received the group intervention also exhibited a significant increase in the number of large granular lymphocytes and NK cells as well as indications of increased NK cell activity. Another group of investigators used a *group behavioral intervention* (relaxation, guided imagery, and biofeedback training) *in patients with breast cancer* to demonstrate increased NK cell activity and lymphocyte mitogen responses in patients receiving treatment compared with controls.

Increasingly, intervention studies in psycho-oncology are focusing on complex variables of disease outcome including neuroendocrine and immune parameters. Investigators have found that psychosocial variables such as *lack of social support and depressive symptoms* may be linked to reduced NK cell activity in women with breast cancer and that more metastatic nodes and decreased NK cell activity are associated with depressive symptoms, emphasizing the need for more research in the area. Addressing psychoneuroimmunological aspects of depression in patients with cancer may have important treatment implications, particularly regarding hypothalamic-pituitary-adrenal axis hyperactivity associated with depression. In fact, hypothalamic-pituitary-adrenal hyperactivity in depressed cancer patients may have important prognostic implications, particularly since *hypothalamic-pituitary-adrenal hyperactivity* induced by exposure of rats to stress is associated with increased tumor growth, especially in older rats. Psychosocial treatment of patients with malignant melanoma has been shown to improve prognoses and enhance certain immune parameters.

30.15 The answer is D

Hans Selye first described the adaptation syndrome in rats exposed to chronic stress, a response characterized by adrenal hypertrophy, gastric ulcers, and thymus and lymph node involution. Since then, psychoneuroendocrinology, the subspecialty that addresses the relationship between hormones and behavior, has continued as an area of study. While earlier researchers in psychosomatic medicine were more interested in endocrine disturbances that produce psychiatric syndromes (Cushing's syndrome, hyperthyroidism, hypothyroidism), exogenous hormone–induced syndromes (glucocorticoid administration), and psychiatric aspects of other endocrine abnormalities (diabetes mellitus), more recent research has focused on the multifaceted role of neuroendocrine modulation and its relation to behavioral disturbances and psychiatric symptomatology.

For example, exposure of rats to stress reliably *increases (not decreases) plasma concentrations of ACTH* and *corticosterone* and *decreases (not increases) secretion of growth hormone* and gonadotropins. Increased secretion of CRF from the hypothalamic-hypophysial portal system mediates a complex cascade. Within the CNS, CRF activates the sympathetic nervous system, raising plasma concentrations of epinephrine and norepinephrine, thereby increasing heart rate, blood pressure, and plasma glucose concentrations. Stress-induced alterations in immune function may also be mediated by increased CRF secretion. *The CRF concentration in the locus ceruleus increases markedly after acute stress.*

When administered directly into the CNS of laboratory animals, CRF produces a number of physiological and behavioral changes similar to the physiological changes observed in stressed animals, which resemble signs and symptoms of depression and anxiety disorders. Centrally administered CRF increases mean arterial pressure, heart rate, oxygen consumption, and plasma glucose and catecholamine concentrations. It also alters locomotor activity, decreases sexual activity, diminishes food consumption, increases emotionality, and induces sleep disturbances.

30.16 The answer is C

Functional gastrointestinal disorders are common syndromes associated with significant subjective distress and abnormalities of bowel function, without evidence of structural abnormalities. Functional gastrointestinal disorders frequently have high rates of psychiatric comorbidity.

Functional heartburn is the most common functional gastrointestinal disorder. Functional heartburn needs to be distinguished from gastroesophageal reflux disease. In functional heartburn, symptoms of acid reflux are present (i.e., heartburn, regurgitation of food), but there is no evidence of anatomical abnormality or esophagitis on endoscopy or radiography.

Emotional distress and anxiety disorders can result in abnormal respiration and air swallowing or aerophagia. Swallowed air produces distension of the stomach and feelings of *abdominal* fullness or *bloating* along with belching.

Chest pain frequently prompts attention for potential cardiac causes. However, functional esophageal motility disorders can produce chest pain and need to be considered in patients with chest pain and no evidence of cardiac abnormalities. Pain related to esophageal motility disturbances can be described as angina-like in location and character. High-amplitude esophageal contractions in the distal esophagus, "nutcracker esophagus," can produce significant pain.

Referral to gastroenterology for evaluation of gastrointestinal causes of chest pain frequently occurs after cardiac causes have been ruled out. It is not unusual for several specialists to see the chest pain patient prior to appropriate psychiatric referral. However, at times psychiatrists may be involved before a comprehensive medical evaluation has been completed. Psychiatrists need to be aware of the possible gastrointestinal causes for chest pain, particularly when there is limited evidence for a psychiatric disorder in an unexplained chest pain presentation (Table 30.3).

Irritable bowel syndrome (IBS) is the prototypical functional gastrointestinal disorder characterized by abdominal pain and diarrhea or constipation. The International Congress of Gastroenterology has developed a standardized set of criteria for IBS:

1. Abdominal pain relieved by defecation or associated with change in frequency or consistency of stool.
2. Disturbed defecation involving two or more of the following:
   - altered stool frequency
   - altered stool form (hard or loose and watery)
   - altered stool passage (straining or urgency, feeling of incomplete evacuation)
   - passage of mucus

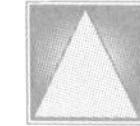

Table 30.3
Common Gastrointestinal Diseases

Disorders of the esophagus
Reflux esophagitis (GERD)
Infectious esophagitis
Esophageal motility disorders
Disorders of the stomach and intestines
Peptic ulcer disease
Gastroparesis
Malabsorption and maldigestion
Inflammatory bowel disease
Crohn's disease
Ulcerative colitis
Diverticular disease
Diseases of the anorectum
Hemorrhoids
Anal fissures
Perirectal abscess
Diseases of the pancreas
Acute pancreatitis
Chronic pancreatitis
Diseases of the liver and gallbladder
Infectious hepatitis
Toxic and drug-induced hepatitis
Primary biliary cirrhosis
Primary sclerosing cholangitis
Metabolic liver disease
Gallstones and cholecystitis
Cancer of the gastrointestinal tract
Colon and rectal cancer
Pancreatic cancer
Esophageal cancer
Stomach cancer
Liver cancer

Irritable bowel syndrome can often be categorized into diarrhea-predominant, constipation-predominant, and mixed subtypes. Medical treatment often targets the predominant symptom. Some studies suggest that irritable bowel syndrome accounts for up to 50 percent of all outpatient evaluations done by gastroenterologists. Comorbid psychiatric disorders appear to increase the likelihood of health-care-seeking behavior for people with symptoms of irritable bowel syndrome.

Some patients with irritable bowel syndrome may demonstrate physiological abnormalities including abnormal intestinal myoelectric activity, gastrointestinal hormonal abnormalities, or allergic responses to some foods. Most clinicians agree that both physiological and psychological factors contribute to the clinical picture of irritable bowel syndrome in most patients.

Globus, the Latin word for lump, indicates a sensation of having a lump in the throat. Alternate terms for globus include *globus pharyngeus*, *globus hystericus*, and *globus syndrome*. Globus must be distinguished from *dysphagia*, or difficulty swallowing. Patients complaining of globus may also report dysphagia and fear of choking, but most patients with globus endorse neither of these other symptoms. Historically, globus constituted one of the symptoms of hysteria and was described by Hippocrates as a symptom related to the wandering uterus putting pressure on the neck. Approximately half of patients complaining of globus have no medical diagnosis after extensive testing. Acid reflux can produce globus and is the most common medical cause of the sensation. Other pharyngeal disorders including pharyngeal cancer can also produce globus.

30.17 The answer is E (all)

Psychocardiology encompasses the spectrum of interactions of psychiatric disorders, cardiac symptoms, and cardiac disease, including associated complicating health behavior. For the past several decades, attention to the psychosocial and behavioral factors in cardiovascular disease has increased significantly. The research has taken two primary pathways: one has examined hypertension and the other has looked generally at coronary artery disease, including myocardial infarction and sudden cardiac death.

Hypertension, one of the originally hypothesized psychosomatic illnesses, is a major risk factor for coronary artery disease and cerebral vascular disease. Psychological factors have been studied closely as part of the pathogenesis of the condition; these factors have been categorized as pressure reactivity and personality and behavioral factors. Physiological hyperactivity to environmental stimuli (pressure reactivity) has been studied many times, and although results are contradictory, some specific commonalities appear. Relatively strong evidence indicates that some persons have greater blood pressure reactivity than do others to a variety of stressors, ranging from experimental stress induced in the laboratory to such social and societal stressful conditions as racism. However, the evidence linking reactivity in normotensive persons with hypertension is equivocal. Perhaps most important, pressure reactivity in hypertensive individuals may exacerbate and even accelerate the disease process.

Other research examining *psychological aspects of hypertension* has focused on personality traits or coping styles. Traits such as submissiveness and distorted expression of anger have emerged as correlates of hypertension. The most consistent correlates have involved anger-coping styles, both *inhibited anger expression and excessive anger expression.* Epidemiological researchers have noted that persons using an active coping style under environmental conditions that are not conducive to success (e.g., low education and socioeconomic status) may be predisposed to hypertension.

As evidence has clarified how psychological factors affect hypertension, investigators have focused on treatment interventions. Various behavioral procedures including biofeedback, relaxation training, and psychotherapy have been used as interventions. Some investigators have reported clinically significant success in controlled studies. For example, studies that used 24-hour monitoring of blood pressure to examine the effects of combined relaxation therapy and medication found the combination to be more effective in controlling blood pressure than medication alone.

Stress causes a sympatheticoadrenal medullary alarm reaction characterized by excess catecholamine secretion. Specifically, excess epinephrine is secreted under what the body interprets as stressful conditions. The *outpouring of epinephrine* raises blood pressure and heart and respiratory rates, enhances neuromuscular transmission, elevates the concentration of blood sugar by glycogenolysis, mobilizes fat, redirects hemodynamic patterns to suit muscular activity, and while increasing blood oxygenation, increases oxygen consumption. More specific β-adrenergically mediated cardiac effects include increased heart rate, *contractility*, and *conduction velocity* and a short arteriovenous refractory period. These catecholamine-mediated cardiac effects are thought to be pathogenically related to adverse cardiac events.

Studies of stress-induced cardiac changes and studies examining stress, arrhythmias, and sudden cardiac death suggest a significant relation in the pathophysiology of coronary artery disease. Early researchers examined temporally related stressful life experiences including stressful states described among patients who had experienced sudden death attributed to arrhythmias. One study found that the *cardiac surgery patients at greatest risk for complications*, including arrhythmias and sudden death, were depressed, anxious, and in denial of their anxiety, or both.

Recent research has examined the direct cardiac effect of controlled stress. For example, in a study of the effects of psychological stress on patients with ventricular arrhythmias, the stress of mental arithmetic and recalling past traumatic events increased the ventricular premature beat frequency in most patients. Other studies have *documented diminished cardiac perfusion during mental stress* via positron emission tomography and radionucleotide ventriculography in patients with coronary artery disease.

30.18 The answer is B

Most of the studies examining the influence of psychosocial and behavioral risk factors in the etiology of coronary artery disease have focused on type A behavior (Fig. 30.1). Individuals with type A behavior exhibit enhanced aggressiveness, ambitiousness, competitive drive, impatience, and a chronic sense of time urgency. Associated speech and motor characteristics are rapid body movements, tense facial and body musculature, explosive conversational speech, and hand or teeth clenching. Three major prospective studies have found the type A behavior pattern to be a risk factor for clinical coronary artery disease; *however, once the disease is present, global type A behavior does not appear to increase the risk of subsequent cardiac morbidity.*

The initial enthusiasm for the global type A concept waned in the middle 1980s, as *hostility was found to be the most toxic element of the syndrome*. Whereas *global type A behavior does not always predict risk* of coronary artery disease, hostility is consistently linked to coronary artery diseases and appears to be pathophysiologically related to the disease by numerous

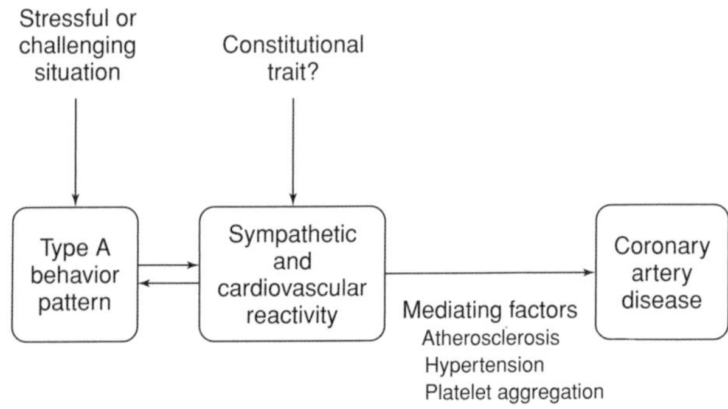

FIGURE 30.1

Conceptual model of type A behavior and the development of coronary artery disease. (Adapted from Goldstein MG, Niaura R. Cardiovascular disease, Part 1: Coronary artery disease and sudden death. In Stoudemire A, ed. *Psychological Factors Affecting Medicial Conditions.* Washington DC: American Psychiatric Press; 1995:117.)

mechanisms. *Expressive hostility and antagonistic interactions* appear to be the subcomponents of type A behavior that *are most strongly (not least strongly) related to the risk of coronary artery disease, especially among female patients* and middle-aged male patients.

Physiological correlates of type A behavior have also been studied with regard to cardiac morbidity. Type A behavior is believed to be part of a stress paradigm. Numerous studies report that persons with type A behavior patterns display large, episodic increases in blood pressure, heart rate, and catecholamine concentrations when confronted by stressful tasks. Interestingly, evidence from primate studies links atherosclerosis in coronary disease and sympathetic nervous system activation. Findings suggest a link between psychological states, physiological activity, and subsequent cardiovascular disease.

A meta-analysis of 18 controlled studies examining effects of psychological treatment on type A behavior concluded that psychological treatment aimed at reducing the behavior had a positive outcome. When type A behavior decreased, treatment had a significant improved effect on coronary events and mortality at 1-year follow-up.

A recent study by Dean Ornish revealed that *lifestyle modification* (e.g., aerobic exercise, stress management, group therapy) *actually promoted revascularization* and improved the prognosis of patients with cardiac disease.

30.19 The answer is C

Obesity refers to an excess of body fat. In healthy individuals body fat accounts for approximately 25 percent of body weight in women and 18 percent in men. Estimating body fat accurately is expensive, although advances in the assessment of body composition may change this picture. Overweight refers to elevated weight above some reference norm, typically standards derived from actuarial or epidemiological data. In most cases, increasing weight reflects increasing obesity, but not always. Muscular individuals may be overweight (weight may be elevated given height) but not obese, and a person might have normal weight but have excess body fat.

Indexes have been developed using height and weight to estimate levels of obesity. The most common of these is the body mass index (BMI). BMI is calculated by dividing weight in kilograms by height squared in meters. Although there is debate about the ideal BMI, it is generally thought that a BMI of 20 to 25 kg/m^2 represents healthy weight; a BMI of 25 to 27 kg/m^2 is associated with somewhat elevated risk; a BMI of above 27 kg/m^2 is where the increase in risk is clear; and a BMI above 30 kg/m^2 is where there is greatly increased risk.

The prevalence of obesity varies greatly by nation, by social groups within nations, and in some cases, within a given nation over time. In the United States, approximately 35 percent of women and 31 percent of men are significantly overweight (BMI 27 or above—about 20 percent overweight). If one defines obesity as BMI over 25, *there are now more obese (not fewer) than nonobese Americans.* Using BMI over 31 (approximately 40 percent overweight), 11 percent of women and 8 percent of men are severely overweight. *The prevalence of obesity in America has tripled (not doubled) since the early 1900s.* Through the 1960s, 1970s, and early 1980s there was a steady rise in prevalence, but the dramatic changes occurred in subsequent years; there has been a 25 percent increase since the 1980s alone.

The prevalence of obesity is highest in minority populations, particularly among women. Fully 60 percent of African-American women ages 45 years and older are overweight, as defined by a BMI of 27 or greater. The high prevalence of *obesity among minorities appears attributable primarily to lower income, type of diet, and educational attainment.* Obesity is six times more prevalent in women of low socioeconomic status than in women of high socioeconomic status.

Weight gain is most pronounced in both sexes between the ages of 25 and 44. During this time, men gain an average of 4 kg and women 7 kg. Pregnancy probably contributes to the greater increase in women, who, on average, begin each successive pregnancy approximately 2.5 kg heavier than at the last. After age 50, weights of men stabilize, and even decline slightly between ages 60 and 74. Women, in contrast, continue to increase in weight until age 60, at which time weight begins to decline.

Obesity is a massive public health problem by any standard. *The prevalence* is extreme, is increasing rather than decreasing, and in what speaks to a bleak future, is *especially high and growing (not stabilized or decreasing) in children.* Obesity rivals the most serious illnesses in the public health toll it takes.

30.20 The answer is A

A patient with an occipital lobe tumor would be least likely to exhibit *paranoid delusions. Visual hallucinations, headache, papilledema, and homonymous hemianopsia* are all reported symptoms and complaints of occipital lobe tumors. Papilledema (edema of the optic disk) may be caused by increased intracranial pressure. Homonymous hemianopsia is blindness in the corresponding (right or left) field of vision of each eye.

30.21 The answer is E (all)

Most chronic pain patients attempt to treat themselves before resorting to medical help. Billions of dollars are spent annually by people seeking relief through *over-the-counter preparations* or other nonmedical means. Those persons often have *alcohol dependence* and other substance-related disorders. Therefore, the physician should be alert for substance toxicity (especially overmedication) and *withdrawal symptoms during the evaluation* and treatment of chronic pain patients. Explaining to the patient and family that sensitivity to pain may greatly increase during substance withdrawal may partially decrease anxiety and increase pain sensitivity. A physician should always remember that a psychiatric diagnosis does not preclude the existence of *an underlying medical illness*. Finally, the clinician should recognize that the patient's pain is not imaginary. It is real and cannot be "willed away."

30.22 The answer is A

Emetogenicity is a measure of the ability to induce vomiting. *Cisplatin* (Platinol) is highly emetogenic. *Doxorubicin* (Adriamycin) is moderately emetogenic, and *vincristine* (Oncovin), *vinblastine* (Velban), and *bleomycin* (Blenoxane) are minimally emetogenic. Table 30.4 summarizes the emetogenic problems with various chemotherapeutic agents.

30.23 The answer is C

Psoriasis is a chronic, relapsing disease of the skin with variable clinical features. Characteristic lesions involve both the vasculature and the epidermis and have clear-cut borders and

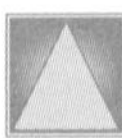

Table 30.4
Emetogenic Potential of Some Commonly Used Anticancer Agents

Highly emetogenic	Cisplatin Dacarbazine Streptozocin Actinomycin Nitrogen mustard
Moderately emetogenic	Doxorubicin Daunorubicin Cyclophosphamide Nitrosoureas Mitomycin-C Procarbazine
Minimally emetogenic	Vincristine Vinblastine 5-Fluorouracil Bleomycin

Courtesy of Marguerite S. Lederberg, M.D., and Jimmie C. Holland, M.D.

noncoherent silvery scales with a glossy, homogeneous erythema under the scales. Some patients also develop nail dystrophy and arthritis. It affects 1 to 2 percent of the United States' general population and is equally common in women and men, with most developing initial lesions in the third decade of life.

Common triggers of psoriasis include cold weather, physical trauma, acute bacterial and viral infections, and drug-related effects associated with corticosteroid withdrawal and with the use of β-adrenergic receptor antagonists and lithium. Lithium-induced psoriasis typically occurs within the first few years of treatment, is resistant to treatment, and resolves after discontinuation of lithium treatment.

The adverse effect of psoriasis on the quality of life can lead to stress that may in turn trigger more psoriasis. In a recent survey of psoriatic patients, 46 percent reported daily problems secondary to psoriasis. The 40 to 80 percent of patients who reported that stress triggered psoriasis often described disease-related stress, resulting mainly from the cosmetic disfigurement and social stigma of psoriasis, rather than stressful major life events. Psoriasis-related stress may have more to do with psychosocial difficulties inherent in the interpersonal relationships of patients with psoriasis than with the severity or chronicity of psoriasis activity. The mechanism of stress-induced exacerbations is unknown but may involve the nervous, endocrine, and immune systems in such a way that descending autonomic information from the CNS is transmitted to sensory nerves in the skin, resulting in relapse of neuropeptides such as substance P into the skin. These neuropeptides help initiate and maintain the inflammatory response in psoriatic lesions.

Controlled studies have found psoriatic *patients to have high (not low) levels of anxiety and depression* and *significant comorbidity with a wide array of personality disorders* from DSM-IV-TR, including schizoid, avoidant, and obsessive-compulsive personality disorders, as well as tendencies toward passive-aggressive traits. Patients' self-reports of psoriasis severity correlated directly with depression and suicidal ideation, and comorbid depression reduced the threshold for pruritus in psoriatic patients. Heavy alcohol drinking (>80 grams of ethanol daily) by male psoriatic patients may predict a poor treatment outcome.

These possible links between mental state and psoriasis have led to the development of *psychosocial interventions* in its

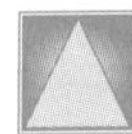

Table 30.5
Summary of Psychoneuroimmunology Factors by Robert Ader

Nerve endings have been found in the tissues of the immune system. The central nervous system is linked to both the bone marrow and the thymus, where immune system cells are produced and developed, and to the spleen and the lymph nodes, where those cells are stored.

Changes in the central nervous system (the brain and the spinal cord) alter immune responses, and triggering an immune response alters central nervous system activity. Animal experiments dating back to the 1960s show that damage to different parts of the brain's hypothalamus can either suppress or enhance the allergic-type response. Recently, researchers have found that inducing an immune response causes nerve cells in the hypothalamus to become more active and that the brain cell anxiety peaks at precisely the same time that levels of antibodies are at their highest. Apparently, the brain monitors immunological changes closely.

Changes in hormone and neurotransmitter levels alter immune responses, and vice versa. The stress hormones generally suppress immune responses. But other hormones, such as growth hormone, also seem to affect immunity. Conversely, when experimental animals are immunized, they show changes in various hormone levels.

Lymphocytes are chemically responsive to hormones and neurotransmitters. Immune system cells have receptors—molecular structures on the surface of their cells—that are responsive to endorphins, stress hormones, and a wide range of other hormones.

Lymphocytes can produce hormones and neurotransmitters. When an animal is infected with a virus, lymphocytes produce minuscule amounts of many of the same substances produced by the pituitary gland.

Activated lymphocytes—cells actively involved in an immune response—produce substances that can be perceived by the central nervous system. The interleukins and interferons—chemicals that immune system cells use to talk to each other—can also trigger receptors on cells in the brain, more evidence that the immune system and the nervous system speak the same chemical language.

Psychosocial factors may alter the susceptibility to or the progression of autoimmune disease, infectious disease, and cancer. Evidence for those connections comes from many researchers.

Immunological reactivity may be influenced by stress. Chronic or intense stress, in particular, generally makes immune system cells less responsive to a challenge.

Immunological reactivity can be influenced by hypnosis. In a typical study. both of a subject's arms are exposed to a chemical that normally causes an allergic reaction. But the subject is told, under hypnosis, that only one arm will show the response—and that, in fact, is often what happens.

Immunological reactivity can be modified by classical conditioning. As Ader's own key experiments showed, the immune system can learn to react in certain ways as a conditioned response.

Psychoactive drugs and drugs of abuse influence immune function. A range of drugs that affect the nervous system—including alcohol, marijuana, cocaine, heroin, and nicotine—have all been shown to affect the immune response, generally suppressing it. Some psychiatric drugs, such as lithium (prescribed for bipolar I disorder), also modulate the immune system.

Adapted from Goleman D., Guerin J. *Mind Body Medicine*. Yonkers, NY: Consumer Reports; 1993.

treatment. Controlled studies have shown *meditation*, hypnosis, *relaxation training*, cognitive-behavioral stress management, and symptom control imagery training to be *effective in reducing psoriasis activity.*

30.24 The answer is E (all)

Pruritus, or itching, is the most common symptom of dermatological disorders and of several systemic diseases including chronic renal disease, hepatic disease, hematopoietic disorders, endocrine disorders, malignant neoplasms, drug toxicity, and neurological syndromes (e.g., multiple sclerosis). Other problems such as advanced age, infections with internal parasites, and viremia can also be associated with pruritus.

Chronic *idiopathic pruritus* and idiopathic pruritus ani (itching in the anal area), vulvae (itching in the vaginal area), and scroti (itching in the scrotum) frequently have been called psychogenic, but more study is needed to determine how psychiatric and other CNS disorders contribute to the development of pruritus. *Antidepressant medications, particularly the tricyclic drugs, can relieve pruritus of many origins.*

Urticaria (also known as hives) is characterized by circumscribed, raised, erythematous, usually pruritic areas of edema that involve the superficial dermis.

Glossodynia (also called burning mouth syndrome) is an unexplained, prolonged sensation of pain, burning, or both inside the oral cavity, most frequently at the tip and lateral borders of the tongue, and often accompanied by other symptoms such as dryness, paresthesia, and changes in taste and smell.

Vulvodynia is chronic vulvar and perineal discomfort of variable severity with burning, stinging, irritation, or rawness.

30.25 The answer is C

The immune system is affected by *conditioning*. According to Ader, immunological reactivity is affected by *hypnosis, lymphocytes* can produce neurotransmitters, *growth hormone* does affect immunity, and *marijuana* does affect the immune system. Robert Ader has summarized the psychoneuroimmunology factors (Table 30.5).

30.26 The answer is A

Phantom limb occurs in *98 percent* of patients—not 10 percent, 50 percent, 80 percent, or 90 percent—who have undergone leg amputation. The experience may last for years. Sometimes the sensation is painful, and a neuroma at the stump should be ruled out. The condition has no known cause or treatment and usually stops spontaneously.

30.27 The answer is A

The most difficult problem in the treatment of psychosomatically ill patients is patients' *resistance to entering psychotherapy* and to recognizing the psychological factors in their illness. Generally, clinicians have difficulty in forming a positive transference with the patients. *An erotic transference to the psychotherapist* usually does not develop, nor is it relevant to the treatment of these patients. The patients *usually react negatively to the interpretation of the physiological meaning of their symptoms* and *do not recognize the psychological correlation with their physiological symptoms.*

Answers 30.28–30.32

30.28 The answer is D

30.29 The answer is C

30.30 The answer is A

30.31 The answer is B

30.32 The answer is E

Wilson's disease, hepatolenticular degeneration, is a familial disease of adolescence that tends to have a long-term course. Its cause is defective copper metabolism leading to excessive copper deposits in tissues. The earliest psychiatric symptoms are *explosive anger and labile mood*—sudden and rapid changes from one mood to another. As the illness progresses, eventual brain damage occurs with memory and intelligence quotient (IQ) loss. The lability and combativeness tend to persist even after the brain damage develops.

Pheochromocytoma is a tumor of the adrenal medulla that causes headaches, paroxysms of severe hypertension, and the physiological and psychological *symptoms of a classic panic attack*—intense anxiety, tremor, apprehension, dizziness, palpitations, and diaphoresis. The tumor tissue secretes catecholamines that are responsible for the symptoms.

Systemic lupus erythematosus is an autoimmune disorder in which the body makes antibodies against its own cells. The antibodies attack cells as if the cells were infectious agents, and depending on which cells are being attacked, give rise to various symptoms. Frequently, the arteries in the cerebrum are affected, causing a cerebral arteritis, which alters the blood flow to various parts of the brain. The decreased blood flow can give rise to psychotic symptoms, such as a thought disorder with paranoid delusions and hallucinations. The symptoms can *resemble steroid psychosis* or schizophrenia.

The diagnosis of *acquired immune deficiency syndrome* (AIDS) includes a *dementia syndrome with global impairment and seropositivity.* The dementia can be caused by the direct attack on the central nervous system by the human immunodeficiency virus (HIV) or by secondary infections, such as toxoplasmosis.

Although any chronic illness can give rise to depression, some diseases, such as *pancreatic cancer*, are more likely causes than are others. The depression of pancreatic cancer patients is often associated with a *sense of imminent doom.*

31

Alternative Medicine and Psychiatry

It has always been important for physicians to ask about and to try to understand the health beliefs and behaviors of their patients. The new and increasing popularity in the United States of alternative therapies means that there are a larger range of health-related behaviors now than most American physicians learned about in medical school. Amazingly, many of the alternative therapies discussed in this chapter pre-date conventional treatments by hundreds and even thousands of years. These therapies have been "conventional" medicine for hundreds of millions of people who have used them throughout the centuries, and people continue to use them today. Unfortunately, alternative methods are not always without their own risk, ranging from simple ineffectiveness to actual harm.

The power of suggestion has been shown to play a significant role in both alternative and more traditional medical and psychiatric treatments. One major difference between traditional and nontraditional methods, however, is that most alternative treatments have not been extensively tested or subjected to controlled studies. Thus, the mechanisms of action, the role of psychology in their effectiveness, and their systemic impact and long-term effects have not been identified adequately. Clinicians may keep an open mind about these treatments until such studies can be performed, but should also refrain from endorsing or recommending treatments with which they are unfamiliar.

In psychiatry, patients often ask questions about alternative treatments, ranging from St. John's Wort to acupuncture. Psychiatrists should feel comfortable indicating which treatments they are familiar with and which they are not, and which treatments they feel comfortable accepting and which they do not. If they are knowledgeable about particular alternative treatments and feel that they might be effective in a specific patient, then this can be discussed. Patients are always free to seek care from practitioners who use alternative methods, and no physician should feel pressured to recommend or support any treatments outside their area of expertise, or that they feel are not indicated, effective, or evaluated sufficiently.

The National Institutes of Health (NIH) established an Office of Alternative Medicine (OAM) in 1991 to attempt to evaluate and test many nontraditional, alternative treatments (Table 31.1).

The student should study this table and the questions and answers below for a useful review of this field.

HELPFUL HINTS

Students should know the following terms.

- acupressure
- acupuncture
- Alexander technique
- allopathy
- aromatherapy
- Ayurveda
- Bates method
- bioenergetics
- biofeedback
- chelation therapy
- chiropractic
- color therapy
- complementary medicine
- dance therapy
- diet and nutrition
- endorphins
- environmental medicine
- essential oils
- Moshe Feldenkrais
- Max Gerson
- Samuel Hahnemann
- herbal medicine
- holistic medicine
- homeopathy
- hypnosis
- light therapy
- macrobiotics
- massage
- meditation
- moxibustion
- naturopathy
- nutritional supplements
- Office of Alternative Medicine (OAM)
- osteopathy
- ozone therapy
- past life
- prana
- psychosomatic approach
- reflexology
- Reiki
- Ida Rolf
- scientific method
- shamanism
- sound therapy
- Rudolf Steiner
- yin and yang
- yoga

Table 31.1
Complementary and Alternative Medicine Practices

Whole Medical Systems	Biologically Based Practices	Manipulative and Body-Based Practice
Anthroposophically extended medicine	Cell treatment	Acupressure or acupuncture
Ayurveda	Chelation therapy	Alexander technique
Environmental medicine	Diet	Aromatherapy
Homeopathy	–Atkins diet	Biofield therapeutics
Kampo medicine	–Macrobiotic diet	Chiropractic medicine
Native American medicine	–Ornish diet	Feldenkrais method
Naturopathic medicine	–Pritikin diet	Massage therapy
Tibetan medicine	–Vegetarian diet	Osteopathic medicine
Mind-Body Interventions	–Zone diet	Reflexology
Art therapy	Dietary supplements	Rolfing
Biofeedback	Gerson therapy	Therapeutic touch
Dance therapy	Herbal products	Trager method
Guided imagery	–Echinacea	**Energy Medicine**
Humor therapy	–St. John's Wort	Blue light treatment and artificial treatment
Meditation	–Ginkgo biloba extract	Electroacupuncture
Mental healing	–Ginseng root	Electromagnetic field
Past life therapy	–Garlic supplements	Therapy
Prayer and counseling	–Peppermint	Electrostimulation and neuromagnetic stimulation
Psychotherapy	Metabolic therapy	Magnetoresonance therapy
Sound, music therapy	Megavitamin	Qi Gong
Yoga exercise	Nutritional supplements	Reiki
Traditional Chinese medicine	Oxidizing agents (ozone, hydrogen peroxide	Therapeutic touch
		Zone therapy

QUESTIONS

Directions

Each of the questions or incomplete statements below is followed by five responses or completions. Select the *one* that is *best* in each case.

31.1 The Alexander technique focuses on improvement of which of the following for better health?

A. Creativity
B. Posture
C. Nutrition
D. Sleep habits
E. Hygiene

31.2 Which of the following statements regarding herbal medicines is *true*?

A. They are subjected to Food and Drug Administration (FDA) approval.
B. Uniform standards for quality control do exist.
C. At least 25 percent of current medicines are derived from the ingredients of plants.
D. Toxic results due to overdose are extremely rare.
E. Herbal medicines originated in the United States.

31.3 Massage therapy is believed to affect the body in all of the following ways *except*

A. Circadian rhythm regulation
B. Increased blood circulation
C. Improved lymph flow
D. Improved muscle tone
E. Tranquilizing effect on the mind

Directions

Each of the three incomplete statements below refers to one of the six lettered terms. Choose the most appropriate term for each statement.

Questions 31.4–31.6

A. Allopathy
B. Homeopathy
C. Osteopathy
D. Biomedicine
E. Technomedicine
F. Herbal medicine

31.4 The medicine taught in U.S. schools
31.5 Similar methods of practice to those of allopathy
31.6 A term coined by Samuel Hahnemann, M.D.

ANSWERS

31.1 The answer is B

The Alexander technique (Fig. 31.1) was developed by F.M. Alexander (1869–1955), who was born in Tasmania and eventually became a well-known stage actor. After developing aphonia, he experimented on himself by changing his body posture and eventually regained his voice. Alexander developed a theory of the proper use of body musculature to help alleviate somatic and mental illness. Techniques involve corrective manipulation of the muscles involving the head and neck, torso, pelvis, and extremities to improve posture. Treatment improves cardiovascular, respiratory, and gastrointestinal functioning as well as mood. A small, devoted group of Alexander practitioners is found in the United States and throughout the world. The Alexander

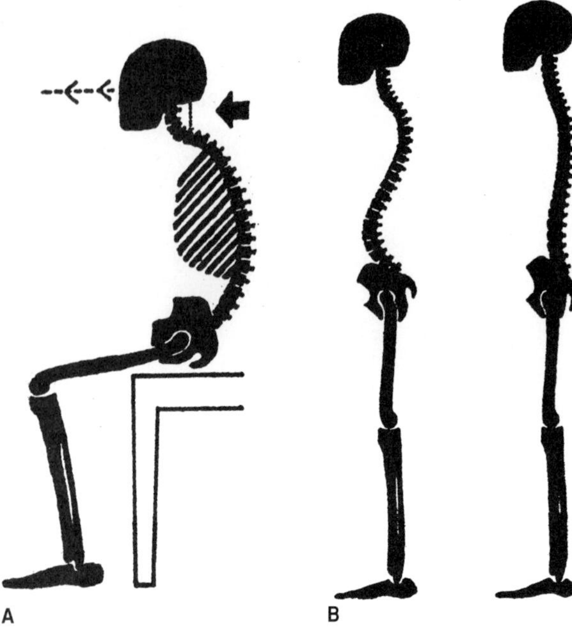

FIGURE 31.1

A. Position of pelvis, back, neck, and head in slumped position. **B.** Standing in hunched position (*left*) and well balanced (*right*). (Reprinted with permission from Barlow W. *The Alexander Principle*. London: Gollancz; 1973.)

technique may deserve consideration if for no other reason than so many persons in the United States have poor posture.

31.2 The answer is C

Herbal medicine relies on plants to cure illness and to maintain health. It is probably the oldest known system of medicine and *originated in China* (not the United States) about 4,000 BC. Like most prescription medicines, these plants contain active compounds that produce physiologic effects. As a result, they *must be used on appropriate doses if toxic results are to be prevented.* About $1.5 billion a year is spent on herbal medicines, which are classified as dietary supplements. They are *not subjected to Food and Drug Administration (FDA) approval*, and there are *no uniform standards for quality control or potency* in herbal preparations. Indeed, some preparations have no active ingredients or are adulterated.

The decline of herbal medicine in the late 20th century was related to scientific and technological advances that led to the use of synthetic pharmaceuticals; nevertheless, according to some estimates, *at least 25 percent of current medicines are derived from the active ingredients of plants.* The examples are many: digitalis from foxglove; ephedrine from ephedra; morphine from the opium poppy; paclitaxel (Taxol) from the yew tree; and quinine from the bark of the cinchona tree.

31.3 The answer is A

Massage is a treatment that involves manipulation of the soft tissues and the surfaces of the body. It was prescribed for the treatment of diseases over 5,000 years ago by Chinese physicians, and Hippocrates considered it to be a method of maintaining health. Massage is believed to affect the body in several ways: *it increases blood circulation, improves the flow of lymph through the lymphatic vessels, improves the tone of the musculoskeletal system, and has a tranquilizing effect on the mind.* Most people who experience massage find it physically and mentally restorative. *Circadian rhythm disturbances* are often treated through the use of light and melatonin therapy, not massage therapy.

Answers 31.4–31.6

31.4 The answer is A

31.5 The answer is C

31.6 The answer is B

Allopathy, from the Greek *Allos* ("other"), is the term for traditional medicine of the kind taught in U.S. medical schools. It is based on the scientific method, the use of experiments to validate a theory or to determine the validity of a hypothesis. In allopathy, the body is a biological and physiological system, and disorders have causes that can be treated with medications, surgery, and other complex methods to produce cures. Traditional medicine incorporates *biomedicine* and *technomedicine*. Allopathy refers to the use of medicine to counteract signs and symptoms of diseases; it remains the most prevalent form of medicine in the Western world.

Homeopathy was derived from the Greek *homos* ("same"); it refers to a form of medicine in which special medicinal remedies, different from allopathic remedies, are used. Homeopathic healing was developed in Germany in the early 1800s by Samuel Hahnemann, M.D., who coined the term *homeopathy*. It is based on the concept that the medicine whose effects in normal people most closely resemble the illness being treated is the one most likely to cure the illness. It treats a disease by the administration of minute doses of a remedy that would in healthy persons, produce symptoms similar to those of the disease. Although traditional medical practitioners doubt its efficacy, homeopathy is increasingly used in this country, in Europe, and throughout the world.

Osteopathy is similar to traditional medicine; doctors of osteopathy are licensed to practice in every state, are qualified to practice in every branch of clinical medicine, and take the same licensure examinations as do medical doctors. Their medical education is identical, except that doctors of osteopathy have additional training in musculoskeletal system disorders.

32 Psychiatry and Reproductive Medicine

The physiological processes associated with menarche, menstrual cycling, pregnancy, postpartum, and menopause occur within the context of a woman's psychological and interpersonal life, interfacing with psychosocial functioning throughout adolescence, young adulthood, midlife, and late life. Reproductive events and processes have both physiological and psychological concomitants. The fields of psychiatry and reproductive medicine are just beginning to elaborate the multiple mechanisms by which psyche and soma interact to determine a woman's gynecological and psychological function.

These issues can include the role of psychogenic stress in reproductive dysfunction, changes in sexuality associated with aging, psychological repercussions of infertility, possible psychogenic causes of pelvic pain, premenstrual dysphoric disorder, and psychological and physiologic responses to menopause. Psychiatry may be helpful in addressing a range of issues related to pregnancy, from the impact of emotional support during labor, to the phenomenon of hyperemesis gravidarum, to the safe utilization of psychiatric medications during pregnancy.

Clinicians must be aware of various postpartum conditions, such as postpartum depression and psychosis, and how to distinguish these very serious and potentially life-threatening disorders from the normal "baby blues" that many women experience.

Disorders of sexual development, such as adrenogenital syndrome, testicular feminization, and Turner's syndrome (XO gonadal dysgenesis), are unusual conditions that can raise a number of complex and painful parental and physician decisions, which may include psychiatric consultation.

The student should study the questions and answers below for a useful review of these issues.

HELPFUL HINTS

Each of the following terms should be defined by the student.

- aging changes in sexuality
- amenorrhea
- anovulation
- artificial insemination
- "baby blues"
- disorders of sexual development
- dyspareunia
- estrogen replacement
- FDA rating of drug safety
- fetal sex steroids
- functional hypothalamic anovulation
- disorders of sexual development
- GnRH secretion
- gonadotropins
- hormone replacement therapy
- hyperemesis gravidarum
- hypothalamic-pituitary-adrenal axis
- infertility
- lesbian and gay parents
- pelvic pain
- postpartum depression
- postpartum psychosis
- pregnancy and labor
- premenstrual dysphoric disorder
- psychogenic stress
- sexual response cycle

QUESTIONS

Directions

Each of the questions or incomplete statements below is followed by five suggested responses or completions. Select the *one* that is *best* in each case.

32.1 Which of the following statements regarding puberty and vulnerability to depression is *true*?

A. Before puberty, boys are more vulnerable to depressive illness than girls.
B. Before puberty, girls are more vulnerable to depressive illness than boys.
C. Depression does not occur in the prepubertal period.
D. After puberty, depressive illness is less prevalent across both sexes.
E. None of the above

32.2 Which of the following statements regarding the changes in sexual response that occur with aging is *true*?

A. Less stimulation is required to achieve an erection.
B. There is a shorter phase of sexual excitement.
C. There is no change in the length of the refractory period following orgasm.
D. Increased intensity of ejaculation occurs.
E. Many changes begin before the 5th decade of life.

32.3 Fetal sex steroid exposure exerts primarily organizational effects upon the fetal

A. central nervous system (CNS)
B. testes
C. ovary
D. neuromuscular system
E. cardiovascular system

32.4 Pseudocyesis is

A. Another name for Braxton-Hicks contractions (i.e., false labor)
B. When the father of a child undergoes a simulated labor as if he were giving birth
C. The development of the classic symptoms of pregnancy in a nonpregnant woman
D. Falsely elevated hCG levels occurring with choriocarcinoma and hydatidiform moles
E. Masking of the symptoms of postpartum depression

32.5 True statements about the relationship between psychogenic stress and reproductive dysfunction include

A. In women with functional amenorrhea, the activity of the hypothalamic-pituitary-adrenal axis is increased.
B. There appears to be a dose-response relationship between the severity and number of stressors and the proportion of women who develop anovulation.
C. Various personality characteristics such as perfectionism and unrealistic expectations have been linked to the development of anovulation.
D. In FHA, pharmacological intervention alone does not lead to spontaneous recovery.
E. All of the above

32.6 Premenstrual dysphoric disorder

A. is associated with hormonally abnormal menstrual cycles
B. is associated with changing levels of sex steroids that accompany an ovulatory menstrual cycle
C. is seen in approximately 50 percent of women
D. is not treated with SSRIs
E. all of the above

32.7 It is generally considered safest to perform a tubal ligation at which of the following times?

A. Immediately postpartum
B. Laparoscopy several weeks after delivery
C. Open procedure several weeks after delivery
D. Open procedure 6 months after delivery
E. Hysterectomy is the safest method of sterilization

32.8 Continuous emotional support during labor reduces

A. the rate of cesarean section
B. the duration of labor
C. the use of anesthesia
D. the use of oxytocin
E. all of the above

32.9 Hyperemesis gravidarum

A. may be associated with women who have histories of anorexia nervosa or bulimia nervosa
B. has a poor prognosis for mother and fetus
C. is rarely chronic or persistent
D. is definitively caused by psychological factors
E. none of the above

Directions

Each group of questions below consists of lettered headings followed by a list of numbered statements. For each numbered statement, select the *one* lettered heading that is most closely associated with it. Each lettered heading may be used once, more than once, or not at all.

Questions 32.10–32.16

A. Postpartum depression
B. "Baby blues"
C. Both
D. Neither

32.10 Occurs in 10 percent of women who give birth
32.11 Can last months to years if untreated
32.12 No association with history of a mood disorder
32.13 Causes tearfulness
32.14 Often associated with thoughts of hurting the baby
32.15 Often associated with anhedonia
32.16 Can include suicidal thoughts

Questions 32.17–32.20

A. Adrenogenital syndrome
B. Turner's syndrome (XO gonadal dysgenesis)
C. Testicular feminization
D. XY gonadal dysgenesis
E. Hermaphroditism

32.17 Masculinized genitalia are usually recognized in the delivery room; however, the internal reproductive tract is normal and puberty usually occurs at the expected time with adequate treatment.
32.18 Ovaries do not contain responsive oocytes because of premature atresia of oocytes or failure of germ cell migration.
32.19 Gonads are testes but the fetus is phenotypically female.
32.20 Caused by a gonad that fails to secrete testosterone; generally the uterus, tubes, and vagina are present.

Questions 32.21–32.25

A. Desire
B. Excitement
C. Orgasm
D. Resolution

32.21 Testes increase in size
32.22 Muscular contractions occur
32.23 Testes descend
32.24 Sexual fantasies
32.25 Vaginal lubrication

ANSWERS

32.1 The answer is A

Before puberty, *boys are more vulnerable than girls are to depressive illness*. Over the course of adolescence, however, a dramatic shift occurs, with girls displaying a precipitous rise in depression rates that far outstrips the negligible (if existent) increase displayed by adolescent boys. By age 15, girls are twice as likely as boys are to have experienced a lifetime episode of major depression. This gender difference persists for the next 35 to 40 years, essentially spanning female reproductive years. Negative life events and chronic psychosocial stressors are known to place individuals at risk for major depressive episodes. A number of theories about the gender difference in depression point to the fact that women are more likely than men are to experience certain types of traumatic life events, such as physical or sexual abuse, or chronic life stressors, such as single parenthood, gender discrimination in the workplace, or financial adversity. In general, however, such theories fail to account for the adolescent onset of the gender difference in depression. Indeed, growing evidence indicates that puberty may sensitize girls to the depressogenic effects of life stress. Specifically, postpubertal women appear to be at heightened risk for experiencing depression when faced with social stressors, such as conflicts, breaches, or losses within interpersonal relationships.

32.2 The answer is E

Aging may be associated with changes in sexuality. *Many changes begin before the fifth decade of life*. In men in particular, significant changes in erections and ejaculation occur with age. As a man gets older, it *usually takes more stimulation* to achieve an erection. In addition, the *phase of sexual excitement is longer* and may not end in ejaculation. When ejaculation occurs, the force of expulsion of semen and the *intensity of ejaculation are lower*. After ejaculation, the erection resolves more quickly and the *refractory period increases*. Many of these changes start gradually and can begin before men are in their 40's and age-associated changes should be anticipated and viewed as normal. Although sexual interest declines to some degree with aging, older men and women who live together are more sexually active than those who are not in a relationship. Because women tend to live longer than men do, many elderly women will be without partners and will have limited opportunities for sexual expression, even if sexual drive is present.

32.3 The answer is A

Sexual differentiation of the central nervous system (CNS) is believed to depend on the presence or absence of circulating levels of testosterone. The *fetal testes* begin to secrete testosterone in the late first trimester in response to placental human chorionic gonadotropin (hCG), whereas the *fetal ovary* does not. The organizational effects of testosterone on the developing CNS are thought to depend primarily upon in situ aromatization (the conversion of androgens to estrogens by the enzyme aromatase) of testosterone to estradiol. In contrast, estrogens from fetal or placental sources do not cross the blood-brain barrier and are not thought to imprint the developing CNS. Also, testosterone may bind directly (without conversion to estradiol) to androgen receptors in the CNS. The behavioral consequences that early exposure to testosterone has upon the developing brain are not clear, but brain areas with high aromatase activity (which thus can convert testosterone to estradiol) and androgen receptors in the nonhuman primate brain include the hypothalamus, amygdala, prefrontal visual, and somatosensory cortices. The asymmetry in exposure to testosterone is also present in early neonatal life. In late pregnancy, gonadotropin secretion is restrained by placental steroid production; when that restraint is lost at the time of birth, gonadotropin secretion rises dramatically in both sexes. In boys but not in girls, the gonadotropin rise is followed by an elevation of testosterone concentrations to adult levels. Thus, by 2 years of age, the brains and bodies of girls and boys have been exposed to dramatically different patterns of sex steroid secretion. The degree to which gender-related behavioral asymmetries are accounted for by those differences in hormone exposure is open to debate, but clearly a mechanism for inducing differences exists. In summary, the *fetal sex steroid exposure exerts primarily organizational effects upon the fetal CNS,* not the neuromuscular or cardiovascular systems.

32.4 The answer is C

Pseudocyesis is the *development of the classic symptoms of pregnancy—amenorrhea, nausea, breast enlargement and pigmentation, abdominal distention, and labor pains—in a nonpregnant woman* (Fig. 32.1). Pseudocyesis demonstrates the ability of the psyche to dominate the soma, probably via central input at the level of the hypothalamus. Predisposing psychological processes are thought to include a pathological wish for and fear of pregnancy; ambivalence or conflict regarding gender, sexuality, or childbearing; and a grief reaction to lost potential after a miscarriage, tubal ligation, or hysterectomy. The patient may have a true somatic delusion that is not subject to reality testing, but, often, a negative pregnancy test result or pelvic ultrasound scan leads to resolution. Psychotherapy is recommended during or after a presentation of pseudocyesis to evaluate and treat the underlying psychological dysfunction. A related event, *couvade*, in which the father of the child undergoes a simulated labor as if he were giving birth, occurs in some cultures.

32.5 The answer is E (all)

The concept that psychogenic stress can induce reproductive dysfunction in women was introduced formally in 1946. The best biochemical evidence in support of the concept that stress impairs GnRH release in women with functional hypothalamic amenorrhea (FHA) is the consistent demonstration that the *activity of the hypothalamic-pituitary-adrenal axis is increased.* Further, a prospective study found that young American women who developed transient amenorrhea while studying in Israel had higher urinary cortisol concentrations upon arrival than those whose menses remained regular.

There appears to be *a dose-response relationship* between the type, severity, and number of stressors on one hand and the proportion of women who develop anovulation. Biological and psychological predispositions may confer resistance or sensitivity to various stressors. Exercise, low weight and weight loss, affective and eating disorders, *personality characteristics* such as perfectionism and unrealistic expectations, drug use, and a variety of external and intrapersonal stresses *have been linked to the development of anovulation.* Most women with FHA, when carefully evaluated, display more than one of these traits or behaviors. Recent evidence suggests synergism between metabolic stressors,

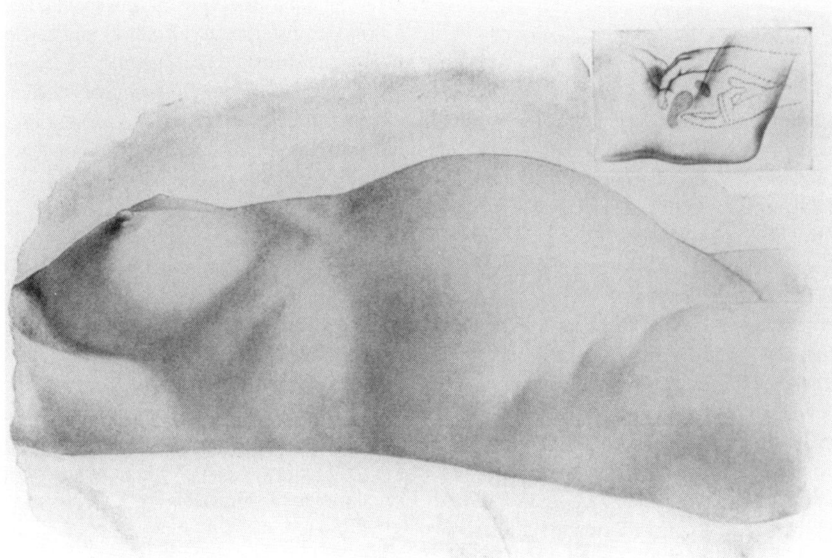

FIGURE 32.1
Patient at 36th (?) week. Bimanual examination revealed uterus normal in size and position.

such as excessive exercise and nutritional restriction, which suppress the hypothalamic-pituitary-thyroidal axis, and psychosocial challenges that activate the hypothalamic-pituitary-adrenal axis.

Recovery is possible if women with FHA develop response patterns to ongoing psychosocial demands that are less likely to activate the central and metabolic processes that disrupt pulsatile GnRH release. The current standard of practice, other than observation, is to offer pharmacological interventions such as oral contraceptives or hormonal replacement if fertility is not desired, and pharmacological ovulation induction if fertility is sought. However, *pharmacological intervention alone does not lead to spontaneous recovery* and cannot be expected to ameliorate stress-induced alterations in central neurotransmission and hypothalamic function, or to reverse ongoing metabolic derangements secondary to exercise or weight loss. For instance, bone accretion does not proceed apace, even if exogenous hormone replacement is given in supraphysiological doses, in the face of metabolic compromise. Although women with FHA frequently do not meet the criteria for eating disorders or depressive disorders given in the revised 4th edition of the *Diagnostic and Statistical Manual of Mental Disorders* (DSM-IV-TR), all of these states are characterized by increased cortisol secretion, which alone can alter thyroid hormone secretion and action and induce metabolic adjustments. Thus, it is not surprising to find that women with amenorrhea due to decreased GnRH drive, regardless of cause, have lower bone mineral density. Further, pharmacological intervention alone may mask recognition of psychological dysfunction and forestall the development of more effective response patterns. Also, ovulation induction may place low-weight women with functional hypothalamic amenorrhea who conceive at risk for premature labor and intrauterine growth retardation. If the parenting skills of women with the disorder are impaired by ongoing stress, their children may be at risk for poor psychosocial development. Clearly, treatment strategies need to consider that stress and mild psychological dysfunction can play an important role in the genesis of this form of anovulation. If an eating disorder is recognized, specialized psychiatric treatment is indicated.

32.6 The answer is B

Premenstrual syndrome (PMS), termed *premenstrual dysphoric disorder* in the DSM-IV-TR, is a somatopsychic illness *triggered by the expected excursions in sex steroids* that accompany *a hormonally normal (not abnormal) ovulatory menstrual cycle.* These somatic changes disturb psychological functioning in predisposed women.

It occurs about one week prior to the onset of menses and is characterized by irritability, emotional lability, headache, anxiety, and depression. Somatic symptoms include edema, weight gain, breast pain, syncope, and paresthesias. *Approximately 5 percent (not 50 percent) of women have the disorder.* Treatment is symptomatic and includes analgesics for pain and sedatives for anxiety and insomnia. *Some cases respond to short courses of SSRIs.* Fluid retention is relieved with diuretics.

32.7 The answer is B

Sterilization can be accomplished by several methods of tubal ligation by hysterectomy with or without oophorectomy in women and by vasectomy in men. *Hysterectomy for sterilization alone is associated with more morbidity and mortality than any method of tubal ligation*; vasectomy is safer than are any of the present methods of tubal ligation. Most studies do not support the contention that tubal ligation carries an increased incidence of gynecological sequelae, but failure rates are high in the first year after tubal ligation. In general, *it is safest to perform a tubal ligation by laparoscopy at least several weeks after delivery.* Tubal ligations immediately after delivery are done because of convenience or because of a woman's unwillingness or inability to return for a later tubal ligation.

32.8 The answer is E (all)

Fears regarding pain and bodily harm during delivery are universal and to some extent, warranted. Preparation for childbirth affords a sense of familiarity and can ease anxieties, which facilitates delivery. Continuous emotional support during labor *reduces the rate of cesarean section* and forceps deliveries, *the need for anesthesia, the use of oxytocin, and the duration of labor.* A technically difficult delivery, however, does not appear to influence the decision to bear additional children.

32.9 The answer is A

Hyperemesis gravidarum is differentiated from morning sickness in that vomiting *is chronic, persistent*, and frequent, leading to ketosis, acidosis, weight loss, and dehydration. *Women with histories of anorexia nervosa or bulimia nervosa may be at risk*. The *prognosis is excellent* for both mother and fetus with prompt treatment. Most women can be treated as outpatients with change to smaller meals, discontinuation of iron supplements, and avoidance of certain foods. In severe cases hospitalization may be necessary. Although the cause is unknown, *there may be a psychological component.*

Answers 32.10–32.16

32.10 The answer is A

32.11 The answer is A

32.12 The answer is B

32.13 The answer is C

32.14 The answer is A

32.15 The answer is A

32.16 The answer is A

About 20 to 40 percent of women report some emotional disturbance or cognitive dysfunction in the postpartum period. Many experience so-called *"baby blues,"* a normal state of sadness, dysphoria, frequent *tearfulness*, and clinging dependence. These feelings, which may last several days, have been ascribed to rapid changes in women's hormonal levels, the stress of childbirth, and the awareness of the increased responsibility that motherhood brings.

Postpartum depression is characterized by a depressed mood, *anhedonia*, excessive anxiety, and insomnia. The onset is within 3 to 6 months after delivery. Table 32.1 differentiates postpartum "baby blues" from postpartum depression.

In rare cases (1 to 2 in 1,000 deliveries), a woman's postpartum depression is characterized by depressed feelings and *suicidal ideation.* In severe cases, the depression may reach psychotic proportions, with hallucinations, delusions, and *thoughts of infanticide.* Although *previous psychiatric problems put women at risk for postpartum disturbances,* there is evidence to suggest that postpartum mood disorder is a specific concept, distinct from other psychiatric diagnoses. Others argue that these mood disorders are not a distinct entity but are part of a bipolar spectrum as reflected in the DSM-IV-TR classification. Women with severe postpartum depressions are at high risk for future episodes, and *failure to treat may contribute to long-term, treatment-refractory mood disorders.*

Answers 32.17–32.20

32.17 The answer is A

32.18 The answer is B

32.19 The answer is C

32.20 The answer is D

Disorders of sexual development in phenotypic girls generally present at birth or at the time of expected puberty. *Adrenogenital syndrome* can be caused by congenital adrenal hyperplasia in female fetuses; the fetal adrenal secretes excess androgens, which then masculinize the external genitalia and possibly the brain. In female infants, the *masculinized genitalia usually are recognized*

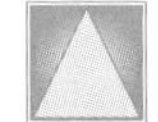

Table 32.1
Comparison of "Baby Blues" and Postpartum Depression

Characteristic	"Baby Blues"	Postpartum Depression
Incidence	50% of women who give birth	10% of women who give birth
Time of onset	3–5 days after delivery	Within 3–6 months after delivery
Duration	Days to weeks	Months to years, if untreated
Associated stressors	No	Yes, especially lack of support
Sociocultural influence	No; present in all cultures and socioeconomic classes	Strong association
History of mood disorder	No association	Strong association
Family history of mood disorder	No association	Some association
Tearfulness	Yes	Yes
Mood lability	Yes	Often present, but sometimes mood is uniformly depressed
Anhedonia	No	Often
Sleep disturbance	Sometimes	Nearly always
Suicidal thoughts	No	Sometimes
Thoughts of harming the baby	Rarely	Often
Feelings of guilt, inadequacy	Absent or mild	Often present and excessive

Reproduced with permission from Miller LJ. How "baby blues" and postpartum depression differ. *Women's Psychiatric Health*, 1995:13.

in the delivery room. Surgery to reduce clitoral size and create or widen the vaginal introitus may be necessary at a later date to restore the external appearance. *However, the internal reproductive tract is normal and puberty generally occurs around the expected time if adrenal replacement therapy is adequate.* Despite medical and surgical interventions, concerns over capacity for sexual function may emerge, particularly in late adolescence or young adulthood.

Turner's syndrome (XO gonadal dysgenesis) may be recognized at birth because of the associated physical stigmata, whereas XX gonadal dysgenesis usually presents at puberty. From a reproductive perspective, the two conditions are similar in that the *ovaries do not contain responsive oocytes* because of premature atresia of oocytes or failure of germ cell migration. Donor oocytes allow the option of pregnancy.

Other disorders of sexual development include *testicular feminization* and its variants; the *gonads in that condition are testes,* but the fetus is phenotypically female in that a defect in the androgen receptor confers androgen insensitivity. Because the testes are normal, they secrete testosterone and müllerian regression occurs (regression of the anlage that would develop into the uterus and tubes). The vagina ends blindly, and the presenting complaint is usually primary amenorrhea. Thelarche (onset of breast development) occurs at the normal time because at puberty the testes secrete testosterone, which then is aromatized to estradiol, which stimulates the growth of breast tissue. Orchiectomy (removal of the testes) is recommended after puberty to avoid the risk of gonadoblastoma, unless there is partial androgen sensitivity, in which case it is performed earlier to prevent the pubertal development of hirsutism and partial masculinization.

There are many types of androgen receptor defects and a spectrum of clinical presentations. Some individuals look phenotypically like men and may present with infertility secondary to azoospermia or oligospermia. A related disorder occurs when there is an inefficiency of the enzyme 5α-reductase, which converts testosterone to dihydrotestosterone (DHT); DHT, in turn, masculinizes the external genitalia. Boys with a deficiency of that enzyme may look phenotypically female or incompletely masculinized at birth. At puberty, further masculinization, including phallic enlargement, may develop, as the increased testicular secretion of testosterone partially overcomes the enzyme deficiency and more dihydrotestosterone is made. Fertility is preserved in this condition, so it is prudent to rear the child as a male if possible. Neonatal treatment with dihydrotestosterone may help to masculinize the external genitalia.

XY gonadal dysgenesis is caused by a gonad that fails to secrete testosterone and MIS; generally the uterus, tubes, and vagina are present. This condition is detected when the menarche does not occur. A karyotype can confirm the XY chromosomal status. Because the gonads are inactive hormonally, they should be removed before puberty to avoid the risk of malignant degeneration. Exogenous hormone replacement is required to stimulate puberty and cause the development of secondary sexual characteristics. If donor oocytes are available, pregnancy is possible following in vitro fertilization and embryo transfer. Telling a young adolescent and her parents about the diagnosis can be difficult, particularly since surgery may be required to remove the gonads.

Answers 32.21–32.25

32.21 The answer is B

32.22 The answer is C

32.23 The answer is D

32.24 The answer is A

32.25 The answer is A

The human sexual response has been described as a cycle with four stages—desire, excitement, orgasm, and resolution. Sexual thoughts or fantasies occur in the appetitive or *desire phase.* Vaginal lubrication in women and penile erection in men are the most noticeable signs of the *excitement phase.* In women, this phase also involves internal vaginal expansion and *nipple erection.* In heightened excitement, the outer portion of the vagina swells, and the external aspects of the female genitalia, the labia, thicken and change to a darker color because of vasocongestion. In men, the *testes increase in size* and are pulled up against the body. A rash called a *sex flush* may develop on the upper torso. In both sexes, *orgasm* involves a series of *muscular contractions* that then diminish in intensity and rapidity. In women, there are muscular contractions of the outer portion of the vagina, the uterus, and the anal sphincter. In men, orgasm begins with contractions in the prostate and seminal vesicles, which cause ejaculation. During the *resolution phase,* the changes reverse to an unaroused state (e.g., *testes descend* as vasocongestion resolves). Men, but not women, have a refractory period after orgasm in which ejaculation and orgasm cannot occur. In women, studies have found the orgasmic response to be the same, regardless of whether there is manual stimulation of the clitoris or penile insertion, although some women report experiencing a different sensation with vaginal orgasm.

33 Relational Problems

Relational disorders require a different clinical approach than other disorders. Instead of focusing primarily on the link between symptoms, signs, and the workings of the individual mind, the clinician must also focus on interactions between the individuals involved and how these interactions are related to the general and other medical or psychiatric symptoms in a meaningful way.

People in intimate relationships with each other often experience problems. This may especially be the case when the relationships are affected by the presence of a mental disorder or medical condition. The revised fourth edition of the *Diagnostic and Statistical Manual of Mental Disorders* (DSM-IV-TR) attempts to formally classify problems in relationships, and this classification is meant to be employed when the focus of clinical attention is the impaired relationship. The specific relational problems indicated in DSM-IV-TR are those between parents and children, and between partners or siblings, as well as those seen in the context of a mental disorder or general medical condition. There is also a category for relational problems not otherwise specified.

An example of a relational problem related to a mental disorder might be the impaired interaction between a mother and her schizophrenic daughter, or the interaction between a brother of normal intelligence and his developmentally delayed sibling. An example of a relational problem related to a general medical condition might be the inability of a husband and wife to have sexual relations because of the husband's diabetes, and the wife's subsequent extramarital affair. A parent–child relational problem might arise in the context of divorce and remarriage, when the child must adjust to a new stepparent or to living for periods of time with each parent.

The student should study the questions and answers below for a useful review of these problems.

HELPFUL HINTS

Each of the following terms should be defined by the student.

- communication problems:
  - negative
  - distorted
  - noncommunication
- day care centers
- divorce and remarriage
- dual obligation
- environmental factors
- family characteristics
- family system
- family therapy
- marital roles
- parent–child problem
- partner relational problem
- physician marriages
- physician's responsibility
- polysomnographic findings
- premature child
- prevention
- psychotherapy
- psychotic symptoms
- racial and religious prejudice
- relational problem due to mental disorder or medical condition
- sibling relational problem
- sibling rivalry

QUESTIONS

Directions

Each of the questions or incomplete statements below is followed by five suggested responses or completions. Select the *one* that is *best* in each case.

33.1 A 15-month-old toddler is observed in a playroom with her mother. The toddler is actively playing with toys and occasionally engages her mother in the play as well. A stranger enters the room, and the child appears hesitant initially, but ultimately plays with the stranger also. When her mother leaves the room, the toddler is visibly upset and cries. When her mother returns to the room, she is happy to see her and gives her mother a hug before returning to play.

This child is exhibiting which type of attachment?

A. Secure attachment
B. Anxious-resistant attachment
C. Anxious-avoidant attachment
D. Insecure attachment
E. Intermediary attachment

33.2 A 26-year-old married woman has recently learned she is pregnant. Her husband is an alcoholic, and has a history of childhood ADHD for which he still takes medication. This is his second marriage. They both work as lawyers in a prestigious law firm and are financially well-off. The woman is concerned about her husband's temper, which she believes stems from his father having physically abused him.

Which of the following does *not* put this woman at an increased risk of domestic violence at this time?

A. Alcoholic husband
B. Pregnancy
C. History of child abuse
D. History of divorce
E. History of ADHD

33.3 Chris is a 13-year-old boy who lives with his parents and 6-year-old sister. His sister was recently diagnosed with leukemia, and has begun chemotherapy treatments. Chris's parents are extremely worried about their daughter and give her constant attention. Chris feels anger toward his sister for getting all the attention and begins playing roughly with her whenever he gets the chance.

Which of the following defense mechanisms best describes this behavior?

A. Acting out
B. Sublimation
C. Projection
D. Denial
E. Repression

33.4 Mr. K is a 43-year-old who owns his own contracting company and loves his job. His father recently helped him expand his business by giving him a generous financial contribution. Because of this contribution, his father now feels he is entitled to more of a say in the day-to-day activities of the company. Mr. K is beginning to feel smothered and questions whether he should have accepted the gift from his father. He now dreads going to work because he knows his father will call with even more changes he would like implemented. He tells you he feels like he is being treated like a child.

Mr. K is being challenged by his father in which of the following areas?

A. Autonomy
B. Triangulation
C. Identity
D. Achievement
E. Financially

33.5 Four-year-old identical twins Mark and Michael are active and rambunctious. Their parents enforce only a few rules in the household, and feel their children should be free to explore their environment as they choose. When the twins do break rules, they are reasoned with and then allowed to continue play, usually without punishment.

Mark and Michael's parents are exhibiting which of the following types of parenting styles?

A. Authoritarian
B. Permissive
C. Authoritative
D. Naturalist
E. Secure

33.6 Based on the above case, Mark and Michael are most likely to exhibit which of the following childhood characteristics?

A. Withdrawn and conflicted
B. Accepting and engaged
C. High social and cognitive functioning
D. Aggressive, impulsive, low achievement
E. Rejecting and neglecting

Directions

For each numbered statement, select the *one* lettered diagnosis that is most closely associated with it. Each lettered heading may be used once, more than once, or not at all.

Questions 33.7–33.10

A. Relational problem linked to a mental disorder or general medical condition
B. Parent–child relational problem
C. Partner relational problem
D. Sibling relational problem
E. Relational problem not otherwise specified

33.7 A 32-year-old recently married man has remained good friends with one of his ex-girlfriends; the man's wife resents this relationship and always starts arguments with the ex whenever she calls their house. Otherwise, things have been very good between the couple.

33.8 A teenage girl is angry with her parents for snooping in her room, and is becoming increasingly withdrawn and rebellious.

33.9 A 60-year-old woman with breast cancer has a radical mastectomy; she and her husband now get into constant fights because she is no longer interested in sex.

33.10 The youngest son in a family of four has a personality just like his oldest brother; as a result, the two have always bickered and gotten into fist fights since they were children.

ANSWERS

33.1 The answer is A

A child who is *securely attached* to its mother will explore freely while the mother is present, will interact with strangers, will be visibly upset when the mother departs, and happy to see the mother return. A child with an *anxious-resistant attachment* style is anxious of exploration and of strangers, even when the mother is present. When the mother departs, the child is extremely distressed. The child will be ambivalent when she returns, seeking to remain close to the mother but resentful, and also resistant when the mother initiates attention. A child with an *anxious-avoidant attachment* style will avoid or ignore the mother–showing little emotion when the mother departs or returns. The child will not explore very much regardless of who is there. Strangers will not be treated much differently from the mother. There is not much emotional range displayed regardless of who is in the room or if it is empty. Both anxious-resistant style and the anxious-avoidant style are types of *insecure attachment*. *Intermediary attachment* is not a recognized attachment style.

33.2 The answer is D

A *history of divorce* is not associated with increased likelihood of violence. However, relational problems are often accompanied by violence. Wife beating is found in every socioeconomic class and culture and at every income level. A pattern of wife beating can indicate individual impulse-control problems (e.g., *history of ADHD*), impaired socialization, being a *victim of child abuse*, and, usually, *alcohol and substance abuse*, the latter enabling impulse dyscontrol to surface. *Pregnancy* is the highest risk time for domestic violence toward the woman. Being subjected to violence often results in depression and learned helplessness across the life cycle. Women, abused as children, often are revictimized in adult significant relationships. The patient too often feels inhibited about divulging the secret of domestic violence and incorrectly blames herself for its occurrence; thus, clinicians must develop an appropriate sensitivity to the possibility of spousal abuse, in which 5 percent of victims are men. Every patient, regardless of gender, must be asked about experiences with violence across his or her life in the first professional interview, apart from age or socioeconomic, educational, racial, or faith background.

33.3 The answer is A

Acting out is the defense mechanism of an action rather than verbal response to an unconscious instinctual drive or impulse that brings about the temporary, partial relief of inner tension. Chris is acting out against his sister in response to not getting attention from his parents. *Sublimation* is an unconscious defense mechanism in which the energy associated with unacceptable impulses or drives is diverted into personally and socially acceptable channels. *Projection* is the unconscious defense mechanism in which a person attributes to another person those unconscious ideas, thoughts, feelings, and impulses that are personally undesirable or unacceptable. *Denial* is a mechanism in which the existence of unpleasant realities is disavowed. *Repression* is a mechanism in which unacceptable mental contents are banished or kept out of consciousness.

33.4 The answer is A

Autonomy is a developmental milestone. Generally, autonomy involves a person's ability to make independent choices. There is no reason to believe Mr. K did not adequately establish autonomy earlier in his life, but his father's insistence on having control of his life and business is now challenging this concept. Mr. K, by becoming a self-sufficient, successful businessman has mastered the development of *achievement*, and this concept is not being challenged here. His *identity* is also not being challenged in this case, as that would indicate Mr. K does not have a clear sense of his own values, beliefs, goals, and expectations. Identity is usually established in adolescence. *Triangulation* refers to the process in which conflicted parents attempt to win the sympathy and support of their child, who is recruited by one parent as an ally in the struggle with the partner. Triangulation is not related to the case in question. *Financially*, Mr. K's father is contributing to the support of his business and has made possible the expansions that recently occurred. However, Mr. K does not feel challenged in this respect, but rather by the changes which have followed the financial contribution.

33.5 The answer is B

Research on parenting skills has isolated two major factors on which parenting styles are judged, first, how permissive versus restrictive parents are, and second, how warm and accepting versus cold and hostile the style is. Parenting lies on a continuum between these two spectrums, and classic types have been defined based on these dimensions. The *permissive* parenting style is minimally restrictive and accepting. The *authoritarian* parenting style is defined as restrictive and cold parenting characteristics. The *authoritative* parenting style is characterized by parents being restrictive as needed, but also warm and accepting. Finally, naturalist and secure types are not recognized parenting styles.

33.6 The answer is D

Children of permissive parents, with their minimally restrictive and accepting style, are likely to be more *aggressive, impulsive, and low achievers* as they develop. Those of authoritarian parents, who are restrictive and cold, tend to be *withdrawn or conflicted*. Those children of authoritative parents that are restrictive as needed, but who are also warm and accepting, seem to *function at the highest level both socially and cognitively*. *Accepting and engaged* describes the permissive parenting style, but not the childhood characteristics that result from this style. *Rejecting and neglecting* describes the uninvolved parenting style that is low in both responsiveness and demands.

Answers 33.7–33.10

33.7 The answer is E

33.8 The answer is B

33.9 The answer is A

33.10 The answer is D

The woman who doesn't get along with her husband's ex-girlfriend is classified as having a *relational problem not otherwise specified*. The teenage girl who is rebelling after her parents snooped in her room is classified as a *parent–child relational problem*. The classification of *relational problem linked to a general medical condition* is best for the woman who is no longer interested in sex after her radical mastectomy. A *sibling relational problem* is the best diagnosis for the son who can't get along with his brother due to their similar personalities.

34

Problems Related to Abuse or Neglect

Abuse and neglect of children and adults are major public health concerns in the United States. According to the U.S. Department of Health and Human Services, there are an estimated 900,000 children who are victims of child abuse or neglect each year. More than 60 percent of child victims experienced neglect. The actual occurrence rates are likely to be higher than estimates, because many maltreated persons go unrecognized, and many are reluctant to report the abuse. Child fatalities are the most tragic consequence of maltreatment, as an estimated 1,500 children died due to abuse or neglect in 2003. Problems related to abuse and neglect are defined as physical abuse of a child or adult, sexual abuse of a child or adult (including rape, sexual coercion, and sexual harassment), and neglect of a child.

More than 50 percent of abused or neglected children were born prematurely or had low birth weight. Many abused children are perceived by their parents as difficult, slow in development or mentally retarded, bad, selfish, or hard to discipline. More than 80 percent of abused children are living with married parents at the time of the abuse and 90 percent of abusing parents were abused by their own parents.

The only sure way of proving infant abuse or neglect, other than catching the perpetrator in the act, is to show that significant recovery occurs when the caretaking is altered. All markedly deprived infants should warrant an investigation of the social and environmental conditions of the family and the psychological status of the parent in order to determine the factors responsible for inadequate and destructive treatment. Parents who abuse substances, who suffer from psychotic or pronounced mood disorders, or who are severely personality disordered are at higher risk for impaired judgment and potentially abusive behavior.

Child abuse and neglect may be suspected when a child appears unduly afraid (especially of the parents), the child is kept confined for overly long periods of time, the child shows evidence of repeated skin or other injuries, the child is undernourished, the child is dressed inappropriately for the weather, the child cries often, and the child has bruising/pain/itching in the genital or anal region or repeated urinary tract infections and vaginal discharges. Unusually precocious knowledge of sexual acts may indicate sexual abuse. Clinicians are required to report suspected cases of child abuse or neglect and must be familiar with the current laws and regulations in their individual states.

Sexual or physical abuse of adults, including the elderly, is also a major problem in the United States. Spouse abuse, for example, is thought to occur in as many as 12 million families in this country, and there are estimated to be almost 2 million battered wives. The age range for rape cases in the United States is reported to be from infancy to the 80s and 90s, and the FBI reports that there are more than 80,000 rapes each year. It has been estimated that only 10 to 25 percent of rapes are ever reported to the proper authorities. About 10 percent of rapes are perpetrated by close relatives, and 50 percent are committed by men known to varying degrees by the victim. Elder abuse is seen in nursing homes and other institutions, as well as in some private households where the demands of caring for a frail, helpless, or demented person can lead individuals to commit acts of physical or sexual abuse.

The student should study the questions and answers below for a useful review of these problems.

HELPFUL HINTS

The student should know the following words and terms.

- annual deaths
- child abuse
- child pornography
- dysthymic disorder
- emotional deprivation
- environmental factors
- family characteristics
- functional impairment
- genetic factors
- hyperactivity
- incest:
  - father–daughter
  - mother–son
- irritable versus depressed mood
- learning disability
- low-birth-weight child
- major depressive disorder
- mania
- mood disorders
- National Committee for the Prevention of Child Abuse
- physician's responsibility
- polysomnographic findings
- precocious sexual behavior
- premature child
- prevention
- psychotic symptoms
- retinal hemorrhages
- secondary complications
- suicide
- symmetrical injury patterns

QUESTIONS

Directions

Each of the questions or incomplete statements below is followed by five suggested responses or completions. Select the *one* that is *best* in each case.

34.1 Workplace violence is documented to be increased in all of the following professions *except*

A. Law enforcement
B. Computer specialists
C. Mental health workers
D. Taxi drivers
E. Bartenders

34.2 Which of the following statements regarding torture is *false*?

A. It is the infliction of physical or mental suffering.
B. It is practiced in 125 countries around the world.
C. It is always used to get victim to reveal compromising information.
D. It is an underrecognized problem.
E. Survivors of torture experience symptoms associated with PTSD and major depressive disorder.

34.3 True statements about typical physical injuries related to abuse include all of the following *except*

A. Less than 50 percent of serious intracranial injuries sustained in the first year of life result from physical abuse.
B. Subdural bleeding ranks among the most dangerous inflicted injuries.
C. Retinal tearing can be caused by shaking injuries.
D. Falls from 1 to 3 feet rarely result in subdural hematomas or clavicle fractures.
E. Bilateral black eyes immediately following facial trauma generally indicates intentional injury.

34.4 Secondary victimization is characterized by all of the following *except*

A. Disbelief and denial
B. Discounting
C. Blaming the victim
D. Verbal abuse
E. Stigmatization

34.5 Which of the following statements about rape is *incorrect*?

A. Rapes are usually premeditated.
B. Rape most often occurs in a woman's own neighborhood.
C. Fifty percent of all rapes are perpetrated by close relatives of the victim.
D. The age range reported for rape cases in the United States is 15 months to 82 years.
E. According to the Federal Bureau of Investigation, more than 80,000 rapes are reported each year.

34.6 Spouse abuse is

A. carried out by men who tend to be independent and assertive
B. a recent phenomenon
C. least likely to occur when the woman is pregnant
D. directed at specific actions of the spouse
E. an act that is self-reinforcing

34.7 Carol, 4 years of age, had a change in her behavior at preschool approximately 3 months after the birth of her sister. Her teacher saw Carol push other children and hit a classmate with a wooden block, causing a laceration of the child's lip. When Carol's teacher took her aside to talk about her behavior, she noticed what seemed to be belt marks on Carol's abdomen and forehead. Carol has also been reluctant to run outside with the other kids when it is time to go home.

Which of the following is the most likely diagnosis in this case?

A. Child abuse
B. Child neglect
C. Normal behavior
D. Conduct disorder
E. Oppositional defiant disorder

34.8 Which of the following forms of incest is most common?

A. Father–son
B. Brother–brother
C. Mother–daughter
D. Father–daughter
E. Uncle–niece

34.9 Which of the following statements about rape is *false*?

A. About 10 to 25 percent of rapes are reported to authorities.
B. The greatest danger of rape exists for women aged 16 to 24.
C. Most men who commit rape are between 25 and 44 years of age.
D. Alcohol is involved in at least 75 percent of forcible rapes.
E. About 50 percent of rapes are committed by strangers.

34.10 Which of the following is the correct order of the five phases of child sexual abuse?

A. Engagement, Secrecy, Sexual Interaction, Suppression, Disclosure
B. Sexual Interaction, Secrecy, Disclosure, Suppression, Engagement
C. Engagement, Sexual Interaction, Secrecy, Disclosure, Suppression
D. Secrecy, Engagement, Sexual Interaction, Suppression, Disclosure
E. Secrecy, Sexual Interaction, Engagement, Disclosure, Suppression

34.11 The parents of a 9-year-old boy were divorced, and he spent the summers visiting his father. When he returned from visitation, the mother noticed injuries: a healing cut on the boy's right ear and a collection of superficial, vertical scratches from his umbilicus to his pubis. She had the boy disrobe and took Polaroid photographs of his abdomen. Several days later, the mother took the boy and the photographs to the boy's regular psychotherapy appointment. She told the therapist that she was concerned that the boy had been physically and sexually abused.

What is the most appropriate next step of the psychotherapist?

A. Notify child protective services
B. Talk to the boy about where the injuries came from
C. Call the boy's father and inquire about abuse
D. Refer the family to a general internist
E. Tell the mother she has nothing to worry about

34.12 Which of the following statements about incest is *true*?

A. About 15 million women in the United States have been the victims of incestuous attacks.
B. One-third of incest cases occur before the age of 9.
C. It is most frequently reported in families of low socioeconomic status.
D. Father–daughter incest is the most common type.
E. All of the above

34.13 Which of the following provides the best proof that child abuse is occurring?

A. Significant recovery when the caretaking is altered
B. Child shows evidence of repeated skin injuries
C. Failure to thrive
D. Child is dressed inappropriately for the weather
E. Unusual knowledge of sexual acts

Directions

The questions below consist of lettered headings followed by a list of numbered statements. For each numbered statement, select:

A. if the item is associated with A only
B. if the item is associated with B only
C. if the item is associated with both A and B
D. if the item is associated with neither A nor B

Questions 34.14–34.17

A. Abuse
B. Neglect

34.14 Father of an 8-year-old boy fails to enforce the boy's school attendance
34.15 Teenage mother repeatedly slaps her toddler and refuses to give him any more to eat after he spills food on the floor
34.16 Twelve-year-old female is kicked out of her home after lying to her mother
34.17 Husband verbally threatens and belittles his wife when she spends too much money

ANSWERS

34.1 The answer is B

Law enforcement is the most common occupation for nonfatal workplace violence, with an average of 234,200 victimizations a year, followed by corrections officers (217.9 per 1,000), *taxi drivers* (183.8 per 1,000), private security guards (117.3 per 1,000), *bartenders* (91.3 per 1,000), mental health professionals (79.5 per 1,000), gas station attendants (79.1 per 1,000), *mental health custodial workers* (63.3 per 1,000), and junior high/middle school teachers (57.4 per 1,000). There is no documented evidence that *computer specialists* are at increased risk for workplace violence.

34.2 The answer is C

Although public perception may be that torture is used to elicit information, more commonly, the purpose of torture is to break the will of the victim and, ultimately, to destroy his or her humanity through the infliction of severe physical or mental suffering in the context of political repression. Torture is defined as the deliberate, systematic, or wanton infliction of *physical or mental suffering*. In their 2001 annual report, Amnesty International reports that torture is practiced in *125 countries around the world.* Those who provide services and treatment for refugees and asylum seekers are aware of the extent of this *under-recognized problem* and of the dearth of funding for services for torture survivors. Survivors of torture experience all of the *symptoms associated with PTSD and major depressive disorder*. The most common psychiatric symptoms found in survivors of torture include memory and concentration impairment, nightmares, intrusive memories, increased startle response, amnesia, flashbacks, sleep disturbance, irritability, and avoidance.

34.3 The answer is A

More than 95 percent (not less than 50 percent) of serious intracranial injuries sustained in the first year of life result from physical abuse. The cause of injury, typically, is violent shaking to-and-fro whiplash, or slamming. *Subdural bleeding* ranks among the most dangerous inflicted injuries, often resulting in death or serious crippling sequelae. *Retinal tearing* and hemorrhage may be caused by shaking injuries. *Falls* are often blamed for injuries, and a fall from 1 to 3 feet can result in linear skull fracture and epidural hematoma. Such falls, however, rarely result in subdural hematomas or clavicle or humerus fractures.

Inflicted black eyes are more common than serious eye injuries. Victims smacked about the eyes with an open or closed hand have both eyelids swollen, with massive bruising. Generally, black eyes sustained from accidents involve trauma to one eye. Although other scenarios are possible, the onset of *bilateral black eyes* immediately following facial trauma generally indicates intentional injury.

Traumatic alopecia and subgaleal hematomas are caused by pulling the hair. Alopecia areata (noninflammatory hair loss) is characterized by loose hairs at the periphery of the bald area and is easily distinguished from inflammation or boggy swelling of the scalp caused by violent lifting of the child by the hair. Subgaleal hematomas may result when the aponeurosis connection between the occipital and frontalis muscles is wrenched off the calvarium, permitting rapid filling of the remaining space with blood.

34.4 The answer is D

Secondary victimization occurs when family, friends, colleagues, or employers respond to a victim of abuse in one of the following ways: (1) *Disbelief and denial*. The incident's description or details provided by the victim(s) are not believed. (2) *Discounting*. The magnitude of the incident and its results are poorly understood or minimized. (3) *Blaming the victim*. Responsibility for the incident is attributed to the victim(s). (4) *Stigmatization*. A judgment is made concerning the psychological consequences for a victim of a traumatic event, such as ridicule for experiencing symptoms or a belief that symptoms result from malingering or for attention or sympathy. *Verbal abuse* is not considered a characteristic of secondary victimization, although it may occur in response to these other characteristics.

34.5 The answer is C

About 10 percent, not 50 percent, of rapes are perpetrated by close relatives. About half of rapes are committed by strangers and half by men known in varying degrees (but unrelated) to the victim. *Rapes are usually premeditated,* although rape often accompanies another crime such as mugging. A rapist frequently threatens a victim with his fists or a weapon and often harms her in nonsexual as well as sexual ways. *Rape most often occurs in a woman's own neighborhood.* It may take place inside or near her home. *The age range reported for rape cases* in the United States is 15 months to 82 years. According to the Federal Bureau of Investigation, *more than 80,000 rapes are reported each year.* The incidence is declining slightly.

34.6 The answer is E

Spouse abuse is an *act that is self-reinforcing*; once a man has beaten his wife, he is likely to do so again. Abusive husbands *tend to be* immature, *dependent, and nonassertive,* and to suffer from strong feelings of inadequacy. Spouse abuse is *not a recent phenomenon*; it is a problem of long standing that is *most likely (not least likely) to occur when the woman is pregnant.* Fifteen to 25 percent of women are physically abused while pregnant, and the abuse often results in birth defects. The *abuse is not directed at specific actions of the spouse;* rather, impatient and impulsive abusive husbands physically displace aggression provoked by others onto their wives.

34.7 The answer is A

The stress of a newborn can cause many changes in household functioning. Physical abuse of other children in the house may be a result of such changes. In many cases, the physical examination and radiological evaluation show evidence of repeated suspicious injuries. These can include belt marks, cigarette burns, and scalding water burns. *Abused children* display behaviors that should arouse the suspicions of the health professional. For example, these children may be unusually fearful, docile, distrustful, and guarded. On the other hand, they may be disruptive and aggressive (e.g., hitting another classmate with a wooden block). They may be wary of physical contact and show no expectation of being comforted by adults, they may be on the alert for danger and continually size up the environment, and they may be afraid to go home. *Conduct disorder* is a childhood behavioral condition involving a pattern of repetitive and persistent conduct that infringes on the basic rights of others or does not conform to established societal norms or rules that are appropriate for a child of that age. *Oppositional defiant disorder* is a recurring pattern of negative, hostile, disobedient, and defiant behavior in a child or adolescent, lasting for at least 6 months without serious violation of the basic rights of others.

34.8 The answer is D

Incest may be defined strictly as sexual relations between close blood relatives, that is, between a child and the father, uncle, or sibling. Because of increased reporting, sibling incest is an area of growing concern. In its broader sense, incest includes sexual intercourse between a child and a stepparent or stepsibling. Incest can involve father and son, mother and daughter, and uncle and niece; however, *father–daughter incest is the most common form.*

34.9 The answer is D

Alcohol is involved in about 35 percent, not 75 percent, of forcible rapes. *The greatest danger of rape exists for women aged 16 to 24,* although victims of rape can be any age. Most men who commit rape are *between the ages of 25 and 44 years old.* It has been estimated that *10 to 25 percent of rapes are reported* to authorities. *About 50 percent of rapes are committed by strangers to the victims,* and the remaining 50 percent are committed by men known by them to varying degrees.

34.10 The answer is C

Child sexual abuse that occurs over a period of time evolves through five phases in this sequence: engagement, sexual interaction, secrecy, disclosure, and suppression.

1. *Engagement Phase:* The perpetrator induces the child into a special relationship. The daughter in father–daughter incest has frequently had a close relationship with her father throughout her childhood and may be pleased at first when he approaches her sexually.
2. *Sexual Interaction Phase:* The sexual behaviors progress from less to more intrusive forms of abuse. As the behavior continues, the abused daughter becomes confused and frightened, because she never knows whether her father will be parental or sexual. If the victim tells her mother about the abuse, the mother may not be supportive. The mother often refuses to believe her daughter's reports or refuses to confront her husband with her suspicions. Because the father provides special attention to a particular daughter, her brothers and sisters may distance themselves from her.
3. *Secrecy Phase:* The perpetrator threatens the victim not to tell. The father, fearful that his daughter may expose their relationship and often jealously possessive of her, interferes with the girl's development of normal peer relationships.
4. *Disclosure Phase:* The abuse is discovered accidentally (when another person walks in the room and sees it), through the child's reporting it to a responsible adult, or when the child is brought for medical attention and an alert clinician asks the right questions.
5. *Suppression Phase:* The child often retracts the statements of the disclosure because of family pressure or because of the child's own mental processes. That is, the child may perceive that violent or intrusive attention is synonymous with interest or affection. Many incest survivors rally around their perpetrators, seeking to capture any modicum of tenderness or interest. At times, affection for the perpetrator

outweighs the facts of abuse, and children recant their statements about sexual assault, regardless of substantiated evidence of molestation.

34.11 The answer is B

Consider the following ending to this case:

The therapist interviewed the boy individually, who explained in a matter-of-fact and believable manner that his ear was cut accidentally when he had his hair cut and that his abdomen was scratched when he went body surfing at a North Carolina beach. The therapist concluded the boy had not been abused and reassured the mother. The therapist did not notify child protective services.

Physicians are required to report abuse when they have reason to believe or to suspect (depending on the jurisdiction) that it occurred; however, they are not required to report other people's beliefs or suspicions. Some clinicians have the mistaken idea that, if a mother expresses a concern that her child may have been abused, the suspected abuse must be reported, even when the clinician has investigated and has no suspicion at all that abuse occurred (e.g., an overly anxious mother who imagines that her child was sexually abused at day care, even though an objective examiner found no indications that abuse had occurred). The negative consequences of overreporting include increasing the load on an already overburdened child protective system and an unnecessary invasion into the lives of families, who are subjected to investigation, suspicion, and criticism.

34.12 The answer is E (all)

About 15 million women in the United States have been the victims of incestuous attacks, and *one-third of incest cases occur before the age of 9*. Incest is *most frequently reported in families of low socioeconomic status*. That finding may be the result of these families' greater than usual contact with welfare workers, public health personnel, law enforcement agents, and other reporting officials; it may not be a true reflection of higher incidence in that demographic group. *Father–daughter incest* is the most common type.

34.13 The answer is A

Other than catching the perpetrator in the act, showing that *significant recovery occurs when the caretaking is altered* can prove a child is being abused or neglected. *Repeated skin injuries* can be the result of physical abuse, but careless play or a medical abnormality such as thrombocytopenia or a dermatologic problem can be the cause as well. *Failure to thrive* can also be the result of abuse, but organic causes also must be investigated. Likewise, *inappropriate dress for the weather* and *unusual knowledge of sexual acts* are suspicious for abuse, but are not definitive as alternative explanations are always possible.

Answers 34.14–34.17

34.14 The answer is B

34.15 The answer is C

34.16 The answer is B

34.17 The answer is A

Physical abuse may be defined as any act that results in a nonaccidental physical injury, such as *slapping*, beating, punching, kicking, biting, burning, and poisoning. Physical abuse may be organized by the site of injury; damage to skin and surface tissue, damage to the head, damage to internal organs, and skeletal damage.

Psychological abuse occurs when a person conveys to someone that he or she is worthless, flawed, unloved, unwanted, or endangered. The perpetrator may spurn, terrorize, isolate, or berate their victim.

Emotional abuse includes *verbal assaults*, unpredictable responses, persistent negative moods, constant family discord, and double-message communications.

Neglect is the most prevalent form of child maltreatment, and is the failure to provide adequate care and protection for children. Children can be harmed by malicious or ignorant withholding of physical, emotional, and educational necessities. Neglect includes *failure to feed children adequately* and to protect them from danger. Physical neglect includes abandonment, *expulsion from home*, disruptive custodial care, inadequate supervision, and reckless disregard for a child's safety and welfare. Medical neglect includes refusal, delay, or failure to provide medical care. Educational neglect includes failure to enroll a child in school and *allowing chronic truancy*.

35

Additional Conditions That May Be a Focus of Attention

There are many types of problems that bring persons into contact with the mental health care system. Once in the system, persons with a condition that may be a focus of clinical attention should have a thorough neuropsychiatric evaluation, which may or may not uncover a mental disorder. The category of conditions that are not diagnosable mental disorders is important to psychiatrists because these conditions may accompany mental illness or may be harbingers of underlying mental disorders. The revised 4th edition of the *Diagnostic and Statistical Manual of Mental Disorders* (DSM-IV-TR) lists and describes 13 such conditions that may or may not be associated with mental disorders, and may or may not be precursors of mental disorders. However, all of these conditions can be identified only when they are not directly attributable to a specific mental or neurological disorder. These 13 conditions are noncompliance with treatment, malingering, adult antisocial behavior, child or adolescent antisocial behavior, borderline intellectual functioning, age-related cognitive decline, bereavement, academic problem, occupational problem, identity problem, religious or spiritual problem, acculturation problem, and phase-of-life problem.

Malingering is the conscious and intentional feigning of physical or psychological symptoms for some clearly definable goal, such as to avoid responsibilities or to receive free compensation. Clinically, it is often crucial to distinguish malingering from true mental illnesses such as factitious, somatoform, or dissociative disorders. Malingering may be associated with child, adolescent, or adult antisocial behavior, which is characterized by engaging in illegal or immoral activities. However, the antisocial behavior in these conditions never reaches the level necessary to diagnose an antisocial personality disorder.

Bereavement is a condition that can become the focus of clinical attention, even if it does not progress to the outright acute mental disorder of depression. The clinician must be aware of the difference between normal bereavement and depression and be alert for the development of more serious symptoms.

Examples of an occupational problem include job dissatisfaction and uncertainty about career choices. A phase-of-life problem might be associated with such major life-cycle changes as starting college, getting married, or having children. Stress during times of cultural transitions, such as moving to a new country or entering the military, can lead to an acculturation problem. Young people who join cults might provide examples of a religious or spiritual problem. Age-related cognitive decline must be distinguished from dementia, while borderline intellectual functioning must be distinguished from diagnosable developmental delays or specific learning disorders. Academic problem, identity problem, and noncompliance with treatment are the remaining conditions addressed in this chapter and the student should be able to describe and recognize their characteristics.

The student should study the questions and answers below for a useful review of these conditions.

HELPFUL HINTS

The students should know the following terms.

- acculturation problem
- adherence
- adoption studies
- age-associated memory decline
- antisocial behavior
- bereavement
- brainwashing
- compliance
- conditioning
- coping mechanisms
- cults
- cultural transition
- culture shock
- dual-career families
- job-related stress
- kleptomania
- malingering
- marital problems
- mature defense mechanisms
- medicolegal context of presentation
- noncompliance
- noncustodial parent
- normal grief
- occupational problem
- patient–doctor match
- phase-of-life problem
- religious or spiritual problem
- sociopathic
- stress
- superego lacunae

QUESTIONS

Directions

Each of the questions or incomplete statements below is followed by five suggested responses or completions. Select the *one* that is *best* in each case.

35.1 Brainwashing

A. is the deliberate creation of cultural shock
B. relies on both mental and physical coercion
C. is often followed by guilt and depression
D. was first practiced on U.S. prisoners
E. All of the above

35.2 Adult antisocial behavior differs from antisocial personality disorder in that:

A. Antisocial behavior does not require a previous diagnosis of conduct disorder
B. Antisocial behavior occurs more often in females
C. Antisocial behavior is considered a mental disorder
D. Antisocial behavior must begin before age 25
E. None of the above

35.3 Malingering should be strongly suspected in all of the following cases *except*

A. When an attorney refers the patient to the clinician
B. When the patient has antisocial personality disorder
C. With a marked discrepancy exists between the claimed stress and objective findings
D. When the patient is incarcerated
E. When there is a lack of cooperation during examination and treatment

35.4 Academic problems

A. cannot be diagnosed if due to a mental disorder
B. can be diagnosed only if they are the result of factors external to the student, such as family difficulties or social stressors
C. are evidenced by a pattern of academic underachievement or a decline from a previous level of functioning
D. intelligence tests are rarely useful in making the diagnosis
E. none of the above

35.5 Occupational problems as defined by DSM-IV-TR can be associated with

A. suicide risk
B. domestic violence
C. working teenagers
D. loss of a job
E. all of the above

35.6 Exit therapy is designed to help people

A. with adult antisocial behavior
B. with acculturation problems
C. who are involved in cults
D. with occupational problems
E. in bereavement

35.7 True statements about compliance include

A. Noncompliance is more common and roughly double among inpatients than among outpatients.
B. Modification in lifestyles is more easily achieved than medication compliance.
C. Compliance is a particular problem in disorders such as glaucoma.
D. Compliance is improved if patients view their disease as not terribly serious.
E. None of the above

35.8 Malingered amnesia is

A. probably the least common clinical presentation of malingering
B. difficult to feign
C. easy to detect
D. more convincing when global rather than spotty and episode-specific
E. none of the above

35.9 Borderline intellectual functioning

A. is defined as an IQ below 70
B. is essentially the same as mental retardation
C. is usually diagnosed after completion of school
D. is present in approximately 14 percent of the general population
E. none of the above

35.10 Which of the following is *not* considered a mental disorder?

A. Factitious disorder
B. Antisocial personality disorder
C. Malingering
D. Hypochondriasis
E. Somatization disorder

35.11 Antisocial behavior is generally characterized by

A. poor intelligence
B. heightened nervousness with neurotic manifestations
C. often successful suicide attempts
D. lack of remorse or shame
E. all of the above

35.12 Which of the following statements involving women in the work force is *false*?

A. More than 50 percent of all mothers in the work force have preschool-aged children.
B. Specific issues that should be addressed are provisions for child care or for care of elderly parents.
C. Managers are more sensitive to crises in women employees' lives than in men employees' lives.

D. Ninety percent of women and girls alive today in the United States will have to work to support themselves.
E. Managers often ignore the stress placed on a worker by the illness of a child.

35.13 A person who malingers

A. often expresses subjective, ill-defined symptoms
B. should be confronted by the treating clinician
C. is usually found in settings with a preponderance of women
D. rarely seeks secondary gains
E. can achieve symptom relief by suggestion or hypnosis

35.14 Causes of workplace distress include all of the following *except*

A. Having too much to do
B. Having too little to do
C. Working for unhelpful managers
D. Being distracted at work by family problems
E. Entering the military

ANSWERS

35.1 The answer is E

First practiced by the Chinese Communists on *U.S. prisoners during the Korean War*, brainwashing is the *deliberate creation of cultural shock*. A condition of isolation, alienation, and intimidation is developed to assault ego strengths and leave the person to be brainwashed vulnerable to the imposition of alien ideas and behavior that he or she would usually reject. Brainwashing *relies on both mental and physical coercion*. All persons are vulnerable to brainwashing if they are exposed to it long enough, if they are alone and without support, and if they are without hope of escape from the situation. Help from the mental health system, in the form of deprogramming, is usually necessary to help persons readjust to their usual environments after the brainwashing experience. Supportive therapy is offered, with emphasis on reeducation, restitution of ego strengths that existed before the trauma, and alleviation of the *guilt and depression that are remnants* of the frightening experience and the lost confidence and confusion in identity that resulted from it.

35.2 The answer is A

The diagnosis of antisocial personality disorder, *in contrast to adult antisocial behavior*, requires evidence of preexisting psychopathology, such as *previous diagnosis of conduct disorder* with onset before age 15, and a longstanding pattern of irresponsible and antisocial behavior since the age of 15. Illegal behavior is not considered the equivalent of psychopathology, and without evidence of preexisting psychological disturbance is not deemed secondary to antisocial personality disorder.

Adult antisocial behavior is *not considered a mental disorder*, but antisocial personality disorder is. Both adult antisocial behavior and antisocial personality disorder *occur more often in males than in females*. Familial patterns for each of the two diagnostic classes have also been reported.

35.3 The answer is D

Malingering is characterized by the voluntary production and presentation of false or grossly exaggerated physical or psychological symptoms for some secondary gain. Malingering should be strongly suspected if any combination of the following is noted:

1. Medicolegal context of presentation (e.g., the *person is referred by an attorney* to the clinician for examination)
2. *Marked discrepancy* between the person's claimed stress or disability and the objective findings.
3. *Lack of cooperation* during the diagnostic evaluation and in complying with the prescribed treatment regimen
4. Presence of *antisocial personality disorder*

While malingering is possible with any patient, incarceration alone should not automatically lead to strong suspicions for malingering, and clinicians should be aware of these sorts of biases.

35.4 The answer is C

DSM-IV-TR describes academic problems as follows:

"This category can be used when the focus of clinical attention is an *academic problem that is not due to a mental disorder or*, if *due to a mental disorder*, is sufficiently severe to warrant independent clinical attention. An example is a pattern of failing grades or of significant underachievement in a person with adequate intellectual capacity in the absence of a Learning or Communication Disorder or another mental disorder that would account for the problem."

Academic problems can result from factors intrinsic as well as external to the student. Psychiatric conditions such as anxiety or mood disorders can impair learning or lead to performance decline. Attention-deficit/hyperactivity disorder, chronic illness, and identity problems can lead to demoralization in school studies apart from any diagnosable mental condition. Family difficulties, social stressors, cultural deprivation, or poor fit between a student and a teacher's temperamental style can also adversely affect scholastic performance.

Academic problems are evidenced by a pattern of *academic underachievement or a decline* from a previous level of functioning. A comprehensive biopsychosocial assessment is fundamental to identification of causal factors. Particular focus should be given to past academic functioning and family and social stressors; concurrent psychopathology must be ruled out. *Intelligence tests*, measures of academic achievement, or language evaluation *may be useful in differentiating academic problems from specific learning or communication disorders*. Review of the medical history and physical examination may be of value in identifying general medical conditions that may adversely affect academic performance, such as hearing loss, poor vision, and chronic illness.

35.5 The answer is E (all)

DSM-IV-TR includes the following statement about occupational problem: "This category can be used when the focus of clinical attention is an occupational problem that is not due to a mental disorder or, if it is due to a mental disorder, is sufficiently severe to warrant independent clinical attention. Examples include job dissatisfaction and uncertainty about career choices." Occupational psychiatry and its expansion to include organizational psychiatry are focused specifically on the psychiatric aspects of work problems, including vocational maladjustment. Symptoms of employment dissatisfaction are varied and include blatant work errors, perceived and verbalized unhappiness and disinterest, absenteeism and tardiness, and passive-aggressive behaviors including accidents and uncooperativeness. Psychiatric symptoms include general signs of distress, anger, resentment about most work assignments, lack of confidence, and lack of interest in carrying out agreed upon and expected work responsibilities.

Occupational problems often arise during stressful changes in work, namely, at initial entry into the work force or when making job moves within the same organization to a higher position because of good performance or to a parallel position because of corporate need. Distress occurs particularly if these changes are not sought and no preparatory training has taken place, as well as during layoffs and at retirement, especially if retirement is mandatory and the person is unprepared for it. Work distress can result if initially agreed-to conditions change to work overload or lack of challenge and opportunity to experience work satisfaction, if persons feel unable to fulfill conflicting expectations or feel that work conditions prevent accomplishing assignments because of lack of legitimate power, and finally if persons believe they work in a hierarchy with harsh and unreasonable superiors.

Some occupations both attract persons with a high *suicide risk* and involve increased chronic distress that may lead to higher suicide rates. Included are health professionals, financial service workers, and police, the first and latter groups because of easier access to lethal drugs and weapons.

Many teenagers work part-time while attending high school. Stress can arise because of reduced parent–teenager interaction and constructive parental control issues about use of earnings and time spent away from home and consequent behaviors in as well as outside the home. When each parent or a single parent works outside the home, as does the teenager, verbal communication must be proactive and clear.

Although occurring in the home, signs and symptoms that interfere with work often trigger identification of *domestic violence* victims. All employees experiencing work distress must be questioned about domestic violence by trained professionals.

Regardless of the reason *for job loss*, most people experience distress, including symptoms of normal grief, loss of self-esteem, anger, and reactive depressive and anxiety symptoms, as well as somatic symptoms and possibly substance abuse and increased (or the onset of) domestic violence. Timely education, support programs, and vocational guidance should be instituted.

35.6 The answer is C

Exit therapy is designed to help people *who are involved in cults*; it works only if their lingering emotional ties to persons outside the cult can be mobilized. Most potential cult members are in their adolescence or otherwise struggling with establishing their own identities. The cult holds out the false promise of emotional well-being and purports to offer the sense of direction for which the persons are searching. Cult members are encouraged to proselytize and to draw new members into the group. They are often encouraged to break with family members and friends and to socialize only with other group members. Cults are invariably led by charismatic personalities, who are often ruthless in their quest for financial, sexual, and power gains and in their insistence on conformity to the cult's ideological belief system, which may have strong religious or quasi-religious overtones.

Exit therapy is not designed to help people with *adult antisocial behavior*, with *acculturation* or *occupational* problems, or in *bereavement*. Occupational problems may bring a person into contact with the mental health field, and psychotherapy may aid in working through some occupational problems.

35.7 The answer is C

The determinants of compliance are kaleidoscopic and ever-changing. There is no stereotypical noncompliant person or situation. Nonetheless, there are areas of consensus.

Noncompliance is more common and *roughly double among outpatients than among inpatients (not vice versa). Medication compliance is more (not less) readily achieved than modification in lifestyle.*

Compliance is a particular problem in disorders that have no symptoms, are persistent, and have no method for self-monitoring such as hypertension, diabetes, and glaucoma. *Glaucoma presents the most difficult problem* because, currently, there is no home tonometer to measure intraocular pressure corresponding to the sphygmometer and glucometer that measure blood pressure and blood sugar concentrations, respectively.

Compliance diminishes across time in disorders that are chronic or long lasting. Compliance generally improves when patients' expectations are met, when they are satisfied, and when they are supervised. *It helps if patients view their disease as a serious one* to which they are susceptible and if they have developed compliance strategies of their own. Supportive family members or friends are important. Factors that generally impede compliance are complicated regimens, troublesome adverse effects, social stress, isolation, and alcohol dependence.

35.8 The answer is D

Amnesia, probably the most (not the least) common clinical presentation of malingering, is claimed by 30 to 55 percent of perpetrators of homicide. *It is easy (not difficult) to feign and is particularly difficult (not easy) to detect.*

At least six possible causes have been suggested for amnesia: (1) conversion disorder; (2) psychosis; (3) alcoholism; (4) head injury; (5) epilepsy; and (6) malingering. Before malingering is ascribed, the clinician should review and eliminate the other five potential causes. A good diagnostic battery would include negative results on skull X-ray, head computed tomography or magnetic resonance imaging, and electroencephalography; normal findings on a neurological examination; a life history inconsistent with either conversion disorder or alcoholism (or other causes of intoxication); and a clinical examination and history inconsistent with either alcoholic amnesia (alcohol-induced persisting amnestic disorder) or psychosis (alcohol-induced psychotic disorder).

If the preceding tests are negative, the clinician faces the difficult task of amassing evidence, albeit inferential, of malingering. Motivation is a key indicator. Previous amnestic episodes without apparent motivational precursors lower the likelihood that the patient is malingering. Similarly, a patient with histrionic personality traits is more likely to be experiencing true dissociative amnesia than one with primarily antisocial traits.

The timing of onset and recovery, and correlation of the alleged amnestic episode with convenience, are other clues to the

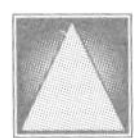

Table 35.1
Clues to the Detection of Malingered Amnesia

1. No history of amnestic episodes
2. Antisocial personality traits more prominent than histrionic personality traits
3. Spotty, episode-specific amnesia rather than global amnesia
4. Self-serving timing of onset and recovery
5. Recent, widely publicized, suspiciously familiar cases involving amnesia

presence of malingering. *Global amnesia is somewhat more convincing than spotty,* patchy, *episode-specific*, and self-serving amnesia. There have been several reported epidemics of copycat amnesias following famous or highly publicized cases; an eye to recent sensational litigation is prudent. Table 35.1 summarizes some guidelines on detecting malingered amnesia.

35.9 The answer is D

DSM-IV-TR describes borderline intellectual functioning as follows:

"This category can be used when the focus of clinical attention is associated with borderline intellectual functioning, that is, *an IQ in the 71–84 range (not an IQ below 70).* Differential diagnosis between Borderline Intellectual Functioning and *Mental Retardation (an IQ of 70 or below*) is especially difficult when the coexistence of certain mental disorders (e.g., schizophrenia) is involved. Coding note: This is coded on Axis II."

The 1959 edition of *Classification in Mental Retardation* defined anyone with an IQ greater than one standard deviation below the mean (IQ below 85) as mentally retarded. This definition was applied without regard to functional impairment, and many individuals who fell within this range had no discernible adaptive difficulties. The 1973 edition of *Classification in Mental Retardation* redefined mental retardation as an IQ greater than two standard deviations below the mean (70 or below) with associated impairments in adaptive functioning. This definition of mental retardation has been retained in subsequent editions and is adhered to in DSM-IV-TR and the 10th revision of *International Statistical Classification of Diseases and Related Health Problems* (ICD-10). An IQ between 71 and 84 was "declassified" as mentally disordered and redefined as borderline intellectual functioning. Because individuals within this IQ range tend to have little impairment outside of educational settings, *the diagnosis is often overlooked after completion of school.* The condition may continue to be a focus of clinical attention if it compromises social functioning, vocational adjustment, or compliance with medical management. *Approximately 14 percent of the general population* has an IQ within this range; borderline intellectual functioning is similarly named and defined in ICD-10.

35.10 The answer is C

Malingering is not considered a mental disorder; it is characterized by the voluntary production and presentation of false or grossly exaggerated physical or psychological symptoms. The patient always has an external motivation, which falls into one of three categories: (1) to avoid difficult or dangerous situations, responsibilities, or punishment; (2) to receive compensation, free hospital room and board, drugs, or haven from the police; and (3) to retaliate when one feels guilt or suffers a financial loss, legal penalty, or job layoff or termination.

Factitious disorder, antisocial personality disorder, hypochondriasis, and *somatization disorder* are all considered mental disorders. The presence of a clearly definable goal is the main factor that differentiates malingering from factitious disorder. Antisocial personality disorder requires evidence of conduct disorder that began before the age of 15. Hypochondriasis and somatization disorder are both somatoform disorders, which are characterized by physical symptoms that suggest physical disease, although no demonstrable organ pathology or pathophysiological mechanism can usually be identified. In hypochondriasis the patient is excessively concerned about disease and health. In somatization disorder, multiple somatic symptoms cannot be explained medically and are associated with psychosocial distress and medical help seeking.

35.11 The answer is D

Antisocial behavior is generally characterized by *lack of remorse or shame.* Other characteristics are *good (not poor) intelligence, an absence of nervousness and neurotic manifestations, (not heightened), and rarely (not often) successful suicide attempts.*

35.12 The answer is C

Studies reveal that managers are more sensitive to crises in men's than in women's lives (not vice versa). Managers respond to such major events as divorce and death of a family member but *ignore the stress placed on a worker by the illness of a child* or a school closing because of a snow day. *More than 50 percent of mothers* in the work force have preschool-aged children. *Specific issues* that should be addressed are *provisions for child care or for the care of elderly parents. Ninety percent of women and girls* alive today in the United States *will have to work to support themselves* and probably one or two other people.

35.13 The answer is A

A person who malingers *often expresses subjective, ill-defined symptoms*—for example, headache; pains in one's neck, lower back, chest, or abdomen; dizziness; vertigo; amnesia; anxiety; and depression—and the symptoms often have a family history, in all likelihood not organically based but extremely difficult to refute. A patient suspected of malingering should be thoroughly and objectively evaluated, and the physician should refrain from showing any suspicion. The patient *should not be confronted by the treating clinician.* If the clinician becomes angry (a common response to malingerers), a confrontation may occur, with two likely consequences: (1) The patient–doctor relationship is disrupted, and no further positive intervention is possible; and (2) the patient is even more on guard, and obtaining proof of deception may become virtually impossible. Preserving the patient–doctor relationship is often essential to accurate diagnosis and effective long-term treatment. Careful evaluation usually reveals the relevant issue without the need for a confrontation.

Malingering *is usually found in settings with a preponderance of men (not women)*, such as the military, prisons, factories, and other industrial settings. The malingerer *always (not rarely) seeks secondary gains*, such as money, food, and shelter. The malingerer *cannot usually achieve symptom relief by suggestion or hypnosis.* Table 35.2 lists malingering features not found in genuine illness.

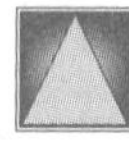

Table 35.2
Malingering Features Usually Not Found in Genuine Illness

Symptoms are vague, ill-defined, overdramatized, and not in conformity with known clinical conditions.
The patient seeks addicting drugs, financial gain, the avoidance of onerous (e.g., jail) or other unwanted conditions.
History, examination, and evaluative data do not elucidate complaints.
The patient is uncooperative and refuses to accept a clean bill of health or an encouraging prognosis.
The findings appear compatible with self-inflicted injuries.
History or records reveal multiple past episodes of injury or undiagnosed illness.
Records or test data appear to have been tampered with (e.g., erasures, unprescribed substances in urine).

Courtesy of Arthur T. Meyerson, M.D.

35.14 The answer is E

Occupational or industrial psychiatry is that area of psychiatry specifically concerned with vocational maladjustment and the psychiatric aspects of problems at work. Persons are particularly vulnerable to occupational problems at several points in their working lives—on entry into the working world, at times of promotion or transfer, during periods of unemployment, and at retirement. Specific situations—such as *having too much or too little to do*, being subjected to conflicting demands, *feeling distracted by family problems*, having responsibility without authority, and *working for demanding and unhelpful managers*—also create occupational distress. *Entering the military* is more accurately defined as an acculturation problem, rather than a cause of workplace distress.

36

Emergency Psychiatric Medicine

Emergency psychiatry refers to the management of disorders of mood, thought, and behavior at a time of crisis. It entails assessment, development of a differential diagnosis of psychiatric and other medical causes of presenting symptoms, and diagnostic-specific pharmacotherapy, medical and surgical therapy, psychotherapy, and sociotherapy. Psychiatric emergencies are often particularly disturbing because they do not just involve the body's reactions to an acute disease state, as much as actions directed against the self or others. These emergencies, such as suicidal acts, homicidal delusions, or a severe inability to care for oneself, are more likely than medical ones to be sensationalized when they end up on the front pages of newspapers. Although the emergency room is a poor substitute for continuing care by a mental health professional in an outpatient setting, many individuals without a usual source of care, particularly the uninsured, use emergency care clinicians for primary care.

Psychiatric emergencies arise when mental disorders impair people's judgment, impulse control, or reality testing. Such mental disorders include all the psychotic disorders, manic and depressive episodes in mood disorders, substance abuse, borderline and antisocial personality disorders, and dementias. There may also be emergencies related to particularly severe reactions to psychiatric medications, such as neuroleptic malignant syndrome or acute agranulocytosis, which must be recognized diagnosed, and treated immediately.

The most common psychiatric emergency is suicide, which is reported to be the eighth leading cause of death in the United States. Clinicians must be aware of the relevant risk factors for suicide (such as age, sex, race, marital status, occupation, family history, physical and mental health, and past suicidal behavior), but must also be aware that the suicidal patient they are evaluating in the emergency room may not necessarily have any of them. Major depressive disorder, alcohol abuse, and schizophrenia are all associated with a higher than usual risk for suicide, as is a positive family history for suicide. Genetic influence in the expression of suicidal behavior has been postulated, and there appears to be substantiating evidence for this in twin and adoption studies. However, a behavior as complex as suicide cannot be reduced to any simplistic biological formulation.

Psychiatrists must learn how to evaluate a suicidal or homicidal patient and must learn how to ask the questions that will help reveal the suicidal or homicidal plan or intent. A skilled clinician will combine this information with a sense of the person's overall risk, based on detailed knowledge of the person's history as well as overall knowledge of suicidal and homicidal behaviors in the context of mental impairment.

The student should study the questions and answers below for a useful review of this subject.

HELPFUL HINTS

These terms relate to psychiatric emergencies and should be defined.

- acute intoxication
- adolescent suicide
- age of suicide
- akinetic mutism
- alcohol dependence
- alcohol withdrawal
- alkalosis
- amnesia
- anniversary suicide
- anorexia nervosa
- bulimia nervosa
- copycat suicides
- delirious state
- delirium
- dementia
- drugs and suicide
- DTs
- Emile Durkheim
- dysmenorrhea
- ECT
- exhaustion syndrome
- grief and bereavement
- headache
- 5-HIAA in CSF
- hyperthermia
- hypertoxic schizophrenia
- hyperventilation
- hypnosis
- hypothermia
- inpatient vs. outpatient treatment
- insomnia
- lethal catatonia
- method
- miosis
- mood disorders
- "Mourning and Melancholia"
- mydriasis
- nystagmus
- opioid withdrawal:
  - anxiolytic
  - hypnotic
  - sedative
- panic disorder
- platelet MAO activity
- posttraumatic stress disorder mania
- premenstrual dysphoric disorder
- prevention center
- psychiatric interview
- psychotic disorders
- psychotic withdrawal
- restraints
- suicidal depression

- suicidal thoughts
- suicidal threats
- suicide:
  - altruistic
  - anomic
  - egoistic
- suicide belt
- suicide rate
- Thanatos
- violence and assaultive behavior
- Wernicke's encephalopathy
- Werther's syndrome

QUESTIONS

Directions

Each of the questions or incomplete statements below is followed by five suggested responses or completions. Select the *one* that is *best* in each case.

36.1 The first task in evaluating violent behavior should be

A. establishing a treatment plan
B. obtaining information from observers
C. ascertaining degree of injuries
D. determination of cause
E. admission to the hospital

36.2 Which of the following most closely represents Freud's theory on suicide?

A. Suicide represents aggression turned inward against an introjected love object
B. Suicide as inverted homicide because of a patient's anger toward another person
C. Suicide as an unconscious wish for revenge
D. Suicide consists of three components: the wish to kill, the wish to be killed, and the wish to die
E. None of the above

36.3 The use of restraints in an emergency setting should include all of the following principles *except*

A. Explanation to the patient why he or she is being placed in restraints
B. Patients should be restrained with legs spread-eagled
C. Patient's head should be raised slightly
D. Leather restraints should be used as they are the safest and surest
E. Once in restraints, there is no need for antipsychotic medications

36.4 Which of the following is *not* an indication for the use of psychotropic medication in the psychiatric emergency room?

A. Assaultive behavior
B. Massive anxiety
C. Extrapyramidal reactions
D. Anticholinergic intoxication
E. None of the above

36.5 Which of the following statements regarding emergency room visits is *true*?

A. More psychiatric emergency visits occur during the night hours.
B. Married persons use psychiatric emergency rooms more often.
C. Approximately 50 percent of the persons using emergency rooms are violent.
D. There are more psychiatric emergency visits on weekends.
E. All of the above

36.6 Which of the following statements correctly defines *anomic suicide*?

A. Suicide among those persons not strongly integrated into any social group.
B. Suicide among those persons whose integration into society is disturbed.
C. Suicide among those whose integration into a group is excessive.
D. Suicide among those who reject society as a whole.
E. None of the above.

36.7 Which of the following neurobiological findings is associated with suicide?

A. increased 5-hydroxyindoleacetic acid (5-HIAA) levels in the cerebrospinal fluid (CSF)
B. changes in the dopaminergic system
C. serotonin deficiency
D. increased levels of platelet monoamine oxidase (MAO)
E. normal findings on electroencephalogram (EEG)

36.8 Among men, suicide peaks after age 45; among women, it peaks after age

A. 35
B. 40
C. 45
D. 50
E. 55

36.9 Figure 36.1 shows the U.S. distribution, according to race and sex, of which of the following?

A. The prevalence of schizophrenia
B. Rates of alcohol-related disorders
C. Rates of suicide attempts (successful and unsuccessful)
D. Death rates for suicide
E. Prevalence of bipolar disorder

36.10 Your patient is a 25-year-old female graduate student in physical chemistry who was brought to the emergency room by her roommates, who found her sitting in her car with the motor running and the garage door closed. The

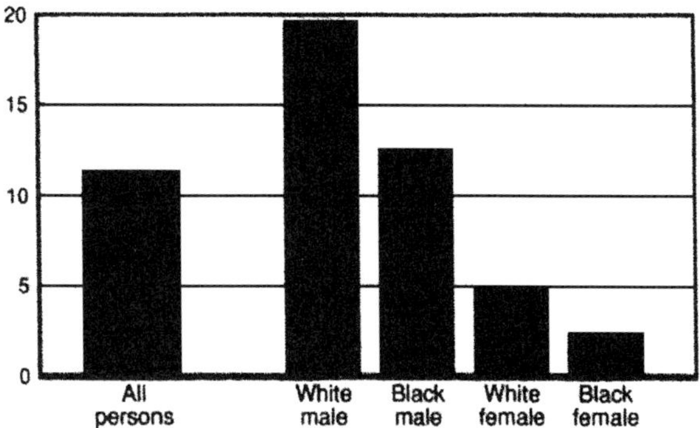

FIGURE 36.1

Reprinted with permission from National Center for Health Statistics. *Health, United States, 1991.* Hyattsville, MD: Public Health Service; 1992.

patient had entered psychotherapy 2 years before, complaining of long-standing unhappiness, feelings of inadequacy, low self-esteem, chronic tiredness, and a generally pessimistic outlook on life. While she was in treatment, as before, periods of well-being were limited to a few weeks at a time. During the 2 months before her emergency room visit, she had become increasingly depressed, had had difficulty in falling asleep and trouble in concentrating, and had lost 10 pounds. The onset of those symptoms coincided with a rebuff she had received from a chemistry instructor to whom she had become attracted.

The treatment of the patient could include

A. hospitalization
B. outpatient psychotherapy
C. antidepressants
D. electroconvulsive therapy
E. all of the above

36.11 Suicide rates

A. have remained relatively stable except for 15- to 24-year-olds, whose rates have decreased two- to threefold
B. have averaged five per 1,000,000 in the 20th century
C. make suicide the 8th leading cause of death in the United States
D. reflect about 10,000 suicides each year in the United States
E. none of the above

36.12 Suicide among schizophrenic patients

A. is low
B. is approximately 10 percent
C. occurs most often in the later years of the illness
D. occurs most often in older, women patients
E. is most frequently secondary to command hallucinations

36.13 Increased rates of suicide attempts occur in patients with

A. panic disorder
B. social phobia
C. personality disorders
D. substance abuse
E. all of the above

36.14 True statements about suicide in the elderly include

A. Compared to other age groups, those 65 and older have the highest risk of committing suicide.
B. The suicide rate for the elderly is more than ten times that of young persons.
C. The least frequent means of committing suicide in the elderly is with a firearm.
D. Alcoholism is less likely to be associated with suicide in the elderly than in younger people.
E. All of the above

36.15 True statements about patients with parasuicidal behavior include

A. About 50 percent are found to have a personality disorder at psychiatric assessment.
B. About 40 percent have made previous attempts.
C. About 1 percent of persons who attempt suicide will commit suicide during the following year.
D. Suicide risk is particularly high during the first year after a suicide attempt.
E. All of the above

36.16 The presence of medical illness should be strongly considered when

A. Psychiatric symptoms appear suddenly in a previously well-functioning person.
B. There is a reported personality change or marked lability of mood.
C. Psychotic symptoms appear for the first time after the age of 30.
D. Temperature, pulse, or respiratory rate is increased.
E. All of the above

36.17 Suicidal behavior

A. tends not to be familial
B. is not associated with a family history of suicide
C. has been found to have the same concordance rate in dizygotic as in monozygotic twins
D. occurs more frequently in the biological relatives of adoptees who commit suicide than in the adoptive relatives
E. none of the above

Directions

The group of questions below consists of lettered headings followed by a list of numbered phrases or statements. For each numbered phrase or statement, select the *one* lettered heading that is most closely associated with it. Each lettered heading may be selected once, more than once, or not at all.

Questions 36.18–36.23

A. Opioid OD

B. Barbiturates
C. Phencyclidine (PCP) OD
D. Monoamine oxidase inhibitors (MAOIs)
E. Acetaminophen (Tylenol) OD

36.18 Treated with propranolol (Inderal)
36.19 Toxic interaction with meperidine hydrochloride (Demerol)
36.20 Phenothiazines contraindicated
36.21 Fever, pancytopenia, hypoglycemic coma, renal failure
36.22 Pale, cyanotic, respiratory depression, pinpoint pupils
36.23 Seizure with withdrawal

Questions 36.24–36.27

A. Delirium, mania, depression, psychosis
B. Marked aggressive and assaultive behavior
C. Alcohol stigmata, amnesia, confabulation
D. Mental confusion, oculomotor disturbances, cerebellar ataxia
E. None of the above

36.24 Bromide intoxication
36.25 Korsakoff's syndrome
36.26 Idiosyncratic alcohol intoxication
36.27 Wernicke's encephalopathy

ANSWERS

36.1 The answer is D

The first task in evaluating violent behavior is to ascertain its cause. Cause directs treatment. Patients with thought disorders characterized by hallucinations commanding them to kill someone require psychiatric hospitalization and anti-psychotic medication. If they are unwilling to accept treatment, certification is necessary to protect the intended victim and the patient. Those who take an extreme civil libertarian perspective fail to recognize that medical certification has evolved legally not only to protect society from violent patients, but also to protect patients from the consequences of their uncontrollable behavior.

Violence and aggressive behavior are difficult to predict, but the fear with which some persons regard all psychiatric patients is completely out of proportion to the few who are an authentic danger to others. The best predictors of potential violent behavior are excessive alcohol intake, a history of violent acts with arrests or criminal activity, and a history of childhood abuse. Although violent patients can arouse a realistic fear in psychiatrists, they can also touch off irrational fears that impair clinical judgment and may lead to premature and excessive use of sedation or physical restraint. Violent patients are usually frightened by their own hostile impulses and desperately seek help to prevent loss of control. Nevertheless, restraints should be applied if there is a reasonable risk of violence.

36.2 The answer is A

Sigmund Freud offered the first important psychological insight into suicide. In his paper "Mourning and Melancholia," Freud stated his belief that suicide represents *aggression turned inward against an introjected, ambivalently cathected love object.* Freud doubted there would be a suicide without an earlier repressed desire to kill someone else.

Building on Freud's concepts, *Karl Menninger* in *Man Against Himself* conceived of suicide as a retroflexed murder, inverted homicide as a result of the patient's anger toward another person, which is either turned inward or used as an excuse for punishment. He also described a self-directed death instinct (Freud's concept of Thanatos). He described *three components of hostility in suicide: the wish to kill, the wish to be killed, and the wish to die.*

36.3 The answer is E

Restraints are used when patients are so dangerous to themselves or others that they pose a severe threat that cannot be controlled in any other way. Patients may be restrained temporarily to receive medication or for long periods if medication cannot be used. Usually, patients in restraints quiet down after a time. On a psychodynamic level, such patients may even welcome control of their impulses provided by restraints. Patients should always *receive an explanation* as to why they are going into restraints; patients should be restrained with *legs spread-eagled* and one arm restrained to one side and the other arm restrained over the patient's head; patient's *head should be raised slightly* to decrease the patient's feelings of vulnerability and to reduce the possibility of aspiration; *leather restraints are the safest and surest* type of restraint; and even in restraints, most patients *still take antipsychotic medication* in a concentrated form.

36.4 The answer is D

The major indications for the use of psychotropic medication in an emergency room include *violent or assaultive behavior, massive anxiety or panic, and extrapyramidal reactions*, such as dystonia and akathisia as adverse effects of psychiatric drugs. Laryngospasm is a rare form of dystonia, and psychiatrists should be prepared to maintain an open airway with intubation if necessary. Conservative measures may suffice for intoxication from drugs of abuse. Benzodiazepines may be used instead of, or in addition to, antipsychotics, however, when a recreational drug has strong anticholinergic properties, *benzodiazepines are more appropriate than antipsychotics.*

36.5 The answer is A

Psychiatric emergency rooms are used equally by men and women and *more by single than by married persons.* About 20 percent of these patients are suicidal and *about 10 percent are violent.* The most common diagnoses are mood disorders (including depressive disorders and manic episodes), schizophrenia, and alcohol dependence. About 40 percent of all patients seen in psychiatric emergency rooms require hospitalization. *Most visits occur during the night hours, but there is no usage difference based on the day of the week or the month of the year.* Contrary to popular belief, studies have not found that use of psychiatric emergency rooms increases during a full moon or the Christmas season.

36.6 The answer is B

The first major contribution to the study of the social and cultural influences on suicide was made at the end of the 19th century by the French sociologist *Emile Durkheim.* In an attempt to explain statistical patterns, Durkheim *divided suicides into three social categories: egoistic, altruistic, and anomic. Egoistic suicide applies to those who are not strongly integrated into any social group*. The lack of family integration can be used to explain why the unmarried are more vulnerable to suicide than are the married and why couples with children are the best-protected group of all. Rural communities have more social integration than do urban areas and thus less suicide. Protestantism is a less cohesive religion than Catholicism is, and so Protestants have a higher suicide rate than do Catholics. *Altruistic suicide applies to those whose proneness to suicide stems from their excessive integration into a group, with suicide being the outgrowth of that integration* (for example, the Japanese soldier who sacrifices his life in battle). *Anomic suicide applies to persons whose integration into society is disturbed, depriving them of the customary norms of behavior.* Anomie can explain why those whose economic situation has changed drastically are more vulnerable than they were before their change in fortune. Anomie also refers to social instability, with a breakdown of society's standards and values.

36.7 The answer is C

A serotonin deficiency, as measured by *decreased (not increased) 5-hydroyindoleacetic acid (5-HIAA) levels in the cerebrospinal fluid* (CSF), has been found in some patients who attempted suicide. In addition, some postmortem studies have reported *changes in the noradrenergic system (not dopaminergic system). Decreased (not increased) levels of platelet monoamine oxidase (MAO)* have been discovered in some suicidal patients. When blood samples from normal volunteers were analyzed, it was found that those with the lowest level of MAO in their platelets had eight times the prevalence of suicide in their families. *Abnormal findings on EEGs (not normal findings)* and ventricular enlargement have been found in a few studies of suicidal patients.

36.8 The answer is E

Among women, suicide peaks after age 55. Rates of 40 per 100,000 population are found in men age 65 and older; the elderly attempt suicide less often than do younger people but are successful more frequently. A decline in suicide in men begins between the ages of 75 and 85. A peak risk among males is also found in late adolescence, when death by suicide is exceeded only by death attributed to accidents and cancer.

36.9 The answer is D

Figure 36.1 represents *death rates for suicide* in the United States according to race and sex. The rate of suicide among whites is nearly twice that among nonwhites, but the figures are being questioned, as the suicide rate among blacks is increasing. In 1989, the suicide rate for white males was 1.6 times that of black males, four times that for white females, and 8.2 times that for black females. Two out of every three suicides are white males. Women are four times as likely to attempt suicide as are men, while overall, men commit suicide more than three times as often as do women.

Schizophrenia is equally prevalent in men and women. *Bipolar I disorder* also has a prevalence that is equal for men and women. The ratio of *alcohol-related disorder* diagnoses for men to women is about 2 to 1 or 3 to 1. Although the rate of alcohol-related disorders has traditionally been highest among young white men, evidence now indicates that young black men and young Hispanic men may have surpassed young white men in their rates of alcohol-related disorders.

36.10 The answer is E (all)

The treatment of the depressed, suicidal 25-year-old female graduate student described could include *hospitalization or outpatient treatment, antidepressants, or electroconvulsive therapy* (ECT). Whether to hospitalize the patient with suicidal ideation is a crucial clinical decision. Not all such patients require hospitalization; some may be treated as outpatients. Indications for hospitalization include the lack of a strong social support system, a history of impulsive behavior, and a suicidal plan of action. Most psychiatrists believe that the young woman described should be hospitalized because she had made a suicide attempt and so was clearly at increased risk. Other psychiatrists believe that they could treat the patient on an outpatient basis provided certain conditions were met, such as (1) reducing the patient's psychological pain by modifying her stressful environment through the aid of a friend, a relative, or her employer; (2) building realistic support by recognizing that the patient may have legitimate complaints and offering alternatives to suicide; (3) securing commitment on the part of the patient to agree to call when she reached a point beyond which she was uncertain of controlling further suicidal impulses; and (4) assuring commitment on the part of the psychiatrist to be available to the patient 24 hours a day until the risk has passed. Because it is difficult to meet many of those conditions, hospitalization is often the safest route.

Many depressed suicidal patients require treatment with antidepressants or ECT. The young woman described had a recent sustained and severely depressed mood that was associated with insomnia, trouble in concentrating, weight loss, and a suicide attempt. Those factors indicate a major depressive episode. There was also evidence of long-standing mild depressive symptoms (pessimism, feelings of inadequacy, and low energy level) that although insufficient to meet the diagnostic criteria for a major depressive episode, do meet the criteria for dysthymic disorder. With those clinical features, the indication for the use of antidepressants is clear; ECT may be necessary if the patient was unresponsive to antidepressants or so severely depressed and suicidal that she required faster-acting treatment than is possible with antidepressants. ECT is a safe and effective procedure that is often misunderstood and even attacked by antipsychiatry forces in society.

36.11 The answer is C

Suicide is a major public health problem: approximately 0.9 percent of all deaths are the result of suicide. About 1,000 persons are estimated to commit suicide each day worldwide. *In the United States suicide ranks as the eighth leading cause of death*, and there are approximately 75 suicides per day, or one every 20 minutes, and *more than 30,000 (not 10,000) each year.* The suicide rate in the United States has *averaged 12.5 per 100,000 (not 5 per 1,000,000) in the 20th century*, with a high of 17.4 per 100,000 during the Great Depression. From 1983 to 1998 the overall suicide rate remained relatively stable whereas the rate *for 15- to 24-year-olds increased (not decreased) two to threefold.* The number one suicide site in the world is the Golden Gate Bridge in San Francisco.

36.12 The answer is B

The suicide risk is high (not low) among schizophrenia patients, and *up to 10 percent die by committing suicide.* Most persons with schizophrenia who commit suicide do so *during the first few years of their illness.* Thus, schizophrenic *suicides tend to be relatively young (not old), and about 75 percent are unmarried males (not older women)*; approximately 50 percent have made a previous suicide attempt. Depressive symptoms are closely associated with their suicide; studies have reported that depressive symptoms were present during the last period of contact in up to two-thirds of schizophrenia patients who committed suicide; *only a small (not a high) percent commit suicide because of hallucinated instructions* or in order to escape persecutory delusions. Up to a third of schizophrenic suicides occur during the first few weeks and months following discharge from hospital; another third commit suicide while they are inpatients.

36.13 The answer is E (all)

Alcoholic persons have an increased risk of suicide, with a lifetime suicide risk of 2.2 to 3.4 percent. More men than women are found among alcoholic suicide victims. Alcoholic persons usually commit suicide after years of alcohol abuse. Comorbidity plays an important role; persons with alcoholism who have comorbid depressive disorders are at particularly high risk. Among 31 alcoholic suicides, 48 percent had lost a loved one during the year before they committed suicide, and 32 percent had experienced such a loss during their last 6 weeks. The St. Louis group examined the lives of 50 other alcoholic suicide victims. Based on the hypothesis that suicide among alcoholics may represent a reaction to life events, the researchers recorded their opinions about the most important reason for suicide in each case (Table 36.1). Loss of a close relationship was the most frequently cited precipitating event; other events included job trouble, financial difficulties, and being in trouble with the law. For only 1 of the 50 suicide victims could no precipitating event be identified.

There is an *increased risk of suicide among substance abusers*. For example, the suicide rate of heroin addicts is about 20 times greater than that of the general population. The availability of lethal amount of drugs, intravenous use, associated antisocial personality disorder, chaotic lifestyle, and impulsivity are some of the factors that predispose drug-dependent persons to suicidal behavior, particularly when they are dysphoric, depressed, or intoxicated.

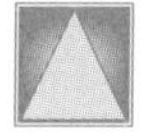

Table 36.1
Presumed Most Important Reason for Suicide Among 50 Alcoholic Suicide Victims

Presumed Reason	Number
Marital separation/divorce	8
Friction with spouse/lover	9
Expectation of loss (realistic)	5
Estrangement from family	2
Bereavement	2
Friction with family	1
Job trouble	4
Financial trouble	3
Trouble with the law	2
Depressed (as principal or only reason)	6
Feeling of disgrace	2
Feared rehospitalization	2
Inability to control drinking	1
Other	2
No provocation identified	1
Total	50

Reprinted with permission from Murphy G. Suicide in alcoholism. In: Roy A., ed. *Suicide*, Baltimore: Willilams & Wilkins; 1986.

It is recognized that patients with borderline personality disorders have an increased risk of suicide. Recently one group reported a psychological autopsy study of suicide victims with personality disorders and found that they were almost always (95 percent) associated with current Axis I depressive disorders, substance use disorders, or both.

The group also reported that *67 of a random sample of 229 suicide victims had an Axis II personality disorder.* About one-fifth (N = 43, 29 percent) of all the 229 suicides had a Cluster B diagnosis (dramatic, emotional, or erratic), compared to the estimated prevalence of 4 to 5 percent in the general population. Ten percent of the sample (N = 23) had a Cluster C diagnosis (anxious or fearful), and only one person had a Cluster A diagnosis (odd or eccentric).

They next compared the personality-disorder suicide victims with sex- and age-matched suicide victims without personality disorder. Suicides with Cluster B personality disorders were more likely than comparison subjects to have substance-use disorders (79 percent versus 40 percent) and previous nonfatal suicide attempts (70 percent versus 37 percent) and were less likely to have Axis III physical disorders (29 percent versus 50 percent). Suicide victims in Cluster B almost always had (98 percent) either comorbid depressive disorders (74 percent), substance-use disorders (79 percent), or both (55 percent). They found no evidence of impulsive suicides that would have occurred without Axis I disorders. In contrast, subjects with Cluster C personality disorders did not differ from their controls on any variable.

Data from the National Institute of Mental Health (NIMH) Epidemiologic Catchment Area (ECA) Study showed that *20 percent of individuals with panic disorder had made a suicide attempt at some time.* This high rate was similar to the rate for individuals with major depression. When patients with panic disorder without comorbidity were examined, the lifetime rate of suicide attempts remained raised at 7 percent. Similarly, individuals *with social phobia have increased rates of suicidal ideation and suicide attempts.* One group found that current panic disorder was rare among completed suicides, being found in only 1.2 percent of all suicides. However, panic disorder suicide victims had superimposed major depression and substance abuse, and associated personality disorders. Thus, clinical assessment of suicide risk in panic and phobia patients should include determination of the presence or absence of major depressive disorder, substance abuse, and personality disorder.

36.14 The answer is A

Compared to other age groups, *those 65 years and older have the highest risk* of committing suicide. For example, the suicide rate for the *elderly is* more than three (not ten) times that of young persons. In the United States, 18 elderly persons commit suicide each day, one every 80 minutes. The majority of elderly suicides are *committed using a firearm.* Some older individuals have a higher suicide risk than others: most at risk are males, whites, the recently widowed, and those aged 75 years or more.

The two psychiatric conditions most associated with suicide in the elderly are depression and alcoholism. Psychological autopsy studies show that approximately 70 percent of elderly suicide victims suffered from depression in the weeks and months before their suicide. Approximately 20 percent of elderly suicides meet the criteria for a substance abuse disorder, usually alcohol abuse or dependence.

Studies show that loss and stress are major etiologic factors in the depression and alcohol abuse found among elderly suicide victims. These include physical losses resulting from poor health, painful illness, sensory deficits, and cognitive decline; social losses like death of a spouse and loss of the work role; and income losses associated with retirement and medical expenses. Such losses may lead to reduced social networks and social isolation, and can produce feelings of despair, loneliness, demoralization, dependency on others, helplessness, and hopelessness, as well as suicidal ideation.

36.15 The answer is E (all)

Persons who attempt suicide also pose a major health problem. *Attempted suicide* is in many ways an unsatisfactory term. For example, most attempters do not actually wish to commit suicide; their motives are different. Thus, the Edinburgh group introduced the term *parasuicide* in an effort to signify that suicide attempts are not just failed suicides but are a very different behavior.

Hospital studies show that about 40 percent of those who attempt suicide have a history of psychiatric treatment. Psychiatric assessments reveal that about *50 percent have a personality disorder*, and up to 40 percent have other psychiatric disorders. The most common diagnoses that are not personality disorders are depressive disorders (up to 40 percent of women and 30 percent of men).

Studies using observer-rated instruments find that although symptoms like tension, depressed mood, hopelessness, irritability, worrying, and poor concentration are present in 40 to 75 percent of attempters, a definite psychiatric disorder can be diagnosed at admission in only about 30 percent of attempters; this percentage decreases rapidly over subsequent weeks. However, workers in Christchurch, New Zealand, have shown that among serious suicide attempters 90 percent had a psychiatric disorder with high rates of mood disorder, substance abuse, and antisocial personality disorder. The incidence of comorbidity was high: 56 percent had two or more disorders. The risk of a serious suicide attempt increased with increasing psychiatric comorbidity.

About 40 percent of suicide attempters have made a previous attempt. Follow-up studies show that between 13 and 35 percent will repeat the attempt during the next 2 years. During this time up to 7 percent will make two or more attempts, 2.5 percent three or more attempts, and 1 percent five or more attempts. Thus, there appear to be three subgroups of repeaters: the very occasional repeater, the person who repeats several times within a short period, and the chronic or habitual repeater.

There are seven main items that may be helpful in identifying the patient at risk of making another suicide attempt: problems with alcohol, antisocial or borderline personality disorder, impulsivity, previous inpatient psychiatric treatment, previous outpatient psychiatric treatment, previous attempt that led to admission, and living alone.

It is recognized that those who attempt and those who commit suicide represent different populations with some overlap. *Approximately 1 percent of persons who attempt suicide will commit suicide during the following year.* For 8 to 50 suicide attempters, one will eventually commit suicide. The risk of subsequent suicide varies with sex and age. For example, at the Karolinska Hospital in Stockholm the suicide risk over the next 5 years after attempting suicide among men (8.3 percent) was nearly twice the suicide risk among women. Both older and younger male suicide attempters are at high risk of suicide (7 percent and 10 percent, respectively), and older women are at higher risk than younger women (6 percent versus 2 percent). The *suicide risk* was *particularly high during the first year after the suicide attempt.*

Follow-up studies show that other factors associated with subsequent suicide include being unemployed or retired; being separated, divorced, or widowed; living alone; having poor physical health; having received medical treatment within the last 6 months; having a psychiatric disorder, including alcoholism; having made many previous attempts by violent methods; the presence of a suicide note; and a history of previous attempts. A subgroup of suicide attempters who have severe personality disorder and interpersonal conflicts, and who often had alcohol or other substance dependence, commit suicide while acutely depressed.

36.16 The answer is E (all)

The presence of medical illness should be strongly considered when *psychiatric symptoms appear suddenly in a previously well-functioning person. A patient over the age of 30 with psychotic symptoms appearing for the first time*, an awareness or conviction that these symptoms are foreign, and especially with concomitant symptoms of cognitive dysfunction should be considered to have a possible organic illness. Clinicians should consider medical and substance-related causes when a patient has a history of a recently diagnosed medical illness, a new prescription, or a change in dosage. *A personality change or marked lability of mood* noticed by friends or relatives also suggests the onset of a serious medical condition.

Vital signs should be obtained on admission to the emergency department, even when the patient appears physically healthy or is intimidating because of disturbed behavior. Psychiatric disorders do not affect vital signs to a significant degree; therefore, abnormal vital signs must be further evaluated by a history, physical examination, and appropriate laboratory tests. *Elevation of temperature, pulse, or respiratory rate* suggests an underlying medical condition. Certain physical findings strongly suggest an organic disorder, including lateralizing neurological symptoms, confusion, and incontinence.

36.17 The answer is D

Suicidal behavior, like other psychiatric disorders, tends to run in families. For example, Margaux Hemingway's 1997 suicide was the fifth suicide among four generations of Ernest Hemingway's family. *In psychiatric patients a family history of suicide increases the risk both of attempted suicide and of completed suicide in most diagnostic groups.* In medicine the strongest evidence for the possibility of genetic factors comes from twin and adoption studies and from molecular genetics.

In 1991, 176 twin pairs in which one twin had committed suicide were investigated. In nine of these twin pairs, both twins had committed suicide. Seven of these nine pairs concordant for suicide were found among the 62 monozygotic pairs, while two pairs concordant for suicide were found among the 114 dizygotic twin pairs. *This twin-group difference for concordance for suicide (11.3 percent versus 1.8 percent) is statistically significant ($P < 0.01$).*

In another study a group of 35 twin pairs of which one twin had committed suicide was collected and the living co-twin was interviewed. It was found that 10 of the 26 living monozygotic co-twins had themselves attempted suicide, compared with zero of the nine living dizygotic co-twins ($P < 0.04$). Although monozygotic and dizygotic twins may have some differing developmental experiences, these results show that monozygotic twin pairs have significantly greater concordance for both suicide and attempted suicide, which suggests that genetic factors may play a role in suicidal behavior.

The strongest evidence suggesting the presence of genetic factors in suicide comes from the adoption studies carried out in Denmark. A screening of the registers of causes of death revealed that 57 of 5,483 adoptees in Copenhagen eventually committed suicide. They were matched with adopted controls. Searches of the causes of death revealed that 12 of the 269 biological relatives of these 57 adopted suicide victims had themselves committed suicide, compared with only 2 of the 269 biological relatives of the 57 adopted controls. This is a highly significant difference for suicide between the two groups of relatives. *None of the adopting relatives of either the suicide or control group had committed suicide.*

In a further study of 71 adoptees with mood disorder, adoptee suicide victims with a situational crisis, impulsive suicide attempt, or both particularly had more biological relatives who had committed suicide than controls. This led to the suggestion that a genetic factor lowering the threshold for suicidal behavior may lead to an inability to control impulsive behavior. Psychiatric disorder or environmental stress may serve as potentiating mechanisms which foster or trigger the impulsive behavior, directing it toward a suicidal outcome.

Answers 36.18–36.23

36.18 The answer is C

36.19 The answer is D

36.20 The answer is C

36.21 The answer is E

36.22 The answer is A

36.23 The answer is B

Substance abuse is one of the many reasons for visits to the psychiatric emergency room. Patients who take overdoses of *opioids* (for example, heroin) tend *to be pale and cyanotic* (a dark bluish or purplish coloration of the skin and mucous membranes), with *pinpoint pupils* and absent reflexes. After blood is drawn for a study of drug levels, those patients should be given intravenous naloxone hydrochloride (Narcan), a narcotic antagonist that reverses the opiate effects, *including respiratory depression*, within 2 minutes of the injection.

The use of *barbiturates* and anxiolytics is widespread, and withdrawal from sedative-hypnotic drugs is a common reason for psychiatric emergencies. The first symptom of withdrawal can start as soon as 8 hours after the last pill has been taken and may consist of anxiety, confusion, and ataxia. *As withdrawal progresses the patient may have seizures;* occasionally, a psychotic state erupts, with hallucinations, panic, and disorientation. Barbiturates are cross-tolerant with all antianxiety agents, such as diazepam (Valium). In the treatment of sedative, hypnotic, or anxiolytic withdrawal, one must take into account the usual daily substance intake.

Phencyclidine (PCP or angel dust) is a common cause of psychotic drug-related hospital admissions. The presence of dissociative phenomena, nystagmus (ocular ataxia), muscular rigidity, and elevated blood pressure in a patient who is agitated, psychotic, or comatose strongly suggests PCP intoxication. In the treatment of PCP overdose, the patient should have gastric lavage to recover the drug, diazepam to reduce anxiety, an acidifying diuretic program consisting of ammonium chloride and furosemide (Lasix), which will enhance PCP excretion, and the treatment of hypertension with *propranolol (Inderal).* Acidification is not recommended with hepatic or renal failure or when barbiturate use is suspected. *Phenothiazines are contraindicated,* because muscle rigidity and seizures, side effects of PCP, can be exacerbated by phenothiazines, as can the anticholinergic effects of PCP.

Monoamine oxidase inhibitors (MAOIs) are useful in treating depression, but a hypertensive crisis can occur if patients have eaten food with a high tyramine content while on their medication. Hypertensive crisis is characterized by severe occipital headaches, nausea, vomiting, sweating, photophobia, and dilated pupils. When a hypertensive crisis occurs, the MAOI should be discontinued, and therapy should be instituted to reduce blood pressure. Chlorpromazine (Thorazine) and phentolamine (Regitine) have both been found useful in those hypertensive crises. MAOIs have *a toxic interaction with meperidine hydrochloride (Demerol)*, which can be fatal. When patients combine the two drugs, they become agitated, disoriented, cyanotic, hyperthermic, hypertensive, and tachycardic.

Acetaminophen (Tylenol) is an analgesic and antipyretic. Overdose with acetaminophen is characterized *by fever, pancytopenia, hypoglycemic coma, renal failure,* and liver damage. Treatment should begin with the induction of emesis or gastric lavage, followed by the administration of activated charcoal. Early treatment is critical to protect against hepatotoxicity.

Answers 36.24–36.27

36.24 The answer is A

36.25 The answer is C

36.26 The answer is B

36.27 The answer is D

Delirium, mania, depression, and psychosis are manifestations of bromide intoxication. If a patient's serum levels are above 50 mg a day, bromide intake should be discontinued; if the patient is agitated, lorazepam (Ativan) may be given for sedation. For severe agitation or psychotic syndromes an antipsychotic dopamine receptor antagonist may be necessary.

Alcohol stigmata, amnesia, and *confabulation* are manifestations of Korsakoff's syndrome. Because this disorder has no effective treatment, the patient must often be institutionalized in a protective environment.

Marked aggression and assaultive behavior are manifestations of idiosyncratic alcohol intoxication. Generally no treatment other than a protective environment is required.

Mental confusion, oculomotor disturbances, and *cerebellar ataxia* are manifestations of Wernicke's encephalopathy.

37 Psychotherapies

The variety of psychotherapies in psychiatry reflects the multi-etiologic theoretical basis of the field in general. Skilled clinicians are aware of all available therapies, but may choose to focus their treatments on just one, or utilize different aspects of the different therapies, depending on the problem or the patient. Most of the important and useful theories recognize that human behavior and emotion cannot be reduced to a simple biological versus psychological equation, and that a true understanding of human functioning begins with adhering to a bio-psycho-social etiologic model.

Students should be aware of the theories that underlie the different therapies, as well as the indications and contraindications proposed for each. The student should be familiar with the most prominent therapies, which include psychoanalytic, supportive, cognitive, behavioral, family, group, brief therapies, and some of the manualized treatments like dialectical behavior therapy for borderline patients.

The psychoanalytic therapies are based on freudian principles of a dynamic unconscious and psychic determinism, and they are all oriented toward the patient's acquisition of insight. Psychoanalysis is a treatment unto itself that differs from psychoanalytic psychotherapy and brief dynamic therapies. Students should understand the differences between these treatments, and their differing goals, techniques, and interventions. Supportive psychotherapy has its roots in analytic theory, but focuses on strengthening healthy defenses to maximize function.

Cognitive therapies or cognitive-behavioral therapies are usually short-term structured treatments that aim to correct illogical or irrational thinking, which can lead to dysfunctional attitudes and behaviors. Behavioral therapies focus on overt, observable behaviors and are unconcerned with underlying causes. These therapies are based on learning theory, which posits that learned behavior is reinforced and conditioned in a variety of ways.

Family therapies are based on general systems theory and focus on patterns of family communication and interaction. Group therapies run the theoretical gamut and may be supportive, psychoanalytic, cognitive, or behavioral in their orientation. Dialectical behavior therapy (DBT) a manualized treatment, cognitive-behavioral in theoretical background, is designed to treat the destructive behaviors associated with borderline personality disorder. There are many other therapies, like biofeedback, eye-movement desensitization and reprogramming (EMDR) and interpersonal psychotherapy for depression with which the student should be familiar.

The student should study the questions and answers below to test his or her knowledge of the subject.

HELPFUL HINTS

The names of the workers, their theories, and the therapy techniques should be known to the student.

- AA, GA, OA
- abreaction
- analyst incognito
- Anna O.
- assertiveness
- authority anxiety
- autogenic therapy
- aversive therapy
- Michael Balint
- Aaron Beck
- behavioral medicine
- bell and pad
- Hippolyte Bernheim
- Murray Bowen
- cognitive rehearsal
- cognitive triad of depression
- cohesion
- combined individual and group psychotherapy
- confidentiality
- countertransference
- crisis intervention
- crisis theory
- day's residue
- disorders of self-control
- disulfiram (Antabuse) therapy
- double and multiple double
- dyad
- early therapy
- ego psychology
- eye-roll sign
- H.J. Eysenck
- family group therapy
- family sculpting
- family systems
- family therapy
- flexible schemata
- flooding
- galvanic skin response
- genogram
- Gestalt group therapy
- graded exposure
- group psychotherapy
- guided imagery
- hierarchy construction
- homogeneous versus heterogeneous groups
- hypnosis
- hypnotic capacity and induction
- hysteria
- identified patient
- implosion

- insight-oriented psychotherapy
- intellectualization, interpretation
- interpersonal psychotherapy
- Jacobson's exercise
- Daniel Malan
- mental imagery
- mirror technique
- Jacob Moreno
- operant conditioning
- parapraxes
- participant modeling
- patient–therapist encounter
- peer anxiety
- positive reinforcement
- psychodrama
- psychodynamic model
- psychotherapeutic focus
- psychotherapy
- reality testing
- reciprocal inhibition
- relaxation response
- resistance
- reward of desired behavior
- Carl Rogers
- role reversal
- rule of abstinence
- schemata
- Paul Schilder
- self-analysis
- self-help groups
- self-observation
- Peter Sifneos
- B.F. Skinner
- splitting
- structural model
- structural theory
- *Studies on Hysteria*
- supportive therapy
- systematic desensitization
- tabula rasa
- testing automatic thoughts
- token economy
- transactional group therapy
- transference, transference neurosis, negative triangulation
- universalization
- ventilation and catharsis

QUESTIONS

Directions

Each of the questions or incomplete statements below is followed by five responses or completions. Select the *one* that is *best* in each case.

37.1 Which of the following is an important patient requisite of suitability for psychoanalysis?

A. high anxiety
B. strong dependency issues
C. the ability to form a relationship
D. poor impulse control
E. alexithymia

37.2 Supportive psychotherapy

A. places major etiological emphasis on intrapsychic events
B. is indicated primarily for patients whose potential for decompensation is low
C. involves genetic interpretations
D. involves the judicious suspension of therapeutic neutrality
E. facilitates a regressive transference

37.3 In the last session of a long-term therapy, the patient talked at great length about car problems he had encountered on the way to the session. The therapist commented, "I think you'd rather talk about your car than face the sadness you're feeling about our last session."

The therapist's intervention is an example of

A. a clarification
B. an empathic validation
C. an affirmation
D. a confrontation
E. an interpretation

37.4 Brief focal psychotherapy

A. is very helpful for self-destructive acting out patients
B. does not focus on transference
C. involves a detached therapist
D. involves setting a termination date in advance
E. usually lasts less than ten to twelve sessions

37.5 Ms. A, a 29-year-old never-married vice president in a successful business, presented with a 9-month history of depression. She described her involvement in a relationship with her superior at work, which they both desired but which work policy forbade. Her symptoms emerged under the pressure she felt to resolve this situation, from which she saw no way out. Neither she nor her boyfriend wanted to leave their jobs, and neither wanted their relationship to end, yet exposure of their secret threatened both their jobs.

The therapist thought the patient would benefit from Interpersonal Psychotherapy to treat her depression. IPT

A. would focus on Ms. A's past relationships as a guide for managing this one
B. is an open-ended treatment
C. would focus on Ms. A's unresolved grief
D. places the patient in the sick role
E. involves a passive therapist

37.6 Dialectical behavior therapy (DBT)

A. is a cognitive behavioral treatment
B. has not been empirically evaluated for efficacy
C. does not directly target suicidal behavior
D. focuses on patient insight
E. favors in-patient treatment when self-destructive risk is high

37.7 A spiritual assessment

A. involves learning about the patient's beliefs
B. addresses issues of meaninglessness
C. empowers the patient to find inner resources of strength
D. is completed during the social history section of the history and physical
E. all of the above

37.8 Flooding

A. is synonymous with "explosion"
B. involves relaxation exercises
C. is a hierarchical exposure technique
D. works best with specific phobias
E. is indicated in anxious patients who are psychologically fragile because of its rapid response rate

37.9 The goals of social skills training include all of the following *except*

A. decreasing social anxiety
B. generalization of the acquired skills to similar situations
C. acquisition of conversational skills
D. acquisition of insight into the social deficit
E. relearning of social skills

37.10 Which of the following methods is *not* used in biofeedback?

A. Electromyography
B. Electroencephalography
C. Galvanic skin response
D. Strain gauge
E. All of the above

37.11 Systematic desensitization is applicable in the treatment of

A. obsessive-compulsive disorder
B. sexual disorders
C. stuttering
D. bronchial asthma
E. all of the above

37.12 All of the following are considered to be possible flexible boundary issues in psychotherapy *except*

A. self-disclosure by the therapist
B. physical contact between therapist and patient
C. sexual contact between therapist and patient
D. gift-giving and receiving
E. extra-analytic contacts

Directions

Each set of lettered headings below is followed by a list of numbered words or statements. For each numbered word or statement, select the *one* lettered heading most closely associated with it. Each lettered heading may be selected once, more than once, or not at all.

Questions 37.13–37.17

A. free association
B. fundamental rule
C. free floating attention
D. resistance
E. working alliance

37.13 Patient's agreement to tell the therapist everything, without selection
37.14 Saying whatever comes to mind
37.15 Analyst's way of listening to the patient
37.16 The relationship between two adults entering into a joint venture
37.17 Unconscious ideas are prevented from reaching awareness

Questions 37.18–37.22

A. contagion
B. altruism
C. ventilation
D. cohesion
E. universalization

37.18 The sense that the group is working together toward a common goal
37.19 The process in which the expression of emotion by one member stimulates the awareness of similar emotions in another member
37.20 The act of one member helping another
37.21 The awareness of the patient that he or she is not alone in having problems
37.22 The expression of suppressed feelings to other group members

Questions 37.23–37.26

A. the Bowen model
B. the structural model
C. the psychodynamic-experiential model
D. the general systems model

37.23 Focuses on a person's differentiation from their family of origin
37.24 Emphasizes individual freedom from unconscious patterns of anxiety and projection rooted in the past in the context of the family system
37.25 Every action in a family produces a reaction in one or more of its members
37.26 Families are viewed as single interrelated systems

ANSWERS

37.1 The answer is C

The capacity to form and maintain, as well as to detach from, a trusting relationship is essential for a patient embarking on an analysis. This treatment cannot begin, be sustained, or terminate properly without such a basis. Patients who cannot establish a viable connection to another human make poor candidates for psychoanalysis. *High anxiety states, strong issues around dependency, and poor impulse control* severely limit the benefits of psychoanalysis. *Alexithymia*, the inability to verbalize feelings, a poverty of fantasy life, and denial of psychic conflict makes a patient a poor candidate for psychoanalysis.

37.2 The answer is D

Supportive psychotherapy aims at the creation of a therapeutic relationship as a temporary buttress or bridge for the deficient patient. Techniques are designed to focus on conscious external events and on the therapist as a largely nontransferential figure. As such, *therapeutic neutrality is judiciously suspended* with much greater direction, disclosure, and gratification offered than would be appropriate in other approaches. The global perspective of supportive psychotherapy *places major etiological emphasis on external rather than intrapsychic events*, particularly on stressful environmental and interpersonal influences on a damaged self. It is indicated generally for those whose *potential for decompensation is high*. It focuses on the here-and-now of the patient's problems; *genetic interpretations relating to the patient's past may cause decompensation*, and are generally contraindicated in this treatment. The therapist works *to diminish the breakthrough of regressive transferences*.

37.3 The answer is D

Confrontation addresses something the patient does not want to accept or identifies the patient's avoidance or minimization. A confrontation may be geared to clarifying how the patient's behavior affects others or to reflecting back to the patient a denied or suppressed feeling. They are not necessarily forceful or hostile, despite the unfortunate connotation in common parlance of being aggressive or blunt. *A clarification* involves a reformulation or pulling together of the patient's verbalizations to convey a coherent view of what is being communicated. It does not address minimization or denial. *An empathic validation* demonstrates the therapist's empathic attunement with the patient's internal state. A typically validating comment is "I can understand why you feel sad about that." *An affirmation* involves succinct comments in support of the patient's comments or behaviors, like "uh-huh." *Interpretation* involves making something conscious that was previously unconscious. It is an explanatory statement that links a feeling, thought, behavior or symptom to its unconscious meaning or origin.

37.4 The answer is D

Brief focal psychotherapy was originally developed in the 1950s at the Tavistock Clinic in London. *In it, the therapist formulates a circumscribed focus and sets a termination date in advance. Contraindications to this treatment include grossly destructive acting out patients*, patients who are chronically dependent on alcohol or other substances of abuse, and *patients with a history of serious suicide attempts*. The therapist identifies the transference early, and interprets it. *Both the patient and the therapist become deeply involved, and therapist does not remain detached*. An experienced therapist *allows about twenty sessions as an average length for the therapy*.

37.5 The answer is D

Interpersonal therapy for depression is a time limited treatment for depressive disorder. *The patient is placed in the sick role.* The therapist is active, explicitly discussing the diagnosis of depression, its attendant symptoms, and is directed toward resolving the problem area. *It deals with current rather than past interpersonal relationships* and focuses on the patient's immediate social context. It assumes a connection between the onset of mood symptoms and the interpersonal context in which they occur. One of four problem areas guides the treatment: *unresolved grief*, social role transitions, interpersonal deficits, and like with Ms. A., role disputes. "What did Ms. A want from her relationship with her boyfriend and what options did she have to negotiate its happening?"

37.6 The answer is A

Dialectical behavior therapy is a cognitive behavioral treatment program that also draws on methods from supportive therapies, as well as some Eastern philosophical schools, like Zen Buddhism. *It does not focus on insight*. It has been developed to treat suicidal patients who meet criteria for borderline personality disorder, and has been evaluated initially in a 1991 randomized trial and follow-up, and subsequently in four published randomized controlled trials across three research centers and in one additional randomized controlled trial of a DBT-oriented treatment. *A recent study has demonstrated that it directly targets suicidal behavior.* An important strategy of DBT is to encourage outpatient use of behavioral skills over inpatient treatment, even when self destructive or suicidal risk is high.

37.7 The answer is E (All)

The spiritual history is taken during the social history section of the history and physical. The goals of the spiritual history are: to invite the patient to share spiritual and religious beliefs if they choose to do so; *to learn about the patient's beliefs and values*; to assess for spiritual distress, like *meaninglessness* as well as for *spiritual resources of strength*; to provide an opportunity for compassionate care whereby the healthcare professional connects to the patient in a deep and profound way; to *empower the patient to find inner resources of healing and acceptance*; to learn about the patient's spiritual and religious beliefs that might affect healthcare decision making.

37.8 The answer is D

Flooding works best with specific phobias, such as a social fear of eating in public. *It is sometimes called "implosion"* and is similar to graded exposure in that it involves exposing the patient to the feared object in vivo, *however there is no hierarchy*. It is based on the premise that escaping from an anxiety-provoking experience reinforces the anxiety through conditioning. Thus, clinicians can extinguish the anxiety and prevent the conditioned avoidance behavior by not allowing the patient to escape the situation. Patients are exposed to the feared situation with no buildup, and *no relaxation techniques are used*. Patients experience fear, which gradually subsides over time. Many patients refuse it because of the psychological discomfort involved, and it is *contraindicated when intense anxiety would be hazardous to a patient, like those who are psychologically fragile*.

37.9 The answer is D

Social skills are interpersonal behaviors required for community survival, for independence, and for establishing, maintaining, and deepening supportive, socially rewarding relationships. Severe mental disorders like schizophrenia disrupt one or more affective, cognitive, behavioral, and verbal domains of functioning and impair the patient's potential for enjoying and sustaining interpersonal relationships. Social skills training is a psychosocial rehabilitative treatment designed to remediate deficits in social behaviors. *It does not address understanding or insight* and focuses on the behaviors themselves. The major goals of social skills training include: *improved social skills in specific situations*; *generalization of the acquired skills* to similar situations; *acquisition or relearning of social and conversational skills*; and *decreased social anxiety*.

37.10 The answer is D

In *electromyography* (EMG), muscle fibers generate electrical potentials that can be measured on an electromyograph. Electrodes placed in or on a specific muscle group—for example, masseter, deltoid, or temporalis—can be monitored for relaxation training. In *electroencephalography* (EEG), the evoked potential of the EEG is monitored to determine relaxation. Alpha waves are generally indicative of meditative states, but wave frequency and amplitude are also measured. In *galvanic skin response* (GSR), skin conductance of electricity is measured as an indicator of autonomic nervous system activity. Stress increases electrical conduction and the GSR; conversely, relaxation is associated with lowered autonomic activity and changes in skin response. Similarly, skin temperature as a measure of peripheral vasoconstriction is decreased under stress and can be measured with thermistors (thermal feedback). A *strain gauge* is a device for measuring nocturnal penile tumescence that is used to determine whether erections occur during sleep. It has no biofeedback applications.

37.11 The answer is E (All)

Systematic desensitization is applicable in the treatment of *obsessive-compulsive disorder, sexual disorders, stuttering, bronchial asthma,* and other conditions. Joseph Wolpe first described systematic desensitization, a behavioral technique in which the patient is trained in muscle relaxation and then a hierarchy of anxiety-provoking thoughts or objects is paired with the relaxed state until the anxiety is systematically decreased and eliminated.

Obsessive-compulsive disorder (recurrent, intrusive mental events and behavior) is mediated by the anxiety elicited by specific objects or situations. Through systematic desensitization, the patient can be conditioned not to feel anxiety when around those objects or situations and thus to diminish the intensity of the obsessive-compulsive behavior. Desensitization has been used effectively with some stutterers by deconditioning the anxiety associated with a range of speaking situations. Some sexual disorders—such as male orgasmic disorder, female orgasmic disorder, and premature ejaculation—are amenable to desensitization therapy.

37.12 The answer is C

Analytic boundaries must build in flexibility. They provide an envelope that creates an optimal environment for the emergence of the analytic process. They must be flexible because different patients require adjustments in the boundaries. Similarly, different patient–analyst dyads find their own optimal conditions under which analysis can be conducted. The relative degree of gratification versus frustration varies given the subjectivities of the two parties. Some patients may benefit from direct *self-disclosure* of the analyst's feelings about a specific situation, while others may deeply resent it and close down as a result. Nevertheless, a variety of boundary considerations serve as guidelines to assist the analyst in maintaining a professional rather than a personal relationship.

Lavish or expensive *gifts from analyst to patient or from patient to analyst* may also violate a professional boundary. Such gifts may serve as an unconscious bribe designed to suppress anger in either party. Small and inexpensive gifts may be accepted by the analyst when the analyst feels that the acceptance might enhance the process. Even when such gifts are accepted, however, the meaning of the gift to the patient may be analyzed as an important part of the work.

As noted previously, self-disclosure is a significant boundary issue that analysts must attend to in their decisions about interventions. Analysis is by nature asymmetrical. Although two subjectivities are in the room and strong feelings are stirred in both parties, the process is designed to focus primarily on the person who is paying for the service. Self-disclosure by the analyst is inevitable, of course, and the analyst is always making decisions about how useful it would be to disclose certain aspects of the analyst's subjectivity to the patient. It may be extraordinarily useful in some cases to talk about areas of common interest with the patient in the service of building a therapeutic alliance. However, self-disclosure of one's personal problems may unduly burden the patient. Analysts who talk about their own problems misuse the patient's time and money. In some cases, the disclosure of here-and-now countertransference feelings may advance the process in a constructive way. However, telling patients, "I have sexual feelings for you" shuts down the process and makes patients feel that they must be the ones to set the boundaries in the relationship. Similarly, disclosing that one hates a patient or is bored by a patient is not useful.

Sexual contact of any form between analyst and patient is unacceptable. This constitutes a firm, inflexible boundary. In the transference, the analyst becomes a parent to the patient so that any form of sexual relations is symbolically incestuous. Moreover, because of the transference and the power differential, the patient cannot provide informed consent to such a relationship, even if the patient is an adult and consciously attracted to the analyst. This absolute abstinence regarding sexual contact facilitates frank and detailed discussion of the patient's sexual desires in a safe environment.

Physical contact such as hugs or pats on the back may also be problematic. In general, a handshake is probably the ordinary limit of physical contact between analyst and analysand. An occasional hug in the midst of a personal tragedy, such as the loss of a child, spouse, or parent, might be appropriate if initiated by the patient. However, when the analyst initiates a hug, the patient may readily misconstrue the analyst's motives. Another basic guideline regarding touch is that the impact of such behavior on the patient may be dramatically different from the analyst's intent. Patients may ask for hugs or even demand them, but psychoanalysis is about the wish to be held or hugged rather than the concrete enactment of such wishes. The patient must be engaged in a mourning process to deal with the grief and resentment about the deprivations of childhood, the frustrations in the present, and the insistence of the analyst that the relationship remain an analytic one. When actual physical contact occurs, especially on a regular basis, the distinction between the symbolic and the concrete is lost, and the patient may feel that powerful childhood longings will finally be satisfied by the analyst. This situation will likely evoke false hopes in the patient that can never be gratified. Table 37.1 lists some of the dimensions of analytic boundaries and boundary violations.

Answers 37.13–37.17

37.13 The answer is B

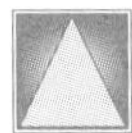

Table 37.1
Analytic Boundaries and Boundary Violations

Dimensions of analytic boundaries	Professional role, time, place and space, money, gifts, business transactions, clothing, language, confidentiality, excessive self-disclosure of personal problems, physical contact, sexual relations
Boundary violations	Egregious enactments that are often repetitive, not subject to analytic scrutiny, pervasive, and harmful to the patient while also destroying the viability of the analysis
Boundary crossings	Benign, and even helpful, countertransference enactments that are attenuated, occur in isolation, are subject to analytic scrutiny, and extend the analytic work in a positive direction

Data from T. Gutheil, M.D., G. Gabbard, M.D., and J. Lester, M.D.

37.14 The answer is A

37.15 The answer is C

37.16 The answer is E

37.17 The answer is D

In free association, *patients say whatever comes to mind.* This is in compliance with the fundamental rule of psychoanalysis, in which *the patient agrees to be completely honest with the analyst and to tell everything without selection.* Inevitably, the patient cannot accomplish this task, and these constitute resistances to the process. *Resistances prevent unconscious ideas or feelings from being experienced consciously.* The *analyst's counterpart to the patient's free association is a particular way of listening*, referred to as free-floating or evenly suspended attention. The *therapeutic or working alliance refers to the relationship established by patient and analyst that involves two adults embarking on a joint venture*, involving mutual trust, cooperation, and an endeavor to explore the patient's symptoms in order to achieve amelioration of those symptoms.

Answers 37.18–37.22

37.18 The answer is D

37.19 The answer is A

37.20 The answer is B

37.21 The answer is E

37.22 The answer is C

Contagion is the process whereby the expression of emotion by one member of a group stimulates the awareness of similar emotions in other group members. Altruism in a group context means helping out another group member. It also involves putting another person's needs before one's own, and learning that there is value in giving to others. *Ventilation is the expression of suppressed feelings, ideas or events to other group members.* It also involves the sharing of personal secrets that ameliorate a sense of sin or guilt. *Cohesion is often referred to as a sense of "we-ness," the sense that the group is working together toward a common goal. Universalization refers to the awareness of the patient that he or she is not alone in their problems*, and that others share similar complaints or difficulties.

Answers 37.23–37.26

37.23 The answer is A

37.24 The answer is C

37.25 The answer is D

37.26 The answer is B

The hallmark of the Bowen model is a person's differentiation from their family of origin. This involves the person's ability to be their true selves in the face of familial or other pressures that threaten the loss of love or social position. In a *structural model, families are viewed as single, interrelated systems*, assessed in terms of significant alliances and splits among family members, hierarchy of power, boundaries between generations, and family tolerance for each other. *Psychodynamic-experiential models emphasize individual maturation in the context of the family system and are free from unconscious patterns of anxiety and projection rooted in the past.* The *general systems model* is based on general systems theory, a model *that holds that families are systems and that every action in a family produces a reaction in one or more of its members.*

38 Biological Therapies

The use of drugs to treat psychiatric disorders is often the foundation for a successful treatment approach that can also include other types of interventions such as psychotherapy or behavioral therapies. As knowledge about the biology of normal and abnormal brain function continues to grow, the practice of clinical psychopharmacology continues to evolve in scope and effectiveness. Those involved in the prescribing and clinical follow-up of psychiatric drug treatments must remain current with the research literature, including the emergence of new agents, the demonstration of new indications for existing agents, and the identification and treatment of drug-related adverse effects. The emergence of new drugs and new indications is one of the most exciting areas of psychiatry.

The practice of pharmacotherapy in psychiatry should not be oversimplified—for example, it should not be reduced to a one-diagnosis-one-drug approach. Many variables affect the practice of psychopharmacology, including drug selection and administration; the psychodynamic meaning to the patient; and family and environmental influences. Some patients may view drug treatment as a panacea; others may view it as an assault. The patient, the patient's relatives, and the nursing staff must be instructed on the reasons for the drug treatment as well as the expected benefits and potential risks. In addition, the clinician may find it useful to explain the theoretical basis for pharmacotherapy to the patient and other involved parties.

Drugs must be used in effective dosages for sufficient periods, as determined by previous clinical investigations and clinical experience. Subtherapeutic doses and incomplete therapeutic trials should not be used simply because the psychiatrist is excessively concerned that the patient will develop adverse effects. The use of dosages that are too low or durations that are too short merely exposes patients to some risk, without providing them the maximum chance of therapeutic benefit. Treatment response and the emergence of adverse effects must be monitored closely; drug dosage should be adjusted accordingly, and appropriate treatments for emergent adverse effects must be instituted as quickly as possible.

Students need to be aware of the pharmacokinetics and pharmacodynamics of psychiatric medications, including absorption, distribution, bioavailability, metabolism, and excretion, as well as receptor affinities, dose-response curves, therapeutic indices, the development of tolerance and withdrawal syndromes, therapeutic indications, adverse effects, drug–drug interactions, and signs and symptoms of overdose. Modifications of dosages or specific drug indications for special populations, such as children, the elderly, suicidal patients, and those with medical conditions, must be understood.

The student should study the questions and answers below for a useful review of these therapies.

HELPFUL HINTS

The student should know these terms and specific drugs.

- adjuvant medications
- adrenergic blockade
- akathisia
- allergic dermatitis
- amantadine (Symmetrel)
- anticholinergic side effects
- anticonvulsants
- antidepressants
- antipsychotics
- anxiolytics
- apnea
- artificial hibernation
- atropine sulfate
- benzodiazepine receptor agonists and antagonists
- Lucio Bini
- biotransformation
- bipolar I disorder, bipolar II disorder
- BPH
- bupropion
- buspirone (BuSpar)
- John Cade
- carbon dioxide therapy
- cardiac effects
- catatonia
- Ugo Cerletti
- cholinergic rebound
- clomipramine (Anafranil)
- clonazepam (Klonopin)
- clonidine (Catapres)
- CNS depression
- combination drugs
- continuous sleep treatment
- CYP enzymes
- D_2 receptors
- DEA
- demethylation
- depot preparations
- distribution volume
- dopamine receptor antagonists
- dose-response curve
- downregulation of receptors
- drug-assisted interviewing
- drug holidays
- drug-induced mania
- drug interactions
- drug intoxications
- drug selection
- dystonias

- eating disorders
- Ebstein's anomaly
- ECT
- ECT contraindications
- EEG, EMG
- electrolyte screen
- electrosleep therapy
- epileptogenic effects
- extrapyramidal side effects
- FDA
- fluoxetine (Prozac)
- fluvoxamine (Luvox)
- generalized anxiety disorder
- geriatric patients
- half-life
- haloperidol (Haldol)
- hematological effects
- hemodialysis
- hydroxylation and glucuronidation
- hypertensive crisis
- idiopathic psychosis
- impulse-control disorders
- informed consent
- insulin coma therapy
- intoxication and withdrawal syndromes
- jaundice
- light therapy
- lipid solubility
- lithium
- MAOIs
- medication-induced movement disorders
- megadose therapy
- megavitamin therapy
- melatonin
- mesocortical
- mesolimbic
- metabolic enzymes
- metabolites
- methadone
- Egas Moniz
- monoamine hypothesis
- mood stabilizers
- movement disorders
- mute patients
- narcotherapy
- narrow-angle glaucoma
- neuroendocrine tests
- neuroleptic malignant syndrome
- noncompliance
- noradrenergic, histaminic, cholinergic receptors
- obsessive-compulsive disorder
- oculogyric crisis
- orthomolecular therapy
- orthostatic (postural) hypotension
- overdose
- panic disorder with agoraphobia
- parkinsonian symptoms
- paroxetine (Paxil)
- pharmacodynamics
- pharmacokinetics
- phosphatidylinositol
- photosensitivity
- physostigmine
- pill-rolling tremor
- pilocarpine
- plasma levels
- positive and negative symptoms
- potency, high and low
- prolactin
- prophylactic treatment
- protein binding
- psychosurgery
- rabbit syndrome
- rapid neuroleptization
- Rauwolfia serpentina
- receptor blockade
- renal clearance
- retinitis pigmentosa
- retrograde ejaculation
- reuptake blockade
- schizoaffective disorder
- schizophrenia
- secondary depression
- secondary psychosis
- serotonin-dopamine antagonists
- sertraline (Zoloft)
- side-effect profile
- sleep deprivation
- SSRIs
- status epilepticus
- stereotactic
- sudden death
- sympathomimetic
- tapering
- tardive dyskinesia
- TD50
- teratogenic
- TFT
- therapeutic index
- therapeutic trial
- tonic, clonic phase
- transcranial magnetic stimulation (TMS)
- treatment-resistant patients
- tricyclic and tetracyclic drugs
- L-Triiodothyronine
- triplicate prescription
- use in pregnancy
- Julius Wagner-Jauregg
- weight gain
- Zeitgebers
- zolpidem

QUESTIONS

Directions

Each of the questions or incomplete statements below is followed by five responses or completions. Select the *one* that is *best* in each case.

38.1 Bupropion

A. does not act on the serotonergic system
B. has an associated withdrawal syndrome linked to its discontinuation
C. is not secreted in breast milk
D. has a 1 percent seizure risk with doses above 400 mg/day
E. is associated with significant drug-induced orthostatic hypotension

38.2 A patient being treated for alcohol dependence is started on acamprosate. Which of the following is *true*?

A. Acamprosate produces aversive side effects if combined with alcohol.
B. Acamprosate is a dopamine antagonist.
C. Abrupt withdrawal of acamprosate is associated with autonomic instability.
D. Acamprosate may be used to treat alcohol withdrawal.
E. Patients with severe renal impairment should not be given acamprosate.

38.3 A 28-year-old man, diagnosed with Psychosis not otherwise specified was started on haloperidol 2 mg by mouth twice a day. On the sixth day of treatment, he developed a high white count, hyperthermia, severe muscular rigidity, confusion, and increased blood pressure and pulse rate. You suspect he has neuroleptic malignant syndrome. Which of the following about this condition is *true*?

A. It usually occurs when patients are neuroleptic naïve.
B. It is more common in the elderly.
C. It is not associated with low-potency neuroleptics.
D. Women are affected more frequently than men.
E. Antiparkinsonian agents have been used to reduce the muscle rigidity.

38.4 Restless leg syndrome

A. is associated with painful dysesthesias

B. peaks in old age
C. responds to SSRIs
D. responds to dopamine receptor agonists
E. abates during sleep

38.5 Which of the following about clonidine is *true*?

A. Patients usually develop tolerance to clonidine-induced sedation.
B. Patients who overdose on clonidine present with dilated pupils.
C. It is primarily a presynaptic alpha-2 adrenergic receptor antagonist.
D. It results in a decrease in the amount of norepinephrine released from the presynaptic nerve terminals.
E. Often causes tachycardia.

38.6 Sildenafil

A. is rapidly absorbed after a fatty meal
B. is mostly excreted in the urine
C. decreases levels of cyclic guanosine monophosphate
D. is a nitric oxide enhancer
E. carries a high risk of priapism

38.7 In treating bipolar disorder

A. lamotrigine is more effective in lengthening the intervals between manic episodes than between depressive episodes
B. lithium exerts its antimanic effects over 1 to 3 weeks
C. lithium prevents relapse of mania in about fifty percent of patients
D. about 10 percent of patients with acute mania respond to valproate
E. carbamazepine is most useful in prior lithium-responders

38.8 Which of the following tricyclic drugs is *least* associated with anticholinergic effects?

A. Amitriptyline (Elavil)
B. Clomipramine (Anafranil)
C. Desipramine (Norpramin)
D. Imipramine (Tofranil)
E. Trimipramine (Surmontil)

38.9 Which of the following is *true*?

A. Lithium is not excreted in breast milk
B. Lithium is unsafe in the elderly
C. Lithium is contraindicated in patients with sick sinus syndrome
D. Lithium cardiotoxicity is more prevalent in people on a high-salt diet
E. Obesity is associated with lower rates of lithium clearance

38.10 Well-controlled studies have supported the use of carbamazepine (Tegretol) for which of the following disorders?

A. Anorexia nervosa
B. Insomnia
C. Neuroleptic-induced parkinsonism
D. Mania
E. Social phobia

38.11 An internist calls you to ask about selecting a serotonin reuptake inhibitor for a patient of hers who is depressed. She tells you that the patient has never been treated with an antidepressant before, is on no other medications, and has no serious medical problems. Which of the following is *true*?

A. Not all the SSRIs are equally effective in treating depression.
B. Most of the SSRIs have similar serum half lives.
C. The SSRIs have a narrow therapeutic index.
D. Paroxetine has significant anticholinergic activity at higher dosages.
E. The metabolites of citalopram have significant pharmacologic activity.

38.12 Which of the following is *true* about monoamine oxidase inhibitors (MAOIs)?

A. The risk of tyramine-induced hypertension is high for someone on moclobemide.
B. White wine together with an MAOI may precipitate a tyramine-induced hypertensive crisis
C. Alkalinization of the urine hastens the excretion of MAOIs.
D. People should continue to restrict tyramine-rich foods for at least one month after they stop MAOI treatment.
E. Lithium together with an MAOI may induce a serotonin syndrome.

38.13 Which of the following is the most common adverse effect of olanzapine (Zyprexa)?

A. Constipation
B. Orthostatic hypotension
C. Sedation
D. Tardive dyskinesia
E. Weight gain

38.14 Potential treatments for the adverse sexual effects of the serotonin-specific reuptake inhibitors include each of the following drugs *except*

A. amantadine (Symmetrel)
B. bromocriptine (Parlodel)
C. cyproheptadine (Periactin)
D. liothyronine (Cytomel)
E. yohimbine (Yocon)

38.15 Which of the following is the most important factor determining a successful response to treatment with naltrexone (ReVia)?

A. Abstinence from opioids during therapy
B. Dosage
C. Duration of therapeutic trials
D. Ability to start and stop naltrexone without physical consequences
E. Psychosocial factors

38.16 The calcium channel blockers

A. are first-line mood stabilizing agents
B. are minimally absorbed after oral use
C. have been shown to be effective in the treatment of depression
D. have been shown to be beneficial in Tourette's disorder
E. cause side effects secondary to their vasodilatory properties

38.17 A 32-year-old woman with a first episode of depression, and no prior treatment history, is started on thyroid hormone after three weeks of partial response to nortryptaline 75 mg/day. Which of the following is *true*?

A. Laboratory values of thyroid hormone will help in assessing response to the hormone.
B. The doctor waited the correct amount of time before beginning his augmentation strategy.
C. Levothyroxine (T4) is the thyroid hormone most used for this purpose.
D. Fifty percent of antidepressant nonresponders become treatment responders using thyroid hormone.
E. She should be advised not to become pregnant on thyroid hormones, as they are associated with multiple serious congenital malformations.

38.18 Which of the following about the rash associated with lamotrigine is *true*?

A. A serious rash may develop in almost 25 percent of patients taking lamotrigine.
B. The development of a rash is not related to how the medication is administered.
C. Approximately 8 percent of patients develop a benign maculopapular rash.
D. There is no evidence to suggest that the rash is age related.
E. Immediate discontinuation of the drug upon development of a rash prevents the subsequent development of a life-threatening rash.

38.19 Carbamazepine may decrease drug plasma concentrations of which of the following agents?

A. Haloperidol (Haldol)
B. Bupropion (BuSpar)
C. Birth control pills
D. Methadone (Dolophine)
E. All of the above

38.20 Factors associated with a more favorable antimanic response to valproate than to lithium include

A. rapid cycling
B. mixed or dysphoric mania
C. mania associated with medical or neurological illness
D. comorbid substance abuse or panic attacks
E. all of the above

38.21 Of the following, the most common adverse effect of valproate is

A. reversible thrombocytopenia
B. hair loss
C. diarrhea
D. persistent elevation of hepatic transaminases
E. ataxia

38.22 Which statement is *not* true about the atypical antipsychotics?

A. They all have proven efficacy as treatments for schizophrenia.
B. They all have low D_2 receptor blocking effects compared with typical antipsychotics.
C. They may have a reduced risk of extrapyramidal side effects compared to older agents.
D. They have proven efficacy as treatments for acute mania.
E. They have similar receptor affinities.

38.23 Which of the following drugs or foods is *not* contraindicated for concurrent administration with triazolobenzodiazepines such as alprazolam (Xanax), based on inhibition of the hepatic enzyme cytochrome P450 (CYP) 3A4?

A. Cisapride (Propulsid)
B. Grapefruit juice
C. Nefazodone (Serzone)
D. Venlafaxine (Effexor)
E. All of the above

38.24 Carbamazepine affects each of the following organ systems *except*

A. dermatological
B. hematopoietic
C. hepatic
D. pulmonary
E. renal

38.25 Which of the following drug interactions is *true*?

A. Nicotine lowers concentrations of tricyclic antidepressants.
B. Clozapine should not be prescribed together with carbamazepine.
C. Indomethacin increases lithium levels.
D. None of the above
E. All of the above

Directions

Each group of questions below consists of lettered headings followed by a list of numbered words or phrases. For each numbered word or phrase, select the *one* lettered heading that is most closely associated with it. Each heading may be selected once, more than once, or not at all.

Questions 38.26–38.30

A. buproprion
B. valproate
C. ziprasidone
D. carbamazepine
E. valproate

38.26 seizures
38.27 ovarian cysts
38.28 QTc prolongation
38.29 diabetes
38.30 Stevens Johnson syndrome

Directions

Each of the questions or incomplete statements below is followed by five suggested responses or completions. Select the *one* that is *best* in each case.

38.31 A 28-year-old woman is brought to the emergency room heavily sedated, with a suspected overdose on sleeping medications. Flumazenil is considered as treatment. Which of the following is *true*?

A. She should be given at least ten minutes of a cumulative dose of flumazenil before you rule out a benzodiazepine as the cause of her sedation.
B. Flumazenil will have no effect if she overdosed on zolpidem.
C. Your biggest concern about giving her flumazenil is that you may precipitate the onset of seizures.
D. Flumazenil will reverse the effects if she took barbiturates.
E. Flumazenil is administered as a rapid bolus injection.

38.32 True statements about pharmacodynamics include

A. Haldol is less potent than chlorpromazine.
B. Haldol is more clinically effective than chlorpromazine.
C. The therapeutic index for Haldol is high.
D. The therapeutic index for lithium is high.
E. None of the above

38.33 Of the following biological treatments the most teratogenic is

A. Electroconvulsive therapy (ECT)
B. Haloperidol (Haldol)
C. Fluoxetine (Prozac)
D. Lithium (Eskalith)
E. Lorazepam (Ativan)

38.34 Blockade of muscarinic acetylcholine receptors causes all of the following side effects *except*

A. mydriasis
B. urinary retention
C. delayed ejaculation
D. photophobia
E. orthostatic hypotension

38.35 True statements about SSRI drug interactions include

A. SSRIs plus phenobarbital leads to increased SSRI concentration.
B. SSRIs plus codeine leads to decreased codeine concentration.
C. SSRIs plus clozapine lead to increased clozapine concentration.
D. Prozac plus alprazolam leads to decreased alprazolam concentration.
E. Prozac plus carbamazepine leads to decreased carbamazepine concentration.

38.36 Increased lithium concentrations are associated with all of the following drug interactions *except*

A. theophylline
B. furosemide
C. salt restriction
D. indomethacin
E. ibuprofen

38.37 Which of the following is *true*?

A. Ramelteon acts on benzodiazepine receptors.
B. Diazepam is short acting.
C. The benzodiazepines modulate gamma-aminobutyric acid activity.
D. Benzodiazepine use in pregnant patients should be confined to the third trimester.
E. Tolerance to the sedative effect of zolpidem occurs often.

38.38 Significant valproate interactions include

A. increased free valproate levels with aspirin
B. decreased concentration of phenobarbital with valproate
C. decreased lamotrigine levels with valproate
D. decreased valproate levels with fluoxetine
E. increased valproate levels with carbamazepine

38.39 Anticholinergic prophylaxis should be used routinely

A. past the second week of treatment with an antipsychotic medication
B. when the equivalent of greater than 12 mg a day of haloperidol is required of high-potency antipsychotics
C. in young women on low-potency antipsychotic medication
D. in elderly patients
E. prior to side effects such as parkinsonism activity

38.40 True statements about gabapentin include

A. Gabapentin is metabolized almost exclusively in the liver.
B. Gabapentin overdose is associated with serious toxicity.
C. Studies suggest that gabapentin may be less useful in the treatment of bipolar II disorder than of bipolar I disorder.
D. Abrupt discontinuation of gabapentin may cause a withdrawal syndrome.
E. Gabapentin interacts with hepatic enzymes and may both inhibit and induce them depending on dose.

38.41 Zolpidem

A. may be used as a muscle relaxant
B. reaches peak plasma levels in about 4 to 6 hours
C. is solely indicated as a hypnotic

D. is generally associated with rebound insomnia after discontinuation of its use for short periods
E. is not contraindicated for use by nursing mothers

38.42 Which of the following statements regarding transcranial magnetic stimulation is *true*?

A. It does not require general anesthesia.
B. Seizures do not appear to be required for therapeutic effects.
C. Optimal stimulation patterns for TMS in psychiatric disorders are not yet known.
D. It is a noninvasive CNS stimulant.
E. All of the above

38.43 Dantrolene is a potentially effective treatment for each of the following disorders *except*

A. acute mania
B. catatonia
C. malignant hyperthermia
D. neuroleptic malignant syndrome
E. serotonin syndrome

38.44 Data supporting the traditional dopamine hypothesis of schizophrenia include each of the following *except*

A. correlation of a decrease in plasma concentrations of homovanillic acid with improvement in symptoms
B. PET scan data correlating D_2 receptor occupancy with antipsychotic efficacy
C. precipitation of psychosis with amphetamines
D. the clinical efficacy of clozapine (Clozaril)
E. correlation of D_2 receptor affinity with the clinical efficacy of dopamine receptor antagonists

38.45 SSRIs are indicated for all of the following *except*

A. Attention-deficit/hyperactivity disorder
B. Premature ejaculation
C. General Anxiety Disorder
D. Panic Disorder
E. Trichotillomania

38.46 Of the following, β-adrenergic receptor antagonists are generally most effective in the treatment of

A. panic disorder
B. generalized anxiety disorder
C. alcohol withdrawal
D. akathisia
E. psychogenic seizures

38.47 Factors that predict a better response to carbamazepine (Tegretol) than to lithium (Eskalith) in bipolar I disorder include each of the following *except*

A. comorbid seizure disorder
B. dysphoric mania
C. first episode of mania
D. negative family history
E. rapid cycling

38.48 Which of the following drugs has the fastest onset of action against acute mania?

A. Carbamazepine (Tegretol)
B. Haloperidol (Haldol)
C. Lithium (Eskalith)
D. Risperidone (Risperdal)
E. Valproate (Depakote)

38.49 Which of the following dopamine receptor antagonists would probably be the safest to use for psychotic symptoms due to a brain tumor?

A. Chlorpromazine (Thorazine)
B. Fluphenazine (Prolixin)
C. Mesoridazine (Serentil)
D. Sulpiride (Dogmatil)
E. Thioridazine (Mellaril)

38.50 Anticholinergic drugs are indicated for treatment of all of the following *except*

A. neuroleptic-induced parkinsonism
B. Huntington's chorea
C. neuroleptic-induced acute dystonia
D. idiopathic Parkinson's disease
E. medication-induced postural tremor

38.51 Which of the following is *true*?

A. Memantine is potent inhibitor of cholinesterase.
B. Tacrine causes relatively few serious side effects.
C. Donepezil selectively inhibits acetyl-cholinesterase within the CNS.
D. Rivastigmine is hepatotoxic.
E. Donepezil is especially indicated in severe stages of Alzheimer's type dementia.

38.52 Mirtazapine

A. is highly sedating
B. decreases appetite
C. causes an irreversible neutropenia
D. lowers the seizure threshold
E. causes nausea

ANSWERS

38.1 The answer is A

Unlike other currently used antidepressants, *bupropion does not act on the serotonin system.* It is a norepinephrine and dopamine reuptake inhibitor for the treatment of major depression. Headache, insomnia, dry mouth, tremor, and nausea are the most common side effects. There is no significant drug-induced orthostatic hypotension, weight gain, daytime drowsiness and anticholinergic effects. *While concern about seizure has deterred some physicians from prescribing it, studies show that at dosages of 300 mg/day or less, the incidence of seizures is 0.05%, no worse than the incidence of seizure with other antidepressants.* The risk increases to 0.1% with dosages of 400 mg/day. *It is secreted in breast milk,* so its use in nursing women should be based on the clinical circumstances of the patient and the clinician's judgment. *No withdrawal syndrome has been linked to the discontinuation of bupropion.*

38.2 The answer is E

Patients with severe renal impairment (creatinine clearance of <30 mL/min) should not be given acamprosate. Acamprosate reduces the craving that is experienced by alcohol-dependent patients. *Its mechanism of action is not fully understood, but it is thought to antagonize neuronal overactivity related to the actions of the excitatory neurotransmitter glutamate, which may in part result from antagonism of NMDA, not dopamine receptors.* The concomitant intake of alcohol and acamprosate does not affect the pharmacokinetics of either alcohol or acamprosate, and it does not produce aversive side effects when combined with alcohol. *It should not be used to treat alcohol withdrawal symptoms*, and should only be started after the patient has been successfully weaned off the alcohol. *There are no adverse events that occur following the abrupt withdrawal of acamprosate, even after long-term use.*

38.3 The answer is E

Neuroleptic malignant syndrome (NMS) is a potentially fatal side effect of dopamine receptor antagonists. *Antiparkinsonian agents may reduce some of the muscle rigidity*, and dantrolene, a skeletal muscle relaxant, may be useful in the treatment of this disorder. *NMS can occur at any time during the course of treatment with dopamine receptor antagonist medications, not just in the neuroleptic-naïve*, and it may also be caused by low potency drugs. *Men are affected more frequently than women, and young people are affected more commonly than the elderly.*

38.4 The answer is D

The dopamine receptor agonist ropinirole, is effective in treating restless leg syndrome whose cause is unknown, but may be a rare side effect of SSRIs. In this syndrome, people feel deep sensations of creeping inside the calves whenever sitting or lying down. The dysesthesias are rarely painful, but are relentless, and cause an irresistible urge to move the legs, so *sleep is regularly interrupted. It peaks in middle age and occurs in 5 percent of the population.*

38.5 The answer is D

Clonidine is a presynaptic alpha-2 adrenergic receptor agonist. *It is not an antagonist.* By working on these receptors in the sympathetic nuclei of the brain, *it results in a decrease in the amount of norepinephrine released from the presynaptic nerve terminals.* This resets the body's sympathetic tone at a lower level, and decreases arousal. The most common side effects are dry mouth and eyes, fatigue, sedation, dizziness, nausea, hypotension, and constipation. It may cause a bradycardia; if this develops, the drug should be discontinued in a gradual taper. Patients usually *do not develop tolerance to the sedation* that may develop. Overdose may result in constricted pupils and coma, with symptoms similar to those of an opioid overdose.

38.6 The answer is D

Sildenafil is a phosphodiesterase-5 (PDE-5) inhibitor. Sexual stimulation causes the release of nitric oxide, which increases the synthesis of cyclic guanosine monophosphate (cGMP), causing smooth muscle relaxation in the corpus cavernosum that allows blood to flow into the penis, resulting in turgidity and tumescence. When the enzyme PDE-5 is inhibited, *there is an increase in cyclic guanosine monophosphate.* This drug works only when there is sexual stimulation; it inhibits PDE-5 allowing an increase in cGMP and enhancing the vasodilatory effects of nitrous oxide. *It is known as a nitric oxide enhancer.* It is highly lipophilic, *so its absorption is delayed after the ingestion of a fatty meal. Excretion of 80 percent of the dose is via feces. There are no cases of priapism reported in premarketing trials.*

38.7 The answer is B

Lithium has a relatively slow onset of action when used and exerts its antimanic effects over 1 to 3 weeks. Often, a benzodiazepine, dopamine receptor antagonist or serotonin-dopamine antagonist is administered for the first few weeks. *It has been reported to control acute mania and prevent relapse in about 80 percent of people with bipolar I disorder. Lamotrigine is indicated in the treatment of bipolar disorder and may prolong the time between episodes of depression and mania. It is more effective in lengthening the intervals between depressive episodes than manic episodes. About two thirds of patients with acute mania respond to valproate.* The majority usually respond within 1 to 4 days after achieving valproate serum levels greater than 50 mcg/mL. *Studies suggest that carbamazepine may be especially effective in people who are not responsive to lithium.*

38.8 The answer is C

Clinicians should warn patients that anticholinergic effects of tricyclic drugs are common but that a patient may develop tolerance for them with continued treatment. *Amitriptyline, imipramine, trimipramine, clomipramine,* and doxepin are the most anticholinergic drugs; amoxapine, nortriptyline, and maprotiline are less anticholinergic; *desipramine* may be the least anticholinergic. Anticholinergic effects include dry mouth, constipation, blurred vision, and urinary retention. Sugarless gum, candy, or fluoride lozenges can alleviate the dry mouth. Bethanechol (Urecholine), 25 to 50 mg three or four times a day, may reduce urinary hesitancy and can be helpful in cases of impotence when the drug is taken 30 minutes before sexual intercourse. Narrow-angle glaucoma can be aggravated by anticholinergic drugs, and the precipitation of glaucoma requires emergency treatment with a miotic agent. Tricyclic and tetracyclic drugs should be avoided in patients with glaucoma, and an SSRI should be substituted. Severe anticholinergic effects can lead to a CNS anticholinergic syndrome with confusion and delirium, especially if tricyclic and tetracyclic drugs are administered with antipsychotics or anticholinergic drugs. Some clinicians have used intramuscular (IM) or intravenous (IV) physostigmine (Antilirium) as a diagnostic tool to confirm the presence of anticholinergic delirium.

38.9 The answer is C

Lithium depresses the pacemaking activity of the sinus node, sometimes resulting in sinus dysrhythmias, heart block and episodes of syncope. *It is therefore contraindicated in people with sick sinus syndrome. Toxicity is more prevalent in people on a low salt diet*, those taking certain diuretics or angiotensin-converting enzyme (ACE) inhibitors, and those with fluid-electrolyte imbalances or any renal insufficiency. *Lithium is excreted into breast milk* and should be taken by a nursing mother only after careful evaluation of potential risks and benefits. *It is safe and effective in the elderly*, but it is important to remember that the treatment of elderly people taking lithium may be complicated by the presence of other medical illnesses, decreased renal function, special diets that affect lithium clearance, and generally increased sensitivity to lithium. *Obesity is associated with higher rates of lithium clearance.*

38.10 The answer is D

Several well-controlled studies have produced data indicating that carbamazepine is effective in the treatment of mania.

The available data indicate that carbamazepine is also an effective treatment for depression in some patients. About 25 to 33 percent of depressed patients respond to carbamazepine. That percentage is significantly smaller than the 60 to 70 percent response rate for standard antidepressants. Nevertheless, carbamazepine is an alternative drug for depressed patients who have not responded to conventional treatments, including electroconvulsive therapy (ECT), or who have a marked or rapid periodicity in their depressive episodes.

Several studies have reported that carbamazepine is effective in controlling impulsive, aggressive behavior in nonpsychotic patients of all ages, from children to the elderly. Other drugs for impulse control disorders, particularly intermittent explosive disorder, include lithium, propranolol (Inderal), and antipsychotics. Because of the risk of serious adverse effects with carbamazepine, treatment with these other agents is warranted before initiating a trial with carbamazepine.

According to several studies, carbamazepine is as effective as the benzodiazepines in the control of symptoms associated with alcohol withdrawal. It may also assist in withdrawal from chronic benzodiazepines in the control of symptoms linked to alcohol withdrawal. Similarly, it may aid in withdrawal from chronic benzodiazepine use, especially in seizure-prone patients. However, the lack of any advantage of carbamazepine over the benzodiazepines for alcohol withdrawal and the risk of adverse effects with carbamazepine limit the clinical usefulness of this application. Carbamazepine has not been shown to be useful in the treatment of *social phobia, insomnia, anorexia nervosa,* or *neuroleptic-induced Parkinsonism.*

38.11 The answer is D

Paroxetine has significant anticholinergic activity at higher dosages, but all of these drugs exert their therapeutic effects through 5-HT reuptake inhibition. The most significant difference among the SSRIs is their broad range of serum half lives. While they are each structurally and chemically distinct from each other, *the SSRIs are all equally effective in the treatment of major depressive disorder.* Citalopram and escitalopram are the most selective inhibitors of serotonin reuptake. Fluoxetine has an active metabolite with a half life of 7 to 9 days. Sertraline's active metabolite has a half life of 3 to 5 days. Citalopram does not have metabolites with significant pharmacologic activity. *These medications have a wide therapeutic index, making them relatively easy to administer.*

38.12 The answer is E

The use of lithium, tryptophan or any serotonergic drug together with an MAOI can trigger a serotonin syndrome, the symptoms of which include tremor, hypertonicity, myoclonus, and autonomic signs, which can the progress to hallucinosis, hyperthermia, and even death. *The most worrisome side effect of MAOIs is the tyramine-induced hypertensive crisis.* Thus, foods rich in tyramine, like cured meats and red wine, or other sympathomimetic amines should be avoided by people who are taking irreversible MOAIs. White wine has no tyramine content. *Patients should be advised to continue the dietary restrictions for two weeks after they stop MAOI treatment to allow the body to re-synthesize the enzyme.* Moclobemide is a reversible inhibitor of MAOa. The risk of a tyramine-induced hypertensive crisis is relatively low for patients taking this medication. *Acidification, not alkalinization of the urine markedly hastens the excretion of MAOIs.*

38.13 The answer is C

The most common adverse effect of olanzapine is *sedation*, which may occur in 30 percent of patients on the usual maintenance dose (10 mg/day). Therefore, patients who take olanzapine should exercise caution when driving or operating dangerous machinery. This side effect may be minimized by giving the dose before sleep. Olanzapine-associated seizures are seen in less than 1 percent of patients. The D_2 receptor antagonism of olanzapine causes a modest rise in prolactin levels for the duration of the therapy. This is a theoretical concern in patients with a history of breast cancer, a tumor that may be dependent on prolactin for growth, although there are no human data establishing such a connection. Dizziness, akathisia, and nonaggressive objectionable behavior have also been reported at frequencies higher than those seen in placebo controls.

No cases of *tardive dyskinesia* have yet been reported in patients taking olanzapine, although experience is limited. No agranulocytosis was reported in more than 3,100 patients taking olanzapine, including 29 who previously had clozapine-induced agranulocytosis.

When olanzapine is first initiated, patients may develop signs and symptoms of *orthostatic hypotension,* such as dizziness, tachycardia, and syncope. The risk of these effects may be minimized by limiting the starting dose to 5 mg a day over a few weeks. Significantly, in 2 percent of patients taking olanzapine, serum ALT (SGPT) elevations more than three times normal were seen. None of these patients developed jaundice. The levels returned to normal whether or not the drug was discontinued. These data indicate that olanzapine should be used with caution by patients with underlying liver disease. *Weight gain* and *constipation* have been associated with olanzapine use. In clinical trials 16 percent of patients gained more than 65 pounds and diabetes has also occurred.

38.14 The answer is D

Serotonergic drugs may cause a reduction in libido, anorgasmia, inhibition of ejaculation, and/or impotence in up to 80 percent of the patients. Many clinicians do not inquire about sexual adverse effects, yet these may be very troubling to patients. Some drugs that may be helpful in reducing these adverse effects are *amantadine, bromocriptine, cyproheptadine,* and *yohimbine.* Amantadine and bromocriptine have dopamine agonist effects; cyproheptadine is a serotonin antagonist; and yohimbine is an α_2-adrenergic antagonist that potentiates release of norepinephrine. Mirtazapine (Remeron), another α_2-adrenergic antagonist, and bupropion (Wellbutrin), an antidepressant with little serotonergic activity, are two antidepressants that are practically free of sexual adverse effects. *Liothyronine* is used as augmentation treatment for SSRI nonresponders, but it has no role in the treatment of sexual adverse effects.

38.15 The answer is E

The success of naltrexone drug and alcohol abstinence programs is more closely associated with *psychosocial factors*, such as educational level, motivation, family support, and continued behavioral therapy, than with factors associated directly with the use of naltrexone, such as dosage or duration of therapeutic trials.

Naltrexone is a pure opioid antagonist, effective in a once-a-day dose that has improved the success of existing behavioral approaches to the treatment of opioid and alcohol addiction. Naltrexone appears to reduce or eliminate the drug craving that torments former addicts by simply eliminating the subjective "high" associated with a return to drug abuse. Abstinence from opioids during therapy is therefore a secondary issue, because users do not experience the usual effects of opioids. Naltrexone must be initiated cautiously in individuals who may still be abusing opioids, because it may induce an acute withdrawal reaction, which may include life-threatening dehydration due to vomiting and diarrhea. It is therefore necessary to ensure an opioid-free state prior to use of naltrexone. Once in use, however, naltrexone may be started and stopped, usually without physical consequences. This feature has unfortunately allowed many less motivated former addicts to withdraw from naltrexone treatment programs, which is an outcome in contrast to that usually seen in methadone programs, where stopping the drug precipitates an unpleasant withdrawal syndrome.

38.16 The answer is D

Calcium channel inhibitors may be beneficial in Tourette's disorder. They are *not effective treatments for depression*, and may in fact prevent response to antidepressants. *They are used as antimanic agents for people who are refractory to, or cannot tolerate treatment with first-line mood-stabilizing agents.* They are *nearly completely absorbed after oral use*, with significant first-pass hepatic metabolism. *The most common side effects associated with these medications are due to vasodilatation: dizziness, headache, tachycardia, nausea, dysesthesias and peripheral edema.*

38.17 The answer is D

The major indication for thyroid hormones in psychiatry is as an adjuvant to antidepressants. *Liothyronine (T3) not levothyroxine (T4)* is the thyroid hormone used as an augmentation agent. *It converts about 50 percent of antidepressant non-responders to responders. There is no clear correlation between the laboratory measures of thyroid function and the response to thyroid hormone supplementation of antidepressants.* Usually, at least a 6-week course of an antidepressant at an adequate dose is tried before beginning supplementation. *Thyroid hormones can be administered safely to pregnant women, provided that laboratory thyroid indexes are monitored.* Thyroid hormones are minimally excreted in the breast milk and have not been shown to cause problems in nursing babies.

38.18 The answer is C

The appearance of a rash in patients taking lamotrigine is a source of concern. *About 8% of patients started on lamotrigine develop a benign maculopapular rash in the first four months of treatment, and the drug should be discontinued if a rash develops.* Estimates of the rate of a *serious rash vary from 0.08 percent to 0.13 percent. The likelihood of a rash increases if the recommended starting dose and speed of dose increase what is recommended. Children and adolescents under age 16 appear more susceptible to a rash with lamotrigine.* The concern about the rash is that it may lead to a Stevens-Johnson syndrome or toxic epidermal necrolysis. *Even if the medication is discontinued immediately upon the development of the rash or other signs of hypersensitivity reaction, this may not prevent subsequent development of a life-threatening rash or permanent disfiguration.*

38.19 The answer is E (all)

Carbamazepine may interfere with the dexamethasone-suppression test and with some pregnancy tests. Carbamazepine increases the metabolism of sex hormones used in *birth control preparations*, so higher-dose formulations of those preparations may be required for the oral contraceptives to maintain their efficacy.

Clinically meaningful drug interactions have occurred with concomitant medications. Most drug interactions result from carbamazepine's induction of hepatic microsomal CYP 2D6, 1A2, 3A4, and 2C9/10, which leads to an accelerated elimination of drugs normally metabolized by this system, including the barbiturates and oral contraceptives. Thus, carbamazepine may decrease the blood levels and efficacy of a variety of drugs. Most notably, *carbamazepine may interact with commonly prescribed agents, such as antidepressants (i.e., bupropion), antipsychotic drugs (i.e., haloperidol), oral contraceptives, methadone,* and anticoagulants. Plasma concentrations of these coprescribed agents may decrease to a clinically significant degree, requiring dosage adjustments to compensate for the lowered plasma concentrations. *Carbamazepine has been reported to decrease levels of haloperidol* by 40 to 60 percent. While administering carbamazepine to refractory excited psychotic patients taking neuroleptic drugs, such as haloperidol, is generally effective, occasional exacerbations may be associated with reduction of serum neuroleptic levels to the undetectable range.

38.20 The answer is E (all)

Several factors may be associated with a more favorable antimanic response to valproate than to lithium, including *rapid cycling* (the occurrence of four or more mood episodes in 1 year) and possibly ultrarapid cycling; mania accompanied by mild, moderate, or severe depressive symptoms, including *mixed or dysphoric mania;* and organic or complicated mania (*mania caused by, or associated with, medical or neurological illness* or drugs). Recent controlled data suggest that acutely manic patients with mixed features or rapid cycling are just as likely to display an antimanic response to valproate as patients with pure mania or slow cycling. Other possible predictors of a better response to valproate than to lithium include *comorbid substance abuse or panic attacks*. Prior response to lithium or other antiepileptic drugs is not associated with valproate response.

38.21 The answer is B

Bothersome side effects of valproate include *hair loss*, reported in 3 to 12 percent of patients. Although the hair loss is often transient, total alopecia has been reported in rare cases. Supplemental treatment with multivitamins containing zinc and selenium may minimize hair loss.

38.22 The answer is E

All the atypical or second-generation antipsychotics have different chemical structures, receptor affinities and side effect profiles. While they all have a higher ratio of serotonin type

2 (5-HT2) to D_2 dopamine receptor blockades than the typical antipsychotics, none is identical in its combination of receptor affinities and the relative contribution of each receptor interaction to the clinical effects is unknown. They all do however share the following characteristics: *they all have a low blocking effect of D_2 dopamine receptors compared with typical antipsychotics; they all have proven efficacy in the treatment of schizophrenia and acute mania; and they may have a reduced risk of causing extrapyramidal side effects compared to the older agents.*

38.23 The answer is D

Venlafaxine (Effexor) may be given with drugs such as alprazolam. Most psychotherapeutic drugs are oxidized by the hepatic cytochrome P450 (CYP) enzyme system.

The CYP genes may be induced by alcohol, certain drugs (barbiturates, anticonvulsants), or by smoking, which increases the metabolism of certain drugs and precarcinogens. Other agents may directly inhibit the enzymes and slow the metabolism of other drugs. In some cases, if one CYP enzyme is inhibited, once the precursor accumulates to a sufficiently high level within the cell, another CYP enzyme may begin to act. Cellular pathophysiology, such as that caused by viral hepatitis or cirrhosis, may also affect the efficiency of the CYP system. With the DNA sequence data available, several genetic polymorphisms in the CYP genes are now recognized, some of which are manifested in a decreased rate of metabolism. Patients with an inefficient version of a specific CYP enzyme are considered "poor metabolizers."

With respect to CYP 2D6, for which 7 percent of whites are poor metabolizers, tricyclic antidepressants, antipsychotics, and type 1C antiarrhythmics should be used cautiously or avoided with selective serotonin reuptake inhibitors (SSRIs). Because of inhibition of the CYP 3A4 enzyme, *nefazodone, cisapride, grapefruit juice*, and fluoxetine should not be used with terfenadine (Seldane), astemizole (Hismanal), carbamazepine (Tegretol), or the triazolobenzodiazepines alprazolam (Xanax) and triazolam (Halcion). Inhibition of CYP 2C9/10 and CYP 2C19 warrants caution for combinations such as fluoxetine plus phenytoin (Dilantin) and sertraline plus tolbutamide (Orinase). It is also important to consider the long half-lives of certain psychiatric drugs, especially fluoxetine, which may extend their inhibition of the CYP enzymes.

38.24 The answer is D

Carbamazepine has *no known effects* on the *pulmonary system*. Besides the effects on the CNS, carbamazepine has its most significant effects on the *hematopoietic* system. Carbamazepine is associated with a benign and often transient decrease in the white blood cell count, with values usually remaining above 3,000. The decrease is thought to be due to the inhibition of the colony-stimulating factor in the bone marrow, an effect that can be reversed by the coadministration of lithium (Eskalith), which activates the colony-stimulating factor. The benign suppression of white blood cell production must be differentiated from the potentially fatal adverse effects of agranulocytosis, pancytopenia, and aplastic anemia.

As reflected by its use to treat diabetes insipidus, carbamazepine apparently has a vasopressin-like effect on the *renal* vasopressin receptor, sometimes causing the development of water intoxication or hyponatremia, particularly in elderly patients. That side effect can be treated with demeclocycline (Declomycin) or lithium. Another endocrine effect associated with carbamazepine is an increase in urinary-free cortisol.

Carbamazepine induces several *hepatic* enzymes and may thus interfere with the metabolism of a variety of other drugs. The effects of carbamazepine on the cardiovascular system are minimal. It does decrease atrioventricular (A-V) conduction, so the use of carbamazepine is contraindicated in patients with A-V heart block.

Carbamazepine may cause a rash, which may be transient even if the drug is continued, but which rarely leads to serious and potentially life-threatening *dermatological* conditions. Other system-specific allergic reactions have been reported, and rarely a lupus-like disorder has been associated with the use of carbamazepine.

38.25 The answer is E (All)

Nicotine may reduce the concentrations of tricyclic antidepressants, and so patients on these medications who smoke, should have close monitoring of their blood TCA levels. *Clozapine should not be used with any other drug that is associated with the development of bone marrow suppression or agranulocytosis, including carbamazepine, phenytoin, sulfonamides, and captopril.* A wide range of nonsteroidal anti-inflammatory drugs (NSAIDS) can decrease lithium clearance and thereby increase lithium concentrations. *This includes indomethacin, ibuprofen and naproxen.*

Answers 38.26–38.30

38.26 The answer is A

38.27 The answer is E

38.28 The answer is C

38.29 The answer is B

38.30 The answer is D

Seizures may occur with *buproprion* at does above 400 mg per day. However, the risk is no worse than with other antidepressants.

Cases of *polycystic ovary disease* have been reported in women using *valproate*.

Prolongation of the QTc complex occurs with ziprasidone and should not be used in patients with a history of cardiac arrhythmias.

Diabetes and weight gain may occur with *olanzapine* and periodic assessment of blood sugar should be obtained.

About 10 to 15 percent of people who take carbamazepine develop a benign maculopapular rash within the first three weeks of treatment. Stopping the medication usually leads to resolution of the rash. Some patients may develop life-threatening dermatologic syndromes, like toxic epidermal necrolysis or *Stevens-Johnson syndrome*.

38.31 The answer is C

Flumazenil is used to reverse the adverse psychomotor, amnestic, and sedative effects of benzodiazepine receptor agonists. *The most common serious side effect associated with its use is the precipitation of seizures*, which is likely to occur in people with seizure disorders, those who are physically dependent on benzodiazepines, or those who have ingested large quantities of benzodiazepines. *It does work to reverse the side effects associated with an overdose of zolpidem and zaleplon*, because they both have benzodiazepine receptor agonistic properties. It does not reverse the effects of ethanol, barbiturates or opioids. *The clinician should not rush its administration, and should be administered as an initial dose of 0.2 mg intravenously over thirty seconds*. Most people with a benzodiazepine overdose respond to a cumulative dose of 1 to 3 mg. If a person has not responded within 5 minutes of a cumulative dose of 5 mg of flumazenil, the major cause of sedation is probably not due to a benzodiazepine agonist.

38.32 The answer is C

The major pharmacodynamic considerations include receptor mechanisms; the dose-response curve; the therapeutic index; and the development of tolerance, dependence, and withdrawal phenomena.

The dose-response curve plots the drug concentration against the effects of the drug (Fig. 38.1). The potency of a drug refers to the relative dose required to achieve certain effects. *Haloperidol (Haldol), for example, is more (not less) potent than chlorpromazine (Thorazine)* because approximately 5 mg of haloperidol is required to achieve the same therapeutic effect as 100 mg of chlorpromazine. However, both these drugs are equal in their clinical efficacy—that is, the maximum clinical response achievable by administration of a drug.

The adverse effects of most drugs are often a direct result of their primary pharmacodynamic effects. *Therapeutic index* is a relative measure of the toxicity or safety of a drug and is defined as the ratio of the median toxic dose to the median effective dose. The *median toxic dose* is the dose at which 50 percent of patients experience a specific toxic effect, and the *median effective dose* is the dose at which 50 percent of patients have a specified therapeutic effect. *The therapeutic index for haloperidol is high,* as evidenced by the wide range of dosages in which haloperidol is prescribed. Conversely, *the therapeutic index for lithium is low (not high)*, thus requiring careful monitoring of serum lithium levels in patients for whom the drug is prescribed. Both interindividual and intraindividual variations can affect the response to a specific drug. An individual patient may be hyporeactive, normally reactive, or hyperreactive to a drug. For example, some patients require 150 mg a day of imipramine (Tofranil), whereas others may require 300 mg a day. Idiosyncratic drug responses occur when a patient experiences a particularly unusual or rare effect from a drug. For example, some patients become quite agitated when given a benzodiazepine, such as diazepam (Valium).

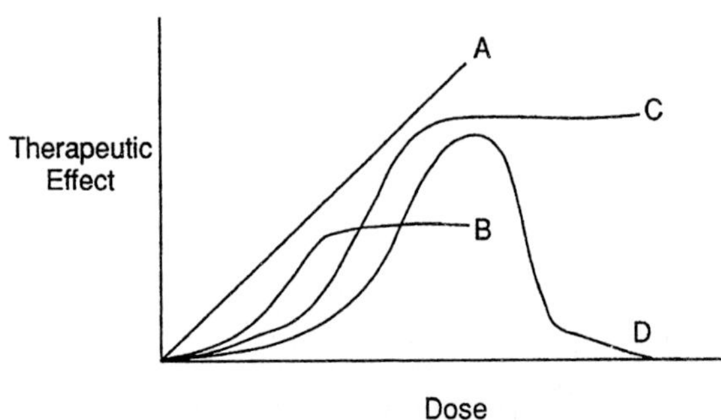

FIGURE 38.1

Dose-response curves plotting the therapeutic effect as a function of increasing the dose often calculated as the log of the dose. Drug A has a linear dose response, drugs B and C have sigmoidal curves, and drug D has a curvilinear dose-response curve. Although doses of drug B are more potent than are equal doses of drug C, drug C has a higher maximum efficacy than does drug B. Drug D has a therapeutic window, such that both low and high doses are less effective than are midrange doses.

38.33 The answer is D

The basic rule is to avoid administering any drug to a woman who is pregnant (particularly during the first trimester) or who is breast-feeding a child. This rule, however, occasionally needs to be broken when the mother's psychiatric disorder is severe. Of the drug treatments listed (Haldol, Prozac, and Ativan), *lithium would be considered the most potentially teratogenic* due to its association with abnormalities such as Ebstein's malformation, a serious abnormality in cardiac development. Anticonvulsant agents, especially valproic acid, are also considered to have high potential teratogenic effects. Other psychoactive drugs (antidepressants, antipsychotics, and anxiolytics) are less clearly associated with birth defects but should also be avoided during pregnancy if at all possible. The most common clinical situation occurs when a pregnant woman becomes psychotic. If a decision is made not to terminate the pregnancy, treatment with antipsychotic drugs or *electroconvulsive therapy (ECT)* may be preferable to lithium.

The administration of psychotherapeutic drugs at or near delivery may cause the baby to be overly sedated, thus requiring a respirator, or to be physically dependent on the drug, requiring detoxification and the treatment of a withdrawal syndrome. Virtually all psychiatric drugs are secreted in the milk of a nursing mother; therefore, mothers on those agents should be advised not to breast-feed their infants.

38.34 The answer is E

Most psychotherapeutic drugs neither affect a single neurotransmitter system nor are their effects localized to the brain. The effects of psychotherapeutic drugs on neurotransmitter systems result in a wide range of adverse effects associated with their use. For example, some of the most common adverse effects of psychotherapeutic drugs are caused by the blockade of muscarinic acetylcholine receptors (Table 38.1). Many psychotherapeutic

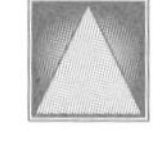

Table 38.1
Potential Adverse Effects Caused by Blockade of Muscarinic Acetylcholine Receptors

Blurred vision
Constipation
Decreased salivation
Decreased sweating
Delayed or retrograde ejaculation
Delirium
Exacerbation of asthma (through decreased bronchial secretions)
Hyperthermia (through decreased sweating)
Memory problems
Narrow-angle glaucoma
Photophobia
Sinus tachycardia
Urinary retention

drugs antagonize dopaminergic, histaminergic, or adrenergic receptors, resulting in adverse effects.

Orthostatic hypotension is caused by the blockade of α_1-adrenergic receptors. It is necessary to warn patients of this possible adverse effect, particularly if patients are elderly. The risk of hip fracture from falls is significantly elevated in patients who are taking psychotropic drugs. With patients at high risk of experiencing orthostatic hypotension, the clinician should choose a drug with low α_1-adrenergic activity. The patient can be instructed to get up slowly and to sit down immediately if dizziness is experienced. The patient can also try support hose to help reduce venous pooling of blood.

The blockade of muscarinic acetylcholine receptors causes *mydriasis (pupillary dilation)* and cycloplegia (ciliary muscle paresis), resulting in presbyopia (blurred near vision). The symptom can be relieved by cholinomimetic eye drops. A 1-percent solution of pilocarpine can be prescribed as one drop in each eye four times daily; bethanechol can be used for dry mouth as an alternative. *Photophobia* is another side effect.

The anticholinergic activity of many psychiatric drugs can lead to *urinary hesitation, dribbling, and retention*, as well as an increased rate of urinary tract infections. Elderly male patients with enlarged prostate glands are at increased risk for such adverse effects; 10 to 30 mg of bethanechol three to four times daily is usually effective in the treatment of the adverse effects on urination.

The use of psychiatric drugs can be associated with sexual dysfunction—decreased libido, *impaired ejaculation* and erection, and inhibition of female orgasm. Although warning patients about these adverse effects may increase their concern, they are not likely to report sexual dysfunction spontaneously to the physician.

38.35 The answer is C

CYP 2D6 isoenzyme inhibition or induction can alter drug metabolism. This has taken on increased importance with the advent of potent inhibitors (e.g., fluoxetine and paroxetine [Paxil]) and potent inducers (e.g., carbamazepine), many of which are commonly used for various psychiatric disorders. Individuals can be genotyped for CYP 2D6 activity by use of polymerase chain reaction (PCR) techniques. *SSRIs plus clozapine lead to increased clozapine concentration.*

38.36 The answer is A

Increased lithium concentrations are associated with drug interactions including *furosemide, salt restriction, indomethacin*, and *ibuprofen*, but not *theophylline*, which decreases lithium concentrations.

38.37 The answer is C

The benzodiazepines share a common effect on benzodiazepine receptors, which in turn modulate gamma-aminobutyric acid (GABA) activity. Diazepam has a very long half life and is, therefore, an example of a long-acting benzodiazepine. *There are some data that suggest benzodiazepines are teratogenic; therefore, their use in pregnancy may be ill-advised.* In addition, they can precipitate a withdrawal syndrome in the newborn, which makes the third trimester an equally complicated time for benzodiazepine administration. *Zolpidem can produce a mild withdrawal syndrome lasting one day after prolonged use at higher therapeutic doses. It is not associated with a development of tolerance to its sedative effects. Ramelteon is a new treatment for insomnia that specifically targets the melatonin MT1 and MT2 receptors in the brain's suprachiasmatic nucleus (SCN).*

38.38 The answer is A

Table 38.2 lists some of the important selected valproate interactions.

38.39 The answer is B

The overuse of prophylactic anticholinergic medications has been the subject of numerous studies, prospective and retrospective. Recent prospective studies using lower doses of antipsychotics demonstrate a 20.9 to 33 percent incidence of acute dystonic reactions in patients receiving no prophylaxis. With increased dosages of higher-potency antipsychotics, the incidence of dystonia rose to 47 percent. Regardless of antipsychotic dosage, over 90 percent of all dystonic reactions reported in various studies occur within the first 3 days of treatment. The trends toward higher incidence among younger patients and those of male sex were observed in most studies. In particular, one retrospective study revealed a markedly higher incidence of acute dystonia in the 10- to 19-year-old group (65 percent) than in 20- to 29-year-olds (46 percent) and 30- to 39-year-olds (32 percent). These combined data suggest that *only when sufficient*

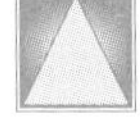

Table 38.2
Selected Valproate Interactions

Drug	Interaction	Type of Data[a]	Management
Phenobarbital	Increased concentration of phenobarbital	1	Reduce dosage of phenobarbital
Mg/Al hydroxide	Increased valproate levels	1	Reduce dosage of valproate if adverse effects occur
Carbamazepine	Decreased valproate levels and potential increased carbamazepine metabolites	1	Dosage adjustments as appropriate
Aspirin	Increased free valproate levels	2	High or chronic dosage of aspirin or naproxen should be used with prudence
Lamotrigine	Increased lamotrigine levels; increased incidence of Stevens-Johnson syndrome	2	Avoid, or use low doses of lamotrigine
Clonazepam	Increased sedation	2	Concurrent use usually uneventful
Fluoxetine	Increased valproate levels	4	Awareness and monitor

[a]1, In vivo studies, well established; 2, multiple case reports and/or based on related compounds; 3, in vitro studies; 4, isolated case report. Adapted from Steffens DC, Krishnan RR, Doraiswamy PM. *Psychotropic Drug Interactions*. New York: MBL Communications; 1998.

dosages (>12 mg a day of haloperidol or its equivalent) of *high-potency antipsychotics are required* in a group at high risk by age and sex—neither *young women* nor *elderly patients*—should anticholinergic prophylaxis be entertained on a routine basis. *The anticholinergic dosage should be tapered during the second week of treatment (not used past the second week)* unless the emergence of further extrapyramidal effects warrants continuation.

A consensus statement of the World Health Organization (WHO) published in 1990 summarizes this position:

On the basis of these considerations, the prophylactic use of anticholinergics in patients on neuroleptic treatment is not recommended and may be justified only early in treatment (after which it should be discontinued and its need should be reevaluated). As a rule, these compounds *should be used only when Parkinsonism has actually developed, (not prior to side effects such as Parkinsonism activity)* and when other measures, such as the reduction on neuroleptic dosage or the substitution of the administered drug by another less prone to induce Parkinsonism, have proven ineffective.

38.40 The answer is D

Case reports and uncontrolled trials suggest that gabapentin facilitates stabilization of mood cycling and helps control manic episodes. In almost all reports, gabapentin is used adjunctively. These reports involve patients with different bipolar disorders (bipolar I disorder, bipolar II disorder, cyclothymic disorder, and bipolar disorder not otherwise specified) who have failed to achieve adequate control with lithium (Eskalith, Lithobid), valproate, or carbamazepine. While there are reports that gabapentin may treat the depressive phase of bipolar disorder with a lower liability for induction of mania or mood cycling than with an antidepressant, apparent mania or cycling has been reported after initiation of gabapentin treatment. Gabapentin may be more (not less) useful in patients with bipolar II disorder than in those with bipolar I disorder.

In contrast to an unusually large amount of highly positive open-label data and many spontaneous case reports, no placebo-controlled trials confirm the efficacy of gabapentin for bipolar disorders as either monotherapy or adjunctive therapy. It has been suggested that the observed benefits of gabapentin therapy in bipolar patients may differ qualitatively from those associated with conventional mood-stabilizing agents, perhaps reflecting secondary anxiolytic or antiagitation properties.

Gabapentin is mildly sedating and normalizes sleep. It can be given at bedtime as an alternative to benzodiazepine agonists or other hypnotic drugs. Withdrawal symptoms and craving that accompany discontinuation of benzodiazepines, alcohol, and cocaine may be helped by gabapentin. *Abrupt discontinuation of gabapentin does not cause a withdrawal syndrome.*

The most frequent side effects of gabapentin are sedation, dizziness, and ataxia, which tend to be mild and transient. Lower-extremity edema has been noted. Because gabapentin is almost exclusively eliminated through the kidneys, patients with renal impairment should be monitored closely. There is no serious toxicity with gabapentin overdose.

Gabapentin does not interact with hepatic enzymes and neither inhibits nor induces them.

38.41 The answer is C

Zolpidem is a hypnotic that acts at the γ-aminobutyric acid (GABA)-benzodiazepine complex as the benzodiazepines do, but it is not itself a benzodiazepine. The drug *lacks* the *muscle-relaxant effects* that are common to the benzodiazepines.

Zolpidem is rapidly and well absorbed after oral administration, and *it reaches peak plasma levels in about 2 to 3 hours (not 4 to 6 hours).* Zolpidem has a half-life of about 2 1/2 hours and is metabolized primarily by conjugation.

The sole indication at this time for zolpidem is as a hypnotic. Several studies have found an absence of rebound REM after the use of the compound for the induction of sleep. The comparatively few data available indicate that *zolpidem may not be associated with rebound insomnia* after the discontinuation of its use for short periods.

Because of the short half-life of zolpidem, clinicians may reasonably evaluate a patient for the possibility of anterograde amnesia and anxiety the day after its administration, although neither of these adverse effects has been reported. Emesis and dysphoric reactions have been reported as adverse effects. Tolerance and dependence have been reported in less than 1 percent of patients, and the withdrawal symptoms are similar to those described for benzodiazepines. Zolpidem is secreted in breast milk and is, therefore, *contraindicated for use by nursing mothers.* The dosage of zolpidem should be reduced in patients with renal and hepatic impairment.

38.42 The answer is E (all)

ECT has multiple effects on brain function that are responsible for both its therapeutic and adverse actions. If changes in only certain regions of the CNS are required for therapeutic benefits, it may be possible to develop stimulation paradigms that target these areas. Such treatments could have great advantages in avoiding many of the unwanted effects of ECT, perhaps including cognitive impairment. Transcranial magnetic stimulation (TMS) is one such treatment. In neurology, TMS has been *developed as a way to stimulate the CNS noninvasively* by application of a focal magnetic field over regions of the cortex. Refinements of magnetic stimulators, including the development of stimulators capable of discharging at frequencies up to 60 Hz (referred to as rapid-rate TMS [rTMS]) have allowed focal stimulation of the CNS to estimate motor thresholds and determine hemispheric language dominance. Interestingly, rTMS was found to benefit some patients with Parkinson's disease, and some Parkinson's disease patients exhibited improved mood following rTMS. Additionally, subjects exposed to rTMS for purposes of determining hemispheric language dominance exhibited affective responses following stimulation of the left frontal cortex.

These observations suggest that rTMS may have therapeutic potential in psychiatry and may allow focal stimulation of areas most involved in affective states. Although experience with rTMS in psychiatry is limited, some evidence suggests that depending on the placement of the magnetic coil, rTMS can improve or worsen affective state. In one of the best studies to date, left dorsolateral prefrontal cortex stimulation significantly improved depression ratings in 11 of 17 patients with psychotic major depression. rTMS appears to be well tolerated and *does not require general anesthesia. Seizures* may be a side effect in some patients but *do not appear to be required for therapeutic effects.*

TMS is performed using a high-speed magnetic stimulator that generates a 1.5 to 2.5 Tesla field for brief periods. This field is similar to that used for nuclear magnetic resonance imaging. rTMS stimulus is delivered at frequencies of 10 to 60 Hz using a figure-8-shaped coil that is placed over the desired region of the skull and cooled continuously with water to prevent overheating. Patients and staff usually wear earplugs because of the noise generated by the stimulator. Stimulation is typically given several times per session and is repeated over several days to weeks. *At present, optimal stimulation patterns for rTMS in psychiatric disorders are not known.*

38.43 The answer is A

Dantrolene (Dantrium) is a direct-acting skeletal muscle relaxant. The only indication for dantrolene in contemporary clinical psychiatry is as one of the potentially effective treatments for *neuroleptic malignant syndrome, catatonia,* and *serotonin syndrome*. It is also used to treat *malignant hyperthermia*, an adverse effect of general anesthesia that bears a clinical resemblance to neuroleptic malignant syndrome. Dantrolene has no other uses in psychiatry and *is not used to treat acute mania.*

Dantrolene produces skeletal muscle relaxation by directly affecting the contractile response of the muscles at a site beyond the myoneural junction. Specifically, dantrolene dissociates excitation-contraction coupling by interfering with the release of calcium from the sarcoplasmic reticulum. The skeletal muscle relaxant effect is the basis of its efficacy in reducing the muscle destruction and hyperthermia associated with neuroleptic malignant syndrome.

The primary psychiatric indication for intravenous (IV) dantrolene is muscle rigidity in neuroleptic malignant syndrome. Dantrolene is almost always used in conjunction with appropriate supportive measures and a dopamine receptor agonist such as bromocriptine (Parlodel). If all available case reports and studies are summarized, about 80 percent of patients with neuroleptic malignant syndrome who received dantrolene apparently benefited clinically from the drug. Muscle relaxation and a general and dramatic improvement in symptoms can appear within minutes of IV administration, although in most cases the positive effects can take several hours to appear. Some evidence indicates that dantrolene treatment must be continued for a period of time, perhaps days to a week or more, to minimize the risk of the recurrence of symptoms, although the data for that clinical opinion are limited. Dantrolene has been used in efforts to treat other psychiatric conditions characterized by life-threatening muscle rigidity, such as catatonia and serotonin syndrome.

38.44 The answer is D

The dopamine hypothesis of schizophrenia grew from the observations that drugs that block dopamine receptors (such as haloperidol) have antipsychotic activity and drugs that stimulate dopamine activity (such as *amphetamines*) can, when given in high enough doses, induce psychotic symptoms in nonschizophrenic persons. The dopamine hypothesis remains the leading neurochemical hypothesis for schizophrenia, but room is being made for a role for serotonin, based on the therapeutic success of the serotonin-dopamine antagonists, such as clozapine. Schizophrenia is now thought to result from misregulation of both dopamine and serotonin function. It is likely that the theories will have to be reconceived several times in the near future as agents become available for modification of particular receptor subtypes. Clozapine has relatively low potency as a dopamine type 2 (D_2) receptor antagonist. Clozapine has much higher potency as an antagonist at D_1, D_3, and D_4, serotonin type 2 (5-HT_2), and noradrenergic α-receptors (especially α_1). Clozapine also has intermediate antagonist activity at muscarinic and histamine type 1 (H_1) receptors. *Clozapine is one of the most effective antipsychotic drugs,* and its unique pharmacodynamic profile has indicated that dopamine is not the only neurotransmitter system involved in the etiology of schizophrenia. In animal models, clozapine appears more active in the mesolimbic system than in the striatonigral system, which correlates with the lack of parkinsonian side effects.

Evidence in support of the dopamine hypothesis of schizophrenia is as follows. The *potency of dopamine receptor antagonist drugs to reduce psychotic symptoms* is most closely correlated with the affinity of these drugs for D_2 receptors. The mechanism of therapeutic action for dopamine receptor antagonist drugs is hypothesized to be through D_2 receptor antagonism, thus preventing endogenous dopamine from activating the receptors. Neuroanatomists have defined two major dopamine tracts, the mesolimbic to cortical (mostly frontal lobe) projection and the substantia nigra to striatum projection. Studies using the *PET technique* in patients who were taking a variety of dopamine receptor antagonists in different dosages have produced data indicating that *occupancy of about 60 percent of the D_2 receptors* in the caudate-putamen is correlated with clinical response and that occupancy of more than 70 percent of the D_2 receptors is correlated with the development of extrapyramidal symptoms.

Another positive association between the clinical efficacy of dopamine receptor antagonists and their dopamine receptor activity is suggested by the effects of the drugs on the plasma concentrations of homovanillic acid, the major metabolite of dopamine. Several studies have reported that high pretreatment concentrations of plasma homovanillic acid are positively correlated with an increased likelihood of a favorable clinical response. Furthermore, *a decrease in plasma homovanillic acid concentrations* early in the course of treatment is correlated with a favorable clinical response.

38.45 The answer is A

Indications for which there is evidence of efficacy for the SSRIs are *general anxiety disorder, panic disorder, trichotillomania,* and *premature ejaculation*. It's main indication is for depression. *It is used in ADHD only to treat a comorbid condition such as depression*. It has also been prescribed for obsessive compulsive disorder, Tourette's disorder, paraphilia, and chronic fatigue syndrome.

38.46 The answer is D

The use of the β-adrenergic receptor antagonists is best supported for neuroleptic-induced acute *akathisia*, lithium-induced postural tremor, and social phobia. The data on the use of these drugs as adjuncts to benzodiazepines for alcohol withdrawal and for the control of impulsive aggression or violence are also promising.

Neuroleptic-induced acute akathisia is recognized in the revised fourth edition of *Diagnostic and Statistical Manual of Mental Disorders* (DSM-IV-TR) as one of the medication-induced movement disorders. Many studies have shown that β-adrenergic receptor antagonists can be effective in the treatment of neuroleptic-induced acute akathisia. The majority of clinicians and researchers believe that β-adrenergic receptor antagonists are more effective for this indication than are anticholinergics and benzodiazepines, although the relative efficacy of those agents may vary among patients. However, the clinician must realize that the β-adrenergic receptor antagonists are not effective in the treatment of such neuroleptic-induced movement disorders as acute dystonia and Parkinsonism. Propranolol has been most studied for neuroleptic-induced acute akathisia, and at least one study has reported that a less lipophilic compound was not effective in the treatment of the disorder. There does not appear to be a clear superiority of β_1-selective versus nonselective agents for this indication.

Propranolol has been reported to be useful as an adjuvant to benzodiazepines but not as a sole agent in the treatment of *alcohol withdrawal.* One study used the following dose schedule: no propranolol for a pulse less than 50; 50 mg propranolol for a pulse between 50 and 79; and 100 mg propranolol for a pulse equal to or greater than 80. The patients who received propranolol and benzodiazepines had less severe withdrawal symptoms, more stable vital signs, and a shorter hospital stay than did the patients who received only benzodiazepines.

Propranolol has been well studied for the treatment of social phobia, primarily of the performance type (for example, disabling anxiety before a musical performance), but data are also available for their use in treatment of social phobia, *panic disorder*, posttraumatic stress disorder, and *generalized anxiety disorder*. Use of β-adrenergic receptor antagonists for panic disorder, generalized anxiety disorder, and *psychogenic seizures* is less efficacious than the use of benzodiazepines or selective serotonin reuptake inhibitors.

38.47 The answer is C

Lithium is the most commonly used agent for treatment of a *first manic episode* because it is generally the most effective drug for this purpose. Almost two dozen well-controlled studies, however, have shown that carbamazepine is effective in the treatment of acute mania, with efficacy comparable to lithium and antipsychotics. About ten studies have also shown that carbamazepine is effective in the prophylaxis of both manic and depressive episodes in bipolar I disorder when it is used for prophylactic treatment. Carbamazepine is an effective antimanic agent in 50 to 70 percent of all patients. Additional evidence from those studies indicates that carbamazepine may be effective in some patients who are not responsive to lithium, such as patients with *dysphoric mania, rapid cycling,* or a *negative family history of mood disorders.* However, a few clinical and basic science data indicate that some patients may experience a tolerance for the antimanic effects of carbamazepine. Because lithium toxicity may produce convulsions, carbamazepine may be a preferred drug for patients with *comorbid seizure disorders.*

38.48 The answer is B

Dopamine receptor antagonists are often used in combination with antimanic drugs to treat psychosis or manic excitement in bipolar I disorder. Although *lithium, carbamazepine,* and *valproate* are the drugs of choice for that condition, these drugs generally have a slower onset of action than do dopamine receptor antagonists, such as *haloperidol*, in the treatment of the acute symptoms. Thus, the general practice is to use combination therapy at the initiation of treatment and to gradually withdraw the dopamine receptor antagonist after the antimanic agent has reached its onset of activity. *Risperidone* lacks the anticholinergic and antihistamine activities that contribute to the calming effects of the dopamine receptor antagonists, and it is not as effective as haloperidol for the treatment of acute mania.

38.49 The answer is B

Secondary psychoses are psychotic syndromes that are associated with an identified organic cause, such as a brain tumor, a dementing disorder (such as dementia of the Alzheimer's type), or substance abuse. The dopamine receptor antagonist drugs are generally effective in the treatment of psychotic symptoms that are associated with those syndromes. The high-potency dopamine receptor antagonists, such as *fluphenazine*, are usually safer than the low-potency dopamine receptor antagonists, such as *chlorpromazine, mesoridazine, sulpiride* (not available in the US or Canada), and *thioridazine*, in such patients because of the high-potency drugs' lower cardiotoxic, epileptogenic, and anticholinergic activities. However, dopamine receptor antagonist drugs should not be used to treat withdrawal symptoms associated with ethanol or barbiturates because of the risk that such treatment will facilitate the development of withdrawal seizures. The drug of choice in such cases is usually a benzodiazepine. Agitation and psychosis associated with such neurological conditions as dementia of the Alzheimer's type are responsive to antipsychotic treatment; high- potency drugs and low dosages are generally preferable. Even with high-potency drugs, as many as 25 percent of elderly patients may experience episodes of hypotension. Low dosages of high-potency drugs, such as 0.5 to 5 mg a day of haloperidol, are usually sufficient for the treatment of those patients.

38.50 The answer is B

Anticholinergics have not been shown to be effective for treatment of *Huntington's chorea.* In the clinical practice of psychiatry, the anticholinergic drugs and amantadine (Symmetrel), like the antihistamines, have their primary use as treatments for medication-induced movement disorders, particularly *neuroleptic-induced Parkinsonism, neuroleptic-induced acute dystonia,* and *medication-induced postural tremor.* The anticholinergic drugs and amantadine may also be of limited use in the treatment of neuroleptic-induced acute akathisia. Before the introduction of levodopa (Larodopa), the anticholinergic drugs were commonly used in the treatment of *idiopathic Parkinson's disease*. The antiparkinsonian effects of amantadine, which was initially developed as an antiviral compound, were discovered when its use improved the parkinsonian symptoms of a patient who was being treated with amantadine for influenza A2.

All of the available anticholinergics and amantadine are equally effective in the treatment of parkinsonian symptoms, although the efficacy of amantadine may diminish in some patients within the first month of treatment. Amantadine may be more effective than the anticholinergics in the treatment of rigidity and tremor. Amantadine may also be the drug of choice if a clinician does not want to add more anticholinergic drugs to a patient's treatment regimen, particularly if a patient is taking an antipsychotic or an antidepressant with high anticholinergic activity—such as chlorpromazine (Thorazine) or amitriptyline (Elavil)—or is elderly and therefore at risk for anticholinergic adverse effects.

Neuroleptic-induced acute dystonia is most common in young men. The syndrome often occurs early in the course of treatment and is commonly associated with high-potency antipsychotics, such as haloperidol. The dystonia most commonly affects the muscles of the neck, the tongue, the face, and the back. Opisthotonos (involving the entire body) and oculogyric crises (involving the muscles of the eyes) are examples of specific dystonias. Dystonias are uncomfortable, sometimes painful, and often frightening to the patient. The onset is often sudden and frequently results in patients complaining about having a thick tongue or difficulty in swallowing. Dystonic contraction can be powerful enough to dislocate joints, and laryngeal dystonias can result in suffocation if the patient is not treated immediately.

38.51 The answer is C

Donepezil, rivastigmine, galantamine and tacrine are cholinesterase inhibitors used for the treatment of mild to moderate cognitive impairment in dementia of the Alzheimer's type. They reduce the inactivation of the neurotransmitter acetylcholine and thus potentiate cholinergic neurotransmission, which in turn produces a modest improvement in memory and goal-directed thought. *Donepezil appears to be selectively active, inhibiting acetyl-cholinesterases within the CNS* and with relatively little activity in the periphery. Memantine is not a cholinesterase inhibitor. It produces its effects by blocking *N*-methyl-D-aspartate (NMDA) receptors. Tacrine is rarely used because of its multiple daily dosing regimen and its potential for hepatotoxicity. It has the potential to cause significant elevations in hepatic transaminase levels in 25 percent to 30 percent of people. Rivastigmine is generally well tolerated and does not appear to cause hepatic, renal or hematologic abnormalities. Only memantine, not donepezil, is approved in the United States for use in moderate to severe Alzheimer's disease.

38.52 The answer is A

Mirtazepine is highly sedating, making it a good choice for use in depressed patients with severe or long-standing insomnia. It also has the tendency to *cause a sometimes ravenous appetite.* It is known to lower the neutrophil count, but this is reversible. *Mirtazapine does not increase the risk for seizures. It is more likely to reduce rather than cause nausea* because of its effects on serotonin 5-HT3 receptors.

39

Child Psychiatry: Assessment, Examination, and Psychological Testing

Psychiatric evaluation of a child is initiated to develop a formulation of the child's overall functioning including long-standing and current behavioral and emotional difficulties. It is essential to assess the developmental patterns of a child during an evaluation, because psychiatric disorders in this age group often emerge as a failure to achieve developmental milestones. Developmental considerations include expected skills in social, motor, language, and intellectual domains. During the evaluation, the clinician must integrate the contributions of many different factors that have affected the child, including biological growth and health, mood and behavioral symptoms, and family, school, and environmental factors. At the end of the evaluation, the extent to which the child's development has not met expectations for his or her chronological age is determined, and the degree of impairment due to behavioral and emotional factors is established. In addition, an assessment of environmental factors that may either exacerbate or improve the child's overall functioning is considered.

A comprehensive evaluation of a child includes interviews with the parents, the child, and other family members; gathering information regarding the child's current school functioning; and often, a standardized assessment of the child's intellectual level and academic achievement. In some cases, standardized measures of developmental level and neuropsychological assessments are useful. Psychiatric evaluations of children are rarely initiated by the child, so clinicians must obtain information from the family and the school to understand the reasons for the evaluation. In some cases, the court, or a child protective service agency may initiate a psychiatric evaluation. Children can be excellent informants about symptoms related to mood and inner experiences such as psychotic phenomena, sadness, fears, and anxiety, but they often have difficulty with the chronology of symptoms and are sometimes reticent about reporting behaviors that have gotten them into trouble. Very young children often cannot articulate their experiences verbally and do better showing their feelings and preoccupations in a play situation.

The student should study the questions and answers below for a useful review of this field.

HELPFUL HINTS

The student should be able to define these terms.

- AAMD
- achievement tests
- adaptive functioning
- Bayley Infant Scale of Development
- borderline intellectual functioning
- Cattell Infant Scale
- Child Behavior Checklist
- chromosomal abnormality
- *cri-du-chat* syndrome
- developmental tests
- DISC-R (Diagnostic Interview Schedule for Children-Revised)
- Down's syndrome
- fragile X syndrome
- intelligence quotient (IQ)
- K-SADS (Kiddie Schedule for Affective Disorders and Schizophrenia)
- Lesch-Nyhan syndrome
- mental deficiency
- mental retardation
- neurofibrillary tangles
- neurofibromatosis
- nondisjunction
- PKU
- Prader-Willi syndrome
- prenatal exposure
- rubella
- Turner's syndrome
- Vineland Adaptive Behavior Scales
- WHO
- WISC-III (Wechsler Intelligence Scale for Children—Third Edition)

QUESTIONS

Directions

Each question or incomplete statement below is followed by five suggested responses or completions. Select the *one* that is *best* in each case.

39.1 Which of the following statements about the distinctive features of child psychopathology is *true*?

A. Co-existence of more than one psychiatric diagnosis is rare in children.
B. Depression commonly presents with excessive guilt, hopelessness, and anhedonia in children.
C. Emotional disturbances in childhood are characterized by specific, pathognomonic symptoms.
D. Fears, tantrums, or moodiness are relatively common in children and occur transiently at different stages.
E. None of the above

39.2 Which of the following tools is considered most appropriate to facilitate the play component of an interview?

A. Stock characters (such as Barbie or Disney figures)
B. Elaborate toys
C. Puppets
D. Chess
E. Video games

39.3 Projective techniques include

A. Picture drawing
B. Asking the child to name three wishes
C. Asking the child to tell about a dream, a book, a movie, or a TV program
D. Sentence completion task
E. All of the above

39.4 Structured assessment instruments for infants and young children

A. yield diagnoses
B. include the Denver Developmental Screening Test (Denver II) and the Bayley Scales
C. are highly reliable in predicting later performance on IQ assessment
D. show only fair reliability and validity
E. all of the above

39.5 Of the following diagnostic laboratory tests used in evaluation of children presenting with psychiatric problems, the one most likely to impact ultimate diagnosis is:

A. Computed Tomography (CT) scan
B. Thyroid Function Test
C. Magnetic Resonance Imaging (MRI)
D. Positron Emission Tomography (PET)
E. Chromosomal Analysis

Directions

Each group of questions below consists of lettered headings followed by a list of numbered phrases or statements. For each numbered phrase or statement, select the *one* lettered heading that is most closely associated with it. Each lettered heading may be selected once, more than once, or not at all.

Questions 39.6–39.10

A. Vineland Adaptive Behavior Scales
B. Children's Apperception Test (CAT)
C. Wide-Range Achievement Test-Revised (WRAT-R)
D. Peabody Picture Vocabulary Test-Revised (PPVT-R)
E. Wechsler Intelligence Test for Children-Third Edition (WISC-III)

39.6 Measures receptive word understanding, with resulting standard scores, percentiles, and age equivalents

39.7 Measures communication, daily living skills, socialization, and motor development, yielding a composite expressed in a standard score, percentile, and age equivalents

39.8 Generates stories from picture cards of animals that reflect interpersonal functioning

39.9 Measures functioning in reading, spelling, and arithmetic, with resulting grade levels, percentiles, and standard scores

39.10 Measures verbal, performance, and full-scale ability, with scaled subset scores permitting specific skill assessment

Questions 39.11–39.15

Which test would be most helpful in the psychiatric evaluation of a child presenting with the symptoms described in the cases below?

A. WISC-III
B. Child Behavior Checklist (CBCL)
C. Children's Apperception Test (CAT)
D. Woodcock-Johnson Psycho-Educational Battery-Revised (W-J)
E. Bayley Scales of Infant Development II

39.11 A 6-year-old boy is highly aggressive and becomes very angry when he doesn't get his way. He has always been prone to severe tantrums and has difficulty with his behavior and mood in school. At home, he is considered manageable, although he seems to have a short attention span. He breaks new toys in a matter of minutes. He is unable to play with peers because of frequent fights.

39.12 A 9-year-old girl is clingy with her mother and will not speak to strangers. She is willing to answer specific questions but not to describe her thoughts or feelings. When she is stressed, she tends to withdraw and become tearful. She seems to be unusually sensitive to criticism and will not join in a group activity.

39.13 A 7-year-old boy has a poor vocabulary and is noted to be unable to follow directions, as well as clumsy and slow. Although he is friendly and good-natured, he has been brutally picked on by peers, who say that he doesn't understand the rules of games. His teacher is concerned about his comprehension.

39.14 A 2-year-old boy has not yet begun to walk, speaks only 2 to 3 words, and often seems disinterested in his surroundings.

39.15 An 11-year-old girl is increasing struggling with academic performance, manifesting particular difficulty with mathematics concepts. She is otherwise functioning well, with excellent social skills and warm relationships with friends and family members. She recently had intelligence testing and scored within normal range in all subsets and in full-scale IQ.

Questions 39.16–39.19

A. Structured interviews
B. Semi-structured interviews
C. Both
D. Neither

39.16 Resemble clinical interviews more closely
39.17 K-SADS (Kiddie Schedule for Affective Disorders and Schizophrenia) and CAS (Child Assessment Scale)
39.18 Particularly appropriate for clinically based research in which subtle diagnostic distinctions may be critical for defining samples
39.19 Investigate issues of prevalence of disorders, developmental patterns of psychopathology, and psychosocial correlates of disorders

Directions

Each question or incomplete statement below is followed by five suggested responses or completions. Select the *one* that is *best* in each case.

39.20 Techniques that are helpful in eliciting information and feelings from a school-aged child include all of the following *except*

A. Asking multiple-choice questions
B. Asking the child to draw a family
C. Using Donald Winnicott's "squiggle game"
D. Using only open-ended questions
E. Using indirect commentary

39.21 Which of the following statements about personality tests for children is *true*?

A. Personality tests and tests of ability have equal reliability and validity.
B. Both the Children Apperception Test (CAT) and the Thematic Apperception Test (TAT) use pictures of people in situations.
C. The Rorschach test has not been developed for children or adolescents.
D. The Mooney Problem Checklist is a self-report inventory.
E. None of the above

39.22 Figure 39.1 is part of a series of drawings used to test children for

A. Response to frustration
B. Psychosis
C. Depression
D. Impulsivity
E. Anxiety

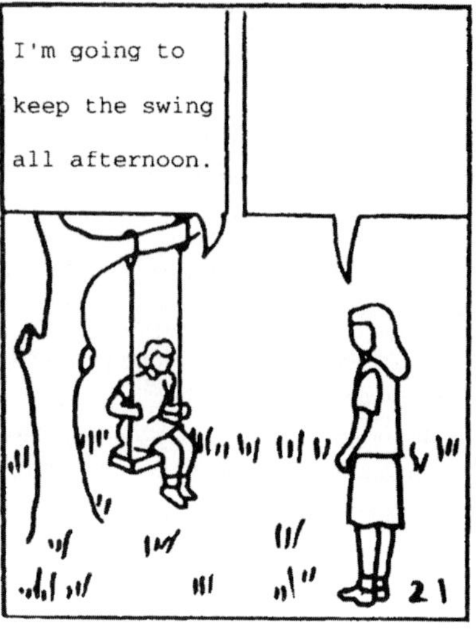

FIGURE 39.1
Courtesy of Saul Rosenzweig.

39.23 Neurological soft signs include all of the following *except*

A. Contralateral overflow movements
B. Learning disabilities
C. Asymmetry of gait
D. Nystagmus
E. Poor balance

39.24 Minor physical anomalies include all of the following *except*

A. Multiple hair whorls
B. Low-set ears
C. High-arched palate
D. Flattened philtrum
E. Persistent Babinski reflex

ANSWERS

39.1 The answer is D

The psychiatric assessment of the child requires a comprehensive approach that evaluates the child's developmental progress in various domains and positive adaptive capabilities, as well as the symptoms of specific disorders. A developmental approach to the assessment of the child is essential because children differ from adults in key respects.

Many children coming to clinical attention have difficulties that cannot be subsumed neatly under the rubric of a single diagnostic label. Thus, *comorbidity is usually not rare, but rather common in childhood disorders*. Even in epidemiological studies of children and adolescents, as many as half of those who meet diagnostic criteria for one disorder also meet criteria for at least one other disorder. This high rate of comborbidity, found even in nonreferred populations, may derive from the fact that predominant diagnostic concepts are drawn from experience with adults, and applicable descriptive boundaries may differ fundamentally in children.

Psychiatric disturbances in children often consist of a lack of developmental progress in one or more domains, rather than the presence of specific symptoms that are pathognomonic in the presentation of adult disorders. Children are typically referred for evaluation when developmental progress is being impeded, as in the case of a school-aged child whose inability to separate from her parents prevents her from participating fully in school.

Children's developmental status has significant impact on the presentation of a given illness. For example, *while adults and older adolescents may present with guilty feelings, hopelessness, and anhedonia as prominent features of a depressive episode, these symptoms are much rarer in depressed children*, who are more likely to manifest irritability, social withdrawal, and somatic complaints.

Oftentimes, clinical conditions represent severe manifestations of symptoms found in milder forms in non-referred children. *Fears, tantrums, and moodiness are relatively common in childhood* and occur transiently at different developmental stages. Assessment may be sought by concerned parents needing guidance in understanding and managing these symptoms. The clinician must judge whether the symptoms are likely to resolve with time and have minimal impact on functioning, or whether the level of distress and likely effect on the child and the family merit clinical intervention.

39.2 The answer is C

Children under 7 years of age have limited capacities to verbally recount their feelings or interpersonal interactions. For these younger children as well as a number of older ones, play is a useful adjunct to direct questioning and discussion and is often a less challenging mode for the child. Some children find it easier to communicate in displacement: thus, *imaginative play with puppets*, small figures, or dolls can provide the interviewer with useful inferential material about the child's concerns, perceptions, and characteristic modes of regulating affects and impulses.

The skilled interviewer will facilitate the child's engagement in play, without prematurely introducing speculations or reactions that might distort or cut short the presentation of certain types of material. During the course of play, the clinician follows the sequences of play content, noting themes that emerge, points at which a child backs away from a story or shifts to a new activity, and situations in which the child gets "stuck" or falls into a repetitive loop. To facilitate the play components of an interview, the interview room should have a supply of human and animal figures or dolls and appropriate props. These should be relatively simple, because *elaborate toys can serve as distractions* rather than as vehicles for expression. *Stock characters (such as Barbie or Disney figures) may impose their own specific story lines and thus limit access to the child's own concerns.*

The content of the child's play provides important details of the mental status examination. During imaginative play, the clinician observes the child's coordination and motor skills, speech and language development, attention, ability to relate, capacity for complex thought, and affective state. Absence of imaginative play or limited, concrete, non-interactive play may indicate a pervasive developmental disorder.

Games such as cards or board games are useful for putting the child at ease and establishing rapport. They also reveal a child's capacity for enjoyment, response to competitive situations, and proneness to cheating. Simple games permit conversation during play while discharging tension and diminishing the pressure of the interview situation. *More complex games such as chess should be avoided given their demand for concentration, which precludes conversation. Video games likewise tend to serve as an impediment to meaningful interaction.*

39.3 The answer is E (all)

Projective techniques, like imaginative play, provide indirect access to concerns that children may be unable or unwilling to express directly. These techniques may improve the child's level of comfort with the clinician, are often experienced as fun, and can provide important information for the diagnostic formulation.

Picture drawing is a commonly used technique. The child may be asked to draw any picture he or she likes, or may be given a specific suggestion. When the picture is nearly finished, the clinician may complement the child's efforts and express interest in the drawing. The child's elaboration often provides information that is not readily apparent in the drawing itself. The content and form of the drawing offer insight into the child's emotional concerns, as well as his/her intellectual and visual-motor capabilities. For example, the relative size, placement, or omission of certain family members may be important indicators of the child's feelings about the family. Aggressive or sexual themes may be more easily expressed in drawings than in words. The clinician should become familiar with developmental norms for depiction of human figures, which can provide a rough estimate of intellectual and visual-motor maturity. The child's behavior during this exercise may also be instructive (e.g., throwing the picture away unfinished and saying that it's no good).

Frequently utilized verbal projective techniques include *asking the child to name three wishes*; if elaboration is needed, the clinician can explain that the wishes could be to have anything, to change the world in any way, or to change themselves in any way. Children's responses are often revealing. Some may impulsively wish for material possessions, while others may reveal longings for distressing circumstances to change (e.g., "For my mom and dad to be together again"). Still others appear uncomfortable wishing for something for themselves, preferring to state altruistic wishes such as "no more wars." These responses may be starting points for further conversation in the interview. *Sentence completion tasks are another verbal projective technique*, in which the child is invited to share thoughts and feelings after being prompted by the clinician speaking the beginning of an open-ended sentence. For example, the clinician might begin, "My favorite thing about my family is . . ." or, "If I could change one thing at school, it would be . . ." The child is asked to complete the sentence, and these responses may provide telling windows into the child's inner life.

Asking the child to tell about a dream, book, movie, or television program can provide information about the child's interests and preoccupations, as well. If the clinician is familiar with the plot of a particular program, any distortions introduced by the child can be informative regarding the child's cognitive and emotional style.

39.4 The answer is B

A variety of instruments exist for the structured assessment of infants and young children, and each has somewhat different goals, theoretical orientation, and psychometric properties. *These instruments do not yield diagnoses*, but rather detail the child's developmental progress in various areas relative to a normative population. For example, the *Denver Developmental Screening Test (Denver II) is suitable for screening use* by pediatricians or trained paraprofessionals to help identify children with significant motor, social, or language delays requiring more complete evaluation. Population-specific norms are also available for assessing children from families of various ethnic or educational backgrounds. The *Bayley Scales of Infant Development II, which are administered by a trained assessor, can be used to evaluate children* 1 to 42 months of age, and include a mental scale (assessing information processing, habituation, memory, language, social skills, and cognitive strategies); a motor scale (assessing gross and fine motor skills); and a Behavior Rating Scale for assessing qualitative aspects of the child's behavior during the assessment. This well-standardized instrument yields standard scores for a Mental Development Index and Psychomotor Development index.

Although *tests like these show good (not fair) reliability and validity, their ability to predict later performance on IQ assessment or later adaptive functioning is highly variable.* Among the reasons for this weakness of prediction are the intervening effects of social and family environment and the heavy emphasis infant tests place on perceptual and motor skills that may have relatively little to do with information-processing abilities.

The mental status examination of the infant and young child may be organized using a schema such as that shown in Table 39.1.

39.5 The answer is E

The clinical utility and cost-effectiveness of routine laboratory and imaging studies of children presenting with psychiatric symptoms has not been thoroughly studied. Most guidelines for performing these tests for children derive from data from adult studies. Adult studies generally suggest that routine laboratory tests are not clinically useful in settings such as outpatient psychiatry clinics or most inpatient units. Diagnostic tests are of greater utility in certain psychiatric settings where patients are at higher risk for medical illness, such as the emergency room, substance abuse treatment settings, AIDS clinics, and geriatric clinics. Additionally, these tests are considered to be worthwhile in patients with first-onset psychosis, depression, mania, or dementia. Furthermore, routine laboratory screening is more likely to yield clinically useful information when signs or symptoms of physical illness are present.

The few studies of the use of routine diagnostic tests in child psychiatry populations have yielded similar conclusions. One review of routine laboratory screenings (*thyroid function tests*, electroencephalograms [EEG], chest X-ray, chemistry panel, urinalysis, complete blood count, electrocardiogram [EKG], and rapid plasma reagin [RPR]) in 100 consecutive adolescent inpatient admissions reported variable rates of abnormal values, depending on the specific test, but in only 1 of these 100 patients did the abnormal test result lead to a change in primary diagnosis. Most laboratory abnormalities in this study were regarded as inconsequential and did not indicate a need for clinical follow-up.

More specialized diagnostic evaluations (CT scan, MRI, EEG*) also appear to provide low yield of clinically useful information.* In a study of 200 consecutive child psychiatric inpatients, these evaluations were done only when "clinically indicated." However, despite their judicious use, the tests provided clinically relevant information in only 7 of 200 patients (3.5 percent). In the same sample population, *chromosomal analysis proved to be the most informative test*, yielding new medical diagnoses in 5 of 32 children on whom these analyses were performed (15.6 percent). A study of 111 putatively high-risk inpatients with new-onset adolescent psychoses produced similar results. In this population, routine endocrine and neuroimaging screening evaluations failed to provide information of diagnostic utility in any patient (although inconsequential laboratory abnormalities were precent in 15.4 percent of the endocrine screens and 11 percent of the neuroimaging screens). *More specialized neuroimaging techniques, such as positron emission tomography (PET),* single photon emission computed tomography (SPECT), and functional MRI (fMRI), *currently have no routine clinical or diagnostic utility in child and adolescent psychiatric populations.*

Answers 39.6–39.10

39.6 The answer is D

39.7 The answer is A

39.8 The answer is B

39.9 The answer is C

39.10 The answer is E

The Vineland Adaptive Behavior Scales are used to measure communication, daily living skills, socialization, and motor development, yielding a composite expressed in a standard score, percentile, and age equivalents. The scales are standardized for normal-intelligence and for mentally retarded individuals. A measure of adaptive functioning such as that derived from the Vineland, as well as a standardized measure of intelligence, is required when a diagnosis of mental retardation is being considered.

The Children's Apperception Test (CAT) is an adaptation for children of the Thematic Apperception Test (TAT). The CAT generates stories from picture cards of animals that reflect interpersonal functioning. The cards show ambiguous scenes related to family issues and relationships. The child is asked to describe what is happening in the scene and to tell a story about the outcome of the scene.

The Wide-Range Achievement Test-Revised (WRAT-R) measures functioning in reading, spelling, and arithmetic, with resulting grade levels, percentiles, and standard scores. It can be used in children 5 years of age and older, and the scores on the test can be compared with the average expected score for the child's chronological age and grade level.

The Peabody Picture Vocabulary Test-Revised (PPVT-R) measures receptive word understanding, with resulting standard scores, percentiles, and age equivalents. It can be used for children 4 years of age and older.

The Wechsler Intelligence Test for Children-Third Edition (WISC-III) measures verbal, performance, and full-scale ability, with scaled subset scores permitting specific skill assessment. In a full-scale intelligence quotient (IQ), 70 to 80 indicates borderline intelligence, 80 to 90 indicates low-average intelligence, 90 to 109 indicates average intelligence, and 110 to 119 indicates high-average intelligence. Table 39.2 lists some commonly used child and adolescent assessment instruments.

Table 39.1
Infant and Toddler Mental Status Exam by Anne L. Benham, M.D.

I. Appearance
Size, level of nourishment, dress and hygiene, apparent maturity compared with age, dysmorphic features (e.g., facies, eye and ear shape and placement, epicanthal folds, digits), abnormal head size, cutaneous lesions.

II. Apparent Reaction to Situation
Note where evaluation takes place and with whom.
- A. Initial reaction to setting and to strangers: explores; freezes; cries; hides face; acts curious, excited, apathetic, or anxious (describe).
- B. Adaptation
  1. Exploration: when and how child begins exploring faces, toys, strangers.
  2. Reaction to transitions: from unstructured to structured activity; when examiner begins to play with infant; cleaning up; leaving.

III. Self-Regulation
- A. State regulation: an infant's state of consciousness ranges from deep sleep through alert stages to intense crying. Predominant state and range of states observed during session; patterns of transition (e.g., smooth versus abrupt capacity for being soothed and self-soothing; capacity for quiet alert state). Some of these categories also apply to toddlers.
- B. Sensory regulation: reaction to sounds, sights, smells, light and firm touch; hyperresponsiveness or hyporesponsiveness (if observed) and type of response, including apathy, withdrawal, avoidance, fearfulness, excitability, aggression or marked behavioral change; excessive seeking of particular sensory input.
- C. Unusual behaviors; mouthing after 1 year of age; head banging; smelling objects; spinning; twirling; hand-flapping; finger-flicking; rocking; toe-walking; staring at lights or spinning objects; repetitive, perseverative, or bizarre verbalizations or behaviors with objects or people; hair-pulling; ruminating; or breath-holding.
- D. Activity level: overall level and variability (note that toddlers are often incorrectly called hyperactive). Describe behavior, e.g., squirming constantly in parent's arms; sitting quietly on floor or in infant seat; constantly on the go; climbing on desk and cabinets; exploring the room; pausing to play with each of six to eight toys.
- E. Attention span: capacity to maintain attentiveness to an activity or interaction; longest and average length of sustained attention to a given toy or activity; distractibility. Infants: visual fixing and following at 1 month; tracking at 2 to 3 months; attention to own hands or feet and faces; duration of exploration of object with hands or mouth.
- F. Frustration tolerance: ability to persist in a difficult task, despite failure; capacity to delay reaction if easily frustrated, e.g., aggression, crying, tantrums, withdrawal, avoidance.
- G. Aggression: modes of expression; degree of control of or preoccupation with aggression; appropriate assertiveness.

IV. Motor
Muscle tone and strength; mobility in different positions; unusual motor pattern (e.g., tics, seizure activity), intactness of cranial nerves (e.g., movement of face, mouth, tongue, and eyes, including feeding, swallowing, and gaze [note excessive drooling]).
- A. Gross motor coordination. Infants: pushing up; head control; rolling; sitting; standing. Toddlers: walking; running; jumping; climbing; hopping; kicking; throwing and catching a ball. (It is useful to have something for the child to climb on, such as a chair.)
- B. Fine motor coordination. Infants: grasping and releasing; transferring from hand to hand; using pincer grasp; banging; throwing. Toddlers: using pincer grasp; stacking; scribbling; cutting. Both fine motor and visual-motor coordination can be screened by observing how the child handles puzzles, shape boxes, a ball and hammer toy, small cars, and toys with connecting parts.

V. Speech and Language
- A. Vocalization and speech production: quality, rate, rhythm, intonation, articulation, volume.
- B. Receptive language: comprehension of others' speech as seen in verbal or behavioral response (e.g., follows commands); points in response to "where is" questions; understands prepositions and pronouns (include estimate of hearing, especially in child with language delay, e.g., response to loud sounds and voice; ability to localize sound).
- C. Expressive language: level of complexity (e.g., vocalization, jargon, number of single words, short phrases, full sentences); overgeneralization (e.g., uses "kitty" to refer to all animals); pronoun use including reversal; echolalia, either immediate or delayed; unusual or bizarre verbalizations. Preverbal children: communicative intent (e.g., vocalizations, babbling, imitation, gestures, such as head shaking and pointing); caregiver's ability to understand infant's communication; child's effectiveness in communication.

VI. Thought
The usual categories for thought disorder almost never apply to young children. Primary process thinking, as evidenced in verbalizations or play, is expected in this age group. The line between fantasy and reality is often blurred. Bizarre ideation; perseveration; apparent loose associations; and the persistence of pronoun reversals, jargon, and echolalia in an older toddler or preschooler may be noted in a variety of psychiatric disorders, including pervasive developmental disorders.
- A. Specific fears: feared object; worry about being lost or separated from parent.
- B. Dreams and nightmares: content is sometimes obtainable in children aged 2 to 3 years. Child does not always perceive it as a dream (e.g., "A monster came in the front door").
- C. Dissociative state: sudden episodes of withdrawal and inattention; eyes glazed; "tuned out"; failure to track ongoing social interaction. Dissociative state may be difficult to differentiate from an absence seizure, depression, autism, or deafness. The context may be helpful (e.g., child with a history of neglect freezes in a dissociative state as mother leaves room). Neurological or audiological evaluation may be warranted.
- D. Hallucinations: extremely rare, except in the context of a toxic or medical disorder, then usually visual or tactile.

(*continued*)

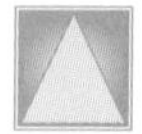

Table 39.1
(*continued*)

VII. Affect and Mood
The assessment of mood and affect may be more difficult in young children because of limited language; lack of vocabulary for emotions; and use of withdrawal in response to a variety of emotions from shyness and boredom to anxiety and depression.
A. Modes of expression: facial; verbal; body tone and positoining.
B. Range of expressed emotions: affect, especially in parent–child relationship.
C. Responsiveness: to situation, content of discussion, play, and interpersonal engagement.
D. Duration of emotional state: need history or multiple observations.
E. Intensity of expressed emotions: affect, especially in parent–child relationship.

VIII. Play
Play is a primary mode of information gathering for all sections of the Infant and Toddler Mental Status Exam. In very young children, play is especially useful in the evaluation of the child's cognitive and symbolic functioning, relatedness, and expression of affect. Themes of play are helpful in assessing older toddlers. The management and expression of aggression are assessed in play as in other areas of behavior. Play may be with toys or with child's own or another's body (e.g., peek-a-boo, roughhousing); verbal (e.g., sound imitation games between mother and infant); interactional or solitary. It is important to note how the child's play varies with different familiar caregivers and with parents versus the examiner.
A. Structure of play (ages approximate).
1. Sensorimotor play.
a. (0–12 months): mouthing, banging, dropping, and throwing toys or other objects.
b. (6–12 months): exploring characteristics of objects (e.g., moving parts, poking, pulling).
2. Functional play.
a. (12–18 months): child's use of objects shows understanding and exploration of their use or function (e.g., pushes car, touches comb to hair, puts telephone to ear).
3. Early symbolic play.
a. (18 months and older): child pretends with increasing complexity; pretends with own body to eat or sleep; pretends with objects or other people (e.g., "feeds" mother); child uses one object to represent another (e.g., a block becomes a car); child pretends a sequence of activities (e.g., cooking and eating).
4. Complex symbolic play.
a. (30 months and older): child plans and acts out dramatic play sequences, uses imaginary objects. Later, child incorporates others into play with assigned roles.
5. Imitation, turn taking, and problem solving as part of play.
B. Content of play. The toddler's choice and use of toys often reflect emotional themes. It is desirable to have on hand toys that tap different developmental and emotional domains. An overfull playroom may be overwhelming or overstimulating and reduce meaningful observations. Young toddlers of both sexes often gravitate to dolls, dishes, animals, and moving toys, such as cars. The examiner's choice of specific materials may facilitate the expression of pertinent emotional themes. For example, a child traumatized by a dog bite may more likely reenact the trauma if a dog and doll figures are available. The child's reaction to scary toys, such as sharks, dinosaurs, or guns, should be noted, especially if they are avoided or dominate the session. Does aggressive pretend play become "real" and physically hurtful? By age $2^1/_2$ to 3 years, a child's animal or doll play can reveal important themes about family life, including reactions to separation, parent–child and sibling relationships, experiences at day care, quality of nurturance and discipline, and physical or sexual abuse. The examiner must use caution in interpreting play, viewing it as a possible combination of reenactment, fears, and fantasy.

IX. Cognition
Using information from all above areas, especially play, verbal and symbolic functioning, and problem-solving, roughly assess child's cognitive level in terms of developmental intactness, delays, or precocity.

X. Relatedness
A. To parents: how in tune do the child and parent seem? Does the child make and maintain eye, verbal, or physical contact? Is there active avoidance by child? Note infant's level of comfort and relaxation being held, fed, "molding" into caregiver's body. Does toddler move away from caregiver and check back or bring toys to show, to put into his or her lap, to play with together or near caregiver? Comment on physical or verbal affection, hostility, reaction to separation and reunion, and use of transitional objects (blanket, toy, caregiver's possession). Describe differences in relating if more than one caregiver is present.
B. To examiner: young children normally show some hesitancy to engage with a stranger, especially after 6 to 8 months of age. Appropriate wariness in young children may result in a period of watching the examiner; staying physically close to a familiar caregiver before engaging; or showing some constriction of affect, vocalization, or play. After initial wariness, does the child relate? Does the child engage too soon or not at all? How does relatedness with a stranger compare to that with a parent? Is the child friendly versus indiscriminately attention-seeking, guarded versus overanxious? Can examiner engage the child in play or structured activities to a degree not seen with caregiver? Does the child show pleasure in successes if the examiner shows approval?
C. Attachment behaviors: observe for showing affection, comfort-seeking, asking for and accepting help, cooperating, exploring, controlling behavior, and reunion responses. Describe age-related disturbances in these normative behaviors. Disturbances often are seen in abused and neglected children, e.g., fearfulness, clinginess, overcompliance, hypervigilance, impulsive overactivity, and defiance; restricted or hyperactive and distractible exploratory behavior; and restricted or indiscriminate affection and comfort-seeking.

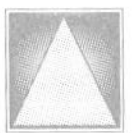

Table 39.2
Commonly Used Child and Adolescent Psychological Assessment Instruments

Test	Age/Grades	Data Generated and Comments
Intellectual ability		
Wechsler Intelligence Scale for Children—Third Edition (WISC-III-R)	6–16	Standard scores: verbal, performance and full-scale IQ: scaled subtest scores permitting specific skill assessment.
Wechsler Adult Intelligence Scale—(WAIS-III)	16–adult	Same as WISC-III-R.
Wechsler Preschool and Primary Scale of Intelligence—Revised (WPPSI-R)	3–7	Same as WISC-III-R.
Kaufman Assessment Battery for Children (K-ABC)	2.6–12.6	Well grounded in theories of cognitive psychology and neuropsychology. Allows immediate comparison of intellectual capacity with acquired knowledge. Scores: Mental Processing Composite (IQ equivalent); sequential and simultaneous processing and achievement standard scores; scaled mental processing and achievement subtest scores; age equivalents; percentiles.
Kaufman Adolescent and Adult Intelligence Test (KAIT)	11–85+	Composed of separate Crystallized and Fluid scales. Scores: Composite Intelligence Scale; Crystallized and Fluid IQ; scaled subtest scores; percentiles.
Stanford-Binet, 4th Edition (SB:FE)	2–23	Scores: IQ; verbal, abstract/visual, and quantitative reasoning; short-term memory; standard age.
Peabody Picture Vocabulary Test—III (PPVT-III)	4–adult	Measures receptive vocabulary acquisition; standard scores, percentiles, age equivalents.
Achievement		
Woodcock-Johnson Psycho-Educational Battery—Revised (W-J)	K–12	Scores: reading and mathematics (mechanics and comprehension), written language, other academic achievement; grade and age scores, standard scores, percentiles.
Wide Range Achievement Test—3, Levels 1 and 2 (WRAT-3)	Level 1: 1–5 Level 2: 12–75	Permits screening for deficits in reading, spelling, and arithmetic; grade levels, percentiles, stanines, standard scores.
Kaufman Test of Educational Achievement, Brief and Comprehensive Forms (K-TEA)	1–12	Standard scores: reading, mathematics, and spelling; grade and age equivalents, percentiles, stanines. Brief Form is sufficient for most clinical applications; Comprehensive Form allows error analysis and more detailed curriculum planning.
Wechsler Individual Achievement Test (WIAT)	K–12	Standard scores: basic reading, mathematics reasoning, spelling (constituting Screener); reading comprehension, numerical operations, listening comprehension, oral expression, written expression. Conormal with WISC-III-R.
Adaptive behavior		
Vineland Adaptive Behavior Scales	Normal: 0–19 Retarded: All ages	Standard scores: adaptive behavior composite and communication, daily living skills, socialization and motor domains; percentiles, age equivalents, developmental age scores. Separate standardization groups for normal, visually handicapped, hearing impaired, emotionally disturbed, and retarded.
Scales of Independent Behavior—Revised	Newborn–adult	Standard scores: five adaptive (motor, social interaction, communication, personal living, community living) and three maladaptive (internalized, asocial, and externalized) areas; General Maladaptive Index and Broad Independence cluster.
Attentional capacity		
Trail Making Test	8–adult	Standard scores, standard deviations, ranges; corrections for age and education.
Wisconsin Card Sorting Test	6.6–adult	Standard scores, standard deviations, T-scores, percentiles, developmental norms for number of categories achieved, perseverative errors, and failures to maintain set; computer measures.
Behavior Assessment System for Children (BASC)	4–18	Teacher and parent rating scales and child self-report of personality permitting multireporter assessment across a variety of domains in home, school, and community. Provides validity, clinical, and adaptive scales. ADHD component avails.
Home Situations Questionnaire—Revised (HSQ-R)	6–12	Permits parents to rate child's specific problems with attention or concentration. Scores for number of problem settings, mean severity, and factor scores for compliance and leisure situations.
ADHD Rating Scale	6–12	Score for number of symptoms keyed to DSM cutoff for diagnosis of ADHD; standard scores permit derivation of clinical significance for total score and two factors (Inattentive-Hyperactive and Impulsive-Hyperactive).

(*continued*)

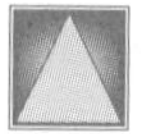

Table 39.2 (*continued*)

Test	Age/Grades	Data Generated and Comments
School Situations Questionnaire (SSQ-R)	6–12	Permits teachers to rate a child's specific problems with attention or concentration. Scores for number of problem settings and mean severity.
Child Attention Profile (CAP)	6–12	Brief measure allowing teachers' weekly ratings of presence and degree of child's inattention and overactivity. Normative scores for inattention, overactivity, and total score.
Projective tests		
Rorschach Inkblots	3–adult	Special scoring systems. Most recently developed and increasingly universally accepted is John Exner's Comprehensive System (1974). Assesses perceptual accuracy, integration of affective and intellectual functioning, reality testing, and other psychological processes.
Thematic Apperception Test (TAT)	6–adult	Generates stories which are analyzed qualitatively. Assumed to provide especially rich data regarding interpersonal functioning.
Machover Draw-A-Person Test (DAP)	3–adult	Qualitative analysis and hypothesis generation, especially regarding subject's feelings about self and significant others.
Kinetic Family Drawing (KFD)	3–adult	Qualitative analysis and hypothesis generation regarding an individual's perception of family structure and sentient environment. Some objective scoring systems in existence.
Rotter Incomplete Sentences Blank	Child, adolescent, and adult forms	Primarily qualitative analysis, although some objective scoring systems have been developed.
Personality tests		
Minnesota Multiphasic Personality Inventory-Adolescent (MMPI-A)	14–18	1992 version of widely used personality measure, developed specifically for use with adolescents. Standard scores: three validity scales, 14 clinical scales, additional content and supplementary scales.
Million Adolescent Personality Inventory (MAPI)	13–18	Standard scores for 20 scales grouped into three categories: Personality styles; expressed concerns; behavioral correlates. Normed on adolescent population. Focuses on broad functional spectrum, not just problem areas. Measures 14 primary personality traits, including emotional stability, self-concept level, excitability, and self-assurance.
Children's Personality Questionnaire	8–12	Generates combined broad trait patterns including extraversion and anxiety.
Neuropsychological screening tests and test batteries		
Developmental Test of Visual-Motor Integration (VMI)	2–16	Screening instrument for visual motor deficits. Standard scores, age equivalents, percentiles.
Benton Visual Retention Test	6–adult	Assesses presence of deficits in visual-figure memory. Mean scores by age.
Benton Visual Motor Gestalt Test	5–adult	Assesses visual-motor deficits and visual-figural retention. Age equivalents.
Reitan-Indiana Neuropsychological Test Battery for Children	5–8	Cognitive and perceptual-motor tests for children with suspected brain damage.
Halstead-Reitan Neuropsychological Test Battery for Older Children	9–14	Same as Reitan-Indiana.
Luria-Nebraska Neuropsychological Battery: Children's Revision (LNNB:C)	8–12	Sensory-motor, perceptual, cognitive tests measuring 11 clinical and two additional domains of neuropsychological functioning. Provides standard scores.
Developmental status		
Bayley Scales of Infant Development—Second Edition	16 days–42 mos	Mental, motor, and behavior scales measuring infant development. Provides standard scores.
Mullen Scales of Early Learning	Newborn–5 yrs	Language and visual scales for receptive and expressive ability. Yields age scores and T scores.

Adapted from Racusin G, Moss N. Psychological assessment of children and adolescents. In: Lewis M, ed. *Child and Adolescent Psychiatry: A Comprehensive Textbook*. Baltimore: Williams & Wilkins; 1991.

Answers 39.11–39.15

39.11 The answer is B

39.12 The answer is C

39.13 The answer is A

39.14 The answer is E

39.15 The answer is D

The Child Behavior Checklist (CBCL) can be very helpful in the evaluation of a child with multiple behavioral problems, especially if the child presents with different symptoms in different settings, such as at school and at home. The CBCL assesses for a broad range of symptoms that relate to academic and social competence. There is a parent version and a teacher version so that the reports of these two observers may be compared. The CBCL can help to systematically identify the problem symptoms related to mood, frustration tolerance, hyperactivity, oppositional behavior, and anxiety. For a child who has a variety of symptoms that span many diagnostic categories, a broad rating scale such as CBCL can be quite helpful.

The Children's Apperception Test (CAT) consists of cards with pictures of animals in ambiguous situations that show scenes related to parent–child and sibling issues. The child is asked to describe what is happening in the scenes. Animals are felt to be less threatening to children who have difficulties speaking about emotional issues. *For this 9-year-old girl who is inhibited and has difficulty disclosing her thoughts and feelings, the use of a projective but structured test such as the CAT can often be a conduit to facilitating these disclosures.*

For a 7-year-old child who appears to be globally slow, unable to understand directions, follow rules, or comprehend tasks in the classroom, a test of intellectual function is indicated. The WISC-III is the most widely used test of intellectual function. Used in children from 6 to 17 years old, it provides information in a variety of verbal areas (vocabulary, similarities, general information, arithmetic, and comprehension), as well as testing abilities in the areas of performance (block design, picture completion, picture arrangement, object assembly, coding, and mazes).

A 2-year-old child manifesting delays in motor skills, language, and social interaction should be screened for developmental delay. One available screening instrument is the Bayley Scales of Infant Development II, which are for children 1 to 42 months of age, and include a mental scale (assessing information processing, habituation, memory, language, social skills, and cognitive strategies); a motor scale (assessing gross and fine motor skills); and a Behavior Rating Scale for assessing qualitative aspects of the child's behavior during the assessment. A more recently developed instrument for assessing children for pervasive developmental disorders is the Autism Diagnostic Observation Schedule-Generic (ADOS-G), a semi-structured assessment of communication skills, social interaction and play or imaginative use of materials.

A school-aged child with emerging difficulties in academic performance should receive academic achievement testing in conjunction with intelligence testing to delineate possible learning disorders. *In an 11-year-old girl who has recently had intelligence testing, an achievement test such as the Woodcock-Johnson Psycho-Educational Battery-Revised (W-J),* which evaluates reading and mathematics mechanics and comprehension, written language, and other academic achievement, is indicated.

Answers 39.16–39.19

39.16 The answer is B

39.17 The answer is B

39.18 The answer is B

39.19 The answer is A

Instruments used in interviews range from highly structured instruments that specify the exact order and wording of all components, to semi-structured interviews that delineate the symptoms to be covered and suggest phrases that may be used but permit much more latitude in the order and phrasing of questions.

Semi-structured interviews resemble clinical interviews more closely than do structured interviews, but they nevertheless differ substantially in style and content from a typical clinical assessment. The flexible structure of the interview allows the clinically informed interviewer some freedom in the manner of inquiry and permits judgments about whether a reported behavior or expression of distress is of the quality and severity required to be considered a symptom. *Interviews of this type include the K-SADS (Kiddie Schedule for Affective Disorders and Schizophrenia) and CAS (Child Assessment Scale). Semi-structured interviews are particularly appropriate for clinically based research in which subtle diagnostic distinctions may be critical for defining samples.*

Structured interviews, on the other hand, provide highly specified protocols that are particularly useful for epidemiological studies with large sample sizes in which non-clinician interviewers are employed. *These studies investigate issues of prevalence of disorders, developmental patterns of psychopathology, and psychosocial correlates of disorders*, topics that often require large sample to provide enough statistical power to test study hypotheses.

39.20 The answer is D

Open-ended questions can overwhelm a school-aged child and result in withdrawal or shrugging of the shoulders; multiple-choice questions may elicit more information from children in this age group. If a child is not adept with verbal skills, asking the child to *draw a family* is often a way to break the ice and to gain information about the child's emotional experience. Activities such as *Winnicott's "squiggle game,"* in which the examiner draws a curved line and then takes turns with the child in continuing the drawing, may also open communication with the child. Using *indirect commentary*, such as, "I once knew a boy about your age who felt very sad when he moved away from all his friends," helps elicit feelings from the child, although the clinician must be wary of leading children into confirming what they believe the clinician wants to hear.

39.21 The answer is D

The Mooney Problem Checklist is a checklist of personal problems and is a self-report inventory, a series of questions concerning emotional problems, worries, interests, motives, values, and interpersonal traits. The primary utility of personality inventories is in the screening and identification of children in need of further evaluation. *Personality tests have lower reliability and validity than tests of ability. The CAT is different from the TAT* in that the CAT uses cards depicting animals whereas the TAT uses images of people. *The Rorschach test*, one of the most widely used projective techniques, has been developed in versions for children between the ages of 2 and 10 years and for adolescents between the ages of 10 and 17.

39.22 The answer is A

Figure 39.1 is part of the Rosenzweig Picture-Frustration Study, in which a series of cartoons is presented in which one character frustrates another. In the blank space provided, the child writes the reply of the frustrated character. From that reply, the clinician assesses the child's *response to frustration*; the response can range from passivity to violence. *The test is not used to measure psychosis, depression, impulsivity, or anxiety.*

39.23 The answer is B

The term "neurological soft signs" was first used by Lauretta Bender in reference to nondiagnostic abnormalities that are seen in some children with schizophrenia. It is now evident that these signs do not indicate a specific neurological or psychiatric disorder, but are relatively common in children with a wide variety of developmental disabilities. *Learning disabilities are not neurological soft signs,* although children with low intellectual function and/or learning disabilities often demonstrate these signs. Soft signs refer to both behavioral findings, such as severe impulsivity or mood instability, and physical findings, such as persistence of infantile reflexes, mild incoordination, *poor balance, contralateral overflow movements, asymmetry of gait, nystagmus,* and mild choreiform movements. The Physical and Neurological Examination for Soft Signs (PANESS), an instrument used in evaluating children up to age 15, consists of 15 questions and 43 physical tasks that assess for presence of these signs.

39.24 The answer is E

Minor physical anomalies or dysmorphic features are most frequently seen in children with *in utero* exposure to toxic substances, chromosomal abnormalities, developmental disabilities, speech and language disorders, learning disorders, and severe hyperactivity. As with neurological soft signs, they are rarely specific in determining a psychiatric or neurological diagnosis, but they are important to document in the evaluation of a child and may prompt further genetic, neurological, and psychiatric investigation. *Minor physical anomalies include multiple hair whorls, low-set ears, high-arched palate, flattened philtrum,* epicanthal folds, hypertelorism, transverse palmar creases, and increased head circumference. *The persistence of the Babinski reflex is a neurological sign rather than a physical anomaly.*

40 Mental Retardation

Accurately defining *mental retardation* has challenged clinicians over the centuries. In the 1800s, the notion that mental retardation was based primarily on a deficit in social or moral reasoning was promoted. Since then, the addition of intellectual deficit was added to the concept of inadequate social function. All current classification systems retain the understanding that mental retardation is based on more than intellectual deficits, that is, it also depends upon a lower than expected level of adaptive function. According to the fourth text revision of *Diagnostic and Statistical Manual of Mental Disorders* (DSM-IV-TR), a diagnosis of mental retardation can be made only when both the IQ, as measured by a standardized test, is subaverage and a measure of adaptive function reveals deficits in at least two of the areas of adaptive function.

According to DSM-IV-TR, mental retardation is defined as significantly subaverage general intellectual functioning resulting in, or associated with, concurrent impairment in adaptive behavior and manifested during the developmental period, before the age of 18. The diagnosis is made regardless of whether the person has a coexisting physical disorder or other mental disorder. Mental retardation diagnoses are coded on Axis II in the DSM-IV-TR.

Approximately 85 percent of persons who are mentally retarded fall within the mild mental retardation category (IQ between 50 and 70). The adaptive functions of mildly retarded persons are effective in several areas, such as communications, self-care, social skills, work, leisure, and safety. Mental retardation is influenced by genetic, environmental, and psychosocial factors, and in past years, the development of mild retardation was often attributed to severe psychosocial deprivation. More recently, however, researchers have increasingly recognized the likely contribution of a host of subtle biological factors including chromosomal abnormalities, subclinical lead intoxication, and prenatal exposure to drugs, alcohol, and other toxins. Furthermore, evidence is increasing that subgroups of persons who are mentally retarded, such as those with fragile X syndrome, Down's syndrome, and Prader-Willi syndrome, have characteristic patterns of social, linguistic, and cognitive development and typical behavioral manifestations. The DSM-IV-TR has included in its text on mental retardation additional information regarding etiological factors and their association with mental retardation syndrome (e.g., fragile X syndrome).

HELPFUL HINTS

The student should define these terms.

- adaptive functioning
- Bayley Infant Scale of Development
- borderline intellectual functioning
- Cattell Infant Scale
- causative factors
- chromosomal abnormality
- *cri-du-chat* syndrome
- CVS (chorionic villi sampling) and amniocentesis
- degrees of mental retardation (mild, moderate, severe, profound)
- Down's syndrome
- fetal alcohol syndrome
- fragile X syndrome
- intelligence quotient (IQ)
- Lesch-Nyhan syndrome
- mental deficiency
- mental retardation
- neurofibrillary tangles
- neurofibromatosis
- PKU
- Prader-Willi syndrome
- prenatal exposure
- primary, secondary, and tertiary prevention
- rubella
- Special Olympics
- Turner's syndrome
- Vineland Adaptive Behavior Scales
- WHO

QUESTIONS

Directions

Each of the questions or incomplete statements below is followed by five suggested responses or completions. Select the *one* that is *best* in each case.

40.1 DSM-IV-TR lists the prevalence of mental retardation in the United States as

A. 1 percent
B. 3 percent
C. 5 percent
D. 6 percent
E. None of the above

40.2 When IQ is used as the sole criterion for mental retardation, the prevalence rate is estimated to be

A. 0.5 percent
B. 1 percent
C. 2 percent
D. 3 percent
E. 10 percent

40.3 A decline in IQ begins at approximately 10 to 15 years in which of the following disorders?

A. Down's syndrome
B. Fragile X syndrome
C. Cerebral palsy
D. Nonspecific mental retardation
E. Fetal alcohol syndrome

40.4 The most common inherited cause of mental retardation is

A. Down's syndrome
B. Fragile X syndrome
C. Fetal alcohol syndrome
D. Prader-Willi syndrome
E. None of the above

40.5 Which of the following disorders is *least* often associated with Fragile X syndrome?

A. Autistic disorder
B. Schizotypal personality disorder
C. Attention-deficit/hyperactivity disorder
D. Bipolar disorder
E. Social anxiety disorder

40.6 Among all known causes of mental retardation, which of the following syndromes is *least* associated with comorbid Axis I psychiatric disorder?

A. Down's syndrome
B. Fragile X syndrome
C. Nonspecific type
D. Fetal alcohol syndrome
E. Prader-Willi syndrome

40.7 Mild mental retardation has been associated with

A. Nonspecific causes
B. Prader-Willi syndrome
C. Females with fragile X syndrome
D. Poor socioeconomic background
E. All of the above

40.8 Moderate mental retardation

A. Reflects an IQ range of 25 to 40
B. Is seen in approximately 3 to 4 percent of persons with mental retardation
C. Has an identifiable organic etiology in the vast majority of cases
D. Usually is associated with the ability to achieve academic skills at the second- to third-grade level
E. All of the above

40.9 Common manifestations of anxiety in persons with mental retardation include

A. Aggression
B. Agitation
C. Repetitive behaviors
D. Self-injury
E. All of the above

Directions

Each group of questions below consists of lettered headings followed by a list of numbered phrases or statements. For each numbered phrase or statement, select the *one* lettered heading that is most closely associated with it. Each lettered heading may be selected once, more than once, or not at all.

Questions 40.10–40.14

A. Prader-Willi syndrome
B. Down's syndrome
C. Fragile X syndrome
D. Phenylketonuria (PKU)

40.10 Attributed to a deletion in chromosome 15
40.11 Most commonly occurs via autosomal recessive transmission
40.12 Abnormalities involving chromosome 21
40.13 Occurs via a chromosomal mutation at Xq27.3
40.14 Example of a genomic imprinting

Questions 40.15–40.18

A. Trisomy 21
B. Autosomal dominant
C. Autosomal recessive
D. X-linked semidominant

40.15 Neurofibromatosis
40.16 Tuberous sclerosis
40.17 Crouzon's syndrome
40.18 Cockayne's syndrome

Questions 40.19–40.23

A. Adrenoleukodystrophy
B. Rett's disorder
C. Acquired immune deficiency syndrome (AIDS)
D. Rubella
E. Cytomegalic inclusion disease/cytomegalic virus (CMV)
F. Toxoplasmosis

40.19 Mental retardation with periventricular intracerebral calcifications, jaundice, microcephaly, and hepatosplenomegaly
40.20 Progressive encephalopathy and mental retardation in 50 percent of children born to mothers with this disorder
40.21 An X-linked mental retardation syndrome that is degenerative and affects only females
40.22 Diffuse demyelination of cerebral cortex leading to visual and intellectual impairment, seizures, and spasticity; accompanied by adrenocortical insufficiency.

40.23 Mental retardation, microcephaly, microphthalmia, congenital heart disease, deafness, and cataracts
40.24 Mental retardation, diffuse intracerebral calcifications, hydrocephalus, seizures, and chorioretinitis

Questions 40.25–40.28

A. Nonspecific mental retardation
B. Boys with fragile X syndrome
C. Down's syndrome
D. Williams' syndrome

40.25 May have particular weakness in expressive communication and grammar
40.26 Particular difficulties in visual-spatial processing skills
40.27 Weaker in sequential processing than in simultaneous processing
40.28 Even or near-even performance across various cognitive domains

Questions 40.29–40.33

A. Fetal alcohol syndrome
B. Down's syndrome
C. Lesch-Nyhan syndrome
D. Prader-Willi syndrome
E. Neurofibromatosis

40.29 High rates of temper tantrums, aggression, excessive daytime sleepiness, emotional lability, obsessions, and compulsions
40.30 Microcephaly, short stature, midface hypoplasia, mild to moderate mental retardation
40.31 Associated with increased incidence of thyroid abnormalities, congenital heart disease, leukemia, and early-onset Alzheimer's disease
40.32 Ataxia, chorea, renal dysfunction, gout, self-mutilation
40.33 Café-au-lait spots, short stature, macrocephaly

Directions

Each of the questions or incomplete statements below is followed by five suggested responses or completions. Select the *one* that is *best* in each case.

40.34 All of the following chromosomal aberrations associated with Down's syndrome lead to a phenotypic expression of the disorder *except*

A. Patients have 45 chromosomes
B. Patients have three copies of chromosome 21
C. Patients have 47 chromosomes
D. Patients have 46 chromosomes, but two, usually 15 and 21, are fused
E. Patients have mosaicism, with normal and trisomic cells in various tissues

40.35 The genetic finding most closely linked to advancing maternal age is

A. Translocation between chromosomes 14 and 21
B. Mitotic non-disjunction of chromosome 21
C. Partially trisomic karyotype
D. Meiotic nondisjunction of chromosome 21
E. All of the above

40.36 Which of the following chromosomal abnormalities is most likely to cause mental retardation?

A. Extra chromosome 21 (trisomy 21)
B. Fusion of chromosomes 21 and 15
C. XO (Turner's syndrome)
D. XXY (Klinefelter's syndrome)
E. XXYY and XXXY (Klinefelter's syndrome variants)

40.37 Mental retardation should be diagnosed when the intelligence quotient (IQ) is below

A. 100
B. 85
C. 70
D. 65
E. 60

40.38 Fragile X syndrome

A. Has a phenotype that includes postpubertal microorchidism
B. Affects only males
C. Usually causes severe to profound mental retardation
D. Has a phenotype that includes a large head and large ears
E. All of the above

40.39 The mentally retarded child shown in Figure 40.1 demonstrates the characteristic facial features and high degree

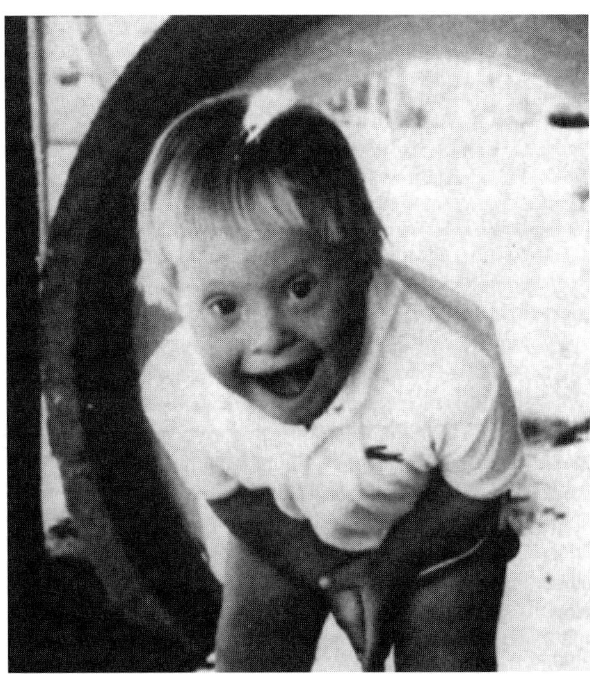

FIGURE 40.1
Courtesy of Ludwik S. Szymanski, M.D.

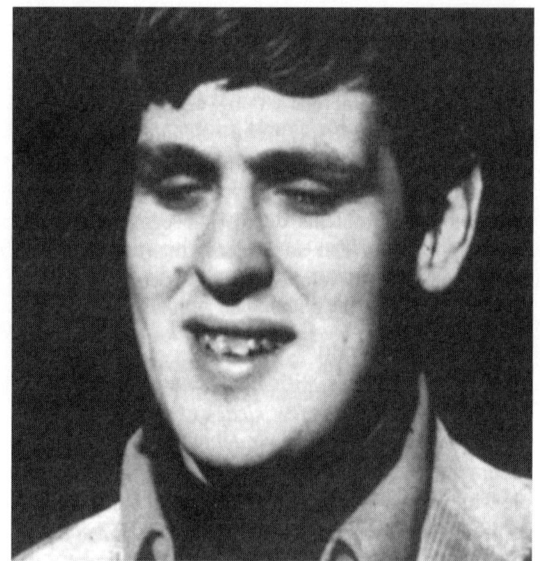

FIGURE 40.2
Courtesy of Ludwik S. Szymanski, M.D.

of social responsiveness suggestive of which of the following etiologies?

A. Autosomal dominant inheritance
B. Prenatal substance exposure
C. Trisomy 21
D. Enzyme deficiency
E. Abnormality in sex chromosomes

40.40 The physical phenotype shown in Figure 40.2, including long facial contour, large anteverted ears, and macroorchidism (not shown) in this young adult with mental retardation is consistent with which of the following diagnoses?

A. Prader-Willi syndrome
B. Down's syndrome
C. Klinefelter's syndrome
D. Fetal alcohol syndrome
E. Fragile X syndrome

ANSWERS

40.1 The answer is A

Most prevalence studies find that approximately 1 percent (not 3, 5, or 6 percent) of the population has mental retardation, and this figure is cited by DSM-IV-TR. The incidence of mental retardation is difficult to calculate because the condition often goes unrecognized until mid-childhood in mild cases. In some cases, even when intellectual function is limited, good adaptive skills exist and the child's deficits are not revealed until greater challenges are confronted in late childhood or early adolescence. The highest incidence is in school-age children with a peak at ages 10 to 14. Mental retardation is about 1.5 times more common among men than women. In older persons, prevalence is lower, as individuals with severe or profound mental retardation have high mortality rates due to the complications of associated physical disorders.

40.2 The answer is D

When the only criterion being used to define mental retardation is IQ less than 70, the prevalence rate for mental retardation is 3 percent (not 0.5, 1, or 2 percent). However, IQ should not be the sole criterion of mental retardation. To be considered to have mental retardation, a person must have an IQ below 70 as well as deficits in adaptive behavior. Although strong correlation between IQ and adaptive skills exists in individuals with severe and profound mental retardation, lower correlation exists for individuals with mild mental retardation. Throughout the entire population of persons with mental retardation, a moderate correlation likely exists between IQ and adaptive skills; to the extent that the two do not correlate perfectly, less than 3 percent of individuals in the population meet full criteria for mental retardation.

40.3 The answer is B

Children with *Down's syndrome show their highest IQ scores during the first year of life, and then decline in IQ* over the early to middle childhood years. *Boys with fragile X syndrome also decline in IQ, but their declines seem to begin at approximately 10 to 15 years of age.* Conversely, *children with cerebral palsy (half of whom have mental retardation) remain remarkably stable in their IQ scores over time, much like groups with mixed or nonspecific etiologies* of mental retardation.

40.4 The answer is B

The most common causes of mental retardation are Down's syndrome, fragile X syndrome, and fetal alcohol syndrome. Together, these three conditions are responsible for about 30 percent of all identified cases of mental retardation. *Down's syndrome is the most common chromosomal abnormality leading to mental retardation.* Fetal alcohol syndrome occurs in up to 15 percent of infants born to mothers who regularly ingested large amounts of alcohol while pregnant. Prader-Willi syndrome is attributed to a small deletion on chromosome 15, and has a prevalence of less than 1 in 10,000.

Fragile X syndrome, the most common inherited cause of mental retardation, results in a wide range of learning and behavioral problems, with males being more often and more severely affected than females. The recently discovered fragile X gene (FRM-1) represents a newly identified type of human disease, caused by amplification (or excessive repetition) of a three-nucleotide repeat sequence (CGG) in DNA. Above a certain threshold number of these repeats, the syndrome occurs. Numbers of repeats between the normal threshold of 50 and the syndromal threshold of 200 are termed "permutations." As many as 1 in 259 women in the general population may carry the permutation, with 1 in 1,000 males and 1 in 2,000 females being fully affected by the syndrome.

40.5 The answer is D

Fragile X syndrome is associated with shyness, gaze aversion, and social difficulties. A number of psychiatric diagnoses commonly co-occur with fragile X, including autistic disorder, schizotypal personality disorder, attention-deficit/hyperactivity disorder, and social anxiety disorder. These difficulties vary in severity in this population, and are found in fragile X individuals across the IQ spectrum, from those with moderate mental retardation to those with mild learning disabilities. Bipolar disorder is less commonly associated with fragile X syndrome than these other disorders.

40.6 The answer is A

Compared to other individuals with mental retardation, persons with Down's syndrome appear to suffer less often and less severely from psychopathology. Rates of psychiatric disorders in children and adolescents with Down's syndrome exceed those in the general population but are significantly lower than in persons with mental retardation due to other etiologies, such as fragile X syndrome, fetal alcohol syndrome, Prader-Willi syndrome, and nonspecific type. Commonly noted psychiatric problems among individuals with mental retardation include attention problems, impulsivity, hyperactivity, and aggression. In contrast to these problems, depression seems to be less common in persons with mental retardation than in the general population.

40.7 The answer is E (all)

Mild mental retardation is associated with certain genetic syndromes, including Prader-Willi syndrome and fragile X syndrome occurring in females. Many cases of mild mental retardation are not attributable to known genetic or other organic syndromes, and nonspecific causes are cited as the etiology of the condition. *Low socioeconomic background is also associated with mild mental retardation*, possibly highlighting the environmental and cultural influences on intellectual attainment.

40.8 The answer is D

Mild mental retardation (IQ 55 to 70) characterizes the largest group of persons with mental retardation, comprising up to 85 percent of the total. These individuals often blend into the general population in the years before and after formal schooling. Many achieve academic skills at the sixth grade level or higher, and some graduate from high school. As adults, many hold jobs, marry, and raise families—yet at times they may appear slow or need extra help negotiating life's challenges.

Moderate mental retardation (IQ 40 to 55) is seen in approximately 10 percent (not 3 to 4 percent) of those with mental retardation, including person with more impaired cognitive and adaptive functioning. Individuals with moderate mental retardation typically are diagnosed in their preschool years, and some (but not the majority) have a clearly identified organic cause for their delay. Persons with Down's syndrome often function in this range, as do many with fragile X syndrome. *Most children with moderate mental retardation require special education services and achieve academic skills at the 2nd to 3rd grade level.* Supportive services are needed throughout life. With proper assistance, many live, work, and thrive in their local communities. One study found that 20 percent of persons with an IQ from 40 to 49 lived independently, 60 percent were considered partially dependent, and 20 percent were totally dependent on others. Similarly, some individuals in this range are employed in the competitive job market and need minimal job supervision, whereas others require more extensive supervision on the job and may work in specialized supportive settings.

Severe mental retardation (IQ 25 to 40) occurs in about 3 to 4 percent of persons with mental retardation. Individuals at this level often have one or more known organic causes for their delay, and many show concurrent motor, ambulatory, and neurological problems as well as poorly developed communication skills. Most persons with severe mental retardation require close supervision and specialized care throughout their lives. Some individuals learn to perform simple tasks or routines that facilitate their self-care or their ability to perform in a sheltered workshop-type vocational setting.

Profound mental retardation (IQ below 25) affects only 1 to 2 percent of individuals with mental retardation and involves pervasive deficits in cognitive, motor, and communication skills. Impaired sensory-motor functioning is often noticeable very early in development and most individuals require extensive training to develop even rudimentary self-care skills. The great majority of people with profound mental retardation have organic causes for their deficits, and most require total care and supervision throughout their lives.

40.9 The answer is E (all)

Anxiety disorders are common and often under-recognized in persons with mental retardation. Reported prevalence varies greatly, likely due to difficulty in eliciting symptoms that enable a diagnosis to be made. Individuals with mental retardation may not be able to identify subjective anxiety as a cause of distress, and a patient's aggression or agitation may be attributed to caregivers as due to poor impulse control rather than to anxiety. *Common manifestations of anxiety in persons with mental retardation include aggression, agitation, repetitive behaviors, self-injury, and insomnia. Panic or phobic symptoms may be expressed as agitation, screaming, or crying, which may be misinterpreted as psychotic behavior.* Furthermore, persons with mental retardation are at increased risk of physical abuse compared to the general population, which may put them at greater risk for posttraumatic stress disorder, another diagnosis that may often be overlooked in this population.

40.10 The answer is A

40.11 The answer is D

40.12 The answer is B

40.13 The answer is C

40.14 The answer is A

Prader-Willi syndrome results from a microdeletion in chromosome 15 and usually occurs sporadically, with prevalence of less than 1 in 10,000. Its clinical manifestations include compulsive eating behaviors, obesity, mental retardation, hypogonadism, hypotonia, and short stature. Disruptive behaviors, including oppositional and defiant behavior with frequent temper tantrums, are also common. *Prader-Willi provides an example of genomic imprinting*, the process whereby specific genes are differentially marked during parental gametogenesis, resulting in differential expression in the individual; Prader-Willi syndrome results when the microdeletion of chromosome 15 occurs in the chromosome inherited from the father, whereas Angelman syndrome, a clinically distinct entity, occurs when the deletion occurs in the chromosome inherited from the mother.

Several chromosomal aberrations may result in Down's syndrome. Trisomy 21 is the most common of these, and results from nondisjunction during meiosis. Nondisjunction after fertilization in any cell division results in mosaicism, in which both normal and trisomic cells can be found. In translocation, usually occurring between chromosomes 15 and 21, fusion of two chromosomes occurs.

Fragile X syndrome is the second most common single cause of mental retardation, and results from a mutation on the X chromosome at the fragile site Xq27.3. The fragile site is expressed only in some cells, and it may be absent in asymptomatic male and female carriers. There is much variation in both the genetic and phenotypic expression. Prevalence rates are 1 per 1,000 males and 1 per 2,000 females, but rates of fully affected individuals are likely closer to 1 per 4,000 males and 1 per 8,000 females. Behaviorally, those with fragile X syndrome often have attention problems, pervasive developmental disorders, and other learning disorders. Intellectual function may deteriorate in adolescence in individuals with fragile X. *Phenylketonuria (PKU) is transmitted via autosomal recessive inheritance of a defect found on chromosome 12, and occurs in 1 in 10,000 births.* The defect transmitted is an inability to convert phenylalanine, an essential amino acid, to paratyrosine due to absence or inactivity of the liver enzyme phenylalanine hydroxylase. The majority of patients with PKU are severely retarded, but some have borderline or normal intelligence. Eczema, hypopigmented hair and eyes, and seizures are other common symptoms. Early detection is crucial, as a low-phenylalanine diet significantly improves both cognitive development and behavior.

40.15 The answer is B

40.16 The answer is B

40.17 The answer is B

40.18 The answer is C

Neurofibromatosis manifests as neurofibromas, café-au-lait spots, seizures, optic and acoustic gliomas, and bone lesions. *Its transmission is autosomal dominant.*

Tuberous sclerosis presents with seizures, intracranial calcifications, pink-brown skins lesions, and bone lesions. *Transmission is autosomal dominant.*

Crouzon's syndrome, also known as craniofacial dysostosis, is manifested by proptosis with shallow orbits, maxillary hypoplasia, and craniosynostosis. *Its transmission is autosomal dominant.*

Cockayne's syndrome presents with hypotrichosis, photosensitivity, thin skin, diminished subcutaneous fat, and impaired hearing. Craniofacial findings include pinched facies, sunken eyes, thin nose, prognathism, and retinal degeneration. Skeletal abnormalities include long limbs with large hands and feet and flexion deformities. *Transmission is autosomal recessive.*

40.19 The answer is E

40.20 The answer is C

40.21 The answer is B

40.22 The answer is A

40.23 The answer is D

40.24 The answer is F

Infants who are exposed to *CMV* in utero may be stillborn; those born alive may be *affected by mental retardation with periventricular intracerebral calcifications, jaundice, microcephaly, and hepatosplenomegaly.* Up to one-half of *infants born to mothers with AIDS develop progressive encephalopathy and mental retardation. Rett's disorder is a syndrome with X-linked dominant inheritance than affects only girls*, and is characterized by developmental arrest and loss of milestones, autistic-like features, mental retardation, and stereotyped hand movements. *Adrenoleukodystrophy* is an X-linked recessive disorder characterized by diffuse *demyelination of the cerebral cortex leading to visual and intellectual impairment, seizures, and spasticity, accompanied by adrenocortical insufficiency.* Onset of the disease typically occurs between the ages of 3 and 10, and the course is usually rapidly progressive and fatal. *Rubella infection in a pregnant woman* leads to grave consequences for the developing fetus, particularly when exposure occurs in the first trimester: *mental retardation, microcephaly, microphthalmia, congenital heart defects, deafness, and cataracts may develop. Congenital toxoplasmosis is associated with mental retardation, diffuse intracerebral calcifications (as opposed to the strictly periventricular lesions seen in congenital CMV), hydrocephalus, seizures, and chorioretinitis.*

40.25 The answer is C

40.26 The answer is D

40.27 The answer is B

40.28 The answer is A

Normal children have a specific, possibly universal, order to their development. For example, in piagetian cognitive development, children proceed from sensorimotor, to preoperational, to concrete operational, to formal operational thought. Even within these four larger stages, smaller orderings hold; within sensorimotor development, normal infants proceed through Piaget's six sub-stages in each of several sub-domains.

Do children with mental retardation also follow a similar sequence in development? Parallel sequences have been identified for children of various cognitive abilities for a variety of developmental tasks. These sequences generally hold for children with genetic or other organic causes for their retardation. The only possible exceptions include some children with uncontrollable seizures (which make accurate testing difficult) and some autistic children, who may show altered development because of their particular disabilities on certain social tasks. These sequences have been noted in many areas: in almost 20 piagetian domains, in symbolic play, and in linguistic grammar and pragmatics. Across the board, it seems that children with mental retardation and other children develop along similar pathways. *With a few exceptions, children with nonspecific mental retardation do show even or near-even performance across various intellectual domains.*

Some important differences are noted in children with various organic forms of mental retardation show specific intellectual strengths and weaknesses. For example, *several groups are weaker in sequential (i.e., serial) processing than in simultaneous (i.e., holistic) processing or achievement abilities. Such sequential deficits are found in boys with fragile X syndrome and children with Prader-Willi syndrome. Children with Down's syndrome may have particular weaknesses in expressive (versus receptive) communication and special problems in grammatical abilities. Children with Williams' syndrome show particular difficulties with visual-spatial processing skills*, and some subsets of these children show heightened abilities in language and music. Different causes of mental retardation thus result in different characteristic intellectual strengths and weaknesses.

40.29 The answer is D

40.30 The answer is A

40.31 The answer is B

40.32 The answer is C

40.33 The answer is E

Prader-Willi syndrome, which occurs due to a defect on chromosome 15, is best known for its symptoms of hyperphagia and obesity. Babies with the disorder show hypotonia and feeding/suckling difficulties, then between ages two and six develop hyperphagia, food seeking, and food hoarding. Hyperphagia is probably related to a hypothalamic abnormality resulting in a lack of satiety. *A high proportion of these children also manifest high rates of temper tantrums, aggression, excessive daytime sleepiness, emotional lability, obsessions, and compulsions.* Often these symptoms are associated with distress and adaptive impairment, indicating the need to consider a diagnosis of obsessive-compulsive disorder when symptoms are severe.

Fetal alcohol syndrome is caused by maternal alcohol consumption during gestation, and prominent symptoms *include physical features such as microcephaly, short stature, midface hypoplasia,* short palpebral fissure, thin upper lip, smooth philtrum, as well as emotional/cognitive features including mild to moderate mental retardation, irritability, inattention, and hyperactivity.

Down's syndrome predisposes individuals to thyroid abnormalities, congenital heart disease, leukemia, and early-onset Alzheimer's disease.

Lesch-Nyhan syndrome, a rare X-linked recessive disorder that involves an inability to metabolize uric acid, causes ataxia, chorea, renal failure, and gout, as well as striking self-mutilatory (particularly self-biting) behavior and mild to moderate mental retardation.

Neurofibromatosis (type 1) is an autosomal dominant disorder caused by a defect in chromosome 17, with a variety of clinical manifestations, including cutaneous neurofibromas, *café-au-lait spots, short stature, macrocephaly, Lisch nodules, and bony dysplasias.* Ten percent of the affected individuals have moderate to profound mental retardation, while half manifest speech and language difficulties. Distractibility, impulsivity, anxiety, and depression are also prominent features.

40.34 The answer is A

Three types of chromosomal aberrations are recognized in Down's syndrome. First, patients with trisomy 21 *(three copies of chromosome 21 rather than the usual two)* represent the overwhelming majority of individuals with Down's syndrome. *They have 47 chromosomes with an extra copy of 21.* The mother's karyotypes are normal. A nondisjunction during meiosis is responsible for the trisomy.

Second, nondisjunction occurring after fertilization in any cell division results in mosaicism, with both normal and trisomic cells found in various tissues.

Third, in translocations there is a fusion of two chromosomes, usually 15 and 21, resulting in a total of 46 chromosomes, despite the presence of an extra chromosome 21. This version of the disorder, unlike trisomy 21, is usually inherited and the translocated chromosome may be found in unaffected parents and siblings, who would have only 45 chromosomes.

40.35 The answer is D

Meiotic non-disjunction of chromosome 21 produces approximately 85 percent of cases of Down's syndrome, and has been most closely linked to advancing maternal age. Paternal age has also been implicated as a factor in some studies.

Translocation events constitute only 5 percent of Down's syndrome cases. In cases in which an asymptomatic parent carries the aberrant chromosome in their genome, subsequent Down's syndrome in an offspring is unrelated to parental age. If the translocation occurs between chromosomes 14 and 21, the proband carries 46 chromosomes, including two normal 21 chromosomes, one normal 14 chromosome, and the 14/21 translocation, which carries parts of both chromosomes. Any asymptomatic parent or sibling who is a carrier of the translocation has only 45 chromosomes, with one 21 chromosome missing, and is thus spared the excessive genetic complement.

Mitotic non-disjunction of chromosome 21, which occurs in 1 percent of all Down's syndrome cases, occurs after fertilization of a presumably healthy ovum and may therefore be considered independent of maternal age. *Partially trisomic karyotype may refer to the mosaicism—some cells normal, others with trisomy 21—seen in mitotic non-disjunction, or to the excessive complement of chromosome 21 produced by translocation.* Neither case is as closely tied to maternal age as is meiotic nondisjunction.

40.36 The answer is A

An extra chromosome 21 is the most common genetic abnormality found in Down's syndrome and the abnormality most likely to cause mental retardation. Abnormalities in autosomal chromosomes are, in general, associated with mental retardation. *The chromosomal aberration represented by 46 chromosomes with fusion of 15 and 21 produces a type of Down's syndrome that, unlike trisomy 21, is usually inherited. Aberrations in sex chromosomes are not always associated with mental retardation: for example, XO (Turner's syndrome), XXY (Klinefelter's syndrome), and XXYY and XXXY (Klinefelter's syndrome variants).* Some children with Turner's syndrome have normal to superior intelligence.

Girls with Turner's syndrome have gonadal agenesis and do not develop secondary sexual characteristics without medical intervention. Another hallmark feature is webbed neck. In Klinefelter's syndrome and its variants, individuals have underdeveloped male genitalia, infertility, and may develop gynecomastia beginning in adolescence.

40.37 The answer is C

Mental retardation should be diagnosed when the intelligence quotient falls below 70. Accepted definitions are as follows: mild (IQ 55 to 70), moderate (IQ 40 to 55), severe (IQ 25 to 40), and profound (IQ below 25).

40.38 The answer is D

Fragile X syndrome has a phenotype that includes a large head with large ears, long and narrow face, short stature, and postpubertal macro-orchidism (not micro-orchidism). The syndrome affects both males and females. *Female carriers are usually less impaired than males but can manifest the typical physical characteristics along with mild mental retardation. In males, the syndrome usually causes moderate to severe mental retardation (not severe to profound).* Those affected by the syndrome may also have attention-deficit/hyperactivity disorder and learning disorders.

40.39 The answer is C

Causative factors in mental retardation include genetic (chromosomal and inherited) conditions, prenatal exposure to infections and toxins, perinatal trauma, acquired conditions, and socio-cultural factors. The child in Figure 40.1 demonstrates the characteristic facial features (epicanthal folds, flattened nasal bridge) and high degree of social responsiveness of Down's syndrome. *In the overwhelming majority of cases, the etiology of Down's syndrome is an abnormality of chromosome 21, known as trisomy 21.*

Autosomal dominant inheritance as the etiology of mental retardation is demonstrated in a number of disorders, including tuberous sclerosis and Sturge Weber syndrome. Prenatal substance exposure as the etiology of mental retardation is demonstrated in fetal alcohol syndrome, which occurs in up to 15 percent of babies born to women who regularly ingest large amounts of alcohol. Enzyme deficiency as the etiology of mental retardation is demonstrated in phenylketonuria (PKU). Abnormality in sex chromosomes as the etiology of mental retardation is demonstrated in fragile X syndrome, the second most common cause of mental retardation, which results from a mutation on the X chromosome.

40.40 The answer is E

Figure 40.2 shows a young adult with fragile X syndrome, the second most common single cause of mental retardation (after trisomy 21, the predominant form of Down's syndrome) and the leading inherited cause of mental retardation. The physical phenotype of Down's includes epicanthal folds, high cheekbones, protruding tongue, single transverse palmar crease, and a number of other associated features including congenital heart defects and gastrointestinal malformations. Prader-Willi syndrome, caused by a micro-deletion on chromosome 15, is characterized by mental retardation, hyperphagia, obesity, hypogonadism, and short stature. Fetal alcohol syndrome consists of mental retardation and a typical phenotypic picture of facial dysmorphism including hypertelorism, microcephaly, short palpebral fissures, smooth philtrum, and thin upper lip. Klinefelter's syndrome is a condition caused by XXY genotype, characterized by male habitus with hypogonadism due to low androgen production.

41 Learning Disorders

Learning disorders refer to a child's or adolescent's deficits in acquiring expected skills in reading, writing, speaking, use of listening, reasoning, or mathematics, compared with other children of the same age and intellectual capacity. Learning disorders are not uncommon; they affect at least 5 percent of school-age children. This represents approximately half of all public school children who receive special education services in the United States. In 1975, Public Law 94-142, the "Education for All Handicapped Children Act," mandated all states to provide free and appropriate educational services to all children. Since that time, the number of children identified with learning disorders has increased, and a variety of definitions of learning disabilities has arisen. The 4th edition of *Diagnostic and Statistical Manual of Mental Disorders* (DSM-IV-TR) introduced the term learning disorders, formerly called academic skills disorders. All of the current learning disorder diagnoses require that the child's achievement in that particular learning disorder is significantly lower than expected and that the learning problems interfere with academic achievement or activities of daily living.

Learning disorders often make it agonizing for a child to succeed in school and, in some cases, lead to eventual demoralization, low self-esteem, chronic frustration, and poor peer relationships. Learning disorders are associated with higher than average risk of a variety of comorbid disorders including attention-deficit/hyperactivity disorder (ADHD), communication disorders, conduct disorders, and depressive disorders. Adolescents with learning disorders are about 1½ times more likely to drop out of school, approximating rates of 40 percent. Adults with learning disorders are at increased risk for difficulties in employment and social adjustment. Learning disorders can be associated with other developmental disorders, major depressive disorder, and dysthymic disorder.

Genetic predisposition, perinatal injury, and neurological and other medical conditions may contribute to the development of learning disorders, but many children and adolescents with learning disorders have no specific risk factors. Learning disorders are, nevertheless, frequently found in association with conditions such as lead poisoning, fetal alcohol syndrome, and in utero drug exposure.

HELPFUL HINTS

The student should be able define these terms related to learning disorders.

- academic skills disorders
- dyslexia
- hearing and vision screening
- phoneme
- right–left confusion
- spatial relations
- visual-perceptual deficits
- word additions
- word distortions
- word omissions

QUESTIONS

Directions

Each of the questions or incomplete statements below is followed by five suggested responses or completions. Select the *one* that is *best* in each case.

41.1 Common elements in the definition of reading disorder include

A. its underlying cause is central nervous system dysfunction
B. an uneven pattern of cognitive functioning
C. a discrepancy between learning potential and actual reading achievement
D. difficulty in single-word decoding
E. All of the above

41.2 A recently proposed definition of dyslexia includes which of the following components?

A. It is one of several distinct learning disabilities not characterized by difficulties in single-word decoding.
B. It does not usually reflect insufficient phonological processing.
C. It is not the result of sensory impairment.

D. It rarely includes a conspicuous problem with acquiring proficiency in writing and spelling.
E. None of the above

41.3 The psychiatric syndrome most often comorbid with mathematical disorder is

A. anxiety
B. depression
C. reading disorder
D. attention-deficit/hyperactivity disorder
E. None of the above

Directions

Each group of questions below consists of lettered headings followed by a list of numbered words or phrases. For each numbered word or phrase, select the *one* lettered heading that is most closely associated with it. Each heading may be selected once, more than once, or not at all.

Questions 41.4–41.7

A. Reading disorder
B. Mathematics disorder
C. Disorder of written expression
D. Learning disorder not otherwise specified

41.4 Used to be known as dyslexia
41.5 Spelling skills deficit is an example
41.6 Usually diagnosed later than the other learning disorders
41.7 Reported to occur frequently in children born in May, June, and July

Questions 41.8–41.12

A. Reading disorder
B. Mathematics disorder
C. Both
D. Neither

41.8 The study of this disorder has been neglected even though it appears to occur with the same frequency as learning disorders in other areas.
41.9 The etiology is unknown.
41.10 Higher monozygotic than dizygotic concordance rates.
41.11 The diagnosis is generally not made until the second or third grade.
41.12 Brain anomalies are inferred but not demonstrated conclusively.

Directions

Each of the questions or incomplete statements below is followed by five suggested responses or completions. Select the *one* that is *best* in each case.

41.13 Reading disorder is characterized by all of the following *except*

A. Impairment in recognizing words
B. Poor reading comprehension
C. Increased prevalence among family members
D. Occurrence in three to four times as many girls as boys
E. Omissions, additions, and distortions of words in oral reading

41.14 Which of the following statements does *not* characterize mathematics disorder?

A. It is more common in boys than girls.
B. The prevalence is estimated to be about 6 percent in school-age children with normal intelligence.
C. It includes impairment in addition, subtraction, multiplication, and division.
D. It is usually apparent by the time a child is 8 years old.
E. All of the above

41.15 Disorder of written expression

A. presents earlier than do reading disorder and communication disorders
B. occurs only in children with reading disorder
C. is not diagnosed until the teenage years
D. includes disability in spelling, grammar, and punctuation
E. is always self-limited

41.16 Disorder of written expression is often associated with

A. reading disorder
B. mixed expressive-receptive language disorder
C. developmental coordination disorder
D. mathematics disorder
E. All of the above

41.17 Janet, age 11, has a long history of school problems. She failed first grade and was removed from a special classroom in second grade after arguing and fighting repeatedly with her peers. She is currently in a regular sixth grade class and is struggling academically: she is failing reading and English and is barely passing in math and science; her performance in art and sports is significantly better. Her teacher describes Janet as "a slow learner with a poor memory," and notes that Janet does poorly in group settings and requires considerable individual attention in class.

Janet has no history of medical problems, and her developmental history was unremarkable—she sat up at 6 months, walked at 12 months, and began speaking at 16 months. Examination revealed an open and friendly girl who bristled at questions about her academic difficulties. She complained of being "teased" and "bossed around" by children at school but described a number of friendships with peers in her neighborhood. Intelligence testing revealed a full-scale IQ of 97. Wide-range achievement testing produced grade-level scores of 2.8 for reading, 3.3 for spelling, and 4.3 for arithmetic.

The most likely diagnosis is

A. disorder of written expression
B. expressive language disorder
C. phonological disorder

D. reading disorder
E. none of the above

ANSWERS

41.1 The answer is E

The definition of reading disorder remains controversial. Five major areas are generally agreed upon in describing the disorder, though debate even on these items continues. First, the underlying cause of reading disorder is *central nervous system dysfunction*. Second, there is an *uneven pattern of cognitive functioning*, meaning that while overall cognitive functioning is intact, specific areas are significantly deficient. Third, there is *difficulty in single-word decoding*, a fundamental skill in the task of learning to read. Fourth, there is a *discrepancy between learning potential and actual reading achievement*. Fifth and finally, there must be exclusion of other causes of reading difficulty.

41.2 The answer is C

Dyslexia is one of several distinct learning disabilities. It is a language-based disorder characterized by *difficulties in single-word decoding*, usually reflecting insufficient phonological processing. These difficulties are unexpected in relation to age and other cognitive and academic abilities. The difficulties are not the result of generalized developmental disability or of *sensory impairment*. Dyslexia is manifested by variable difficulty with different forms of language, often (not rarely) including *problems with reading, writing, and spelling*. This recently proposed definition reflects two important advances. First, instead of defining reading disorders generally, it focuses on one type of reading disorder dyslexia. Second, it localizes the difficulty associated with dyslexia at the single-word level and pinpoints the cause as *insufficient phonological processing*. Although this definition has not gained universal acceptance, it represents a significant step forward in addressing some of the previous confusion and disagreement surrounding previous definitions of learning disabilities.

41.3 The answer is D

Other developmental and learning disorders are often linked with mathematics disorder. Reading disorder, disorder of written expression, expressive language disorder, mixed receptive-expressive language disorder, and developmental coordination disorder, have all been reported in association with mathematics disorder. Specific cognitive processing difficulties (e.g., auditory-verbal deficits, visual-spatial deficits, motor deficits, memory deficits, and attention deficits) may be associated features.

Social immaturity, school and peer problems, social skills deficits, anxiety, and depression likewise have been reported as associated problems. However, the psychiatric syndrome that is most often found comorbid with mathematics disorder is attention-deficit/hyperactivity disorder. The precise nature of the relationship is unclear; however, recent studies suggest that specific symptoms of *ADHD* (inattention, distractibility, decreased vigilance) *may strongly correlate with deficiencies in mathematics performance*.

41.4 The answer is A

41.5 The answer is D

41.6 The answer is C

41.7 The answer is A

Reading disorder used to be known as dyslexia; as described in the answer to question 41.2, the term dyslexia has recently taken on a more specific meaning. *Reading disorder is reported to occur most frequently in children born in May, June, and July*, a finding that has sparked theories of a relationship between the disorder and maternal infections during the winter months that might affect the developing fetus' brain. *Disorder of written expression is usually diagnosed later than other learning disorders*, as writing skills are acquired at a later age than are reading skills. Learning disorder not otherwise specified is a category of learning disorders that do not meet criteria for any of the specific learning disorders; *spelling skills deficit is an example of a condition that would fall under the heading of learning disorder not otherwise specified*. Mathematics disorder includes deficits in linguistic skills related to understanding mathematical terms, converting written problems into mathematical symbols, and perceptual skills such as the ability to recognize and understand symbols and to order clusters of numbers.

41.8 The answer is B

41.9 The answer is C

41.10 The answer is C

41.11 The answer is C

41.12 The answer is C

Although not definitively studied, the prevalence of mathematics disorder in school-age children has been estimated at 6 percent. *The study of mathematics disorder has been neglected despite a prevalence that is similar to other learning disorders*. Several researchers have asserted that this reflects a cultural bias that prioritizes literacy skills over mathematics skills.

The etiologies of reading disorder and mathematics disorder are unknown. Both likely involve biological dysfunctions that results in impairment of or delay in development of cognitive skills required for these operations. Many of the theories of brain dysfunction in children with reading disorder are based on observations of associated symptoms. For example, because language and speech problems are often related, abnormalities in the left hemisphere and in the frontal speech regions in both hemispheres have been cited as possible etiological factors. Similarly, insofar as motor problems with balance and equilibrium are often linked with reading difficulties, abnormalities in cerebellar-vestibular function have been postulated. *Thus brain anomalies are inferred but have not been definitively demonstrated in reading disorder*. In mathematics disorder, the finding that adults with acquired right parietal-occipital hemispheric lesions developed a loss of arithmetical skills has prompted *speculation that abnormalities in the same region might underlie mathematical disorder in children; this, too, remains to be convincingly demonstrated*.

Twin studies have consistently found higher concordance rates for reading disorder in monozygotic twin pairs than in dizygotic pairs; estimates of genetic influence on acquisition of reading disorder have been between 30 and 60 percent, with environmental factors also contributing significantly. *Mathematics disorder also has evidence of genetic influence, with higher rates of concordance in monozygotic versus dizygotic twins.*

Although symptoms of reading disorder may appear as early as age 5, as manifested by inability to distinguish between letters or to associate phonemes with letter symbols, referral for evaluation and formal diagnosis typically occur later. *Many children are first diagnosed when they fail to respond to formal instruction in second grade.* Others, especially those with high intelligence, may not be diagnosed until fourth or fifth grade. Similarly, although difficulties with counting and number concepts may be apparent in kindergarten, a *diagnosis of mathematics disorder is not often made prior to second or third grade.*

41.13 The answer is D

Reading disorder occurs in three to four times as many boys as girls (not vice versa). This rate in boys may be falsely elevated, as boys with reading disorders commonly also have behavioral problems, and the latter symptoms often prompt scrutiny of boys' psychological and learning issues.

Reading disorder is characterized by *impairment in recognizing words*, slow and inaccurate reading, and *poor reading comprehension. Omissions, additions and distortions of words are made in oral reading.* Reading achievement is below that expected for the individual's age on standardized testing. While no causal factor has been identified in the disorder, *increased prevalence in family members* suggests a genetic contribution.

41.14 The answer is A

Unlike reading disorder, in which the prevalence appears to be higher in boys, there is *no demonstrated gender difference* in mathematics disorder, and the problem may be more common in girls than in boys. The *prevalence of mathematics disorder is estimated at 6 percent of school-age children with normal intelligence.* Mathematics disorder includes *impairment in addition, subtraction, multiplication, and division.* The disorder is usually *apparent by age 8*, though it may present as early as 6 or as late as 10 years of age. Mathematics disorder commonly coexists with reading disorder.

41.15 The answer is D

Disorder of written expression includes *disability in spelling, grammar, and punctuation.* The disorder is characterized by writing skills that are significantly below the expected level given the child's age and intelligence (as measured by standardized testing). Because children learn to speak and read prior to learning to write, disorder of written expression *presents later (not earlier)* than do reading disorder and communication disorders. Disorder of written expression *can occur in children both with and without concomitant reading disorder.* The disorder should be diagnosed in the school-age years; in severe cases problems are evident by age 7, whereas in milder cases the disorder may not be apparent until age 10 or later. *The disorder is not self-limited*; children with mild to moderate problems do well with timely remedial work around writing skills, while more severely affected children may require ongoing, extensive remediation through high school and even into college. Remedial treatment involves direct practice in spelling, sentence construction, and rules of grammar.

41.16 The answer is E (all)

Reading disorder, mixed expressive-receptive language disorder, developmental coordination disorder, mathematics disorder, attention-deficit/hyperactivity disorder, and other disruptive behavior disorders often co-occur with disorder of written expression. The ability to transfer one's thoughts into effective written communication requires multimodal sensorimotor coordination and information processing. Disorder of written expression is an academic skills disorder that presents during childhood and is characterized by poor performance in spelling, grammar, and punctuation.

41.17 The answer is D

The most likely diagnosis for Janet is *reading disorder.* Reading disorder is characterized by marked impairment in the development of word recognition skills and reading comprehension that cannot be explained by mental retardation, inadequate schooling, visual or hearing defect, or a neurological disorder. Reading-disordered children make many errors in their oral reading, including omissions, additions, and distortions of words. Janet's difficulties, apparently, were limited to reading and spelling. She had average intelligence and normal scores on achievement tests of arithmetic but markedly low scores for spelling and reading.

Disorder of written expression is characterized by poor performance in writing and composition. *Expressive language disorder* is characterized by serious impairment in age-appropriate expressive language. *Phonological disorder* is characterized by frequent and recurrent misarticulations of speech sounds, resulting in abnormal speech. The case described does not meet the criteria for any diagnosis other than reading disorder.

42

Motor Skills Disorder: Developmental Coordination Disorder

Developmental coordination disorder is a condition characterized by low performance in daily activities that require coordination below what is expected for age and intellectual level. According to the text revision of the 4th edition of *Diagnostic and Statistical Manual of Mental Disorders* (DSM-IV-TR), the disorder may present with delays in achieving motor milestones such as sitting, crawling, and walking.

Developmental coordination disorder may also be manifested by clumsy gross and fine motor skills, resulting in poor performance in sports and even poor handwriting. A child with developmental coordination disorder may bump into things more often than siblings or drop things. In the 1930s, the term *clumsy child syndrome* began to be used in the literature to denote a condition of awkward motor behaviors that could not be correlated with any specific neurological disorder or damage. This term continues to be used to identify imprecise or delayed gross and fine motor behavior in children, resulting in subtle motor inabilities, but often significant social rejection. Currently, there are indications that perinatal problems such as prematurity, low birth weight, and hypoxia may contribute to the emergence of developmental coordination disorders. Children with developmental coordination disorder are at higher risk for language and learning disorders. There is a strong association between speech and language problems and coordination problems, as well as an association of coordination difficulties with hyperactivity, impulsivity, and poor attention span.

The student should study the questions and answers below for a useful review of this disorder.

HELPFUL HINTS

The student should be able to define the terms listed here.

- attention-deficit/hyperactivity disorder
- Bender Visual Motor Gestalt test
- Bruininks-Oseretsky Test of Motor Development
- catching a ball
- cerebral palsy
- clumsiness
- conduct disorder
- deficits in handwriting
- delayed motor milestones
- expressive language disorder
- eye–hand coordination
- fine motor skills
- finger tapping
- Frostig Movement Skills Test Battery
- Gerstmann syndrome
- graphemes
- gross motor skills
- informal motor skills screening
- learning disorders
- linguistic, perceptual, mathematical, and attentional skills
- perceptual motor training
- psychoeducational tests
- remedial treatments
- shoelace tying
- social ostracism
- temperamental attributes
- unsteady gait

QUESTIONS

Directions

Each of the questions or incomplete statements below is followed by five suggested responses or completions. Select the *one* that is *best* in each case.

42.1 Manifestations of developmental coordination disorder include:

A. delays in reaching motor milestones such as sitting and crawling
B. avoidance of participation in sports activities with peers
C. messy or illegible writing

D. difficulty learning feeding skills
E. all of the above

42.2 Which of the following tests is *not* helpful in demonstrating developmental coordination disorder?

A. Bender Visual Motor Gestalt test
B. Verbal subsets of the Wechsler Intelligence Scale for Children—Third Edition (WISC-III)
C. Bruiniks-Oseretsky Test of Motor Development
D. Frostig Movement Skills Test Battery
E. None of the above

42.3 Which of the following is a risk factor for developmental coordination disorder?

A. Birth in May, June, or July
B. Borderline intellectual functioning
C. Frequent episodes of *otitis media* in the first two years of life
D. Prematurity
E. Dysfunctional family

42.4 Which of the following statements is *false*?

A. Children with developmental coordination disorder may resemble younger children motorically.
B. Developmental coordination disorder commonly occurs in conjunction with a communication disorder.
C. Children with developmental coordination disorder during early childhood typically develop age-expected fine motor and gross motor coordination skills by early adolescence.
D. Prematurity, low birth weight, neonatal malnutrition, and perinatal hypoxia are all risk factors for developmental coordination disorder.
E. Medical causes of motor deficits such as cerebral palsy or muscular dystrophy must be ruled out prior to making a diagnosis of developmental coordination disorder.

Directions

The group of questions below consists of lettered headings followed by a list of numbered words or statements. For each numbered word or statement, select the *one* lettered heading that is most closely associated with it. Each lettered heading may be selected once, more than once, or not at all.

Questions 42.5–42.8

A. Dyspraxia
B. Synkinesia
C. Impersistence
D. Asymmetries
E. Hypertonus

42.5 Facial grimaces when child is asked to make hand movements

42.6 Clinician tracks how long a child can stick out his tongue

42.7 Child tends to throw a ball too hard and inaccurately at short distances

42.8 Inability to follow directions to hold a comb with the right hand, pass it to the left hand, and use it to comb hair from front to back

ANSWERS

42.1 The answer is E (all)

Children with developmental coordination disorder perform motor coordination tasks at levels markedly below those expected for their chronological ages and intelligence. The motor deficits significantly interfere with academic achievement and social integration. Specific manifestations may include *delays in achieving motor milestones, difficulty acquiring feeding skills, poor handwriting, and poor performance in sports (leading to avoidance of sports activities).*

42.2 The answer is B

Children with developmental coordination disorder often have below-normal scores on the performance subsets of the WISC-III, but *do not tend to have below-normal scores on the verbal subsets of the WISC-III.* A number of other tests are useful for detecting motor coordination difficulties, including the *Bender Visual Motor Gestalt test, the Bruiniks-Oseretsky Test of Motor Development, and the Frostig Movement Skills Test Battery.*

42.3 The answer is D

Risk factors postulated to contribute to developmental coordination disorder include *prematurity*, perinatal hypoxia, neonatal malnutrition, low birth weight, and prenatal exposure to nicotine, alcohol, and cocaine. *Although reading disorder has been associated with birth in May, June, or July,* suggesting a possible link between winter maternal infectious illness and reading disorder in the child, no such link has been found in developmental coordination disorder. *Borderline intellectual functioning* (an IQ between 70 and 90) is not an identified risk factor for developmental coordination disorder, *nor is a dysfunctional family.* There is *no documented relationship between frequent episodes of otitis media and onset of developmental coordination disorder.*

42.4 The answer is C

Children with developmental coordination disorder may resemble younger children motorically. Follow-up studies of children with developmental coordination disorder in early childhood indicate that *these individuals continue to have deficits in most motor skills well into adolescence and young adulthood*; they also tend to have persistently poorer educational achievement and significantly lower perceived social competence than their peers. These related problems may be attributable to the finding that children with developmental coordination disorder frequently suffer from other developmental-learning difficulties: *the disorder is frequently seen in conjunction with communication disorders* as well as learning disorders. Secondary complications are also common in developmental coordination disorder: socialization problems commonly arise when these children struggle with sports and games and are subsequently rejected by peers.

As noted in the answer to question 42.3, a number of risk factors have been associated with developmental coordination disorder, including *prematurity, low birth weight, neonatal malnutrition, and perinatal hypoxia.* As specified in the DSM-IV-TR diagnostic criteria for developmental coordination disorder, *the disturbance in coordination must not be due to a general medical condition (such as cerebral palsy, muscular dystrophy*, or hemiplegia) and must not occur in the context of a pervasive developmental disorder.

Answers 42.5–42.8

42.5 The answer is B

42.6 The answer is C

42.7 The answer is E

42.8 The answer is A

The essential feature of developmental coordination disorder is poor motor coordination. Motor skills tend to be imprecise or clumsy rather than globally impaired. Impairments affect fine and gross motor coordination skills, and can be observed clinically when the patient is engaged in tasks requiring the use of various muscle groups. There are seven diagnostic categories which describe these impairments: dyspraxia, synkinesia, hypotonus, hypertonus, tremors, impersistence, and asymmetries.

Dyspraxia describes the child's inability to produce correctly sequenced, coordinated motor movements when presented with a demonstration or oral command*; an example would be the inability to follow directions to hold a comb with the right hand, pass it to the left hand, and use it to comb hair from front to back.* Synkinesia is a phenomenon involving unintentional muscle movements, or muscle overflow; *a child with synkinesia might make a facial grimace when asked to make hand movements.*

Hypotonus and hypertonus describe abnormalities in muscle tone. Hypotonus is characterized by flaccid muscle tone; these children often appear lazy and sleepy. *Hypertonus* involves excessive muscle tone, leading to poor modulation of muscle activity and observed *behaviors such as throwing a ball too hard and inaccurately at short distances.*

Tremors are characterized by irregular unsteadiness in muscle movements, leading to difficulties in activities such as writing or walking. *Impersistence* refers to the child's inability to sustain body postures for reasonable periods of time; clinicians may determine *how long a child is able to stick out his or her tongue* to check for this symptom. Asymmetries are motor behaviors affecting only one side of the body, such as weakness or abnormal muscle flexion or extension.

43 Communication Disorders

Spoken language is an essential part of communicating ideas, social interactions, and academic understanding. Effective communication for a child or adolescent includes proficiency in both language and speech skills. The text revision of the 4th edition of *Diagnostic and Statistical Manual of Mental Disorders* (DSM-IV-TR) includes four specific communication disorders and one residual category. Two of the communication disorders (expressive and mixed receptive-expressive communication disorder) are language disorders; the other two (phonological disorder and stuttering) are speech disorders. A child with a language disorder may have a limited vocabulary, speak in short simple sentences, and tell stories in a disorganized and incomplete manner. A child with a speech disorder may attempt to use appropriate descriptive words but has difficulty pronouncing the speech sounds correctly and may either omit sounds or pronounce sounds in an unusual way. A child with stuttering generally has acquired a normal vocabulary, but speech fluency is disrupted by pauses, sound repetitions, or sound prolongations.

Language usage includes four components: phonology, grammar, semantics, and pragmatics. Phonology refers to the ability to produce sounds that constitute words in a given language and the skills to discriminate the various phonemes (sounds that are made by a letter or group of letters in a language). To imitate words, a child must be able to produce the sounds of a word. Grammar designates the organization of words and the rules for placing words in an order that makes sense in that language. Semantics refers to the organization of concepts and the acquisition of words themselves. A child draws from a mental list of words to produce sentences. Pragmatics has to do with skill in the actual use of language and the "rules" of conversation, including pausing so that a listener can answer a question and knowing when to change the topic when there is a break in a conversation. By age 2 years, toddlers may know up to 200 words, and by age 3 years, most children understand the basic rules of language and can converse effectively.

The student should study the questions and answers below for a useful review of these disorders.

HELPFUL HINTS

These terms relate to communication disorders and should be known by the student.

- ambilaterality
- articulation problems
- audiogram
- baby talk
- cluttering
- comprehension
- decoding
- developmental coordination disorders
- dysarthria
- encoding
- expressive language disorder
- fluency of speech
- language acquisition
- lateral slip and palatal lisp
- maturational lag
- misarticulation
- mixed receptive-expressive language disorder
- neurodevelopmental delays
- omissions
- phoneme
- phonological disorder
- semantogenic theory of stuttering
- sound distortion
- spastic dysphonia
- speech therapy
- standardized language test
- stuttering
- substitution
- time patterning of speech

QUESTIONS

Directions

Each of the questions or incomplete statements below is followed by five responses or completions. Select the *one* that is *best* in each case.

43.1 Normal development in a 3-year-old child includes:

A. Use of 900 to 1,000 words
B. Speech is usually understood by strangers
C. Follows three-step commands
D. Use of conjunctions (e.g., if, but, because)
E. Discusses feelings

43.2 Which of the following is a true statement about diagnosis of communication disorders?

A. Substantial deficits in receptive language do not preclude the diagnosis of expressive language disorder.

B. Substantial deficits in nonverbal intelligence do not preclude the diagnosis of expressive language disorder.
C. If both expressive and receptive deficits occur in the absence of nonverbal deficits, the diagnosis of mixed receptive-expressive language disorder is not appropriate.
D. If language and nonverbal functioning are both substantially below age-level expectations, the diagnosis of mental retardation should be made.
E. None of the above

43.3 Which of the following is a true statement about presentation and course of developmental expressive language deficits?

A. Less than 20 percent of "late talkers" achieve language skills within the normal range during the preschool years.
B. Most "late talkers" who recover during preschool appear to be at relatively high risk for severe learning and behavioral problems during their early school years.
C. Expressive language disorder often appears in the absence of comprehension problems, whereas receptive dysfunction generally diminishes proficiency in expressive language.
D. There is clear consensus among experts that intervention to improve expressive language should only be provided for children whose problems persist to age 4 or 5.
E. None of the above

43.4 Children with expressive language disorder are distinguishable from children with pervasive developmental disorders in that they

A. appropriately use gestures to communicate
B. are noted to use symbolic or imaginary play
C. readily form meaningful and warm social relationships
D. show significant frustration with the inability to communicate verbally
E. All of the above

Directions

Each group of questions below consists of lettered headings followed by a list of numbered phrases or statements. For each numbered phrase or statement, select the *one* lettered heading that is most closely associated with it. Each lettered heading may be selected once, more than once, or not at all.

Questions 43.5–43.9

A. Expressive language disorder
B. Phonological disorder
C. Voice disorder
D. Verbal apraxia
E. None of the above

43.5 Disturbance in the programming of speech movements associated with a primary insult to the left cerebral hemisphere

43.6 Organic causes include endocrine dysfunction and laryngeal papillomas

43.7 Use of sentences that are short, incomplete, or ungrammatical

43.8 In DSM-IV-TR, this category encompasses speech sound problems that have no known cause and presumably reflect developmental difficulties in acquiring the sound system of a language

43.9 Associated with cleft lip and palate

Questions 43.10–43.12

A. A child sings normally
B. A child cannot understand language
C. A child has an abnormally loud voice
D. A child substitutes and omits speech sounds
E. None of the above

43.10 Phonological disorder

43.11 Stuttering disorder

43.12 Mixed receptive-expressive language disorder

Questions 43.13–43.17

A. Expressive language disorder
B. Mixed receptive-expressive language disorder
C. Phonological disorder
D. Stuttering
E. All of the above

43.13 This disorder may include dysarthria and apraxia when occurring in the context of neurological disorders such as cerebral palsy or head injury.

43.14 A child with this disorder may appear to be deaf.

43.15 This disorder is most commonly seen in males.

43.16 Cluttering, a dysrhythmic speech pattern with jerky spurts of words, is often an associated feature of this disorder.

43.17 This disorder has two peaks of onset: between 2 and $3^1/_2$ years and between 5 and 7 years.

ANSWERS

43.1 The answer is A

Expressive language disorder is diagnosed when a selective deficit in expressive language development occurs in the presence of intact nonverbal intelligence and receptive language skills. Children with expressive disorders do acquire language, albeit at a slower rate than their peers. Accordingly, the specific manifestations of expressive language disorder change over the course of development. Affected children often show expressive language characteristics that resemble those of younger children who are developing language at a normal rate. Table 43.1 provides an overview of typical milestones in language and nonverbal development. *Normal development in a 3-year-old child includes use of 900 to 1,000 words*; speech understood by family members (*not necessarily by strangers*); ability to follow two-step (*not three-step*) commands; and three-to-four word sentences composed mainly of nouns and verbs (*not conjunctions*). *The age at which children begin discussing feelings*

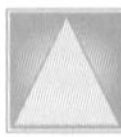

Table 43.1
Normal Development of Speech, Language, and Nonverbal Skills in Children

Speech and Language Development	Nonverbal Development
1 yr	
Recognizes own name	Stands alone
Follows simple directions accompanied by gestures (e.g., bye-bye)	Takes first steps with support
Speaks one or two words	Uses common objects (e.g., spoon, cup)
Mixes words and jargon sounds	Releases objects willfully
Uses communicative gestures (e.g., showing, pointing)	Searches for object in location where last seen
2 yrs	
Uses 200–300 words	Walks up and down stairs alone but without alternating feet
Names most common objects	Runs rhythmically but is unable to stop or start smoothly
Uses two-word or longer phrases	Eats with a fork
Uses a few prepositions (e.g., in, on), pronouns (e.g., you, me), verb endings (e.g., -ing, -s, -ed), and plurals (-s), but not always correctly	Cooperates with adult in simple household tasks Enjoys play with action toys
Follows simple commands not accompanied by gestures	
3 yrs	
Uses 900–1,000 words	Rides tricycle
Creates three- to four-word sentences, usually with subject and verb but simple structure	Enjoys simple "make-believe" play Matches primary colors
Follows two-step commands	Balances momentarily on one foot
Repeats five- to seven-syllable sentences	Shares toys with others for short periods
Speech is usually understood by family members	
4 yrs	
Uses 1,500–1,600 words	Walks up and down stairs with alternating feet
Recounts stories and events from recent past	Hops on one foot
Understands most questions about immediate environment	Copies block letters
Uses conjunctions (e.g., if, but, because)	Role-plays with others
Speech is usually understood by strangers	Categorizes familiar objects
5 yrs	
Uses 2,100–2,300 words	Dresses self without assistance
Discusses feelings	Cuts own meat with knife
Understands most prepositions referring to space (e.g., above, beside, toward) and time (e.g., before, after, until)	Draws a recognizable person Plays purposefully and constructively
Follows three-step commands	Recognizes part-whole relationships
Prints own name	
6 yrs	
Defines words by function and attributes	Rides a bicycle
Uses a variety of well-formed complex sentences	Throws a ball well
Uses all parts of speech (e.g., verbs, nouns, adverbs, adjectives, conjunctions, prepositions)	Sustains attention to motivating tasks Enjoys competitive games
Understands letter-sound associations in reading	
8 yrs	
Reads simple books for pleasure	Understands conservation of liquid, number, length, etc.
Enjoys riddles and jokes	Knows left and right of others
Verbalizes ideas and problems readily	Knows differences and similarities
Understands indirect requests (e.g., "It's hot in here" understood as request to open window)	Appreciates that others have different perspectives
Produces all speech sounds in an adult-like manner	Categorizes same object into multiple categories

Adapted from Owens RE. *Language Development: An Introduction.* 4th ed. Needham Heights, MA: Allyn & Bacon; 1996.

in the course of normal development is five years old (not three years old).

43.2 The answer is D

Differential diagnosis of developmental expressive language disorder requires standardized evaluations of expressive language, receptive language, and nonverbal intellectual functioning. Expressive language development must fall significantly below (1) the range of normal expressive performance expected for a child's age, (2) the child's receptive language performance, and (3) the child's nonverbal intellectual performance. Furthermore, the expressive language difficulties must be severe enough to impair academic performance or social communication. This severity criterion is assessed by direct observation of the child and analysis of spontaneous language use, supplementing standardized testing.

Substantial deficits in either receptive language or nonverbal intelligence preclude the diagnosis of expressive language disorder. If both expressive and receptive deficits occur in the absence of nonverbal deficits, the diagnosis of mixed receptive-expressive language disorder is appropriate. However, *if language and nonverbal functioning are both substantially below age-level expectations, the diagnosis of mental retardation should be made.*

43.3 The answer is C

Developmental expressive language disorder is characterized by considerable variability in severity, course, and outcome. *Expressive language disorder commonly appears in the absence of comprehension problems, whereas receptive language dysfunction generally diminished proficiency in expressive language.* Experts disagree on whether "late talkers," children with normal cognitive functioning who use fewer than 50 words and no word combinations at age 2, meet criteria for a diagnosis of expressive language disorder. Irrespective of diagnosis, language delays often provoke parental concern and professional referral. *Studies indicate that 50 to 80 percent (not less than 20 percent) of these children achieve language skills within the normal range during the preschool years.* Additionally, *"late talkers" who "catch up" during the preschool years are at low (not high) risk for severe learning and behavioral problems during their early school years.* Prognosis tends to be less favorable for children whose expressive language problems persist into late preschool or early school-age years. Language development proceeds at a slower rate in these children than in their normally developing peers, and they are also at elevated risk of associated problems including reading disorder and attention-deficit/hyperactivity disorder. By adolescence, most children with expressive language disorder acquire sufficient language skills to function reasonably well in daily communication activities, though subtle residual deficits may be apparent in demanding speaking tasks.

Experts disagree on when intervention is warranted for expressive language disorder. Some favor a wait-and-see approach for young children with early expressive delays ("late talkers") because most will acquire language functioning within the normal range during their preschool years. According to this view, intervention to improve expressive language should only be provided to children whose problems persist to age 4 or 5. However, others argue that earlier intervention may serve to prevent or minimize long-term language, academic, and behavioral difficulties.

43.4 The answer is E (all)

When evaluating children with problems with expressive language, the differential diagnosis may include expressive language disorder and pervasive developmental disorders (PDD). Several key features help to distinguish these diagnoses. *Children with expressive language disorder typically appropriately use gestures to communicate, engage in symbolic and imaginary play, readily form meaningful and warm social relationships, and show significant frustration with the inability to communicate verbally.* By contrast, children with PDD tend not to use gestures, do not develop imaginary play or use of symbolism, show little interest in most social relationships, and appear less disturbed by their inability to communicate verbally.

Answers 43.5–43.9

43.5 The answer is D

43.6 The answer is C

43.7 The answer is A

43.8 The answer is B

43.9 The answer is B

Verbal apraxia (also called apraxia of speech) is a disturbance in the programming of movements that produce speech. It is differentiated from voice disorder by its association with a *primary insult to the left cerebral hemisphere.* Additionally, verbal output in apraxic patients is often normal in automatic or overlearned speech (e.g., automatic social greetings, singing "Happy Birthday").

A voice disorder, as described in the DSM-IV-TR, is any "abnormality of vocal pitch, loudness, quality, tone or resonance." Given the complexity and sensitivity of the process of voice production, it is unsurprising that these disorders may arise from myriad factors, including medical disease and psychological distress. *Voice disorders of organic cause among children and adolescents include laryngeal papillomas,* vocal fold nodules, laryngomalacia, laryngeal webbing (congenital or traumatic), vocal polyps, vocal hemorrhage, vocal fold paralysis or paresis, endocrine dysfunction, and laryngeal cancer. Premature infants and children with a history of prolonged endotracheal intubation are at high risk for development of a number of laryngeal pathologies. Reflux esophagitis and irritation of the larynx are observed in patients with bulimia and may be accompanied by hoarse voice. Because persistent hoarseness in a child or adolescent may be a sign of malignancy or another serious medical condition, otolaryngological evaluation is warranted.

Children with expressive language disorders have difficulty communicating via spoken language. They commonly (1) have limited speaking vocabularies; (2) *speak in short, incomplete, or ungrammatical sentences*; and (3) related stories and events in a disorganized or unsophisticated manner. These problems are evident despite performance within normal ranges on measures of hearing acuity, nonverbal intelligence, and comprehension of spoken language.

Children with phonological disorders have difficulties producing speech sounds that are appropriate for their ages and dialects. They may omit sounds, substitute sounds for other sounds, or distort sounds by producing them incorrectly. Typically, the abnormal sounds occur in systematic patterns—e.g., omitting final consonants, pronouncing /s/ or /z/ sounds with the tongue protruded. Listeners may be unable to understand the speech of children with severe phonological disorders.

The DSM-IV-TR uses terminology for speech sound production disorders that differs from what is commonly used in the clinical and scientific literature. *In DSM-IV-TR, the category of phonological disorders includes difficulties in speech sounds production that have no known cause as well as those that arise from hearing impairment, structural abnormalities of the speech mechanism (e.g., cleft lip or palate), or neurological conditions (e.g., head injury, cerebral palsy).* In the literature, the terms articulation disorder and speech sound production disorder may be used to label this inclusive group of disorders. The terms *dysarthria* and *dyspraxia* are typically used to refer to speech sound production difficulties that have a neurological basis. The term phonological disorder is usually reserved for speech sound problems that have no known cause and presumably reflect developmental difficulties in acquiring the regularities of phonology (the sound system of a language).

The speech of children with cleft palate may be characterized by excessive nasality and by the inability to produce the many consonants that require the oral cavity to be closed off from the nasal passage by the palate. Children may develop unusual way of articulating certain sounds in an attempt to compensate for structural deficits. Even after corrective surgery, these unusual patterns may persist.

Answers 43.10–43.12

43.10 The answer is D

43.11 The answer is A

43.12 The answer is B

In phonological disorder, children substitute and omit speech sounds. The misarticulation of speech in this disorder may resemble baby talk. The omissions, substitutions, and distortions typically occur with late-learned phonemes. *A child who stutters may sing normally. A child with mixed receptive-expressive language disorder cannot understand language.* Although his or her nonverbal intellectual performance is age-appropriate, a child with this disorder struggles with speech and cannot mimic sounds.

Answers 43.13–43.17

43.13 The answer is C

43.14 The answer is B

43.15 The answer is E

43.16 The answer is A

43.17 The answer is D

Phonological disorder is characterized by poor sound production or articulation. There may be substitutions of one sound for another, omissions of certain sounds, or an inability to reproduce a sound accurately. Often children with phonological disorder appear to be using "baby talk." *In certain neurological conditions, phonological disorder may be characterized by dysarthria and apraxia.*

Mixed receptive-expressive language disorder is an impairment both in the understanding and production of language. Deficits in receptive language are most often accompanied by impairments in expressive language. Children with mixed receptive-expressive language disorder show a markedly delayed ability to comprehend verbal or sign language, despite normal intellectual functioning. *Children with this disorder may appear to be deaf,* as they don't respond normally to language; however, they do tend to respond to non-language sounds in their environment. When these children begin to use language, their speech contains numerous errors in articulation and substitutions of phonemes. *All of the communication disorders are two to four times more common in boys than girls.* This striking gender difference implies a genetic basis for these disorders.

Cluttering is a disordered speech pattern in which speech is erratically produced, with bursts of rapid and jerky words and phrases. Children with this speech pattern are typically unaware that their speech is abnormal. *Cluttering is often an associated feature of expressive language disorder.* Cluttering differs from stuttering in that the disturbance in fluency in stuttering is characterized by sound repetitions, pauses within words, prolongations, and audible or silent word blocking. Stutterers are generally aware of their stuttering and many experience anxiety before speaking. *Stuttering usually appears before the age of 12; two peaks of onset exist at 2 to $3^1/_2$ years and 5 to 7 years.* In the preschool age group, children tend to stutter most often when they are excited or have a lot to say; stuttering at this age is often a passing phase. In the elementary school years, stuttering may become more chronic and may characterize the child's everyday speech. Later in childhood, stuttering is often an intermittent event that manifests itself in the course of a specific situation. Stutterers often display fear, embarrassment, and anxious anticipation of speaking in public, or avoid certain words and phrases that they associate with their stuttering.

44

Pervasive Developmental Disorders

The pervasive developmental disorders include a group of conditions in which there are delay and deviance in the development of social skills, language and communication, and behavioral repertoire. Children with pervasive developmental disorders often exhibit idiosyncratic intense interest in a narrow range of activities, resist change, and are not appropriately responsive to the social environment. These disorders affect multiple areas of development, manifest early in life, and cause persistent dysfunction. Autistic disorder, the best known of these disorders, is characterized by sustained impairment in comprehending and responding to social cues, aberrant language development and usage, and restricted, stereotypical behavioral patterns. According to the text revision of the 4th edition of *Diagnostic and Statistical Manual of Mental Disorders* (DSM-IV-TR), to meet criteria for autistic behavior, abnormal functioning in at least one of the above areas must be present by age 3. More than two thirds of children with autistic disorder have mental retardation, although it is not required for the diagnosis.

DSM-IV-TR includes five pervasive developmental disorders: autistic disorder, Rett's disorder, childhood disintegrative disorder, Asperger's disorder, and pervasive developmental disorder not otherwise specified. Rett's disorder appears to occur exclusively in girls; it is characterized by normal development for at least 6 months, stereotyped hand movements, a loss of purposeful motions, diminishing social engagement, poor coordination, and decreasing language use. In childhood disintegrative disorder, development progresses normally for the first 2 years, after which the child shows a loss of previously acquired skills in two or more of the following areas: language use, social responsiveness, play, motor skills, and bladder or bowel control. Asperger's disorder is a condition in which the child is markedly impaired in social relatedness and shows repetitive and stereotyped patterns of behavior without a delay in language development. In Asperger's disorder, a child's cognitive abilities and adaptive skills are normal.

The student should study the questions and answers below for a useful review of these disorders.

HELPFUL HINTS

The student should know the following terms related to pervasive developmental disorders.

- abnormal relationship
- acquired aphasia
- Asperger's disorder
- attachment behavior
- autistic disorder
- brain volume
- childhood disintegrative disorder
- childhood schizophrenia
- communication disorder
- concordance rate
- congenital deafness
- congenital physical anomaly
- congenital rubella
- CT scan
- dermatoglyphics
- disintegrative (regressive) psychosis
- dread of change
- echolalia
- echolalic speech
- educational and behavioral treatments
- EEG abnormalities
- ego-educative approach
- encopresis
- enuresis
- extreme autistic aloneness
- eye contact
- failed cerebral lateralization
- grand mal seizure
- haloperidol (Haldol)
- Heller's syndrome
- hyperkinesis
- hyperserotonemia
- hyperuricosuria
- "idiot savant"
- insight-oriented psychotherapy
- islets of precocity
- Leo Kanner
- language deviance and delay
- low-purine diet
- mental retardation
- monotonous repetition
- organic abnormalities
- pain threshold
- parental rage and rejection
- perinatal complications
- pervasive developmental disorder
- physical characteristics
- PKU
- play
- prevalence
- pronominal reversal
- psychodynamic and family causation
- Purkinje's cells
- Rett's disorder
- ritual
- rote memory
- seizures
- self-injurious behavior
- separation anxiety
- sex distribution
- social class
- splinter function
- stereotypy
- tardive and withdrawal dyskinesias
- temporal lobe
- tuberous sclerosis
- vestibular stimulation
- voice quality and rhythm

QUESTIONS

Directions

Each of the questions or incomplete statements below is followed by five suggested responses or completions. Select the *one* that is *best* in each case.

44.1 Which of the following features does *not* distinguish autistic disorder from mixed receptive-expressive language disorder?

A. Echolalia
B. Stereotypies
C. Imaginative play
D. Associated deafness
E. Family history of speech delay

44.2 Neurological-biochemical abnormalities associated with autistic disorder include

A. grand mal seizures
B. ventricular enlargement on computed tomography (CT) scan
C. electroencephalogram (EEG) abnormalities
D. increased total brain volume
E. all of the above

44.3 True statements about autistic disorder include which of the following?

A. Girls outnumber boys in individuals with autism without mental retardation.
B. There is an established and conclusive association between autism and upper socioeconomic status.
C. Prevalence rates may be as high as 1 in 1000 children.
D. Abnormalities in functioning must be present by age 2 to meet DSM-IV-TR diagnostic criteria.
E. All of the above

44.4 True statements about the role of genetics in autistic disorder include which of the following?

A. Twin studies indicate only moderate concordance for monozygotes.
B. Family studies show a prevalence of approximately 2 to 3 percent of autism among siblings of children with autism.
C. Unaffected siblings are not at increased risk for language problems.
D. It is clear that what is inherited is a specific predisposition to autistic disorder.
E. The role of genetic factors in autistic disorder is not well established.

44.5 The most frequent *presenting* complaint of parents about their autistic child is

A. their lack of interest in social interaction.
B. their lack of usual play skills.
C. their difficulty tolerating change and variations in their routines.
D. delays in the acquisition of language.
E. stereotyped movements.

44.6 Relative strengths of autistic children in psychological testing include which of the following?

A. Block design and digit recall
B. Verbal concept formulation
C. Integration skills
D. Similarities and comprehension
E. Abstract reasoning

44.7 What percentage of autistic individuals exhibits special abilities or splinter (savant) skills?

A. Less than 1 percent
B. 10 percent
C. 25 percent
D. 50 percent
E. 80 percent

44.8 Rett's disorder

A. is seen only in boys.
B. does not involve motor abnormalities.
C. is associated with normal intelligence.
D. shows no loss of social skills.
E. none of the above

44.9 Childhood disintegrative disorder is

A. characterized by behaviors markedly different than those seen in autistic disorder
B. more common in boys than girls
C. always characterized by a gradual onset
D. notable in that acquired self-help skills do not deteriorate
E. all of the above

44.10 Asperger's disorder is characterized by delays in

A. self-help skills
B. curiosity about the environment
C. nonverbal communication
D. receptive language
E. none of the above.

44.11 James, a 4-year-old boy, is referred for a psychiatric evaluation at the suggestion of his preschool teacher, who noticed unusual interactions with other children. He is an only child who started preschool 4 months ago. He seldom plays with other children, preferring to play with a specific toy truck or toy dog. He spends much of the morning with the toy, moving it back and forth in a repetitive pattern. If he is unable to find the toy, or if another child is playing with it, he sits on the floor and wails until it is found and given to him. On the occasions when he approaches another child, it is in a blunt, verbose way, devoid of give-and-take, and other children tend to avoid him. The teacher never observes reciprocal interactions, and James never seems to catch on to what is happening in games. He approaches adults in a similar blunt, one-sided manner.

James was the product of a full-term vaginal delivery without complications. His mother describes him as a fussy baby who did not like being held. She and his father cannot remember James smiling as a baby or ever wanting to play peek-a-boo, despite their efforts to engage him. He talked before he walked and was speaking two to three word sentences by age 2. Because of his early and rich vocabulary, his parents assumed that he was probably gifted. He achieved bowel control at 3 years and bladder control at 4 years, with the exception of occasional nighttime accidents. He is able to dress and bathe himself with minimal help. He enjoys looking at pictures in his parents' art books and tends to return to the same pages again and again. His parents say that James's play at home is similar to what his teacher describes at school. He almost never initiates an activity or engages in reciprocal play. They assumed that his preference for being left alone was due to his superior intelligence. He sleeps and eats well. They have never observed or heard anything that would lead them to believe that James was experiencing hallucinations.

On examination James is found to be at the 30th percentile for height and weight for his age. He is well-developed and there are no facial abnormalities. His vocabulary is above average for his age, and he talks freely but without engaging in back-and-forth conversation. He avoids eye contact with the examiner and tends not to respond to questions or commands. When he is allowed to choose a toy, he selects a truck and spends several minutes spinning one of the wheels backward and forward.

Which of the following is the most likely diagnosis in the case described above?

A. Fetal alcohol syndrome
B. Autistic disorder
C. Down's syndrome
D. Childhood schizophrenia
E. Asperger's disorder

44.12 What is the most likely cause of James' difficulties?

A. Neurodevelopmental abnormalities
B. Maternal neglect
C. Autosomal recessive inheritance
D. Lead poisoning
E. Chromosomal nondisjunction

44.13 Based on the case above, which of the following interventions is most likely to be helpful?

A. Risperidone therapy
B. Psychodynamic play therapy
C. Social skills training
D. Methylphenidate therapy
E. Interpersonal psychotherapy

Directions

Each group of questions below consists of lettered headings followed by a list of numbered statements. For each numbered word or statement, select the *one* lettered heading that is most closely associated with it. Each lettered heading may be selected once, more than once, or not at all.

Questions 44.14–44.18

A. Autistic disorder
B. Childhood disintegrative disorder
C. Pervasive developmental disorder not otherwise specified
D. Asperger's disorder
E. Rett's disorder

44.14 Normal development for the first 6 months, followed by a progressive encephalopathy
44.15 A better prognosis than other pervasive developmental disorders because of the lack of delay in language and cognitive development
44.16 Some but not all of the features of autistic disorder
44.17 Several years of normal development followed by a loss of communication skills, a loss of reciprocal social interaction, and a restricted pattern of behavior
44.18 Occurrence at a rate of two to ten cases per 10,000 and characterized by impairment in social interaction, communicative language, or symbolic play before age 3.

Questions 44.19–44.22

A. Risperidone (Risperdal)
B. Haloperidol (Haldol)
C. Naltrexone (ReVia)
D. Selective serotonin reuptake inhibitors

44.19 This opiate antagonist is being investigated in the treatment of autism.
44.20 This drug has both dopamine (D_2) and serotonin (5-HT) antagonist properties.
44.21 This drug has been shown to reduce lability and stereotypic behaviors, but is also associated with withdrawal dyskinesias.
44.22 This drug is used to decrease obsessive-compulsive and stereotypic behaviors.

Questions 44.23–44.27

A. Autistic disorder
B. Asperger's disorder
C. Both
D. Neither

44.23 Onset is usually later and outcome involved less impairment
44.24 Motor clumsiness is more common
44.25 Qualitative impairments in social interaction and restricted patterns of interest
44.26 Withdrawn in the presence of others
44.27 Aggression and self-injurious behaviors are more common

ANSWERS

44.1 The answer is E

Family history of speech delay is found in about 25 percent of children with autistic disorder, and is found at similar rates in children with mixed receptive-expressive language disorder. *Echolalia* occurs commonly in children with autistic disorder and is not a typical feature of children with receptive-expressive language disorder. Similarly, *stereotypies* are more common and more severe among autistic children, and absent or less severe in children with the language disorder. *Imaginative play* is typically absent or rudimentary in children with autism, while it is usually present in some form in children with mixed receptive-expressive language disorder. *Deafness* is very uncommon in autistic children but is not unusual in children with language disorder.

44.2 The answer is E (all)

An abundance of evidence exists demonstrating associations between autistic disorder and a variety of biological abnormalities. Estimates of lifetime occurrence of *grand mal seizures* ranges between 4 and 32 percent. Alterations in volume of the total brain and specifically the cerebellum, frontal lobe, and limbic system have been identified. Recent neuroimaging studies suggest a pattern of increased and then decreased rate of brain growth over time; *increased total brain volume* is noted in many individuals with autism. *Ventricular enlargement on CT* scan is observed in 20 to 25 percent of autistic individuals. While no EEG findings are specific for autism, abnormalities are common in the disorder: *estimates of prevalence of EEG abnormalities range from 10 to 83 percent*, and failure of cerebral lateralization is a typical finding. One-third of autistic children demonstrate elevated serum serotonin levels; the significance of this finding is uncertain, particularly given similar rates of hyperserotoninemia in children with severe mental retardation.

44.3 The answer is C

Autistic disorder is characterized by marked and sustained impairment in social interaction, delayed and aberrant communication skills, and restricted repertoire of activities and interests. In order to meet criteria for diagnosis, *abnormal functioning in at least one of these areas must begin by age 3 (not 2) years*. Mental retardation is the most common comorbid condition with autism: approximately 75 percent of autistic children are also mentally retarded.

Prevalence rates as assessed in population studies have ranged from 0.7 to 21.1 per 10,000; the median prevalence estimate for studies conducted since the 1960s is approximately 4 to 5 per 10,000. Variability among studies may reflect methodological issues such as sample size, definition of the syndrome, and aspects of screening and ascertainment. Recent studies have reported higher prevalence rates. Possible explanations for this increase include: (1) broader definitions of the syndrome, (2) smaller target populations (smaller studies have tended to yield higher rates), (3) better detection of cases in the extreme ranges of the syndrome (i.e., severally mentally retarded children with autism, nonretarded children with autism). Some studies reporting higher rates have also included other diagnoses in the autism spectrum (Asperger's disorder, PDD NOS, etc.). Accumulating evidence indicates that *prevalence rates for autistic disorder may be as high as 1 in 1,000 children*.

Autistic disorder is 4 to 5 times more likely in boys than in girls. Girls with autism are more likely to have severe mental retardation than boys with autism. *Among autistic children with normal intelligence, the ratio of boys:girls may be as high as 6:1*, whereas among autistic children with moderate to severe mental retardation the ratio of boys:girls may be as low as 1.5:1. There is no clear explanation for females' underrepresentation among nonretarded autistic children; one hypothesis suggests that more severe brain dysfunction is required to cause autism in girls.

Although early work on the epidemiology of autism suggested an association between the disorder and higher socioeconomic status, more recent and methodologically sophisticated studies have failed to confirm this relationship. Nevertheless, families from disadvantaged backgrounds appear underrepresented in clinically referred samples. Outreach initiatives are needed to provide children from all socioeconomic backgrounds access to crucial diagnostic and treatment services.

44.4 The answer is B

While early theories focused upon now-discredited theories of faulty parenting as etiologic factors in autism, current evidence strongly supports biological and genetic factors as causal. *Studies of twins indicate high (not moderate) concordance among monozygotic twins*, with reduced concordance for dizygotic twins. Recent genetics research suggests that as many as 15 or more genes may be involved. However, environmental influences are also important, as concordance in monozygotic twins is less than 100 percent and the phenotypic expression of the disorder varies widely, even within monozygotic twins. Among monozygotic twins in which one twin is autistic, there are elevated rates of cognitive disorders in the non-autistic twin. Additionally, there are higher rates of perinatal complications in the autistic monozygotic twin as compared to the non-autistic monozygotic twin. These findings suggest a role for combined risk factors in the etiology of autism: genetic liability combined with perinatal insult or other environmental factor.

Family studies have shown a prevalence of approximately 2 to 3 percent of autism in siblings of autistic children, which represents a 50- to 100-fold increase in risk compared with the general population. Parents of children diagnosed with autism may decide against having additional children; this phenomenon, called "stoppage," may indicate that the risk in siblings is even higher than that observed. Even when not affected with autism, *siblings of autistic children are at increased risk for various developmental problems, particularly language and cognitive difficulties*. It is *unclear whether what is inherited is a specific predisposition to autism or a more general predisposition to developmental issues*. Recent family studies reveal increased rates of mood disorders, anxiety disorders, and social difficulties among first-degree relatives of autistic individuals. Although *the influence of genetic factors on autistic disorder is now well established*, specific modes of inheritance are unknown. Current research seeks to elucidate further details of the genetics of the disorder.

44.5 The answer is D

As many as 50 percent of all individuals with autism never develop speech. *Delays in the acquisition of language are the most frequent presenting complaints of parents of children later diagnosed with autism*. Usual patterns of language acquisition (babbling, practicing sounds, etc.) are often absent. Infants and young children with autism may take the parent's hand to obtain a desired object without initiating eye contact (as though the hand, and not the person, is responsible for obtaining the item). In contrast to children with language disorder, these children do not appear to be very motivated to engage in communication or exclusively attempt to communicate via nonverbal means. When autistic individuals do use speech, their language is remarkable. They often echo words and sounds they've heard (echolalia). They struggle with flexibility in language; for example, they don't recognize that changes in perspective of speaker require pronoun changes, leading to pronoun reversal ("You want juice," rather than "I want juice.") Speech is often *nonreciprocal*, a term that indicates speech not intended to produce communication with another person. While the syntax and morphology of their speech are relatively spared, vocabulary and semantic skills are slow to develop, and aspects of social uses of language (pragmatics) are particularly difficult for autistic individuals. Thus humor and sarcasm frequently confuse children with autism, who make overly literal interpretations of language and miss the speaker's intent. Additionally, autistic individual commonly speak with monotonic and robotic intonation.

Deficits in play may include a failure to develop usual patterns of symbolic-imaginative play. Children with autism may preferentially explore non-functional aspects of play materials (e.g., taste or smell) or use elements of toys exclusively for self-stimulation (e.g., spinning the wheels on a toy truck rather than "driving" the truck).

Autistic children fail to develop social relatedness to their parents and other people. They may lack a social smile as infants and their eye contact is limited. Human faces hold little interest for autistic infants and children, which likely relates to *disturbances in development of joint attention, attachment, and other aspects of social interaction*. Along these lines, the child may not engage in normative games of infancy, and may struggle with imitation and other play skills. When they reach school age, their lack of "theory of mind" skills leave them unable to interpret the social behavior of others and significantly impairs their ability to interact meaningfully with peers. These deficits are highly distinctive of autism.

Children with autistic disorder often have difficulty tolerating changes and variations in routine. For example, an attempt to alter the sequence of some activity may be met with what appears to be catastrophic distress on the part of the child. Parents may report that children insist upon engaging in activities in very particular ways. Meanwhile, autistic children do not tend to engage in spontaneous exploratory play. Toys and objects are not used in symbolic play, and the play they do initiate tends to be rigid and monotonous. The child may develop an interest in a repetitive activity such as collecting strings, memorizing numbers, or repeating certain words and phrases. In younger children, attachment to objects, when they occur, tends to differ from more normative transitional objects. They often spin, bang, or line up their favored objects.

Movement abnormalities are common in autism, particularly in children who are also mentally retarded. *Stereotyped movements* may include toe walking, finger flicking, body rocking, arm flapping, and other mannerisms, which are engaged in for pleasurable or self-soothing purposes. They may be intensely preoccupied with spinning objects, and may, for example, spend long periods of time watching a ceiling fan rotate.

44.6 The answer is A

Approximately 75 percent of autistic children are mentally retarded; 30 percent are in the mild-to-moderate range and 45 percent are severely-to-profoundly mentally retarded. On psychological testing, typical profiles of autistic children reveal *significant deficits in abstract reasoning, verbal concept formulation, integration skills*, and tasks requiring social understanding. Therefore, on the Intelligence Scale for Children, for example, *weaknesses are observed on the Similarities and Comprehension subtests*. In contrast, relative strengths tend to exist in areas of rote learning, memory skills, and visual-spatial problem solving, particularly on tasks that can be completed piecemeal and don't require understanding of the context of the task. Therefore, *performance on the Block Design and Digit Recall subtests of the Wechsler scales are usually the areas of highest achievement* for autistic children. This tendency among autistic individuals to prefer rote and sequential tasks over reasoning and integrative tasks carries the implication that individuals with autism fail to "see the forest for the trees," a characteristic that creates difficulties across functioning modalities, from cognitive testing to communication to social interactions. Given the ubiquity of verbal deficits in autistic disorder, these individuals usually have higher performance than verbal scores on intelligence testing, particularly those falling in the mentally retarded range. Interestingly, the opposite pattern has been found in individuals with Asperger's disorder.

44.7 The answer is B

One of the most fascinating cognitive phenomena in autistic disorder is the presence of so-called "islets of precocity" or "splinter skills," preserved or highly developed skills in particular areas which contrast with the individual's overall cognitive deficits. For example, autistic children may have great facility in decoding numbers and letters, sometimes at early stages of development (hyperlexia), despite very limited comprehension of what is read. *Approximately 10 percent of individuals with autism exhibit splinter skills*—high performance on a specific skill in the presence of mild or moderate mental retardation. This phenomenon tends to occur among a narrow range of skills—memorizing lists or other trivial information, calculations, visual-spatial skills such as drawing, musical skills such as perfect pitch or ability to memorize a piece of music after hearing it once.

44.8 The answer is E (none)

Rett's disorder is a progressive condition that develops after some months of apparently normal development after birth. Head circumference at birth is normal and early developmental milestones, including social interactions, are unremarkable. Between 6 and 48 months, most commonly between 6 and 12 months, a progressive encephalopathy develops. Head growth begins to decelerate, with resultant microcephaly. *Motor abnormalities occur*: purposeful hand movements are lost, and characteristic midline hand movements, such as hand wringing, emerge. Gait and truncal apraxia, ataxia, and poor coordination develop in the preschool years. Expressive and receptive language skills deteriorate and are associated with *marked mental retardation (not normal intelligence)*. *A loss of social interactional skills* is observed during the preschool year. The etiology of the disease is unknown. A genetic basis for the condition is likely; *Rett's disorder occurs only in girls,* and case reports indicate complete concordance in monozygotic twins. Associated features include seizures (occurring in up to 75 percent of affected patients) and irregular respiration, with episodes of hyperventilation, apnea, and breath holding.

44.9 The answer is B

Childhood disintegrative disorder is a rare condition characterized by a marked regression in multiple areas of development occurring after several years of normal development. The disorder was first described in 1908 by Theodore Heller, an Austrian educator. He reported on a series of children who displayed a marked and persisting developmental regression after 3 to 4 years of normal development. He first termed the condition dementia infantilis; subsequently it has also been named disintegrative psychosis or Heller's syndrome. *The gender ratio of affected children has been estimated at between 4 and 8 boys to 1 girl*; prevalence is estimated at one case in 100,000 boys.

According to diagnostic criteria, early development must proceed normally for at least the first 2 years, including normal communication, social relationships, play, and adaptive behavior. Then prior to age 10, there occurs a significant loss of previously acquired skills in at least two of the following areas: expressive or receptive language, social interaction, motor skills, play, and bowel or bladder control. Additionally, *patients develop symptoms similar to those seen in autistic disorder*—in addition to the aforementioned abnormalities in language, social interaction, and play, they may develop stereotyped behaviors, problems with transitions and changes in routine, and nonspecific hyperkinesis. *Onset is usually between the ages of 3 and 4 and may be gradual or acute*. There may be nonspecific agitation or anxiety prior to the emergence of developmental deterioration. *Deterioration in self-help skills occurs and is in marked contrast to observed behaviors in autism*, in which such skills are acquired later that usual but then typically are not lost.

44.10 The answer is C

Asperger's disorder is characterized by impairments in social interaction and restricted interests and behaviors as seen in autism, but its *early developmental course is characterized by no significant delays in spoken or receptive language, cognitive development, self-help skills, or curiosity about the environment.* All-absorbing and circumscribed interests and motor clumsiness are often characteristic of the condition but are not required for diagnosis.

In 1944, Hans Asperger, an Austrian pediatrician with an interest in special education, described four children who had difficulty integrating socially into peer groups. Unaware of Kanner's description of "infantile autism" published a year previously, Asperger called the condition he observed "autistic psychopathy," indicating a stable personality disorder marked by social isolation. Despite preserved intellectual capacity, the children showed a *marked paucity of nonverbal communication* involving both gestures and affective tone of voice; poor empathy and a tendency to intellectualize emotions; an inclination to engage in one-sided, long-winded, and sometimes incoherent speech (Asperger called them "little professors"); all-absorbing interests involving unusual topics, which dominate their conversation; and motoric clumsiness. The etiology of Asperger's is unknown; family studies suggest a relationship to autistic disorder.

44.11 The answer is E

Fetal alcohol syndrome and Down's syndrome include characteristic facial and other features that James does not have. In addition, he does not appear to be impaired cognitively: He is able to function at a level of independence (dressing, bathing) appropriate to his age. *Schizophrenia in children* can be difficult to diagnose because of their limitations in describing inner experiences and the sometime difficulty in distinguishing normal childhood fantasy from hallucinations and delusions. However, unlike James, children who have schizophrenia almost always develop symptoms after a period of normal childhood development. James's unwillingness to be held, failure to make eye contact, and lack of pleasure in playing peek-a-boo all suggest impaired social interactions from very early on. These are core feature of both *autistic disorder* and *Asperger's disorder*. The difference between them is that language is impaired in autistic disorder and normal in Asperger's disorder. James's language is normal or perhaps even a little advanced. The experience of his parents is not uncommon among parents and teachers of children with Asperger's disorder, for whom good language skills may mask the social deficits. James is lucky in having a teacher astute enough to recognize the limitations behind his verbosity.

44.12 The answer is A

The etiology of Asperger's disorder (as with autism) is unknown. There is *no evidence that it is caused by parental neglect* or any other pattern of parenting. There is a slight familial trend to the disorder—the prevalence among first- and second-degree relatives is greater than the prevalence for the population at large—but whether or not this represents a genetic factor is not established. There is a growing consensus among clinicians and researchers that both autism and Asperger's disorder *are the result of neurodevelopmental abnormalities*, but no specific neuroanatomic or neurofunctional deficit has been identified.

44.13 The answer is C

There is no definitive treatment for Asperger's disorder. *Pharmacotherapy will not treat the underlying disorder* but may be helpful for ancillary symptoms such as aggression or depression. *Psychodynamic and interpersonal psychotherapy are inappropriate* because of the problems with social understanding and empathy. *Therapy that focuses on social and communications skills, problem solving, and deriving strategies for dealing with novel situations has the greatest likelihood of being helpful.* In addition, many adults with Asperger's disorder benefit from self-support groups in which they can meet and learn from other people with similar disabilities.

Answers 44.14–44.18

44.14 The answer is E

44.15 The answer is D

44.16 The answer is C

44.17 The answer is B

44.18 The answer is A

Rett's disorder is characterized by normal development for at least the first 6 months, followed by a progressive encephalopathy. *Asperger's disorder may have a better prognosis than other pervasive developmental disorders* because of the preservation of normal language and cognitive development. *Pervasive developmental disorder not otherwise specified includes atypical autism—presentations that include some but not all of the features of autistic disorder. Childhood disintegrative disorder is characterized by several years of normal development* followed by a loss of communication skills, a loss of reciprocal social interaction, and a restricted pattern of behavior. *Autistic disorder occurs at a rate of two to ten cases per 10,000* and is characterized by impairment in social interaction, communicative language, or symbolic play before age 3.

Answers 44.19–44.22

44.19 The answer is C

44.20 The answer is A

44.21 The answer is B

44.22 The answer is D

No specific medications exist to target the core symptoms of autistic disorder. However, a number of drugs have proven useful in ameliorating associated behavioral symptoms, including aggression, self-injurious behaviors, mood lability, irritability, obsessive-compulsive behaviors, hyperactivity, stereotypic behaviors, and social withdrawal. *Naltrexone, an opiate antagonist,* has been tried with the hope that by blocking endogenous opioid activity, stereotypic behaviors in autism will decrease. *Risperidone, an antipsychotic medication with blocking activity at both dopamine (D_2) and serotonin (5-HT) receptors*, has been shown to be effective in diminishing aggression, irritability, and self-injurious behaviors in autism. *Haloperidol, a high-potency dopamine-blocking antipsychotic, has been useful in reducing irritability and improving sociability among autistic children.* Approximately one-quarter of children given haloperidol develop withdrawal dyskinesias, a troubling but generally self-limited symptom, when this drug is stopped. The *selective serotonin reuptake inhibitors*, which are effective medications for obsessive-compulsive symptoms among adults, have also been employed for the treatment of obsessions, compulsions, and stereotypic behaviors among autistic children and adolescents.

Answers 44.23–44.27

44.23 The answer is B

44.24 The answer is B

44.25 The answer is C

44.26 The answer is A

44.27 The answer is A

Most children with autism have significant early delays and disruption in language acquisition and cognitive development. *The differential diagnosis between autistic disorder without mental retardation and Asperger's disorder can be difficult, but is made clearer by the findings that the latter condition tends to have later onset and less overall impairment.* In addition, Asperger's disorder is distinguished by less severe social and communication deficits, *less prominent aggression and self-injurious behaviors*, absent or minor sterotypies, more conspicuously circumscribed interests, and *more frequent motor clumsiness*, compared to autistic disorder.

Diagnosis of Asperger's disorder requires demonstration of qualitative impairments in social interaction and restricted patterns of interest, identical criteria to those for autistic disorder. In contrast to autism, however, criteria differ in that there should be no clinically significant delay in language acquisition, cognitive development, or self-help skills. *While autistic children tend to be socially withdrawn, children with Asperger's do not tend to withdraw socially*, but nevertheless struggle socially because of their tendency to approach and interact with others in awkward or inappropriate ways. They often are interested in friendship and socializing, but are thwarted due to their eccentric styles of interaction and insensitivity to the other person's feelings, motivations, and nonverbal implied communications. Their poor intuition and lack of adaptability are accompanied by reliance of formalistic rules of behavior, leading to the impression of social naiveté and behavioral rigidity that these individuals convey so strongly.

45

Attention-Deficit Disorders (ADHD)

Attention-deficit/hyperactivity disorder (ADHD) consists of a persistent pattern of inattention and/or hyperactive and impulsive behavior that is more severe than expected in children of that age and level of development. To meet the criteria for the diagnosis of ADHD, some symptoms must be present before the age of 7 years, although many children are not diagnosed until they are older than 7 years when their behaviors cause problems in school and other places. To meet diagnostic criteria for ADHD, impairment from inattention and/or hyperactivity-impulsivity must be present in at least two settings and interfere with developmentally appropriate functioning socially, academically, and in extracurricular activities. The disorder must not take place in the course of a pervasive developmental disorder, schizophrenia, or other psychotic disorder and must not be better accounted for by another mental disorder.

The disorder has been identified in the literature for many years under a variety of terms. In the early 1900s, impulsive, disinhibited, and hyperactive children—many of whom had neurological damage caused by encephalitis—were grouped under the label hyperactive syndrome. In the 1960s, a heterogeneous group of children with poor coordination, learning disabilities, and emotional lability but without specific neurological damage were described as having minimal brain damage. Since then, other hypotheses have been put forth to explain the origin of the disorder, such as genetically based condition involving abnormal arousal and poor ability to modulate emotions. This theory was initially supported by the observation that stimulant medications help produce sustained attention and improve these children's ability to focus on a given task. Currently, no single factor is believed to cause the disorder, although many environmental variables may contribute to it and many predictable clinical features are associated with it.

Students should test their knowledge by addressing the following questions and answers.

HELPFUL HINTS

The student should know the following terms.

- adult manifestations
- ambidexterity
- antidepressant
- body anxiety
- clonidine (Catapres)
- developmentally inappropriate attention
- disinhibition
- disorganized EEG pattern
- distractibility
- EEG findings
- emotional lability
- genetic-familial factors
- growth suppression
- hyperactivity-impulsivity
- hyperkinesis
- impaired cognitive performance
- inattention
- learning disorders
- locus ceruleus
- matching familiar faces
- minimal brain damage
- nonfocal (soft) signs
- perceptual-motor problems
- PET scan
- poor motor coordination
- rebound effect
- right–left discrimination
- school history
- secondary depression
- soft neurological signs
- sympathomimetic

QUESTIONS

Directions

Each of the questions or incomplete statements below is followed by five suggested responses or completions. Select the *one* that is *best* in each case.

45.1 Which of the following statements regarding ADHD is *true*?

A. ADHD occurs in about 1 percent of prepubertal elementary school children in the United States.
B. ADHD remains one of the least-validated disorders in psychiatry.
C. Parents of children with ADHD show increased incidence of alcohol use disorders.
D. Symptoms of ADHD rarely appear before the age of 5.
E. None of the above

45.2 Findings from neuroimaging studies of subjects with ADHD include which of the following?

A. Reduced perfusion in bilateral frontal areas on PET scan
B. Increased perfusion in prefrontal, striatal, and thalamic regions in response to methylphenidate administration on PET scan

C. Dorsal anterior cingulate cortex (DACC) dysfunction on functional MRI scan
D. abnormalities in fronto-striatal brain regions on various imaging techniques
E. All of the above

45.3 Which of the following statements describing the genetics of ADHD is *true*?

A. The risk of ADHD for a sibling of a child proband with ADHD increases up to five times in some studies.
B. Children with ADHD are at no greater risk of developing conduct disorder than children of similar ages without ADHD.
C. Concordance rates for ADHD range from 25 to 40 percent for monozygotic twins.
D. Concordance rates for ADHD range from 5 to 10 percent for dizygotic twins.
E. The heritability of inattention-related behaviors is estimate to range between 40 and 55 percent.

45.4 Possible acquired etiological influences in ADHD include

A. low socioeconomic status
B. elevated intake of sugar-containing foods during early childhood
C. high birth weight (above 4,000 g)
D. prenatal exposure to alcohol and/or nicotine
E. all of the above

Directions

Each set of lettered headings below is followed by a list of numbered words or statements. For each numbered word or statement, select the *one* lettered heading most closely associated with it. Each lettered heading may be selected once, more than once, or not at all.

Questions 45.5–45.9

A. Methylphenidate (Ritalin)
B. Dextroamphetamine (Dexedrine)
C. Bupropion (Wellbutrin)
D. Clonidine (Catapres)
E. None of the above

45.5 This drug is favored in children with ADHD and a history of severe tic disorders and may be particularly helpful when ADHD symptoms are pronounced in the late afternoon or evening.
45.6 This drug has a short half-life, and has been shown to improve symptoms in approximately 75 percent of ADHD-diagnosed children.
45.7 This drug may be favored in children who suffer significant rebound symptoms from stimulants, or in children with comorbid ADHD and depression.
45.8 This drug has a half-life of 8-12 hours and is approved in children as young as 3-years-old for treatment of ADHD.
45.9 Growth suppression occurs during treatment with this drug, but studies indicate that children recoup the growth when given "drug holidays" over weekends and vacations.

Questions 45.10–45.13

A. ADHD, inattentive type
B. ADHD, hyperactive-impulsive type
C. ADHD, combined type
D. All of the Above
E. None of the above

45.10 Most common
45.11 Least common
45.12 Most children identified as having this subtype were 3 to 4 years younger than children diagnosed with other subtypes.
45.13 These children are often described as sluggish, anxious, and sleepy.

45.14 Which of the following statements about ADHD is *false*?

A. Children with ADHD can have inattention with no hyperactivity or impulsivity.
B. Children with ADHD may have symptoms of hyperactivity but not inattention.
C. The disturbance in behavior must occur in at least two settings.
D. Children can meet the criteria for ADHD with impulsive symptoms only.
E. Many children with ADHD have many symptoms of inattention, hyperactivity, and impulsivity.

45.15 The first symptom of ADHD to remit is usually

A. hyperactivity
B. distractibility
C. careless mistakes in schoolwork
D. impulsivity
E. learning difficulties

45.16 The hyperactive and impulsive child is often

A. accident prone
B. explosively irritable
C. unable to resist blurting out answers
D. excessively talkative
E. all of the above

45.17 Diana is a 9-year-old girl brought in for her first psychiatric consultation by her parents, who were troubled by Diana's behavior during the Thanksgiving holiday. Diana's mother described Diana's propensity toward interrupting others' conversations, her inability to stay seated at the dinner table for longer than several minutes at a time, and her frequent, brief, but very noticeable bouts of sullen mood.

Both parents reported that Diana's "quirks" have been observable throughout her life. They described her as "moody," "stubborn," "turbo-charged," "impulsive," and "a bit aggressive with others," traits which they've noticed since she was an infant. They've also been concerned among themselves about Diana's limited friendships, noting, "She doesn't seem to get many invitations for play dates." They wondered whether Diana's tendencies toward bossiness and quick bursts of temper, which they'd long observed at home, were impairing her ability to form strong ties with peers.

Academically, Diana thrived in certain classes, particularly those in which she was immediately engaged with the material, but she also struggled mightily with certain subjects, particularly reading and writing. She seemed to grasp new concepts at first before falling off and losing interest in the task. She was frequently frustrated with herself and openly self-critical. She left materials scattered around the classroom and frequently forgot necessary papers or books at home. Distractibility also caused significant problems; teachers frequently commented on the need to seat Diana away from the windows and at the front of the class in an effort to maintain her focus on the lesson. The teacher also commented that Diana rarely stayed in her seat for more than a few minutes at a time and made frequent visits to the bathroom and drinking fountain.

At home, she and her sister frequently argued, and Diana at times was physically aggressive with her sister, though never harmed her in any significant way. Diana was noted to be quick to anger and quick to cry, and had "bad afternoons" in which she sulked and didn't respond to consoling. She was described as somewhat uncoordinated by her parents; sports at school were always difficult for her.

Diana was resistant to meeting with the psychiatrist and was feeling "grouchy" when the interview began. She expressed frustration over her difficulties at school and acknowledged her struggles with paying attention and with sitting still; she volunteered feeling that "I'm stupider than the other kids and I hate it." She spoke of several friends at school but also acknowledged, "We fight sometimes" and expressed her hope that she might "get a best friend someday." During the interview, after initially sitting in a chair with her arms crossed, she walked around the psychiatrist's office, examining objects within reach, and at one point perching perilously on the edge of an end table in an effort to reach a book, responding only to the psychiatrist's repeated insistence that she not climb on the furniture.

The diagnosis in the case above is

A. ADHD
B. Anxiety Disorder
C. Bipolar I Disorder
D. Conduct Disorder
E. Expressive Language Disorder

ANSWERS

45.1 The answer is C

First-degree biological relatives of children with ADHD, for example siblings, are at increased risk of having ADHD, as well as other psychiatric disturbances, including disruptive behavior disorders, anxiety disorders, and depressive disorders. *Parents of children with ADHD show an increased incidence of alcohol use disorders, in addition to sociopathy and hyperkinesis.* Parents of ADHD probands not uncommonly meet criteria for ADHD themselves.

Significant strides have been made in the last 30 years in (1) identifying core deficits associated with ADHD, (2) developing empirically tested and reliable diagnostic criteria, and (3) validating the diagnosis of ADHD based upon natural history, symptom profiles, neurobehavioral and functional neuroanatomical findings in the laboratory, family and genetic influences, and response to treatment. With these developments, *ADHD has become one of the best- (not least-) validated disorders in psychiatry.* Recent trends in research into ADHD have emphasized two distinct dimensions of behavior: inattentive and hyperactive/impulsive. The increased number of both children and adults receiving treatment for the condition indicates advancing public acceptance of the need to diagnose and treat ADHD.

While prevalence data has varied as definitions of ADHD have evolved, community samples of children and adolescents have consistently found ADHD to be a common disorder, with *conservative estimates of prevalence ranging from 3 to 7 percent (not 1 percent) of prepubertal elementary school children.* A strong male predominance, ranging from 2 to 1 to as high as 9 to 1, has been consistently observed in studies of ADHD prevalence among school-aged children.

Although diagnostic criteria outlined in DSM-IV-TR specify that onset of symptoms must occur prior to age 7, *symptoms of ADHD commonly (not rarely) appear before the age of 5.* However, diagnosis is not commonly made until the child has entered a structured school setting, when teachers' observations assist in distinguishing a child's difficulties with attention, hyperactivity, or impulsivity from more normative behaviors that characterize the child's non-ADHD peers.

45.2 The answer is E (all)

Structural and functional neuroimaging techniques have contributed significantly to the evolving understanding of the etiology of ADHD. Across a range of techniques, including PET, SPECT, fMRI, and MRS, a consistent finding has been *abnormalities in fronto-striatal brain regions.* These discoveries are in keeping with clinical observations of ADHD patients that suggest deficits in attention, self-regulation, cognition, working memory, motor control and other functions which are principally mediated by fronto-striatal structures, particularly dorsolateral prefrontal cortex (DLPFC), ventrolateral prefrontal cortex (VLPFC), dorsal anterior cingulated cortex (DACC), caudate, and putamen. In general, underactivity in implicated areas, for example *reduced perfusion in bilateral frontal areas on PET scan* and *dorsal anterior cingulate cortex (DACC) dysfunction on functional MRI scan* is thought to correspond to key behavioral and emotional difficulties that characterize ADHD. Further evidence for the connection between fronto-striatal dysfunction and ADHD symptoms and treatment is provided by the observation of *increased perfusion in prefrontal, striatal, and thalamic regions in response to methylphenidate administration,* as measured on PET scan.

45.3 The answer is A

There is ample and compelling evidence for a genetic basis for ADHD. Most published controlled family studies report significantly higher risks of ADHD in first- and second-degree relatives of pro bands with ADHD compared with normal controls. For example, *the risk of ADHD in siblings of child probands is increased by between 1.8 and 5 times.* Analyses of twin studies have provided further evidence of a genetic influence in ADHD: *concordance rates for monozygotic twins range from 51 to*

80 percent (not 25 to 40) and for dizygotic twins range from 29 to 33 percent (not 5 to 10). Individual symptom domains of inattention and hyperactivity have also been tracked in terms of heritability. *The heritability of inattention-related behaviors is estimated to range between 76 and 98 percent (not 40 and 55),* and the heritability of hyperactivity-related behaviors is judged to range between 64 and 77 percent. These very high rates of behavioral trait heritability provide convincing evidence that the cardinal behaviors of ADHD are highly influenced by genetics. The presence of ADHD in a proband indicate an increase risk of other disorders in both the probrand and biological relatives; one example of this increased risk is the *significant increase in risk of developing conduct disorder in children with ADHD compared with normal controls.*

45.4 The answer is D

A number of acquired influences have been identified as etiologic factors in the development of ADHD in some individuals, including pregnancy and delivery complications, *low birth weight (not high birth weight),* traumatic brain injury, and *prenatal exposure to substances including alcohol and nicotine.* The impact of these factors appears to be more limited than familial/genetic factors within groups of subjects with ADHD; they likely are most salient in the etiology of nonfamilial forms of ADHD.

Several studies have reported associations between complications during pregnancy and delivery and later development of disruptive behavior disorders, including ADHD. Low birth weight similarly appears to present a risk factor for later development of ADHD and other disruptive behavior disorders that is independent of other pre-and perinatal factors commonly associated with prematurity. These adverse pre- and perinatal events may be associated with particular forms or subgroups of ADHD, such as ADHD with comorbid conduct disorder. However, not all studies of pre-or perinatal adversity have found associations with ADHD; therefore, these factors appear to function as nonspecific risk factors for psychopathology in children.

Supporting evidence for the association between traumatic brain injury and later development of ADHD has been mixed. The relationship between brain injury and ADHD symptoms is influenced by factors such as location of injury, severity of tissue damage, and age at time of injury. The strongest relationship between brain injury and ADHD has been found for severe, frontal lobe injuries occurring in younger subjects. These findings have been interpreted to suggest that earlier injuries may compromise ongoing brain development and disrupt executive functioning, whereas individuals who have achieved greater cognitive development prior to injury may adapt better to loss of skills.

Substance exposure in utero has long been implicated in childhood problems with behavioral control and emotional regulation. Prenatal exposure to alcohol and nicotine has been strongly associated with the development of ADHD, as well as other difficulties with cognition and behavior. Although these exposures to substances may often co-occur with other environmental factors that influence development, alcohol and nicotine have generally been found to independently increase the risk of ADHD. Meanwhile, *low socioeconomic status does not independently increase risk of developing ADHD.* Similarly, despite the common misperception in the public, *sugar intake at any age has not been found to play a role in the etiology of ADHD.*

Answers 45.5–45.9

45.5 The answer is D

45.6 The answer is A

45.7 The answer is C

45.8 The answer is B

45.9 The answer is A

CNS stimulants have long records of significant efficacy and excellent safety profiles in the treatment of ADHD. These medications, including methylphenidate, dextroamphetamine, and mixed amphetamine salts, exist in both short-acting and sustained-release preparations; the longer-acting versions are increasingly preferred both for ease of dosing (especially as children no longer have to take second doses in the middle of the school day) and for decreased concerns about rebound symptoms. *Tic disorders can be exacerbated by stimulant use, and therefore clonidine, an agent effective both in treating ADHD symptoms and in diminishing tic symptoms*, is a good choice when these conditions coexist. Clonidine commonly causes sedation, a beneficial effect in children who become particularly hyperactive in the evening. *Methylphenidate reaches peak blood level 1–2 hours after administration and has a half-life of 3–4 hours,* the shortest of the stimulant medications. *Efficacy rates of methylphenidate are approximately 75 percent in most studies.* This short duration of action may lead to rebound symptoms, including irritability and enhanced hyperactivity, in some children. These symptoms *are intolerable in some children*; *bupropion may be a good choice for these patients, and also is useful in patients with comorbid depression* who benefit from the antidepressant effects of this medication. *Dextroamphetamine* is approved by the U.S. Food and Drug Administration *for use in the treatment of ADHD in children 3 years old and older*. Its *half-life is 8 to 12 hours*, after which significant rebound may be experienced. *Growth suppression may occur in children taking methylphenidate*. While growth may be suppressed when the drug is being taken, evidence suggests that final height of children prescribed methylphenidate is unchanged, provided that "drug holidays" are given on weekends and summer vacations. Table 45.1 presents commonly prescribed medications for ADHD.

Answers 45.10–45.13

45.10 The answer is C

45.11 The answer is B

45.12 The answer is B

45.13 The answer is A

The DSM-IV-TR subtypes of ADHD describe some of the symptom variability found in ADHD: ADHD, inattentive type; ADHD, hyperactive-impulsive type; and ADHD, combined type. Among children referred to clinics for diagnosis and treatment, *the combined type is most common,* followed by the inattentive type; *the hyperactive-impulsive type is least common.* While by definition individuals diagnosed with ADHD must present with a history of symptoms prior to the age of 7, the average age at

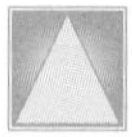

Table 45.1
Medications for the Treatment of ADHD and Suggested Monitoring

Medication	Preparation	Approximate Dosage Range
First-line agents		
Methylphenidate (Ritalin)	5-, 10-, and 20-mg scored tablets	0.3–1.0 mg/dose, t.i.d.; total daily dose <60 mg
	SR (sustained release): 20-mg tablet	
Dextroamphetamine (Dexedrine)	5- and 10-mg scored tablets Spansules (sustained release): 5-, 10-, and 15-mg capsules	0.15–0.5 mg/kg/dose, b.i.d.; total daily dose <40 mg
Dextroamphetamine and amphetamine salts (Adderall)	5-, 10-, 20-, 30-mg tablets	0.15–0.5 mg/kg dose, q.a.m. or b.i.d.; total daily dose <4 mg
Second-line agents		
Pemoline (Cylert)	18.75-, 37.5-, and 75-mg tablets; 37.5-mg chewable tablets	1–3 mg/kg/day
Bupropion (Wellbutrin; Zyban)	50-, 75-, 150-mg tablets, 150 mg	150–300 mg/day (3–6 mg/kg)
Venlafaxine (Effexor)	25-, 37.5-, 50-, 100-mg tablets	25–150 mg/day, b.i.d.
Clonidine (Catapres)	0.1-, 0.2-, and 0.3-mg scored tablets	3–10 μg/kg given t.i.d. or q.i.d. (average 0.1 mg q.i.d.)
Monitoring		
Baseline	Physical examination within 6 months Height, weight, blood pressure, and pulse	
Every 3–4 mo	Height, weight, blood pressure, and pulse	
Annual	Physical examination, laboratory studies as indicated	

diagnosis is approximately 7 to 9 years old. Among the subtypes, *the hyperactive-impulsive subtype is notable in that most children with this subtype were diagnosed 3 to 4 years before children diagnosed with other subtypes.* ADHD children with the inattentive subtype tend to be diagnosed later, perhaps because they tend to exhibit fewer of the oppositional, defiant, and aggressive behavior that often occurs in the hyperactive-impulsive subtype and that tends to prompt early referral for evaluation. While symptoms often overlap across subtypes of ADHD, and while there is significant correlation between hyperactive-impulsive and inattentive behaviors, some notable differences are observed between the subtypes. For example, *children with the inattentive subtype are often described as sluggish, anxious, sleepy,* and prone to daydreaming.

45.14 The answer is D

Children cannot meet criteria for ADHD with impulsive symptoms alone; they must exhibit either hyperactivity or inattention as well. Children with ADHD *can have inattention with no hyperactivity or impulsivity if at least six symptoms of inattention are present.* Children with ADHD may have *hyperactivity without inattention*, but they must have four symptoms of hyperactivity or four symptoms of a combination of hyperactivity and impulsivity. *The disturbance must be present in at least two settings.* Many children with ADHD have *multiple symptoms including inattentive, hyperactive, and impulsive symptoms.*

45.15 The answer is A

Hyperactivity is usually the first symptom of ADHD to remit in the natural course of the disorder. Overall the course of ADHD is highly variable: for example, symptoms may remit at puberty, or they may persist into adolescence and adulthood; alternatively, hyperactivity may remit, but *decreased attention span, careless mistakes in school work, poor impulse control, and learning difficulties often persist.* Remission prior to age 12 is rare; when remission does occur, it tends to do so between the ages of 12 and 20. Studies suggest, however, that the majority of individuals with ADHD experience only partial improvement in symptoms, contributing to vulnerabilities in adult life to professional/vocational difficulties, mood disorders, and substance abuse disorders.

45.16 The answer is E (all)

Hyperactive children are often *accident prone, explosively irritable, excessively talkative,* and reluctant to engage quietly in leisure activities. In school they may begin an assignment eagerly but then quickly lose interest; *they blurt out answers prematurely,* have difficulty waiting for their turn, and struggle socially as a result of their tendency toward interrupting conversations and intruding on the activities of their peers. At home they are demanding and impatient, and irritable reactions may be provoked by seemingly innocuous stimuli; these reactions often seem to puzzle and dismay the child as well as the parents. They are emotionally labile, and their performances at various tasks tend to be variable and unpredictable.

45.17 The answer is A

Many children with *ADHD* have secondary depression in reaction to their continuing frustration over their failure to learn and their consequent low self-esteem. This condition must be distinguished from a primary depressive disorder, which is likely to be characterized by hypoactivity and withdrawal. Mania and ADHD share many core features such as excessive verbalization, motoric hyperactivity, and high levels of distractibility. Additionally, in children with mania, irritability seems to be more common than euphoria. Although mania and ADHD can coexist, children with *bipolar I disorder* exhibit more waxing and waning of symptoms than those with ADHD. Recent follow-up data for children who met the criteria for ADHD and subsequently developed bipolar disorder suggest that certain clinical features occurring during the course of ADHD predict future mania. Children with ADHD who had developed bipolar I disorder at 4-year follow-up had a greater co-occurrence of additional disorders and a greater family history of bipolar disorders and other mood disorders than children without bipolar disorder.

Frequently, *conduct disorder* and ADHD coexist, and both must be diagnosed. Learning disorders of various kinds must also be distinguished from ADHD; a child may be unable to read or do mathematics because of a learning disorder, rather than because of inattention. ADHD often coexists with one or more learning disorders, including reading disorder, mathematics disorder, and disorder of written expression.

46

Disruptive Behavior Disorders

Oppositional and aggressive behaviors during childhood are among the most frequent reasons that a given youth is referred for mental health evaluation. Many youth who exhibit negativistic or oppositional behaviors will find other forms of expression as they mature and will no longer demonstrate these behaviors in adulthood. However, children who develop enduring patterns of aggressive behaviors that begin in early childhood and violate the basic rights of peers and family members may be destined to an entrenched pattern of conduct disorder behavior over time. Controversy has arisen as to whether a set of "voluntary" antisocial behaviors can be construed as a psychiatric disorder, or can be better accounted for as maladaptive responses to overly harsh or punitive parenting, or strategies that have survival value in chronically threatening environmental situations. Longitudinal studies have demonstrated that for some youth, early patterns of disruptive behavior may become a lifelong pervasive repertoire culminating in adult antisocial personality disorder. The origin of stable patterns of disruptive behavior is widely accepted as a convergence of multiple contributing factors including biological, temperamental, learned, and psychological conditions.

Disruptive behavior disorders can be divided into two distinct constellations of symptoms categorized as oppositional defiant disorder and conduct disorder, both of which result in impaired social or academic function in a child. Some defiance and refusal to comply with adult requests is developmentally appropriate and marks growth in all children, yet children with certain disorders are themselves impaired by the frequency and severity of their disruptive behaviors.

The student should study the questions and answers below for a useful review of these disorders.

HELPFUL HINTS

The student should be able to define the following terms.

- ADHD
- autonomy
- child abuse
- CNS dysfunction
- comorbid disorders
- harsh child-rearing structure
- issues of control
- mood disorders
- negativistic relationships
- normative oppositional stages
- parental psychopathology
- poor peer relationships
- poor self-esteem
- socioeconomic deprivation
- temperamental predispositions
- terrible twos
- truancy
- violation of rights

QUESTIONS

Directions

Each of the questions or incomplete statements below is followed by five suggested responses or completions. Select the *one* that is *best* in each case.

46.1 Oppositional defiant disorder

A. is associated with major antisocial violations
B. is defined as part of a developmental stage
C. is limited to a particular age group
D. most commonly emerges in late-preschool– or early-school–aged children
E. diagnosis implies less circumscribed disturbances of greater severity than in conduct disorder

46.2 In oppositional defiant disorder

A. The average age of onset is 3 years.
B. Boys always outnumber girls, regardless of age range.
C. Occurrence is mostly in cohorts of middle to higher socioeconomic status.
D. Point prevalence has been reported to average around 6 percent.
E. All of the above

46.3 True statements about oppositional defiant disorder include

A. In one study, about one-third of boys with the disorder progress to develop conduct disorders.
B. Ninety percent of boys with conduct disorder have

fulfilled criteria for oppositional defiant disorder previously in their lives.
C. The disorder has been linked to the presence of anxious-avoidant parental attachment.
D. Twenty-five percent of children with this disorder will have no further diagnosis.
E. All of the above

46.4 The most common comorbidity with oppositional defiant disorder is

A. attention-deficit/hyperactivity disorder
B. dysthymic disorder
C. major depressive disorder
D. early-onset bipolar I disorder
E. anxiety disorders

46.5 In conduct disorder

A. Symptoms are clustered in two areas.
B. Subtyping is allowed based on the age of onset of symptoms.
C. At least five of a list of 15 antisocial behaviors must be present.
D. All behaviors must have been present in the last 6 months.
E. All of the above

46.6 Factors associated with conduct disorder include

A. chronic illness
B. disturbed laterality and language performance
C. viewing televised or other media violence
D. temperament
E. all of the above

46.7 The most virulent comorbid condition of conduct disorder is considered to be

A. paranoid psychotic disorders
B. substance-use disorders
C. oppositional defiant disorder
D. attention-deficit/hyperactive disorders
E. major depressive disorder

46.8 Oppositional defiant disorder is characterized by all of the following *except*

A. negativistic behavior
B. placing blame on others
C. physical aggression
D. difficulty in school
E. theft

Directions

These lettered headings are followed by a list of numbered statements. For each numbered statement, select the *one* lettered heading most closely associated with it. Each lettered heading may be used once, more than once, or not at all.

Questions 46.9–46.11

A. Oppositional defiant disorder
B. Conduct disorder

46.9 It may be diagnosed when symptoms occur exclusively with attention-deficit/hyperactivity disorder, learning disorders, and mood disorders.
46.10 It may be equally prevalent in adolescent boys and adolescent girls.
46.11 The patient often bullies, threatens, or intimidates others.

ANSWERS

46.1 The answer is D

Oppositional defiant disorder consists of negativistic, hostile, or defiant behavior creating disturbances in one of three domains of functioning (academic, occupational, or social) and lasting at least 6 months. The diagnosis also refers to angry and vindictive behavior and problems with control of temper. Most of the behaviors are directed at someone—usually an authority figure. However, *there are no major antisocial violations.* The behavior is also *not part of a developmental stage* (i.e., oppositional behavior around ages 2 to 3 years and in early adolescence). The diagnosis is not limited to a particular age group, but *most commonly emerges in late-preschool– or early-school–aged children. The diagnosis implies more (not less) circumscribed disturbances of lesser (not greater) severity* than in conduct disorder but represents more troublesome behavior than normative oppositionality. Behaviors of the oppositional defiant disorder type, on the average, appear 2 to 3 years earlier than those of conduct disorder. The latest factor analysis suggests that there is significant coherence of the oppositional defiant disorder behaviors as outlined in the diagnostic criteria. However, support for the diagnosis has not been uniform; some authors question its status as a separate diagnosis or even as any kind of taxonomy at all, and there have been some negative public reactions categorizing oppositional defiant disorder as an attempt to characterize normative behavior as pathological.

46.2 The answer is D

The epidemiological data for oppositional defiant disorder needs to be regarded with some caution because of the recent modifications of the diagnostic criteria. *The point prevalence* of the disorder has been reported to vary between 1.7 to 9.9, with *a weighted average of around 6 percent. The average age of onset is about 6 (not 3) years. Boys outnumber girls in the prepubertal age range, after which the two genders are more equal. The disorder occurs mostly in cohorts of lower (not middle to higher) socioeconomic status.*

46.3 The answer is E (all)

Very little is known regarding the role of psychological factors in oppositional defiant disorder. Attachment theorists have noted the similarities between the behavioral manifestations of insecure attachment and disruptive behavior disorders. In their view, antisocial behavior is seen as a special signal to an unresponsive parent. Oppositional defiant disorder has been *linked to the presence of anxious-avoidant parental attachment* in particular. Insecure attachment also predicts aggression in elementary school in boys and multiple behavior problems in the classroom. Given the inconsistency in the data, most experts believe that multivariate transactional pathways will be found in this area of research.

Another important research area includes the work of Kenneth Dodge, who focused on aggressive children's deficient information processing in regard to social stimuli. Aggressive children have shown deficits at every phase of this multistage process: They underutilize pertinent social clues, misattribute hostile intent to peers, generate fewer solutions to problems, and expect to be rewarded for aggressive responses.

One of the main explanatory problems in developmental psychopathology is the simultaneous existence of stability in behavior paired with its protean appearance. Nowhere is this as apparent as in the area of antisocial behavior and its syndromal disturbances. Models need to be developed that do justice to this heterotypic continuity. The underlying process may remain stable, but manifest disturbances can change, depending on the context of the situation and the developmental phase of a given individual. One of the crucial issues for the diagnostic category of oppositional defiant disorder is the demonstration of its continuity with conduct disorder and antisocial personality disorder. One longitudinal study establishes such a link: researchers have demonstrated that *about one-third of boys* with oppositional defiant disorder *progress to suffer conduct disorders*. Conversely, *90 percent of boys with conduct disorder previously fulfilled criteria for oppositional defiant disorder.* Thus, the syndrome has considerable sensitivity for the prediction of conduct disorder from oppositional defiant disorder, but the positive predictive power is much less. One-half of the sample retained oppositional defiant disorder diagnoses while one-quarter desisted from oppositional defiant disorder at 3-year follow-up. It is an open issue whether children with oppositional defiant disorder who do not go on to develop conduct disorder will develop other psychiatric diagnoses.

With the exception of one 3-year prospective study there is no information about the naturalistic progression or response to treatment in these children. Most will not develop conduct disorders or antisocial personality disorder. One-half will show stable signs of oppositional defiant disorder after 3 years; *25 percent will have no further diagnosis.* Extrapolating from studies on conduct disorder and oppositional defiant disorder, about one-quarter of the initial total will go on to develop conduct disorders and about 10 percent will progress to antisocial personality disorder.

46.4 The answer is A

Differentiation of oppositional defiant disorder from normative oppositional behavior, transient antisocial acts, and conduct disorder is of paramount importance. Oppositional defiant disorder is not transient, leads to significant impairment, but does not involve major violations of the law and the rights of others. *Attention-deficit/hyperactivity disorder is the most common comorbidity*: Between 25 to 60 percent of children with oppositional defiant disorder also fulfill criteria for attention-deficit/hyperactivity disorder by parental report, and half of attention-deficit/hyperactivity disorder children have oppositional defiant disorder. As with conduct disorder, the association of oppositional defiant disorder and attention-deficit/hyperactivity disorder confers poor prognosis. Youngsters tend to be more aggressive, show a greater range and persistence of problem behaviors, are rejected at higher rates by peers, and underachieve more severely in the academic domain. Furthermore, attention-deficit/hyperactivity disorder facilitates the early appearance of oppositional defiant disorder and conduct disorder. Antagonistic behavior is commonly found in internalizing disorders in this age group: *dysthymic disorder, major depressive disorder*, and *early-onset bipolar I disorder* should be considered. *Anxiety disorders*, especially separation anxiety disorder, can present with predominant temper control problems. Pervasive developmental disorders also can demonstrate oppositionality, but the underlying bizarre problems with relating to others are usually absent in oppositional defiant disorder children.

46.5 The answer is B

Conduct disorder is a clinical term referring to the clustering of persistent antisocial acts of children and adolescents. The condition is thought to be due to underlying psychopathology leading to significant impairment in one or more domains of functioning. *The symptoms are clustered in four (not two) areas:* aggression to people and animals, destruction of property, deceitfulness and theft, and serious violations of rules. *Subtyping is allowed based on the age of onset of symptoms.* Severity can be specified as mild, moderate, or severe. The category is currently conceived of as a polythetic diagnosis in that no one specific criterion is necessary for and any combination of criteria will suffice to establish the diagnosis. There is no formal provision for evaluating the context in which these antisocial clusters occur. Both these features contribute to the fact that the category is inherently heterogenous. The current criteria require that *at least three (not five) of a list of 15 antisocial behaviors* be *present over a period of 12 months; one of them (not all) has to be present in the past 6 months.* Exclusion criteria for antisocial personality disorder are added. In epidemiological studies, this category has been robust, especially in its most recent, more stringent versions. Its inherent heterogeneity has made conduct disorder less useful for causal and treatment studies.

46.6 The answer is E (all)

One important model of conduct disorder posits that it is the gradual accumulation of risk as well as the absence or weak presence of protective factors and their interactions that lead ultimately to the conduct disorder, rather than single risk factors operating in isolation. Rolf Loeber has illustrated the gradual stacking of factors in the genesis of conduct disorder. An expanded model would include a parallel pyramid of resilience or protective factors, balancing the aggregation of risk as it accumulates over time. Figure 46.1 portrays the predominance of risks in ecological (e.g., poverty), constitutional (e.g., difficult temperament), and parenting (e.g., poor response to coercive behaviors, abuse) factors. This results in poor internal self-regulation, which becomes manifest especially during school age. School performance is also affected because these children lack skills needed to deal with authority and cannot fulfill their academic potential. Peer relationships suffer, as the child tends to find acceptance only from similarly socially inept peer groups. As there is an increasing aggregation of risk, it takes more and stronger protection to offset the risk, and more domains may be adversely affected. Empirical data also show that as risks accumulate in number, the greater is the chance that conduct disorder will develop via multiple interactive loops among risks.

Difficult *temperament has been repeatedly implicated* in the genesis of the disorder. It may work in at least two ways: It can

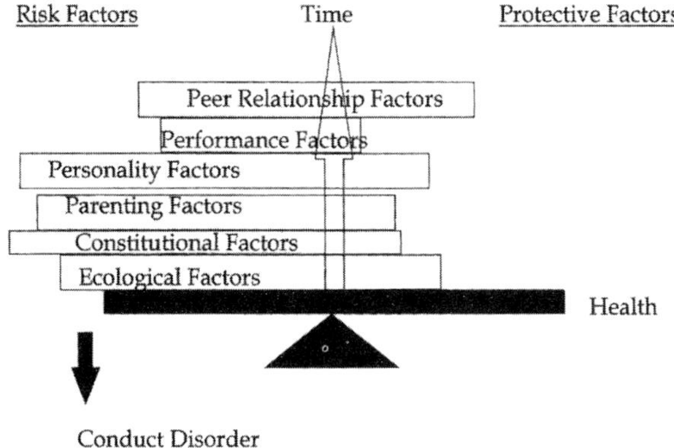

FIGURE 46.1
Developmental pathways to disruption behavior disorders.

make children more likely targets of parental anger and thus of poor parenting, or it may be linked directly to behavior problems later on. Inappropriate aggression at an early age, especially in combination with shyness, predicts later conduct disorder. *Chronic illness* and disability also have been known to increase the prevalence of conduct disorder, especially if the primary illness affects the central nervous system (CNS). Chronically ill children have three times the incidence of conduct problems of their healthy peers; if chronic illness affects the CNS, the risk is about five times as high.

Conduct disorder is more likely to be paired with diverse and complex disturbances in psychological domains. The origin of these disturbances is not clear, but their presence implies that many risks for conduct disorder are retained and internalized and independent of specific environments. Academic underachievement, learning disabilities, and problems with attention span and hyperactivity are all associated with conduct disorder. Hyperactivity, especially in the presence of poor parental functioning, is a risk; it seems to facilitate rapid development of conduct disorder. Neuropsychological deficits have been documented, implicating frontal and temporal lobe dysfunctions. *Laterality and language performance are disturbed.* Higher personality functions are also affected: In complex social situations, children with conduct disorder have been shown to perceive fewer appropriate responses, lack the skills to negotiate conflict, and lose their ability to restrain themselves when stressed emotionally.

Poor family functioning, familial aggregation of drug and alcohol abuse, psychiatric problems, marital discord, and especially poor parenting are all associated with conduct disorder. Abusive, neglectful parenting, and child maltreatment are unusually high-risk factors for the development of conduct disorder. The specific parenting patterns contributing to the development of conduct disorder have been described as training in noncompliance by inconsistent responses to coercive behavior of the child, and by capitulating to demands in response to the child's coercion. There is substantial evidence that *viewing televised or other media violence* and violence in the child's community contributes to conduct disorder problems, especially in children who are at special risk for other reasons. Socioeconomic disadvantage as manifested in poor housing, crowding, and poverty all exert consistently negative influences.

46.7 The answer is D

Conduct disorder has to be distinguished, first and foremost, from antisocial behavior without underlying psychopathology, *oppositional defiant disorder*, antisocial personality disorder, and impulse-control disorders. *Substance-use disorders* are extremely common in conduct disorder and can be the primary diagnostic reason for antisocial conduct. *Attention-deficit/hyperactivity disorder* is the next most common differential. The association with conduct disorder has been so frequent that there has been a debate over combining the diagnoses, but empirical data finds that the disorders differ in terms of premorbid risk and their respective predictive power for adult criminal outcomes. Divergent validity for conduct disorder from *attention-deficit/hyperactive disorders* is generally considered as established. The latter disorder is *considered the most virulent comorbid condition*: It facilitates the early appearance of conduct disorder, which is a strong predictor of adverse outcome. *Psychotic disorders, especially those with paranoid processes,* can be mistaken for conduct disorder. Internalizing disorders, such as mood disorders, posttraumatic stress disorder, and dissociative disorder can be confused with conduct disorder, although less commonly. Age under 18 generally prevents the diagnosis of personality disturbances, but in some cases borderline, narcissistic, and antisocial personality disorders should be considered. DSM-IV-TR allows for extensive comorbidities, as no exclusion criteria are provided. Conduct disorder is usually accompanied by a wide range of comorbid conditions. These comorbidities contribute independently and interactively to prognosis and outcome. Internalizing and externalizing comorbidities become increasingly common as the disorder becomes more severe. Repeated studies have shown that complex diagnostic patterns are the rule in this population, resulting in compound psychopathology requiring special management and treatment. Loeber's data provide a unique opportunity to examine the developmental unfolding of various comorbid states: Prior to adolescence, attention-deficit/hyperactivity disorder is most frequently associated with conduct disorder, especially in boys, declining in importance thereafter. The typical sequence seems to be attention-deficit/hyperactivity disorder—opposition defiant disorder—conduct disorder; alcohol and substance abuse follow. Each additional comorbidity adds to the poor prognosis in boys. The picture is different for girls: They also have a greater chance of getting conduct disorder when they suffer from attention-deficit/hyperactivity disorder, but it is not clear that the prognostic implications are as grave. Internalizing disorders, most commonly mood and anxiety disorders, but also somatization disorders, seem to appear during adolescence when conduct disorder is firmly entrenched. *Depression* in particular affects both sexes but especially girls, especially after they have reached pubertal maturation. Evidence on the prognostic impact of internalizing comorbidity and conduct disorder is mixed.

46.8 The answer is C

Oppositional defiant disorder is characterized by *enduring patterns of negativistic*, disobedient, and hostile behavior toward authority figures as well as the inability to take responsibility for mistakes, leading to *placing blame on others*. Children with oppositional defiant disorder frequently argue with adults and become easily annoyed by others, leading to a state of anger and resentment. Children with oppositional defiant disorder may have *difficulty in the classroom and with peer relationships but generally do not resort to physical aggression or significantly destructive behavior.*

In contrast, children with conduct disorder engage in severe repeated acts of aggression that may cause physical harm to themselves and others and frequently violate the rights of others. Children with conduct disorder usually have behaviors characterized by aggression to persons or animals, destruction of property, deceitfulness or *theft*, and multiple violations of rules such as truancy from school. These behavior patterns cause distinct *difficulties in school life* as well as in peer relationships. Conduct disorder has been divided into a childhood-onset subtype, in which at least one symptom has emerged repeatedly before age 10 years, and adolescent-onset type, in which there were no characteristic persistent symptoms until after age 10 years. While some young children show persistent patterns of behavior consistent with violating the rights of others or destroying property, the diagnosis of conduct disorder in children appears to increase with age.

Answers 46.9–46.11

46.9 The answer is B

46.10 The answer is A

46.11 The answer is B

Conduct disorder may be diagnosed when symptoms occur exclusively with attention-deficit/hyperactivity disorder, learning disorders, and mood disorders, whereas oppositional defiant disorder cannot be diagnosed when symptoms occur solely during a mood disorder. *Oppositional defiant disorder* may be equally prevalent in adolescent boys and adolescent girls, but conduct disorder is generally present more often in adolescent boys than adolescent girls. In *conduct disorder,* the patient often bullies, threatens, or intimidates others.

47 Feeding and Eating Disorders of Infancy or Early Childhood

Feeding and eating disorders of infancy or early childhood include persistent symptoms of inadequate food intake, recurrent regurgitation and rechewing of food, or repeated ingestion of nonnutritive substances. Because very young children depend upon parents or caregivers to feed them and provide meals, these disorders are often conceptualized as reflecting, in part, an interaction between the child and parent. The text revision of the 4th edition of *Diagnostic and Statistical Manual of Mental Disorders* (DSM-IV-TR) includes three distinct disorders of feeding and eating in this age group: pica, rumination disorder, and feeding disorder of infancy or early childhood. There is a high rate of spontaneous recovery from all of these feeding disorders, although a subset of infants refuses to eat and has persistent eating problems throughout childhood.

In DSM-IV-TR, pica is described as persistent eating of nonnutritive substances for at least 1 month. The behavior must be developmentally inappropriate, not culturally sanctioned, and sufficiently severe to merit clinical attention. Pica is diagnosed even when these symptoms occur in the context of another disorder such as autistic disorder, schizophrenia, or Kleine-Levin syndrome. Pica appears much more frequently in young children than in adults; it also occurs in persons who are mentally retarded. Among adults, certain forms of pica, including geophagia (clay eating) and amylophagia (starch eating), have been reported in pregnant women.

In DSM-IV-TR, rumination disorder is described as an infant's or child's repeated regurgitation and rechewing of food, after a period of normal functioning. The symptoms last for at least 1 month, are not caused by a medical condition, and are severe enough to merit clinical attention. The onset of the disorder generally occurs after 3 months of age; once the regurgitation occurs, the food may be swallowed or spit out. Infants who ruminate are observed to strain to bring the food back into their mouths and appear to find the experience pleasurable. The infants are often brought for evaluation because of failure to thrive. The disorder is rare in older children, adolescents, and adults. It varies in severity and is sometimes associated with medical conditions, such as hiatal hernia, that result in esophageal reflux. In its most sever form, the disorder can be fatal.

According to DSM-IV-TR, feeding disorder of infancy or early childhood is a persistent failure to eat adequately, reflected in significant failure to gain weight or in significant weight loss over 1 month. The symptoms are not better accounted for by a medical condition or by another mental disorder and are not caused by lack of food. The disorder has its onset before the age of 6 years.

The student should study the questions and answers below for a useful review of these disorders.

HELPFUL HINTS

The student should know the following terms.

- amylophagia
- anemia
- behavioral interventions
- cultural practices
- esophageal reflux
- failure to thrive
- geophagia
- hiatal hernia
- impoverished environments
- intestinal parasites
- iron deficiency
- lead poisoning
- mental retardation
- nutritional deficiencies
- overstimulation
- parental neglect and deprivation
- positive reinforcement
- psychosocial dwarfism
- regurgitation
- self-stimulation
- spontaneous remission
- zinc deficiency

QUESTIONS

Directions

Each of the questions or incomplete statements below is followed by five responses or completions. Select the *one* that is *best* in each case.

47.1 Feeding disorder of infancy or early childhood

A. has narrow DSM-IV-TR diagnostic criteria that address the specificity of various feeding disorders
B. has been reported in 1 to 2 percent of infants and toddlers
C. may have an age of onset after 6 years
D. does not necessarily result in significant failure to gain weight
E. none of the above

47.2 Pica

A. is usually diagnosed most easily when the child is under two years of age
B. decreases in prevalence with increasing severity of mental retardation
C. is not diagnosed if symptoms occur in the context of another disorder, including schizophrenia and autistic disorder
D. is diagnosed even if symptoms are culturally accepted
E. none of the above

47.3 Behaviors which may be related to pica include

A. Nail biting
B. Thumb sucking
C. Delays in speech and psychosocial development
D. Bulimia nervosa
E. All of the above

47.4 A diagnosis of rumination disorder

A. is commonly made in older children and adolescents
B. cannot be made in individuals with mental retardation or a pervasive developmental disorder
C. cannot be due to an associated gastrointestinal condition
D. is not made in children with a prior period of normal functioning.
E. occurs more often in females than in males

47.5 Susan was admitted to the hospital at age 6 months for evaluation of failure to gain weight. She had been born into an impoverished family after an unplanned, uncomplicated pregnancy. During her first 4 months of life, she gained weight steadily. Beginning in her 5th month, she was noted to regurgitate milk after feedings, in the following manner: she would open her mouth and elevate her tongue after feedings, thrust her tongue forward and backward, after which milk would appear at the back of her mouth. She would then vigorously suck her thumb and other fingers, and milk would continue to be regurgitated into her mouth. Her weight leveled off and then began to decrease during this time. In the two months prior to the onset of this behavior, Susan had multiple caregivers and received little attention from her parents. Nevertheless, she smiled often and was responsive to all of her caregivers.

The most likely diagnosis is

A. Rumination disorder
B. Reactive attachment disorder
C. Pica
D. Failure to thrive
E. None of the above

47.6 All of the following behaviors are association with the disorder *except*

A. sucking noises
B. rechewing food
C. reswallowing food
D. mutism
E. appearance of satisfaction

Directions

The questions below consist of lettered heading followed by a list of numbered phrases. For each numbered phrase, select the correct heading.

Questions 47.7–47.14

A. Rumination disorder
B. Pica
C. Both
D. Neither

47.7 May lead to lead poisoning and toxoplasmosis.
47.8 This disorder falls under the ICD-10 diagnostic category of "Feeding Disorders of Infancy and Childhood," but forms its own diagnostic category in DSM-IV-TR.
47.9 The onset may occur at any age in life, including adolescence and adulthood.
47.10 High rate of spontaneous remission
47.11 Reinforcement by pleasurable self-stimulation
47.12 Associated with failure to thrive
47.13 Associated with adolescent- and adult-onset eating disorders
47.14 Associated with pregnant women

ANSWERS

47.1 The answer is B

According to DSM-IV-TR criteria, feeding disorder of infancy or early childhood is a persistent failure to eat adequately, *resulting in significant failure to gain weight* or in significant weight loss over at least one month. The symptoms are not better accounted for by a medical condition, another mental disorder, or lack of food, and *the disorder's onset must occur before (not after) age 6.* The *DSM-IV-TR criteria are broad (not narrow)* and do not address the specificity of feeding disorders that are not separately included in the DSM-IV or ICD-10.

An estimated 15 to 35 percent of infants and young children have feeding difficulties; common problems include eating too little, refusing certain foods, objectionable mealtime behaviors, and bizarre food habits. However, these problems tend to be mild and do not significantly impact the child's growth. Severe feeding problems associated with poor weight gain are reported in *1 to 2 percent of infants and toddlers*. Several studies indicate that infants who exhibit food refusal in the first year of life continue to have feeding problems when followed up later in childhood. Picky eating and gastrointestinal symptoms in early childhood have been linked to anorexia nervosa in adolescence, while pica and disruptive mealtime behaviors have been associated with bulimia nervosa in adolescence.

47.2 The answer is E (none)

DSM-IV-TR describes pica as the persistent eating of non-nutritive substances for at least one month. The behavior must be developmentally inappropriate, not culturally sanctioned, and sufficiently severe to merit clinical attention. Under these circumstances, *pica is diagnosed even when symptoms occur in the context of another mental disorder,* such as schizophrenia, autistic disorder, or Kleine-Levin syndrome.

Pica occurs more frequently in young children than in adults, and is more common in individuals with mental retardation. Forms of pica, including geophagia (clay eating) and amylophagia (starch eating) do occur among adults, particularly pregnant women. In certain geographic regions and cultures, such as Australian aborigines, high rates of pica among pregnant women are reported. *According to DSM-IV-TR criteria, if such practices are culturally sanctioned, diagnostic criteria for pica are not met.*

Because infants commonly mouth objects as part of their exploration of their environment, it is *difficult (not easy) to diagnose pica in children under age 2*. Among individuals with mental retardation, *the prevalence of pica appears to increase with the severity of the retardation*. The occurrence of pica among institutionalized mentally retarded individuals has been estimated to range from 10 to 33 percent.

47.3 The answer is E (all)

Many children with pica engage in other oral activities that likely have self-soothing effects, including *thumb sucking* and *nail biting*. Typically pica occurs for several months and then remits. However, a minority of cases continues through childhood and adolescence and even into adulthood. Several authors have highlighted significant impact associated with longstanding pica, including *delays in speech and psychosocial development*, depression, ongoing disturbed oral activities (thumb sucking, nail biting), and tobacco and other substance abuse. Additionally, some authors have identified a relationship between pica during early childhood and *bulimia nervosa* during adolescence.

47.4 The answer is C

DSM-IV-TR describes rumination disorder as behavior by an infant or child in which food is repeatedly regurgitated or rechewed. The behavior must occur *after a period of normal functioning*, take place for at least 1 month, and *not be attributable to a gastrointestinal or other medical condition*. The onset of the disorder typically occurs after 3 months of age. Infants who ruminate are observed to strain to bring food back into their mouths and appear to derive pleasure from the behavior. After regurgitation the food is swallowed, chewed, or spit out. The infants often come to clinical attention due to failure to thrive. *Even in the context of other mental disorders, such as mental retardation or pervasive developmental disorders, the diagnosis of rumination disorder may be made if the symptoms are sufficiently severe to warrant clinical attention.* The disorder is *rare (not common) in older children and adolescents*, and occurs *more often in males than in females (not vice versa)* and individuals with mental retardation.

Answers 47.5–47.6

47.5 The answer is A

47.6 The answer is D

Failure to gain weight or weight loss in an infant, once general medical conditions have been ruled out, suggests Rumination Disorder of Infancy, Feeding Disorder of Infancy or Early Childhood, or Reactive Attachment Disorder of Infancy or Early Childhood. The child in this case is not gaining weight because of the regurgitation of food after each feeding, indicating *a diagnosis of Rumination Disorder of Infancy*. Typically, the child strains and makes *sucking noises* with the tongue in order to regurgitate food, *then re-chews or re-swallows the food. Often the child gives the impression of deriving considerable satisfaction from the behavior*. The disorder usually occurs between 3 and 12 months of age. There is a suggestion in this case that parental care may be inadequate, but the absence of evidence of inappropriate social relatedness rules out the diagnosis of Reactive Attachment Disorder of Early Childhood. Because the cause of the weight loss is the regurgitation, the general diagnosis of Feeding Disorder of Infancy or Early Childhood is not made. *Reactive attachment disorder* is the severe impairment of the ability to relate, beginning before age 5. *Pica* is the craving and eating of nonfood substances, such as paint, clay, and dirt. In *failure to thrive*, an infant shows physical signs of malnourishment and does not exhibit the expected developmental motor and verbal milestones.

Answers 47.7–47.14

47.7 The answer is B

47.8 The answer is A

47.9 The answer is C

47.10 The answer is C

47.11 The answer is A

47.12 The answer is C

47.13 The answer is C

47.14 The answer is B

Young children with pica typically eat plaster, paper, paint (which may cause *lead poisoning*), cloth, hair, animal droppings (which may cause *toxoplasmosis*), sand, pebbles, or dirt.

Rumination disorder is included under "Feeding Disorders of Infancy and Childhood" in ICD-10, but forms its own diagnostic category in DSM-IV-TR. Pica is a diagnosis under both ICD-10 and DSM-IV-TR.

Although rumination disorder and pica most commonly occur in infancy and early childhood, *both may have their onset at any age in life, including adolescence and adulthood.* Rumination disorder has been reported to start later in life in adults with eating disorders. In individuals with mental retardation and developmental disorders, these conditions may have onset later in life.

Both rumination disorder and pica have high rates of spontaneous remission. Rumination disorder appears to be reinforced by pleasurable self-stimulation. Frequently, vomiting secondary to acute illness or to gastroesophageal reflux precedes the onset of rumination; presumably, the infant learns to initiate vomiting and finds self-soothing, tension-relieving, or self-stimulating effects from the behavior. Once the infant has developed rumination as means of self-regulation and gratification, it becomes a difficult habit to break. *Both pica and rumination are associated with failure to thrive*; in severe cases life-threatening malnutrition may occur with rumination. *Both rumination and pica are associated with adolescent- and adult-onset eating disorders. Pica may occur in pregnant women* and is especially prevalent during pregnancy in certain cultures.

48 Tic Disorders

Tics are defined as rapid and repetitive muscle contractions resulting in movements or vocalizations that are experienced as involuntary. Children and adolescents may exhibit tic behaviors that occur after a stimulus or in response to an internal urge. Tic disorders are a group of neuropsychiatric disorders that generally begin in childhood or adolescence and may be constant or wax and wane over time. Although tics are not volitional, in some individuals they may be suppressed for periods. The most widely known and most severe tic disorder is Gilles de la Tourette syndrome, also known as Tourette's disorder. The text revision of the 4th edition of the *Diagnostic and Statistical Manual of Mental Disorders* (DSM-IV-TR) includes several other tic disorders such as chronic motor or vocal tic disorder, transient tic disorder, and tic disorder not otherwise specified. While tics have no particular purpose, they often consist of motions that are used in volitional movements.

Motor and vocal tics are divided into simple and complex types. Simple motor tics are those composed of repetitive, rapid contractions of functionally similar muscle groups—for example, eye blinking, neck jerking, shoulder shrugging, and facial grimacing. Common simple vocal tics include coughing, throat clearing, grunting, sniffing, snorting, and barking. Complex motor tics appear to be more purposeful and ritualistic than simple tics. Common complex motor tics include grooming behaviors, the smelling of objects, jumping, touching behaviors, echopraxia (imitation of observed behavior), and copropraxia (display of obscene gestures). Complex vocal tics include repeating words or phrases out of context, coprolalia (use of obscene words or phrases), palilalia (a person's repeating his or her words), and echolalia (repetition of the last-heard words of others).

Some persons with tic disorders can suppress the tics for minutes or hours, but others, especially young children, either are not cognizant of their tics or experience their tics as irresistible. Tics may be attenuated by sleep, relaxation, or absorption in an activity. Tics often, but not always, disappear during sleep.

According to DSM-IV-TR, tics in Tourette's disorder are multiple motor tics and one or more vocal tics. The tics occur many times a day for more than 1 year. Tourette's disorder causes distress or significant impairment in important areas of functioning. The disorder has an onset before the age of 18 years, and it is not caused by a substance or by a general medical condition.

Georges Gilles de la Tourette first described a patient with what was later known as Tourette's disorder in 1885, while he was studying with Jean-Martin Charcot in France. De la Tourette noted a syndrome in several patients that included multiple motor tics, coprolalia, and echolalia.

The student should study the following questions and answers for a useful review of these disorders.

HELPFUL HINTS

The terms that follow relate to tic disorders and should be known by the student.

- attention-deficit/hyperactivity disorder
- barking
- behavioral treatments
- benztropine (Cogentin)
- Jean Charcot
- clonidine (Catapres)
- compulsions
- coprolalia
- dopamine antagonists and stimulants
- dystonia
- echokinesis
- echolalia
- echopraxia and copropraxia
- encephalitis lethargica
- eye blinking
- facial grimacing
- Gilles de la Tourette
- grunting
- Hallervorden-Spatz disease
- hemiballism
- Huntington's chorea
- hyperdopaminergia
- Lesch-Nyhan syndrome
- motor tic
- neck jerking
- obsessive-compulsive disorder
- palilalia
- Pelizaeus-Merzbacher disease
- pimozide (Orap)
- poststreptococcal syndromes
- shoulder shrugging
- simple or complex tic
- stereotypy
- Sydenham's chorea
- tardive dyskinesia
- torsion dystonia
- Tourette's disorder
- transient tic disorder
- tremor
- vocal tic
- Wilson's disease

QUESTIONS

Directions

Each of the questions or incomplete statements below is followed by five responses or completions. Select the *one* that is *best* in each case.

48.1 Which of the following symptoms is required for diagnosis of Tourette's disorder according to DSM-IV-TR criteria?

A. Vocal tic
B. Multiple motor tics
C. Symptoms occurring for at least 1 year
D. Onset before age 18
E. All of the above

48.2 Which of the following statements about the epidemiology of Tourette's disorder is true?

A. The lifetime prevalence of Tourette's disorder is estimated at one per 10,000.
B. The average age of onset of the motor component of the disorder is 7 years old.
C. The average age of onset of the vocal component of the disorder is 7 years old.
D. Prevalence of Tourette's disorder is similar in boys and girls.
E. All of the above

48.3 In Tourette's disorder, the initial tics are in the

A. Face and neck
B. Arms and hands
C. Body and lower extremities
D. Respiratory system
E. Alimentary system

48.4 True statements about Tourette's disorder include which of the following?

A. The most frequent initial symptom is mental coprolalia.
B. Coprolalia usually begins around 6 to 8 years of age and occurs in about 5 percent of cases.
C. Most complex motor and vocal symptoms emerge virtually simultaneously with the initial symptoms.
D. Attention-Deficit/Hyperactivity Disorder (ADHD) is rarely diagnosed in children who are later diagnosed with Tourette's disorder.
E. Typically, behavioral symptoms, such as hyperactivity, are evident several years before or concurrent with the initial symptoms.

48.5 If onset is after age 18, which of the following tic disorders may be diagnosed?

A. Transient tic disorder
B. Chronic motor or vocal tic disorder
C. Tourette's disorder
D. Tic disorder not otherwise specified
E. All of the above

48.6 The dopamine system has been hypothesized to be involved in the development of tic disorders because:

A. Haloperidol (Haldol) suppresses tics
B. Pimozide (Orap) suppresses tics
C. Methylphenidate (Ritalin) exacerbates tics
D. Pemoline (Cylert) exacerbates tics
E. All of the above

48.7 Which of the following statements concerning evidence supporting genetic factors as likely to play a role in the development of Tourette's disorder is *false*?

A. Concordance for Tourette's disorder is significantly higher in monozygotic than in dizygotic twins.
B. Sons of men with Tourette's disorder are at highest risk of developing the disorder.
C. First-degree relatives of probands with Tourette's disorder are at higher-than-average risk for developing Tourette's disorder and chronic tic disorder.
D. First-degree relatives of probands with Tourette's disorder are at higher-than-average risk for developing obsessive-compulsive disorder, and up to 40 percent of patients with Tourette's disorder also have obsessive-compulsive disorder.
E. None of the above

48.8 Which of the following distinguishes transient tic disorder from chronic motor or vocal tic disorder and Tourette's disorder?

A. age of onset
B. the presence of motor tics only
C. the presence of vocal tics only
D. the presence of both motor and vocal tics
E. temporal progression of the tic symptoms

48.9 Which of the following is *not* an appropriate pharmacologic treatment for tic disorders?

A. Methylphenidate
B. Guanfacine
C. Risperidone
D. Clonidine
E. Haloperidol

Directions

Each group of questions below consists of lettered headings followed by a list of numbered phrases. For each numbered phrase, select the *one* lettered heading most associated with it. Each heading may be used once, more than once, or not at all.

Questions 48.10–48.12

A. tonic tic
B. dystonic tic
C. clonic tic
D. simple phonic tic
E. complex tic

48.10 May be mistaken for a volitional act.

48.11 Sniffing, grunting, or yelping.
48.12 Brisk movements.

Questions 48.13–48.17

A. Tourette's disorder
B. Sydenham's chorea
C. Both
D. Neither

48.13 Associated with obsessive-compulsive behavior.
48.14 Possible autoimmune response to streptococcal antigens.
48.15 Self-limiting syndrome.
48.16 Chronic illness with a waxing and waning course.
48.17 More common in males.

Questions 48.18–48.21

A. Tic disorders
B. Non-tic movement disorders
C. Both
D. Neither

48.18 Repetitive vocalizations
48.19 Premonitory sensation
48.20 Description of movements as intentional in response to urges or sensations
48.21 Association with mental retardation or dementing process

ANSWERS

48.1 The answer is E (all)

To make a diagnosis of Tourette's disorder, clinicians must obtain a history of *multiple motor tics* and at least *one vocal tic*. The tics must occur many times a day nearly every day or intermittently throughout a period of *at least 1 year*, during which time there was never a tic-free period of more than 3 consecutive months. The onset must occur *prior to age 18*, and must not be attributable to the physiological effects of a substance (such as stimulants) or a general medical condition.

48.2 The answer is B

The lifetime prevalence of Tourette's disorder is estimated to be *four to five per 10,000* (not one per 10,000). *The motor component of the disorder has an average age at onset of seven years old; the onset of the vocal component occurs later, at an average of 11 years of age* (not seven years). Tourette's disorder is at least *three times as common in boys as in girls* (not equal prevalence).

48.3 The answer is A

In Tourette's disorder, the most commonly observed tics affect the face and head, arms and hands, trunk and lower extremities, and the respiratory and alimentary systems. *The first tics tend to appear in the face and neck.* Tics may take the following forms: grimacing; forehead puckering; eyebrow raising; eye blinking; eye winking; nose wrinkling; nostril trembling; mouth twitching; displaying the teeth; biting the lips or tongue; tongue extruding; protracting the lower jaw; nodding, jerking or shaking the head; twisting the neck; looking sideways; head rolling; hand shaking; arm jerking; finger plucking; finger writhing; fist clenching; shoulder shrugging; foot, knee or toe shaking; peculiar walking; body writhing; jumping; hiccupping; sighing; yawning; grunting; blowing through the nostrils; whistling; belching; making sucking or smacking sounds; and clearing the throat.

48.4 The answer is E

Prodromal behavioral symptoms (irritability, hyperactivity, inattention, and poor frustration tolerance) very commonly precede or coincide with the onset of tics. ADHD is *commonly (not rarely) diagnosed* in children who are later diagnosed with Tourette's. The most frequent initial symptoms of Tourette's are eye-blink tics, facial grimaces, and head tics (*not mental coprolalia*, a later-occurring symptom of Tourette's in which a patient experiences a sudden, intrusive thought of a socially unacceptable word or idea). Most complex motor and vocal symptoms emerge several years after (*not simultaneously with*) the initial symptoms. Coprolalia (speaking obscene words or phrases) usually begins in adolescence (*not around 6 to 8 years of age*) and occurs in approximately one third (*not 5 percent*) of cases of Tourette's.

48.5 The answer is D

All tic disorders with onset after age 18 must be diagnosed as tic disorder not otherwise specified, a residual category for tics that do not meet the criteria for a specific tic disorder. Transient tic disorder, chronic motor or vocal tic disorder, and Tourette's disorder all specify onset before age 18.

48.6 The answer is E (all)

Evidence that supports a role for the dopamine system in the etiology of tic disorders includes: dopamine antagonists such as *haloperidol and pimozide suppress tics;* agents that increase central dopamine activity, such as cocaine, dextroamphetamine, *methylphenidate, and pemoline, exacerbate tics*. However, there is a not a straightforward relationship between dopamine and tics, as dopamine antagonists do not always suppress tics, and agents that increase central dopamine activity, such as stimulants, may not exacerbate tics. Complex interactions between dopamine and other neurotransmitters, particularly norepinephrine, as well as the contribution of other neurochemical systems, such as endogenous opiates, likely contribute to the phenomenon of tics.

48.7 The answer is B

There is convincing evidence of genetic factors influencing risk of Tourette's disorder. *Sons of women (not men) with Tourette's disorder appear to be at highest risk of developing the disorder*; there is evidence of transmission in a bilinear mode, indicating an autosomal pattern intermediate between dominant and recessive. *Concordance for Tourette's disorder is significantly higher in monozygotic versus dizygotic twins. First-degree relatives of probands with Tourette's disorder are at increased risk for developing Tourette's disorder, and also for developing chronic tic disorder and obsessive-compulsive disorder*; this finding, in conjunction with the observation that up to 40 percent of patients with Tourette's disorder also have OCD, strongly suggests a genetic link between these conditions.

48.8 The answer is E

Transient tic disorder cannot be distinguished from chronic tic disorders or from Tourette's disorder on the basis of age of onset, presence of motor tics or vocal tics alone, or presence of both motor and vocal tics. Only the *temporal progression of the tic symptoms is significant in differentiating among these conditions.* All three diagnoses specify onset before age 18. Transient tic disorder refers to single or multiple motor and/or vocal tics occurring for up to 1 year. Chronic motor or vocal tic disorder specifies that only one type of tic be involved, and must occur for over 1 year. Tourette's disorder refers to multiple motor and at least one vocal tic occurring for over 1 year.

48.9 The answer is A

Methylphenidate and other psychostimulants do not treat tics and may occasionally cause tics as an adverse effect; tics that first emerge during treatment with stimulants generally resolve promptly with dose reduction or drug discontinuation. *Guanfacine and clonidine, alpha-2 agonist agents, are effective and well-tolerated medications for the treatment of tics*; they are increasingly becoming first-line agents in the treatment of Tourette's and other tic disorders. These medications reduce central noradrenergic activity, likely producing secondary effects upon dopamine transmission, which may explain their efficacy in ameliorating tics. *Risperidone and haloperidol are two medications with proven efficacy in reducing tics,* likely acting through dopamine antagonism.

Answers 48.10–48.12

48.10 The answer is E

48.11 The answer is D

48.12 The answer is C

Tics are defined as rapid, repetitive muscle contractions or sounds that are usually experienced as beyond volitional control and that often resemble aspects of normal movement or behavior. They can be elicited by particular stimuli, and are often preceded by an urge or sensation. Tics are classified as motor or vocal and as simple or complex. Simple motor tics involve one or several muscle groups and include eye blinking, facial grimacing, and shoulder shrugging. Simple motor tics can be further divided into clonic, tonic, or dystonic subtypes. *Clonic tics are very brisk movements*; tonic and dystonic tics involve more sustained muscle contractions such as arm extension, muscle tensing, oculogyric movements, and torticollis.

Complex motor tics may be mistaken for volitional acts; they may involve multiple muscle groups and mimic normal coordinated movements, such as jumping, hopping, knee bends, simultaneous extension of upper and lower extremities, and less commonly obscene gesturing or copropraxia.

Phonic tics may also take simple form (as in coughing, *sniffing, grunting, or yelping*), or complex form, including words and phrases that uncommonly include coprolalia.

Answers 48.13–48.17

48.13 The answer is C

48.14 The answer is C

48.15 The answer is B

48.16 The answer is A

48.17 The answer is A

Sydenham's chorea is a self-limiting syndrome consisting of a variety of abnormal movements including choreiform movements, tics, and compulsive behavior, which occurs as a result of autoimmune response to streptococcal antigens. *Recent evidence has emerged linking autoimmune response to streptococcal infection with Tourette's disorder* and with obsessive-compulsive disorder; in these patients, elevated titers of autoantibodies may be detected. The proposed autoimmune process in these cases of Tourette's and OCD, which likely represent a significant minority of the overall prevalence of these conditions, may suggest an environmental insult exposing an underlying genetic vulnerability. *Obsessive-compulsive behaviors are common in both Sydenham's chorea and in Tourette's disorder*; up to 40 percent of patients with Tourette's disorder also meet diagnostic criteria for OCD. *Tourette's disorder is more common in males*, whereas Sydenham's chorea is more common is females. While Sydenham's chorea is a self-limited illness, Tourette's disorder is chronic, with waxing and waning symptoms, and the condition often persists into adulthood.

Answers 48.18–48.21

48.18 The answer is A

48.19 The answer is A

48.20 The answer is A

48.21 The answer is B

Differentiating tics from abnormal movements associated with non-tic movement disorders is accomplished by clinical history and examination. *Repetitive vocalizations are characteristic of tic disorders and occur rarely in non-tic movement disorders. Premonitory sensations are very commonly described by patients with tic disorders*, who report a variety of sensations or experiences including urges, itches, feelings or tightness or tingling, and feelings of irritation or worry. Patients often describe a crescendo of urge or discomfort leading up to the tic, and may report feelings of relief following the tic. Another common feature is the perceived need to repeat tic behaviors until relief is achieved or until the individual feels "just right." *Patients with tics often acknowledge their tic movements as intentional, carried out in response to an urge or sensation.* The complex mental processes preceding and succeeding tics often make it difficult to distinguish tics from obsessive-compulsive thoughts and behaviors, which are likely closely linked biologically. *All of these features are very uncommon in non-tic movement disorders.*

Additional features that assist in differentiating tics from non-tic movement disorders include age of onset (average age of 7 in Tourette's and other tic disorders; younger in autistic disorder, athetoid cerebral palsy, Pelizaeus-Merzbacher disease, and Lesch-Nyhan syndrome; older in Huntington's disease, Wilson's disease, spastic torticollis), and the *lack of a common association between tic disorders and mental retardation or dementing processes* (in contrast to autistic disorder, cerebral palsy, Lesch-Nyhan syndrome, Wilson's disease, and Huntington's disease).

49 Elimination Disorders

Enuresis and encopresis are the two elimination disorders described in the text revision of the 4th edition of *Diagnostic and Statistical Manual of Mental Disorders* (DSM-IV-TR). These disorders are considered only when a child is chronologically and developmentally beyond the point at which it is expected that these functions can be mastered. Normal development encompasses a range of time in which a given child is able to devote the attention, motivation, and physiological skills to exhibit competency in elimination processes. Encopresis is defined as a pattern of passing feces into inappropriate places, whether the passage is involuntary or intentional. The pattern must be present for at least 3 months; the child's chronological age must be at least 4 years. Enuresis is the repeated voiding of urine into clothes or bed, whether the voiding is involuntary or intentional. The behavior must occur twice weekly for at least 3 months or must cause clinically significant distress or impairment socially or academically. The child's chronological or developmental age must be at least 5 years.

Bowel and bladder control develops gradually over time. Toilet training is affected by many factors, such as a child's intellectual capacity and social maturity, cultural determinants, and the psychological interactions between child and parents. The normal sequence of developing control over bowel and bladder functions is the development of nocturnal fecal continence, diurnal fecal continence, diurnal bladder control, and nocturnal bladder control.

The student should study the questions and answers below for a useful review of these disorders.

HELPFUL HINTS

The student should know the following terms.

- abnormal sphincter contractions
- aganglionic megacolon
- behavioral reinforcement
- bell (or buzzer) and pad
- diurnal bowel control
- ego-dystonic enuresis
- fluid restriction
- functionally small bladder
- genitourinary pathology and other organic disorders
- Hirschsprung's disease
- imipramine
- intranasal desmopressin (DDAVP)
- laxatives
- low nocturnal antidiuretic hormone
- neurodevelopmental problems
- nocturnal bowel control
- obstructive urinary disorder abnormality
- olfactory accommodation
- overflow incontinence
- poor gastric motility
- psychosocial stressors
- rectal distention
- regression
- thioridazine
- toilet training

QUESTIONS

Directions

Each of the questions or incomplete statements below is followed by five suggested responses or completions. Select the *one* that is *best* in each case.

49.1 According to DSM-IV-TR enuresis can be defined as repeated voiding of urine into bed or clothes in children over the age of

A. 2 years
B. 3 years
C. 4 years
D. 5 years
E. no defined age

49.2 True statements about enuresis include

A. The majority of enuretic children wet intentionally.
B. There is a correlation between enuresis and psychological disturbance that increases with age.
C. Children with enuresis are no more likely to have developmental delays than other children.
D. There is no evidence for a genetic component to enuresis.
E. Children living in socially disadvantaged environments do not have an increased incidence of enuresis.

49.3 In DSM-IV-TR, qualifiers to the diagnosis of enuresis include

A. Minimum duration of symptom
B. Diurnal vs. nocturnal enuresis

C. Combined nocturnal and diurnal pattern
D. Physical causes such as bladder infection must be excluded
E. All of the above

49.4 The incidence of obstructive urinary tract lesions in children with enuresis has been reported at approximately

A. 1.5 percent
B. 3.5 percent
C. 10 percent
D. 15 percent
E. 25 percent

49.5 True statements about enuresis include

A. The vast majority of enuretic children experience spontaneous resolution of the problem.
B. Medications are generally the first step in the treatment of childhood enuresis.
C. Psychotherapy is never indicated as part of the treatment of enuresis.
D. The success rate for behavioral interventions is nearly 40 percent.
E. Classical conditioning methods (bell and pad) are ineffective in children with concomitant psychiatric disorders.

49.6 True statements about encopresis include

A. No significant relationship exists between encopresis and enuresis.
B. Less than 25 percent of children with encopresis have constipation.
C. Psychological factors are often relevant when encopresis occurs after a previous period of fecal continence.
D. The symptom must occur at least once weekly for 3 months as part of DSM-IV-TR criteria for the diagnosis of encopresis.
E. None of the above

Directions

The lettered headings below are followed by a list of numbered phrases. For each numbered phase, select

A. if the item is associated with A only
B. if the item is associated with B only
C. if the item is associated with both A and B
D. if the item is associated with neither A nor B

Questions 49.7–49.8

A. primary encopresis
B. secondary encopresis

49.7 More likely to have developmental delays and associated enuresis
49.8 More often diagnosed with conduct disorder

Questions 49.9–49.15

A. encopresis
B. enuresis

49.9 This disorder is more common in females.
49.10 Psychopharmacological intervention for this disorder often provides symptomatic improvement, but is of limited utility as relapse tends to occur as soon as the drug is withdrawn.
49.11 Although physiological factors likely play a significant role in this disorder, structural abnormalities are rarely the cause of symptoms.
49.12 At age 7 years, approximately 1.5 percent of boys have this disorder.
49.13 At age 5 years, approximately 7 percent of boys have this disorder.
49.14 To be diagnosed with this disorder, a child must have a chronological or developmental age of 5 years.
49.15 To be diagnosed with this disorder, a child must have a chronological or developmental age of 4 years.

Directions

The statement below is followed by five suggested responses. Select the *one* that is *best*.

49.16 Tim, age 6, was referred to the clinic by his pediatrician because of persistent soiling. Tim's mother reported that he had never gained control of his bowel habits. After a febrile illness at age 2, he developed constipation, and required laxatives and suppositories as treatment. Following this episode, there was an alternating pattern of constipation, when he did not move his bowels for several days, and diarrhea, when he soiled his pants many times a day. At age 4, he again took laxatives for a period of time and his stools became softer and more regular. His mother began to toilet train him at that time. He was made to sit on the toilet each evening until he "performed." Although he usually managed to produce a tiny amount of stool during these sessions, he continued to soil his pants frequently during the day. This pattern continued until the time of referral.

Tim himself had been distressed about his soiling since starting school, fearing that others would notice when he stained his clothes or when he smelled after a soiling episode. He was anxious when sitting on the toilet in the evenings and insisted that his mother stay in the bathroom with him. He was also enuretic at night. He became dry by day at age 3 but continued to wet at night; because waking him at night has not prevented his wetting, his mother still put him in diapers to sleep.

Apart from the problems of soiling and wetting, his mother felt that Tim was a normal little boy who was happy and outgoing. His developmental milestones were all a little behind those of his older sisters. He sat at 7 months, walked at 18 months, and spoke his first words at about 18 months as well.

In the interview Tim was shy at first, clinging to his mother. However, he allowed her to leave the room after a short period and became more assertive and outgoing in her absence. He played with family figures in the dollhouse and portrayed the little boy figure on the toilet and all the other members of the family observing his efforts.

The pediatrician's report indicated that a full medical workup revealed no general medical condition that could account for the soiling. On physical exam, a fecal mass was palpated in Tim's lower abdomen, and soft feces were present in his rectum.

The diagnosis in this case is

A. encopresis
B. enuresis
C. conduct disorder
D. Hirschsprung's disease
E. childhood schizophrenia

ANSWERS

49.1 The answer is D

Enuresis is defined as the repeated voiding of urine into bed or clothes, whether involuntary or intentional, in *children over the age of 5 years* (or equivalent developmental level). These children fail to inhibit the reflex to pass urine when it occurs during waking hours, and fail to awake on their own when the process occurs during sleep.

49.2 The answer is B

There is a correlation between enuresis and psychological disturbance that increases with age. Additionally, there is increasing evidence for the role of physiological factors in enuresis. Although the DSM-IV-TR definition of enuresis includes both voluntary and unintentional wetting, *the vast majority of enuretic children do not wet intentionally.* Bladder control is achieved gradually and is influenced by neuromuscular and cognitive development, as well as by emotional factors and toilet training; difficulties in one or more of these areas may delay acquisition of urinary continence. There is also accumulating evidence for a genetic role in enuresis; one large study found that a child's risk of being enuretic was increased 5.2 times if the mother had been enuretic as a child and 7.1 times if the father had been enuretic. Additionally, the concordance rate is higher in monozygotic than in dizygotic twins, and 75 percent of enuretic children have a first-degree biological relative with enuresis. A small minority of children with enuresis wet intentionally; these children often manifest oppositional defiant disorder or a psychotic disorder. *Children living in socially disadvantaged circumstances and children experiencing significant psychosocial stress have a greater incidence of enuresis than other children.* The behavioral disturbances that co-occur with enuresis are quite variable and nonspecific, and may represent either coincidental rather than causal correlations with enuresis. *Children with enuresis have significantly higher rates of developmental delays than nonenuretic children,* including both children in psychiatric clinic populations and normal controls.

49.3 The answer is E (all)

According to the DSM-IV-TR criteria for enuresis, *the wetting must occur at least twice a week for at least three consecutive months, or if less frequent, must cause significant distress or functional impairment. Physical etiologies such as bladder infections must be excluded.* Most children have only *nocturnal enuresis,* which is specified in contrast to *daytime (diurnal) pattern or a combined nocturnal and diurnal pattern.* Primary enuresis (in which continence has never been achieved), as distinguished from secondary enuresis (in which previously acquired continence is lost), is not specified in the DSM-IV-TR.

49.4 The answer is B

Clinicians must rule out organic factors that may predispose a child to enuresis, such as urinary tract infections; urinalysis should be part of every evaluation. Structural abnormalities may be the cause of the symptom, but this is a relatively rare causal factor–*a large study in a pediatric primary care setting found that* 3.7 *percent of children with enuresis had obstructive lesions.* Given the low diagnostic yield and invasive nature of the sophisticated radiographic procedures necessary for the investigation of anatomical causes of enuresis, these studies are usually deferred in cases of enuresis with no signs of repeated infections or other medical problems.

49.5 The answer is A

The natural history of enuresis is significant because it impacts upon treatment decisions, insofar as *enuresis is a self-limiting disorder that will eventually spontaneously remit.* Diagnosis is not made until age 5 to account for children who undergo toilet training at a later stage in the accepted age range (2 to 5 years of age). The prevalence of enuresis is relatively high between the ages of 5 and 7 and then substantially declines. By age 14 only 1.1 percent of boys wet once a week or more, and very few persist into adulthood with the problem.

Behavioral and pharmacological treatments have well established efficacy in treating enuresis, but *medications are not the first line of treatment* given risks of side effects and high likelihood of recurrence of the problem when the drugs are discontinued. *Psychotherapy is often useful for ameliorating behavioral disturbances that often accompany enuresis, especially secondary enuresis;* however, studies indicate that psychotherapy alone does not tend to have a high success rate in the treatment of enuresis.

A comprehensive review of several studies determined the success rate for behavioral treatment of enuresis to be 75 *percent (not 40 percent).* The primary method of behavioral treatment is the bell and pad method of conditioning. A pad is placed on the bed, with a wire connected to a bell. When the child wets, the moisture completes a circuit in the pad, ringing the bell and waking the child. With repeated use the child learns to awaken before wetting occurs. *This treatment is equally effective in children with and without concomitant psychiatric disorders.*

49.6 The answer is C

Encopresis may *be precipitated by stressful life events; when the disorder begins after a prior sustained period of fecal continence,* the behavior may represent a regression precipitated by stressors such as birth of sibling, parental separation, or the start of school. *Significant relationship exists between encopresis and enuresis; the two disorders commonly co-occur.* Encopresis involves a complicated interplay between physiological and psychological factors. Inadequate or inappropriate toilet training, ineffective sphincter control, and a variety of emotional reasons may all contribute to the development of the disorder. Regardless of the origin of the symptom in a given individual, bowel functioning tends to be disturbed: *up to 75 percent of children with encopresis are constipated* and have excessive fluid overflow.

The *DSM-IV-TR specifies one event per month for at least 3 months* as part of the criteria for encopresis.

49.7 The answer is A

49.8 The answer is B

In both enuresis and encopresis, the distinction between primary and secondary has bearing upon the likelihood of associated psychopathology. One study of 63 boys found that *boys with primary encopresis were more likely to have developmental delays and associated enuresis,* while *those with secondary enuresis were more likely to have experienced high level of psychosocial stress and to have been diagnosed with conduct disorder.*

49.9 The answer is D

49.10 The answer is B

49.11 The answer is C

49.12 The answer is A

49.13 The answer is B

49.14 The answer is B

49.15 The answer is A

Both enuresis and encopresis are three to four times more common in males than in females. Several medications have been used with some success in the treatment of enuresis. Imipramine has FDA approval for the treatment of childhood enuresis on a short-term basis. However, tolerance typically develops within 6 weeks of beginning treatment, and *relapse at former frequencies of wetting predictably occurs after discontinuing the drug.* Desmopressin (DDA VP), an antidiuretic hormone available in intranasal spray form, is useful in preventing enuresis while being used, but also does not seem to maintain its effect after discontinuation. Thus, behavioral techniques are the first line of treatment for enuresis. For treatment of encopresis, combined behavioral and family intervention is the recommended treatment. Accurate evaluation of the patterns of encopresis is necessary for successful treatment. Constipation with overflow incontinence should be identified if present. The degree to which the child is aware of the passage of feces is significant as well. If encopresis is a behavior through which the child expresses anger or attracts negative parental attention, the treatment approach is altered. Psychopharmacological interventions are not typically part of the treatment of encopresis, although they may be indicated in cases of chronic constipation in order to regulate stool consistency and improve bowel regularity.

While structural abnormalities are rare causes of enuresis or encopresis, physiological factors are important contributors to both conditions. For example, children with encopresis who have chronic constipation and overflow incontinence are often found to have abnormal sphincter contractions. Physiological characteristics, some of which are likely heritable, also contribute to enuresis: three-quarters of children with enuresis have a first-degree relative with enuresis. Furthermore, children with enuresis are twice as likely to have concomitant developmental delay as other children.

Bowel control is established in 95 percent of children by the 4th birthday and in 99 percent of children by the 5th birthday. *At age 7, the frequency of encopresis is 1.5 percent in boys* and 0.5 percent in girls. The prevalence of enuresis declines with age: 82 percent of 2-year-olds, 49 percent of 3-year-olds, 26 percent of 4-year-olds, and *7 percent of 5-year-olds have enuresis.* To be diagnosed as having enuresis, a child must have a chronological or developmental age of 5 years; the cutoff for encopresis is a chronological or developmental age of 4 years.

49.16 The answer is A

Encopresis is defined by DSM-IV-TR as a pattern of passing feces into inappropriate places, whether the passage is involuntary or intentional. The pattern must be present for at least 3 months; the child's chronological age must be at least 4 years.

Enuresis is the repeated voiding of urine into clothes or bed, whether the voiding is involuntary or intentional. The behavior must occur twice weekly for at least 3 months or must cause clinically significant distress or impairment socially or academically. The child's chronological or developmental age must be at least 5 years.

Conduct disorder is an enduring set of behaviors that evolves over time, usually characterized by aggression and violation of the rights of others. Conduct disorder is associated with many other psychiatric disorders including attention-deficit/hyperactivity disorder, depression, and learning disorders, and it is also associated with several psychosocial factors such as low socio-economic level; harsh, punitive parenting; family discord; lack of appropriate parental supervision; and lack of social competence. The DSM-IV-TR criteria require three specific behaviors of the 15 listed, which include bullying, threatening, or intimidating others and staying out at night despite parental prohibitions, beginning before 13 years of age.

Hirschsprung's disease, also known as congenital megacolon, is the congenital dilation and hypertrophy of the colon due to absence (aganglionosis) or marked reduction (hypoganglionosis) in the number of ganglion cells of the myenteric plexus of the rectum.

Schizophrenia in prepubertal children is exceedingly rare; it is estimated to occur less frequently than autistic disorder. In adolescents, the prevalence of schizophrenia is estimated to be 50 times that in younger children, with probable rates of 1 to 2 per 1,000.

50 Other Disorders of Infancy, Childhood, or Adolescence

Reactive attachment disorder (RAD) is a clinical disorder characterized by aberrant social behaviors in a young child reflecting an environment of maltreatment that interfered with the development of normal attachment behavior. Unlike most disorders in the text revision of the 4th edition of the *Diagnostic and Statistical Manual of Mental Disorders* (DSM-IV-TR), a diagnosis of RAD is based on the presumption that the etiology is directly linked to environmental deprivation experienced by the child. The diagnosis of reactive attachment disorder is a relatively recent entity, added to the 3rd edition of DSM (DSM-III) in 1980. The formation of this diagnosis is largely based on the building blocks of attachment theory, which described the quality of a child's generalized affective relationship with primary caregivers, usually parents. This basic relationship is the product of a young child's need for protection, nurturance and comfort and the interaction of the parents and child in fulfilling these needs.

Stereotypic movements are repetitive voluntary, often rhythmic movements that occur in normal children, and occur with increased frequency in children carrying the diagnoses of pervasive developmental disorder and mental retardation syndromes. These movements appear to be purposeless but in some cases, such as body rocking, head rocking or hand flapping, they may be either self-soothing or self-stimulating. In other cases, stereotypic movements such as head banging, face slapping, eye poking, or hand biting may cause significant self-harm. Nail biting, thumb sucking, and nose picking are generally not included as symptoms of stereotypic movement disorder since they rarely cause impairment.

The student should study the questions and answers below for a useful review of these disorders.

HELPFUL HINTS

The student should know the following terms.

- anticipatory anxiety
- behavioral inhibition
- delayed language acquisition
- desensitization
- driven, nonfunctional behavior
- dyskinetic movements
- emotional and physical neglect
- external life stressors
- failure to respond socially
- failure to thrive
- generalized anxiety
- head banging and nail biting
- indiscriminate familiarity
- inhibition to speak
- lack of stable attachment
- Lesch-Nyhan syndrome
- major attachment figure
- multimodal treatment approach
- nonverbal gestures
- panic disorder
- pathogenic caregiving
- psychopharmacologic interventions
- "psychosocial dwarfism"
- school phobia
- school refusal
- selective mutism
- self-injurious stereotypic acts
- sensory impairments
- separation anxiety
- shyness
- social anxiety
- social phobia
- specific phobia
- stereotypic movements
- stress anxiety
- temperamental constellation

QUESTIONS

Directions

Each of the questions or incomplete statements below is followed by five suggested responses or completions. Select the *one* that is *best* in each case.

50.1 Stereotypic movement disorder

A. Includes trichotillomania
B. Includes stereotypy that is part of a pervasive developmental disorder
C. Is not diagnosed if mental retardation is present
D. Includes tics and compulsions
E. None of the above

50.2 Which of the following accurately describes head banging, one example of a stereotypic movement?

A. Has a prevalence of approximately 1 percent in child populations
B. Affects males three times more commonly than females

C. Typically begins after the age of 12 months
D. Is relatively common after the age of 3 years
E. Is rarely self-limiting

50.3 The most widely used intervention in the treatment of stereotypic movements is

A. Clomipramine (Anafranil)
B. Desipramine (Norpramin)
C. Haloperidol (Haldol)
D. Chlorpromazine (Thorazine)
E. Behavioral modification

50.4 Figure 50.1A shows a 3-month-old baby boy whose weight is 1 ounce over birth weight. His history of care taking had been characterized by persistent disregard for his basic needs for comfort, affection, stimulation, and nourishment. Upon his hospitalization, the infant's head circumference was normal, as was his bone age. While he failed to show normal spontaneous activity, his growth hormone levels were in the normal range. This infant's symptoms typify a classic disorder of infancy. Which, if any, symptom is at odds with the diagnosed disorder?

A. Insufficient spontaneous activity
B. Normal head circumference for age
C. Normal bone age
D. Normal levels of growth hormone
E. None of the above

Directions

Each group of questions below consists of lettered headings followed by a list of numbered phrases or statements. For each numbered phrase or statement, select the *one* lettered heading that is most closely associated with it. Each lettered heading may be selected once, more than once, or not at all.

Questions 50.5–50.6

A. Reactive attachment disorder, inhibited type
B. Reactive attachment disorder, disinhibited type
C. Both
D. Neither

50.5 Linked to institutionalization or exposure to multiple caregivers prior to age 5
50.6 Linked to early childhood maltreatment

Questions 50.7–50.10

A. Reactive attachment disorder
B. Stereotypic movement disorder
C. Both
D. Neither

50.7 Pervasive developmental disorder must be ruled out in order for the diagnosis to be made.
50.8 Includes some symptoms, such as rocking or thumb sucking, that are considered developmentally normal self-comforting behaviors in very young children.
50.9 May be associated with multiple foster care placements in early childhood.

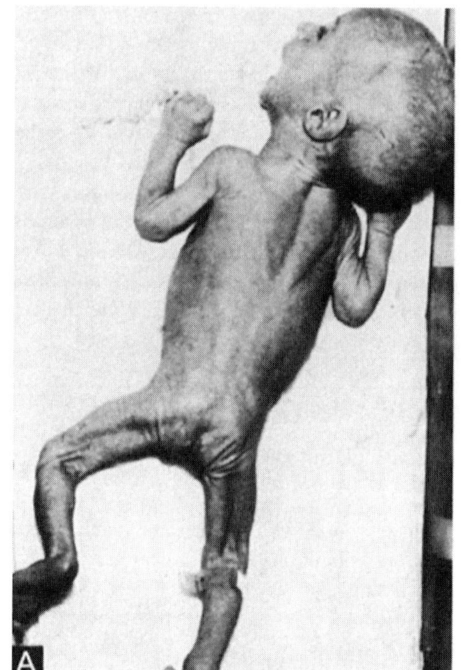

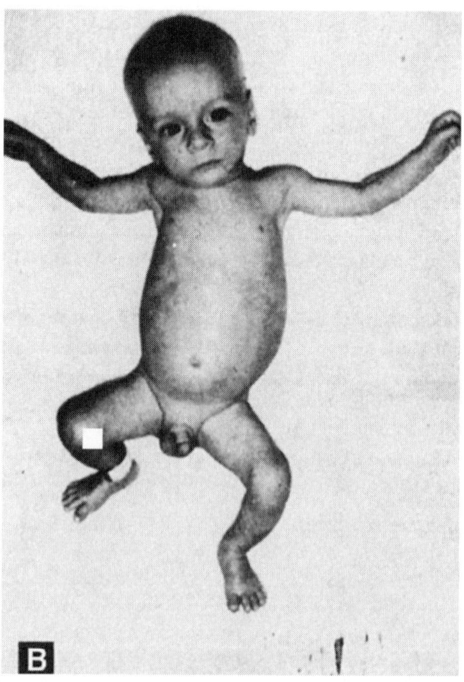

FIGURE 50.1
Reprinted with permission from Barton Schmitt, M.D., Children's Hospital, Denver, CO.

50.10 Clearly indicate increased risk of future psychotic disorder.

ANSWERS

50.1 The answer is E (none)
Stereotypic movement disorder has undergone some modification with the evolution of the DSM system. DSM-III contained

a broader definition of the disorder than does DSM-IV-TR. The DSM-III criteria described voluntary, nondistressing, nonspasmodic movements and specified that the behaviors were associated with psychosocial deprivation, mental retardation, or pervasive developmental disorder, but could occur independently of these conditions. In DSM-III-R, *the diagnosis was renamed stereotypy/habit disorder, and was a broadened category that included periodic and persistent nonfunctional behaviors, such as nail biting.* DSM-III-R also specified functional impairment—the behavior had to either cause physical injury or interfere with normal activities—and excluded diagnosis in the presence of tic disorder or pervasive developmental disorder. *DSM-IV-TR continues with these specifications, and further excludes specific behaviors such as trichotillomania* (hair pulling), tics, and compulsions, since they are thought to fit more coherently into other diagnostic categories.

When stereotypic movements occur as part of another general neurological, medical, or psychiatric condition, an additional diagnosis of stereotypic movement disorder is not required. *Stereotypic movement disorder can be diagnosed in the presence of mental retardation when the movements are severe enough to warrant clinical attention.*

50.2 The answer is B

Although the prevalence of stereotypic movement disorders in the general population is unknown, some data exist on the prevalence of individual stereotyped behaviors in certain populations. The prevalence of self-injurious behaviors is higher among children with mental retardation than among the general population. *Head banging is estimated to have a prevalence of approximately 5 percent (not 1 percent) in child populations*, with *males affected three times more frequently than females*. The behavior is *usually (not rarely) self-limiting*, and typically occurs in the first three years of life, with *typical age of onset between 5 and 12 months (not after 12 months)*. It is *relatively rare (not relatively common) after age 3*. Similarly, breath holding is rare after the 3rd birthday and occurs most commonly between 12 and 18 months of age; this behavior is also more common in boys than girls.

50.3 The answer is E

No specific treatment has been shown to be effective for stereotypic movement disorder in general; however, a small number of double-blind studies have investigated the efficacy of pharmacological treatments for specific behaviors. For example, investigations have suggested the superiority of *clomipramine over desipramine* for severe nail biting; more recent clinical practice has favored SSRI medications over tricyclic antidepressants for these symptoms given their more benign side-effect profile. Neuroleptics are also frequently used and may demonstrate significant clinical benefit; both *haloperidol and chlorpromazine* have demonstrated efficacy in randomized placebo-controlled trials of patients with stereotyped movements associated with mental retardation and autistic disorder.

Despite some established efficacy of pharmacological agents, *behavioral modification techniques have been the most widely used interventions* for the treatment of stereotypic movements. These techniques include both positive and negative reinforcement and have shown success in diminishing the severity and frequency of the movements.

50.4 The answer is C

The infant suffers from reactive attachment disorder of infancy, presenting with the typical clinical picture of nonorganic failure to thrive. *In such infants, hypokinesis, dullness, apathy, and paucity of spontaneous activity are usually seen.* Most of the infants appear malnourished and many have protruding abdomens, as indicated in this photograph. Although many such infants' weights are below the third percentile and markedly below appropriate weight for height, *head circumference is usually normal for age. Bone age is usually retarded (not normal). Growth hormone levels are usually normal or elevated*, suggesting that growth failure is secondary to malnutrition. The children improve physically and gain weight rapidly after hospitalization, as evident in Figure 50.1B.

Answers 50.5–50.6

50.5 The answer is B

50.6 The answer is A

Reactive attachment disorder of infancy and early childhood is described in DSM-IV-TR as behavior characterized by "markedly disturbed and developmentally inappropriate social relatedness in most contexts." These findings must be consistent with "grossly pathogenic care." *The disorder must begin before 5 years of age to meet criteria and cannot be accounted for "solely by developmental delay."* Children who are mentally retarded are thus difficult to diagnose; those who meet criteria for pervasive developmental disorder are explicitly excluded from consideration for reactive attachment disorder.

Two subtypes are spelled out in the DSM-IV-TR criteria. *The first pattern, generally linked in the literature to early childhood maltreatment, is characterized by inhibition of the normal developmental tendency to seek comfort from a select group of caregivers.* Responses to social interactions are "excessively inhibited, hypervigilant, or highly ambivalent," reflecting the overall inhibition of the attachment system in affected children. *The second pattern, linked to institutionalization or exposure to multiple caregivers prior to age 5, is characterized by a relative hyperactivation of the attachment system*, resulting in "diffuse" and nonselective attachments, and patterned behavior labeled "indiscriminate sociability."

Answers 50.7–50.10

50.7 The answer is C

50.8 The answer is B

50.9 The answer is A

50.10 The answer is D

Pervasive developmental disorders are marked by significant impairments in social interactions as well as repetitive and stereotyped movements; as a result, *neither reactive attachment disorder nor stereotypic movement disorder diagnoses are made in the presence of a pervasive developmental disorder. Neither reactive attachment disorder nor stereotypic movement disorder has been established as a risk factor for future development of a psychotic disorder.*

As many as 80 percent of normal children show rhythmic activities such as thumb sucking or rocking that seem purposeful and soothing and tend to disappear by 3 to 4 years of age; it is only when these symptoms persist beyond normal developmental expectations, and markedly interfere with normal activities or cause bodily injury, that a diagnosis of stereotypic movement disorder is considered.

Reactive attachment disorder results from grossly pathogenic care of an infant or young child. Likelihood of the disorder increases with a variety of circumstances including parental mental retardation; parenthood during adolescence; institutionalization; repeated lengthy hospitalizations; and *multiple foster care placements*.

51

Mood Disorders and Suicide in Children and Adolescents

Mood disorders appear in children of all ages, and may consist of enduring patterns of disturbed mood; diminished enthusiasm in play activities, sports, friendships, or school; and a general feeling of worthlessness. The core features of major depression are similar in children, adolescents, and adults, with the expression of these features modified to match the age and maturity of the individual.

Mood disorders among children and adolescents have been increasingly diagnosed and treated with a variety of modalities. Although clinicians and parents have always recognized that children and adolescents may experience transient sadness and despair, it has become clear that persistent disorders of mood occur in children of all ages and under many different circumstances. Two criteria for mood disorders in childhood and adolescence are a disturbance of mood, such as depression or elation, and irritability.

Although diagnostic criteria for mood disorders in the text revision of the 4th edition of *Diagnostic and Statistical Manual of Mental Disorders* (DSM-IV-TR) are almost identical across all age groups, the expression of disturbed mood varies in children according to their age. Young, depressed children commonly show symptoms that appear less often as they grow older, including mood-congruent auditory hallucinations, somatic complaints, withdrawn and sad appearance, and poor self-esteem. Symptoms that are more common among depressed youngsters in late adolescence than in young childhood are pervasive anhedonia, severe psychomotor retardation, delusions, and a sense of hopelessness. Symptoms that appear with the same frequency regardless of age and developmental status include suicidal ideation, depressed or irritable mood, insomnia, and diminished ability to concentrate.

Developmental issues, however, influence the expression of all symptoms. For example, unhappy young children who exhibit recurrent suicidal ideation are generally unable to think of a realistic suicide plan or to put their ideas into action. Children's moods are especially vulnerable to the influences of severe social stressors, such as chronic family discord, abuse and neglect, and academic failure. Many young children with major depressive disorder have histories of abuse or neglect. Children with depressive disorders in the midst of toxic environments may have remission of some or many depressive symptoms when the stressors diminish or when the children are removed from the stressful environment. Bereavement often becomes a focus of psychiatric treatment when children have lost a loved one, even when a depressive disorder is not present.

Depressive disorders and bipolar I disorder are generally episodic, although their onset may be insidious. Manic episodes are rare in prepubertal children but fairly common in adolescents. Attention-deficit/hyperactivity disorder (ADHD), oppositional defiant disorder, and conduct disorder may occur among children who later experience depression. In some cases, conduct disturbances or disorders may occur in the context of a major depressive episode and resolve with the resolution of the depressive episode. Clinicians must clarify the chronology of the symptoms to determine whether a given behavior (such as poor concentration, defiance, or temper tantrums) was present before the depressive episode and is unrelated to it or whether the behavior is occurring for the first time and is related to the depressive episode.

The student should study the questions and answers below for a useful review of these disorders.

HELPFUL HINTS

The student should study the following terms.

- academic failure
- anhedonia
- antisocial behavior and substance abuse
- bereavement
- boredom
- copycat suicides
- cortisol hypersecretion
- developmental symptoms
- double depression
- environmental stressors
- family history
- hallucinations
- inpatient vs. outpatient treatment
- insidious onset
- irritable mood
- lethal methods
- poor concentration
- poor problem solving
- precipitants of suicide
- psychosocial deficits
- REM latency
- sad appearance
- social withdrawal
- somatic complaints
- temper tantrums
- toxic environments

QUESTIONS

Directions

Each of the questions or incomplete statements below is followed by five suggested responses or completions. Select the *one* that is *best* in each case.

51.1 Which of the following statements about the epidemiology of mood disorders in children and adolescents is *true*?

A. Major depressive disorder in preschool-age children is fairly common; a typical estimate of prevalence in epidemiologic studies is three percent.
B. Depression is more common among boys than girls among school-age children.
C. Major depression is more common than dysthymia among school-age children.
D. Dysthymia rarely progresses to major depression among children and adolescents.
E. Among adolescents, about 15 to 20 percent of community samples have major depressive disorder.

51.2 True statements about the phenomenology of bipolar disorder in children and adolescents include all of the following *except*

A. Prepubertal children very rarely exhibit discrete episodes of mania or depression.
B. Some clinicians ascribe symptoms such as extreme mood variability, aggressive behavior, and high rates of distractibility and impulsivity to pediatric bipolar disorder, though controversy exists over this diagnosis.
C. Psychotic symptoms such as hallucinations and delusional thought content are rare in adolescent mania.
D. Among adolescents, depressive episodes characterized by severely depressed mood, psychosis, psychomotor retardation, and hypersomnia may be predictive of later development of bipolar disorder.
E. Antidepressant medications may trigger hypomania or mania in children and adolescents with no known history of bipolar disorder.

51.3 Major depressive disorder in school-aged children

A. may present as irritable mood rather than depressed mood
B. usually includes pervasive anhedonia
C. includes mood-congruent auditory hallucinations less commonly than in adults with the same disorder
D. is never diagnosed in the context of bereavement
E. none of the above

51.4 Which of the following statements is *true* of suicide in adolescence?

A. Completed suicide decreases in incidence with increasing age.
B. Completed suicide is more common in girls than in boys.
C. Suicide attempts are always associated with a mood disorder.
D. Suicide attempts often precipitated by arguments with family members, girlfriends, or boyfriends.
E. The most common method used in completed suicide among adolescents in the United States is toxic ingestion.

51.5 Which of the following is *not* a true statement regarding suicide among children and adolescence?

A. Suicide is the third leading cause of death among persons 15 to 24 years of age in the United States.
B. Risk factors for completed suicide include family history of suicidal behavior, exposure to family violence, impulsivity, substance use, mood disorder, and availability of lethal means.
C. High levels of serotonin and its metabolites have been found postmortem in the brains of individuals who completed suicide.
D. One-third of individuals who complete suicide had at least one prior attempt.
E. A history of aggressive behavior is an important predictor of increased risk for suicide.

51.6 Which of the following symptoms presents with similar frequency among children, adolescents, and adults with major depressive disorder?

A. Suicidal ideation
B. Somatic complaints
C. Mood-congruent auditory hallucinations
D. Pervasive anhedonia
E. None of the above

51.7 Which of the following treatments have demonstrated efficacy in treating adolescent depression based upon controlled clinical trials?

A. Cognitive-behavioral psychotherapy
B. Interpersonal psychotherapy
C. Fluoxetine
D. All of the above
E. None of the above

ANSWERS

51.1 The answer is B

Mood disorders among children and adolescents are characterized by increasing prevalence with increasing age. *Among preschool age children, major depressive disorder is uncommon, with prevalence rates estimated at approximately 0.3 percent (not 3 percent)* in community samples. The prevalence increases slightly among school-age children, with prevalence estimates of two percent for major depressive disorder; in contrast to findings among adolescents, *school-age boys are more likely to be affected than girls (not vice-versa).* The rates continue to *increase in adolescence, with estimates of prevalence approximating five percent (not 15 percent to 20 percent).* Dysthymia occurs in children and adolescence as well; as with adults, among adolescents major depressive disorder is more common than dysthymia, but *in school-age children the reverse is true: dysthymia is more prevalent than major depression.* Additionally, *dysthymia among school-age children commonly (not rarely) progresses to major depression.*

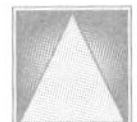

Table 51.1
Prevalence (Point or 1-year)

Major depression	
Preschoolers	0.3%
Children	0.4%–3.0%
Adolescents	0.4%–6.4%
Dysthymic disorder	
Children	0.6%–1.7%
Adolescents	1.6%–8.0%
Bipolar I disorder	
Children	0.2%–0.4%
Adolescents	1%
Attempted suicide	
Children	1%
Adolescents	1.7%–5.9%
Completed suicide	
5–9-year-old boys	0.04/100,000
5–9-year-old girls	0
10–14-year-old boys	2.4/100,000
10–14-year-old girls	0.96/100,000
15–19-year-old males	18.25/100,000
15–19-year-old females	3.48/100,000

Prevalence rates for mood disorders among children and adolescents vary significantly between genders, as do rates of attempted and completed suicide. Epidemiological studies have reported a range of prevalence estimates, with differences attributed to sampling methods, measurement instruments, and sources of information. See Table 51.1 for prevalence rates.

51.2 The answer is C

Bipolar disorder is being diagnosed with increasing frequency in prepubertal children, despite the fact that in this age group "classic" manic episodes are extremely rare, and that *prepubertal children very infrequently exhibit discrete episodes of mania or depression.* While an ongoing controversy exists over the diagnosis of bipolar disorder in this age group, *increasing numbers of clinicians diagnose bipolar disorder based upon findings of extreme mood variability, aggression, distractibility, impulsivity,* and depressive symptoms, particularly in the context of a family history of bipolar disorder. Whether or not these children will go on to develop more discrete mood cycling later as they mature, or whether their presentations will differ from adult bipolar disorder, remains under investigation. Adolescent-onset bipolar disorder much more closely parallels in its presentation the characteristics of bipolar disorder in adults. *Psychotic symptoms, such as hallucinations and delusions, are common (not rare) in adolescent mania*; indeed, some authors suggest that psychosis as part of a manic state is more common in adolescents than in adults. *Adolescents with depressive episodes characterized by severely depressed mood, psychosis, psychomotor retardation, and hypersomnia may be at increased risk of going on to develop bipolar disorder*, compared with adolescents whose major depressive episodes are not so characterized. As in adults, *antidepressant medications may trigger hypomania or mania in children and adolescents with no known history of bipolar disorder.*

51.3 The answer is A

Major depression in school-aged children does not commonly present with findings typical among adults, such as depressed mood and neurovegetative symptoms; instead, somatic complaints, psychomotor agitation, and *irritable mood are more common. Additionally, mood-congruent auditory hallucinations are much more (not less) common among prepubertal children with major depression than among adults* with the same condition. *Pervasive anhedonia, a common finding in depressed adults, is less typical (not usually present) among school-aged children* with major depression. A diagnosis of major depressive disorder is not usually made within 2 months of the loss of a loved one; *however, in the event of marked functional impairment, morbid preoccupation with worthlessness or guilt, psychomotor retardation, suicidal ideation, or psychosis, a diagnosis of major depression, and appropriate treatment, is indicated.*

51.4 The answer is D

Suicide in adolescents is often precipitated by arguments with family members, girlfriends, or boyfriends. Suicidal adolescents often lack the ability to synthesize solutions to vexing problems, and lack coping skills to manage acute stressors. A narrow view of available options for dealing with family discord, rejection, or failure seems to contribute to a decision to commit suicide. *Both suicide attempts and completions increase (not decrease) in incidence with increasing age through childhood and adolescence*, peaking in the 15 to 19 year old age range. *Completed suicide is five times more common in boys than girls (not vice versa)*, though girls attempt suicide at three times the rate of boys. While presence of a mood disorder, particularly, depression, is an important risk factor for attempted suicide, other important risk factors have also been identified; *suicide attempts often (not always) are associated with a mood disorder. The most common method of completed suicide in the United States is the use of firearms (not toxic ingestion)*, which accounts for two-thirds of suicides in boys and one-half of suicides in girls.

51.5 The answer is C

Suicide is the third leading cause of death among persons 15 to 24 years of age in the United States, and the second leading cause among white males in the same age range. *Risk factors for completed suicide include family history of suicidal behavior, exposure to family violence, impulsivity, substance use, mood disorder, and availability of lethal means*, as well as prior suicide attempts, other mental illnesses (particularly psychotic disorders), *history of aggressive behavior*, and losing a parent prior to age 13. *One-third of individuals who complete suicide had at least one prior attempt.* Neurochemical findings in the study of suicide indicate some overlap between patients who commit suicide and patients with other impulsive and aggressive behaviors: a suggestive finding is *low (not high) levels of serotonin and its major metabolite, 5-HIAA, found postmortem in the brains of individuals who completed suicide.*

51.6 The answer is A

Although the core symptoms of major depressive disorder overlap considerably among children, adolescents, and adults, different symptoms predominate in each age group. *Suicidal ideation is a symptom that occurs with similar frequency among depressed individuals of all ages.* Psychomotor agitation, irritable mood, *somatic complaints, and mood-congruent auditory hallucinations are common manifestations of major depression among school-age children. Pervasive anhedonia is less common among children, but is frequently present in depressed adolescents and adults.* Adolescents with depression also present more commonly with irritability, aggression, sulkiness, withdrawal from social activities, and a desire to leave home than do depressed patients from other age groups. Changes in sleep and appetite are more common in adults with major depression than in children or adolescents with the disorder.

51.7 The answer is D (all)

A number of studies have demonstrated the *efficacy of cognitive-behavioral psychotherapy in treating major depressive disorder in adolescents. Interpersonal therapy has also shown good results* in the treatment of depressed adolescents. Recent controversies surrounding potential side effects of the selective serotonin reuptake inhibitors (SSRIs) among children and adolescents, including the possible increase in suicidal ideation, have complicated the use of these medications to treat adolescents with major depressive disorder; nevertheless, *fluoxetine has been to shown to effectively treat the condition in this age group.*

52 Anxiety Disorders of Infancy, Childhood, and Adolescence

There are four categories of anxiety disorder in children. The first is obsessive-compulsive disorder (OCD). OCD is characterized by the presence of recurrent intrusive thoughts associated with anxiety or tension and/or repetitive purposeful mental or physical actions aimed at reducing fears and tensions caused by obsessions. It has become increasingly clear that the majority of cases of OCD begin in childhood or adolescence. The clinical presentation of OCD in childhood and adolescence is similar to that in adults and the only alteration in diagnostic criteria in the text revision of the 4th edition of *Diagnostic and Statistical Manual of Mental Disorders* (DSM-IV-TR) for children is that they do not necessarily demonstrate awareness that their thoughts or behaviors are unreasonable.

The second category is posttraumatic stress disorder (PTSD). PTSD is characterized by a set of symptoms such as reexperiencing symptoms, distressing recollections, persistent avoidance, and hyperarousal in response to exposure to one or more traumatic events. PTSD is the only disorder described in DSM-IV-TR in which the etiologic factors, exposure to an extreme traumatic stressor either directly or as a witness, is the first diagnostic criterion of the disorder. Many children and adolescents are exposed to traumatic events ranging from direct experiences with physical or sexual abuse, domestic violence, motor vehicle accidents, severe medical illnesses or natural or human created disasters, leading to full PTSD in some, and at least some PTSD symptoms in many others. Although the presence of posttraumatic stress symptoms has been described among adults for more than a century, it was first officially recognized as a psychiatric disorder in 1980 with the publication of DSM-III. Recognition of its frequent emergence in children and adolescence has broadened over the last decade.

The third category includes separation anxiety disorder, generalized anxiety disorder and social phobia. Separation anxiety disorder is diagnosed when developmentally inappropriate and excessive anxiety emerges related to separation from the major attachment figure. Generalized anxiety disorder is characterized by chronic generalized anxiety not limited to any particular idea, object, or event.

The fourth category is selective mutism. Selective mutism is characterized in a child by persistent failure to speak in one or more specific social situations most typically including the school setting. The most recent conceptualization of selective mutism highlights the relationship between underlying social anxiety and the resulting failure to speak. Most children with the disorder are completely silent during the stressful situations, while some may verbalize almost inaudibly single-syllable words. Children with selective mutism are fully capable of speaking competently when not in a socially anxiety-producing situation.

The student should study the questions and answers below for a useful review of these disorders.

HELPFUL HINTS

The student should be able to define the following terms.

- adoption studies
- age of onset
- anticipatory
- aphonia
- asthma
- attention-deficit/hyperactivity disorder (ADHD)
- β-adrenergic receptor antagonists
- cannabis-induced
- central noradrenergic system
- cognitive-behavioral
- comorbid disorders
- EEG
- exposure therapy
- family studies
- free-floating
- genetics
- impulse control
- kleptomania
- life events
- neurochemical
- neuroimaging
- panic disorder
- performance
- psychotherapy
- rating scales
- religious ritual
- self-cutting
- separation
- separation anxiety disorder
- serotoninergic system
- situational
- startle reflex
- stranger
- striatum
- substance abuse
- temperament
- thalamus
- Tourette's syndrome
- trait

QUESTIONS

Directions

Each of the questions or incomplete statements below is followed by five suggested responses or completions. Select the *one* that is *best* in each case.

52.1 OCD in children is characterized by all of the following *except*

A. intrusive thoughts
B. anxiety
C. awareness that thoughts are unreasonable
D. response to serotonergic agents
E. male predominance

52.2 Which of the following is *not* a true statement about the genetics of OCD?

A. There is an increased risk of OCD in first degree relatives.
B. Subclinical syndromes occur in family pedigrees.
C. OCD is related to Tourette's disorder.
D. There is a linkage to chromosome 21.
E. Tics are highly correlated to OCD.

52.3 Pediatric autoimmune neuropsychiatric disorders associated with streptococcus (PANDAS) are characterized by all of the following *except*

A. an autoimmune process
B. inflammation of the basal ganglia
C. thalamo-cortical dysfunction
D. obsessive thinking
E. lower limb paralysis

52.4 Habit disturbances that stem from separation anxiety include

A. nail biting
B. thumb sucking
C. masturbation
D. temper tantrums
E. all of the above

52.5 Separation anxiety in children is characterized by

A. fears that a loved one will be hurt
B. fears about getting lost
C. irritability
D. animal and monster phobias
E. all of the above

52.6 An 8-month-old infant who is separated from his mother for the first time goes through three well-defined sequential stages. In order they are

A. Protest, detachment, and despair
B. Protest, despair, and detachment
C. Detachment, despair, and protest
D. Despair, protest, and detachment
E. Detachment, protest, and despair

52.7 Psychoanalytic bases for anxiety in the child has been ascribed to

A. dependency
B. fear of the superego
C. symbiosis
D. castration fears
E. all of the above

52.8 There is clinical evidence to support which of the following as predisposing toward overanxious disorders in children

A. Large families
B. First-born children
C. Low socioeconomic status
D. Low expectations
E. Last-born children

52.9 Which of the following statements is *not* true about separation anxiety in infants?

A. It is not a universal phenomenon in infants.
B. It emerges in infants less than one year of age.
C. It has survival value.
D. It peaks between 9 months and 18 months.
E. It is pathological in about 15 percent of infants.

52.10 Which of the following statements is *true* about preschoolers?

A. Approximately 10 percent will meet criteria for an anxiety disorder
B. About 6 percent will suffer from generalized anxiety disorder
C. Approximately 3 percent will suffer from separation anxiety disorder
D. About 2 percent will suffer from social phobia
E. All of the above

52.11 Extremely shy children show all of the following *except*

A. high resting heart rate
B. low cortisol levels
C. insecure attachment
D. elevated urinary catecholamines
E. dilation of the pupil during cognitive tasks

52.12 Fear in children may be produced by which of the following?

A. Direct modeling by the parents
B. Parental overprotection
C. Anger
D. Temperamental predisposition
E. All of the above

52.13 Separation anxiety disorder

A. is a developmental phase
B. affects up to 4 percent of school-aged children
C. has its most common onset at 1 to 2 years of age
D. it less serious when it occurs in adolescence
E. always involves refusal to go to school

52.14 In the differential of PTSD the clinician should consider which of the following conditions?

A. Obsessive-compulsive disorder
B. Social phobia
C. Bereavement
D. Disruptive behavior disorder
E. All of the above

52.15 Conditions associated with PTSD in children include all of the following *except*

A. decreased intracranial volume
B. increased corpus callosum area
C. low IQ
D. depression
E. physical abuse

52.16 Selective mutism

A. has an age of onset from 2 to 3 years old
B. rarely manifests outside of the home
C. may develop gradually or suddenly
D. is unrelated to temper tantrums
E. all of the above

Questions 52.17–52.20

Directions

Each set of lettered headings below is followed by a list of numbered words or statements. For each numbered word or statement, select the *one* lettered heading most closely associated with it. Each lettered heading may be selected once, more than once, or not at all.

A. Parental treatment
B. Gradual exposure
C. Cognitive processing
D. Stress inoculation

52.17 Thought stopping
52.18 Physical sensations experienced
52.19 Inaccurate thought processing
52.20 Support

ANSWERS

52.1 The answer is C

Obsessive-compulsive disorder (OCD) is characterized by the presence of recurrent *intrusive thoughts* associated with *anxiety* or tension and/or repetitive purposeful mental or *physical actions* aimed at reducing fears and tensions caused by obsessions. It has become increasingly evident that the majority of cases of OCD begin in childhood or adolescence. The clinical presentation of OCD in childhood and adolescence is similar to that in adults and the only alteration in diagnostic criteria in the DSM-IV-TR for children is that they *do not necessarily demonstrate awareness that their thoughts or behaviors are unreasonable*. Pediatric OCD has been investigated with respect to treatment with placebo-controlled trials of pharmacologic agents and cognitive-behavior therapy (CBT) and to date, it is the only childhood anxiety disorder with data showing optimal treatment to include a combination of *serotonergic agents* and CBT treatment.

52.2 The answer is D

OCD is a heterogeneous disorder that has been recognized for decades to run in families. Family studies have documented an *increased risk of at least fourfold in the first-degree relatives* of early-onset OCD. In addition, presence of *subclinical symptom constellations in family members appears to breed true*. Molecular genetic studies have suggested *linkage to regions of chromosomes 2 and 9 (not 21)*, in certain pedigrees with multiple members exhibiting early-onset OCD. Candidate gene studies have been inconclusive thus far. Family studies have pointed to a *relationship between OCD and tic disorders such as Tourette's syndrome*. OCD and tic disorders are believed to share susceptibility factors. The concept of a broader "obsessive-compulsive spectrum" including eating disorders, and somatoform disorders may account for the expression of repetitive and stereotyped symptoms.

52.3 The answer is E

The association of emergence of OCD syndromes following a documented exposure to or infection with group A beta hemolytic streptococcus in a subgroup of children and adolescents has led to studies of immune response in OCD. Cases of infection-triggered OCD have been termed pediatric autoimmune neuropsychiatric disorders associated with streptococcus (PANDAS) and are *believed to signify an autoimmune process* such as that of Sydenham's chorea during rheumatic fever. It is hypothesized that exposure to streptococcal bacteria activate the immune system leading to inflammation of the basal ganglia and resulting disruption of *cortical-striatal-thalamo-cortical function*. MRI has documented a proportional relationship between *the size of the basal ganglia and the severity of OCD symptoms*. The presentation of OCD in children and adolescents *due to acute exposure to group A beta hemolytic streptococcus* represents a minority of OCD cases in this population.

52.4 The answer is E (all)

Many habit disturbances, such as *nail biting, thumb sucking, temper tantrums,* eating problems, *masturbation*, and stuttering, stem from a common base of separation anxiety. Transient experiences of separation anxiety are quite frequent, and as the child cannot tolerate anxiety for any length of time, the anxiety tends to crystallize into other kinds of disorders. The transformation of anxiety into compulsive mechanisms, phobias, and other symptoms occurs frequently.

Nail biting is also known as onychophagy and is a habitual manipulation in which one's inner tension is released. *Thumb sucking* is one of the earliest and most common manipulations of one's body used by young children. During the first month, thumb sucking is common, but it is not a universal characteristic of the infant. It is classified as abnormal if it continues to persist through early childhood. *Masturbation* is a self-stimulation of the genitals for sexual pleasure. A *temper tantrum* is an outburst of crying, screaming, and kicking produced by a child in response to frustrations.

52.5 The answer is E (all)

Morbid fears, preoccupations, and ruminations are characteristic of separation anxiety in children. Children become fearful that *someone close to them will be hurt* or that something terrible will happen to them when they are away from important caring figures. Many children worry that accidents or illness will befall their parents or themselves. *Fears about getting lost* and about being kidnapped and never again finding their parents are common. Young children express less specific, more generalized concerns because their immature cognitive development precludes the formation of well-defined fears. In older children, fears of getting lost may include elaborate fantasies around kidnappings, being harmed, being raped, or being made into slaves.

When separation from an important figure is imminent, children show many premonitory signs, such as *irritability,* difficulty in eating, and complaints such as vomiting and headaches are common when separation is anticipated or actually happens. These difficulties increase in intensity and organization with age because the older child is able to anticipate anxiety in a more structured fashion. Thus, there is a continuum between mild anticipatory anxiety before a threatened separation and pervasive anxiety after the separation has occurred.

Animal and monster phobias are common, as are concerns about dying. The child, when threatened with separation, may become fearful that events related to muggers, burglars, car accidents, or kidnapping may occur.

52.6 The answer is B

Attachment disorder of the anaclitic type may be seen in any infant between the ages of 6 months and 36 months. The primary symptoms consist of depressive-anxious affect and the dropping out of attachment behaviors that had been achieved before separation from the mother.

The infant's reaction to such a loss occurs in several well-defined stages after the age of 6 months. In order, these stages are: *protest, despair, and detachment*. The attitude of detachment refers to the infant's failure to make new attachments after the loss of the mother; detachment occurs generally a few days after such a loss. Other major symptoms include psychosocial retardation, avoidance of others, gastrointestinal disturbances without organic cause, and depressive withdrawal.

52.7 The answer is E (all)

In the course of development, various stresses were conceptualized by Freud as triggers for the occurrence of anxiety in a child. Each period of the individual's life has its appropriate determinant of anxiety. Thus, the danger of physical helplessness is appropriate to the period of life when his or her ego is immature; the danger of loss of object, *to early childhood when he or she is still dependent on others*; *the danger of castration to the phallic phase*; *and the fear of his or her superego*, to the latency period. Nevertheless, all these danger-situations and determinants of anxiety can persist side by side and cause the ego to react to them with anxiety at a period later than the appropriate ones; or, again, several of them can come into operation at the same time.

These views have been elaborated conceptually and clinically by a number of workers. During the period of *symbiosis* described by Mahler as occurring between 3 to 18 months of age, the mother functions as an auxiliary ego and helps the infant develop ego boundaries that define and de-limit reality testing, frustration tolerance, and impulse control. The traumatic loss of a mothering figure or the rejection of the infant by the mothering figure early in life may result in a fear of total annihilation, followed later by a fear of the loss of the mothering figure or object. These anxieties must border on panic and be among the most powerful and terror-ridden ones experienced by a human. Anna Freud emphasized the concept of anxiety in the recognition of the strength of the instincts of the infant. In this dim, early developmental period, the strength of the infants rage and destructive impulses may leave them with a feeling of overwhelming anxiety.

During the maximal development of early self-awareness or object constancy, the 2-year-old child has internalized experiences of goodness and badness from the mother and is able to retain an internalized memory of the mothering figure and of others in a rudimentary way. Under stress, the child may regress and lose this sense of self-awareness or object constancy, resulting in terror and panic. These fears of the loss of boundaries and of annihilation are in many ways similar to the overwhelming adult anxiety at loss of identity and loss of impulse control.

A fear of loss of body parts and loss of body functions, often conceptualized as castration fears, can be demonstrated most clearly in the child who is 3 to 6 years old. As the sense of self develops, the 3- to 6-year-old child, under the stress of dealing with oedipal transformations, gradually encompasses a beginning sense of personal responsibility. An internalized superego develops, and the child becomes prone to anxiety and dread at the internalized anger and harsh thoughts directed toward the self.

52.8 The answer is B

Some clinical evidence suggests that overanxious disorder is most common in small families of upper socioeconomic status, *in first-born children*, and in situations in which there is unusual concern about performance, even when the child is functioning at an adequate level. In such families, children who develop the overanxious disorder come to feel that they must earn their acceptance in the family by high-level, conforming behavior. They tend to be goody-two-shoes children. Although both boys and girls develop this disorder, it has been seen more frequently in girls than in boys.

52.9 The answer is A

Anxiety disorders are among the most common disorders in youth, affecting more than ten percent of children and adolescents at some point in their development. *Separation anxiety is a universal human developmental phenomenon emerging in infants less than 1 year of age* and marking a child's awareness of a separation from his or her mother or primary caregiver. Normative separation anxiety *peaks between 9 months and 18 months* and *diminishes by about 2 1/2 years of age* enabling young children to develop a sense of comfort away from their parents in preschool. Separation anxiety or stranger anxiety as it has been termed most likely *evolved as a human response that has survival value*. The expression of transient separation anxiety is also normal in young children entering school for the first time. *Approximately 15 percent of young children display intense and persistent fear, shyness, and social withdrawal when faced with unfamiliar settings and people*. Young children with this pattern of behavioral inhibition are at a higher risk for the development of separation anxiety disorder, generalized anxiety disorder, and social phobia. Behaviorally inhibited children, as a group, exhibit characteristic physiologic traits including higher than average resting heart rates, higher morning cortisol levels than average, and low heart rate variability.

52.10 The answer is E (all)

The prevalence of anxiety disorders has varied with the age group of the children surveyed and the diagnostic instruments used. Lifetime prevalence of any anxiety disorder in children and adolescents ranges from 8.3 percent to 27 percent. A recent epidemiologic survey using the Preschool Age Psychiatric Assessment (PAPA) found that *9.5 percent of preschoolers met DSM-IV-TR criteria for any anxiety disorder, with 6.5 percent exhibiting generalized anxiety disorder, 2.4 percent meeting criteria for separation anxiety disorder, and 2.2 percent meeting criteria for social phobia.*

52.11 The answer is B

There is neurophysiological correlation of behavioral inhibition (extreme shyness); children with this constellation are shown to have a higher resting heart rate and an acceleration of heart rate with tasks requiring cognitive concentration. Additional physiological correlates of behavioral inhibition include *elevated (not lowered) salivary cortisol levels, elevated urinary catecholamine levels, and greater pupillary dilation during cognitive tasks.* The quality of maternal attachment also appears to play a role in the development of anxiety disorder in children. Mothers with anxiety disorders who are observed to show insecure attachment to their children tend to have children with higher rates of anxiety disorders. It is difficult to separate the contribution of the relationship between mother and child from the mother's potential genetic contribution to anxiety. Families in which a child manifests separation anxiety disorder may be close-knit and caring, and the children often seem to be the objects of parental overconcern. External life stresses often coincide with development of the disorder. The death of a relative, a child's illness, a change in a child's environment, or a move to a new neighborhood or school is frequently noted in the histories of children with separation anxiety disorder. In a vulnerable child, these changes probably intensify anxiety.

52.12 The answer is E (all)

Fear, in response to a variety of unfamiliar or unexpected situations, may be unwittingly communicated from parents to children by *direct modeling*. If a parent is fearful, the child will probably have a phobic adaptation to new situations, especially to a school environment. Some parents appear to teach their children to be anxious by *overprotecting them from expected dangers or by exaggerating the dangers*. For example, a parent who cringes in a room during a lightning storm teaches a child to do the same. A parent who is afraid of mice or insects conveys the affect of fright to a child. *Conversely, a parent who becomes angry with a child* when the child expresses fear of a given situation, for example when exposed to animals, may promote a phobic concern in the child by exposing the child to the intensity of the anger expressed by the parent. Social learning factors in the development of anxiety reactions are magnified when parents have anxiety disorders themselves. These factors may be pertinent in the development of separation anxiety disorder as well as in generalized anxiety disorder and social phobia. In a recent study, there was no association between psychosocial hardships and behavioral inhibition among young children. *Temperamental predisposition to anxiety disorders likely results from a heritable constellation of traits, and is not directly caused by psychosocial stressors.*

52.13 The answer is B

Separation anxiety disorder accounts for most of the anxiety in children, *affecting up to 4 percent of school-aged boys and girls.* Unlike many other childhood psychiatric disorders, it has been reported to occur in boys and girls equally. While separation anxiety is a developmentally appropriate response to various situations, especially in young children, separation anxiety disorder *is not a developmental stage.* It is characterized by impaired function and *has its most common onset at 7 to 8 (not 1 to 2) years of age.* Separation anxiety disorder *is usually more serious (not less serious) in adolescence* than in childhood. Separation anxiety disorder consists of persistent worry about losing a parent or harm befalling a child's major attachment figure. Separation anxiety disorder *sometimes, but not always, involves refusal to go to school* to avoid separating from the parent.

52.14 The answer is E (all)

OCD, phobias, bereavement and disruptive behavior disorder all have to be considered in the child who is being worked up for posttraumatic stress disorder (PTSD) because many of the symptoms overlap.

Obsessive-compulsive disorder is an anxiety disorder which is characterized by the persistent recurrence of obsessions and compulsions.

A *phobia* is the persistent, pathological, unrealistic, intense fear of an object or situation; the phobic person may realize that the fear is irrational but is, nonetheless, unable to dispel it. Some examples are: acrophobia (high places), agoraphobia (open places, leaving familiar setting of home), algophobia (pain), claustrophobia (closed or confined places), zoophobia (animals).

Bereavement is the feeling of grief or desolation, especially at the death or loss of a loved one.

Disruptive behavior disorder is characterized by inattention, overaggressiveness, delinquency, destructiveness, hostility, feelings of rejection, negativism, or impulsiveness.

Finally, the clinician should remember that PTSD can be superimposed on any of the above disorders.

52.15 The answer is B

The area of the corpus *callosum is decreased (not increased)* in children with PTSD. In addition, there are a variety of other serious comorbidities and psychobiological abnormalities associated with PTSD. In one study, children and adolescents with severe PTSD evidenced *decreased intracranial volume, diminished corpus callosum area and lower intellectual quotients compared to children without PTSD.* Children and adolescents with histories of physical and sexual abuse have been found to exhibit *elevated rates of depression* and suicidality. This highlights the importance of early recognition and treatment of PTSD among youth that may significantly improve their long term outcome.

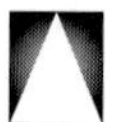

Table 52.1
DSM-IV-TR Diagnostic Criteria for Selective Mutism

A. Consistent failure to speak in specific social situations (in which there is an expectation for speaking, e.g., at school) despite speaking in other situations.
B. The disturbance interferes with educational or occupational achievement or with social communication.
C. The duration of the disturbance is at least 1 month (not limited to the first month of school).
D. The failure to speak is not due to a lack of knowledge of, or comfort with, the spoken language required in the social situation.
E. The disturbance is not better accounted for by a communication disorder (e.g., stuttering) and does not occur exclusively during the course of a pervasive developmental disorder, schizophrenia, or other psychotic disorder.

Reprinted with permission from *American Psychiatric Association. Diagnostic and Statistical Manual of Mental Disorders.* 4th ed. Text rev. Washington, DC: American Psychiatric Association; 2000.

52.16 The answer is C

The diagnostic criteria from DSM-IV-TR appears in Table 52.1. The diagnosis of selective mutism is not difficult to make after it is clear that a child has adequate language skills in some environments but not in others. The mutism *may have developed gradually or suddenly* after a disturbing experience. *The age of onset can range from 4 to 8 years.* Mute periods are *most commonly manifested in school or outside the home*; in rare cases, a child is mute at home but not in school. Children who exhibit selective mutism may also have symptoms of separation anxiety disorder, school refusal, and delayed language acquisition. Because social anxiety is almost always present in children with selective mutism, behavioral disturbances, such as *temper tantrums and oppositional behaviors, may also occur in the home.*

Answers 52.17–52.20

52.17 The answer is D

52.18 The answer is B

52.19 The answer is C

52.20 The answer is A

Various treatments exist for PTSD in children: in *stress inoculation*, children are guided to utilize muscle relaxation, focused breathing, affective modulation, thought stopping and cognitive coping techniques in order to diminish feelings of helplessness and distress. *Gradual exposure* is a technique for a child to recall, first in small segments and then in increasing amounts, the details of the traumatic exposure and describe the thoughts, feelings and physical sensations experienced during the trauma as well as in the retelling of the event. *Cognitive processing* is used in identifying those associated thoughts, feelings and ideas that may be inaccurate and serving to cause additional impairment to the victim, so that reframing of the thoughts and feelings can help the sense of being incapacitated by them. *Parental treatment component* provides parent management strategies in order for the parent to enhance the child's ability to communicate proactively and elicit support from the parents. The above set of therapeutic strategies is designated by experts as the currently accepted first line of treatment for PTSD symptoms. They can be adapted for use in group settings in school, with entire families who have been traumatized, and in groups of adolescents. A variant of trauma-focused cognitive-behavioral therapy for PTSD is called eye movement desensitization and reprocessing (EMDR) in which an exposure and cognitive reprocessing interventions are paired with directed eye movements. This technique is not as well accepted as the more extensive trauma-focused cognitive behavior therapy detailed above.

53 Early-Onset Schizophrenia

Schizophrenia usually has its onset in late adolescence or early adulthood, but it does (rarely) present in children 10 years of age or younger. Schizophrenia with childhood onset is conceptually the same as schizophrenia in adolescence and adulthood. When schizophrenia occurs in prepubertal children, it more commonly occurs in males. Psychosocial stressors are known to influence the course of schizophrenia, and the same stressors may possibly interact with biological risk factors in the emergence of the disorder. Schizophrenia in prepubertal children includes the presence of at least two of the following: hallucinations, delusions, grossly disorganized speech or behavior, and severe withdrawal for at least 1 month. Social or academic dysfunction must be present, and continuous signs of the disturbance must persist for at least 6 months. The diagnostic criteria for schizophrenia in children are identical to the criteria for the adult form, except that instead of showing deteriorating functioning, children may fail to achieve their expected levels of social and academic functioning.

Before the 1960s, the term childhood psychosis was applied to a heterogeneous group of pervasive developmental disorders without hallucinations and delusions. In the 1960s and 1970s, children with evidence of a profound psychotic disturbance early in life often were observed to be mentally retarded, socially dysfunctional with severe communication and language impairments, and without a family history of schizophrenia. In children with psychoses that emerged after the age of 5, however, auditory hallucinations, delusions, inappropriate affects, thought disorder, and normal intelligence were manifest, and these children often had a family history of schizophrenia; they were viewed as exhibiting schizophrenia, whereas the younger children were identified as having a pervasive developmental disorder.

In the 1980s, schizophrenia with childhood onset was formally separated from autistic disorder. This change reflected evidence accrued during the 1960s and 1970s that the clinical picture, family history, age of onset, and course of the two disorders differed. However, some researchers remained of the opinion that a subgroup of autistic children would eventually develop schizophrenia. In general, schizophrenia is easily differentiated from autistic disorder. Most children with autistic disorder are impaired in all areas of adaptive functioning from early life onward. The onset is almost always before 3 years of age, whereas the onset of schizophrenia usually is in adolescence or young adulthood. Schizophrenia in prepubertal children is much rarer than in adolescence and young adulthood, and there are practically no reports of an onset of schizophrenia before 5 years of age. According to the text revision of the fourth edition of the *Diagnostic and Statistical Manual of Mental Disorders* (DSM-IV-TR), schizophrenia can be diagnosed in the presence of autistic disorder.

The second controversy concerned applying adult diagnostic criteria for schizophrenia to children. Several reports indicate that some children do have hallucinations, delusions, and thought disorders typical of schizophrenia, but normal developmental immaturities in language development and in separating reality from fantasy sometimes make it difficult to diagnose schizophrenia in children ages 5 to 7 years.

The student should study the questions and answers below for a useful review of the condition.

HELPFUL HINTS

The student should understand these terms.

- agranulocytosis
- autistic disorder
- childhood psychosis
- clozapine (Clozaril)
- comorbidity
- delayed motor development
- developmental level and age-appropriate presentations
- diagnostic stability
- disturbed communication
- expressed emotion
- family support
- haloperidol (Haldol)
- high-risk children
- hypersalivation
- persecutory delusions
- pervasive developmental disorders
- premorbid disorders
- premorbid functioning
- risperidone (Risperdal)
- schizotypal personality
- sedation
- social rejection
- tardive dyskinesia
- transient phobic hallucinations
- visual hallucinations

QUESTIONS

Directions

Each of the questions or incomplete statements below is followed by five suggested responses or completions. Select the *one* that is *best* in each case.

53.1 Which of the following statements about schizophrenia among prepubertal children is *true*?

A. Abnormalities on CT and EEG are found in children with schizophrenia but cannot be used to make the diagnosis.
B. Childhood-onset schizophrenia is not associated with social withdrawal.
C. Marked deterioration in functioning is required to make the diagnosis.
D. Childhood-onset schizophrenia is more common than autistic disorder.
E. None of the above

53.2 Predictors of poor prognosis in schizophrenia with childhood onset include all of the following *except*

A. Misdiagnosed schizophrenia in a child with bipolar I disorder
B. Onset before 10 years of age
C. Premorbid diagnoses of attention-deficit/hyperactivity disorder (ADHD) and learning disorders
D. Lack of family support
E. Delayed motor milestones and delayed language acquisition

53.3 Which of the following is helpful in distinguishing childhood-onset schizophrenia from autistic disorder?

A. Age of onset of symptoms
B. Intelligence
C. Presence of formal thought disorder
D. Family history of schizophrenia
E. All of the above

53.4 All of the following statements regarding hallucinations in prepubertal children are true *except*

A. Auditory and visual hallucinations occur commonly in childhood-onset schizophrenia.
B. Auditory hallucinations occur in childhood mood disorders.
C. Auditory hallucinations may occur in children exposed to extreme stress.
D. Childhood-onset schizophrenia cannot be diagnosed in the absence of hallucinations.
E. Visual hallucinations are pathognomonic in childhood schizophrenia

53.5 Schizophrenia

A. is rare prior to age 13
B. has a rate of onset that increases sharply in adolescence
C. occurs predominantly in males among children with the disorder
D. appears to be essentially the same heterogeneous disorder in children as in adults
E. all of the above

53.6 Which of the following statements regarding childhood-onset schizophrenia is *true*?

A. Command hallucinations do not occur among children with schizophrenia.
B. Rates of schizophrenia are less common among parents of patients with childhood-onset schizophrenia that among parents of patients with adult-onset schizophrenia.
C. Among children with schizophrenia, there is often a premorbid history of behavioral disturbances, delayed motor milestones, and delayed language acquisition.
D. Symptoms of childhood schizophrenia respond more robustly to antipsychotic medication than do symptoms of adult-onset schizophrenia.
E. Childhood-onset schizophrenic patients are usually mildly to moderately mentally retarded.

53.7 All of the following are true statements about the course and prognosis of depression in children and adolescents *except*

A. Early onset predicts a poorer prognosis.
B. There is no increased risk of later developing bipolar disorder among adolescents with a major depressive episode as compared with nondepressed teens.
C. Depressive disorders are associated with long-term peer relationship difficulties.
D. Risk of suicide is significant among adolescents with major depressive disorder.
E. Short-term complications include poor academic achievement

ANSWERS

53.1 The answer is E (none)

While various abnormal findings have been reported on imaging and EEG studies of children with schizophrenia, *no reliable findings have emerged that would allow CT or EEG to be used diagnostically in this disorder*. Schizophrenia with prepubertal onset is exceedingly rare, with estimated prevalence of approximately 2 to 3 in 10,000 children, making this illness, which is estimated to occur in as many as 1 in 1000 children, *less common (not more common) than autistic disorder.* As in adults, delusions, hallucinations, grossly disorganized speech or behavior, and *social withdrawal may be present in childhood-onset schizophrenia; at least two of these symptoms must occur for the diagnosis to be made*. While adults are required to demonstrate deteriorating function to meet diagnostic criteria for schizophrenia, *children may show either deterioration in functioning or failure to achieve expected developmental gains socially or academically.*

53.2 The answer is A

In children with bipolar I disorder, mania with psychotic features, with no prior history of depressive episodes, may be mistaken for schizophrenia; the distinction is crucial, as *bipolar I disorder has a better prognosis that an accurate schizophrenia diagnosis in children*. Factors that appear to be related to poor prognosis in childhood schizophrenia include: *onset before 10 years of age*, *premorbid ADHD and learning disorders*, *lack of family support*, and developmental delays including *delays in acquiring motor milestones and language*.

53.3 The answer is E (all)

Schizophrenia with childhood onset can be differentiated from autistic disorder based upon a number of key diagnostic and epidemiological features. *Age of onset* distinguishes the two: autistic children must display delays or abnormal functioning prior to age 3, whereas schizophrenia is considered not to present prior to age 5. *Intelligence* is another factor to consider: autistic children most often have impaired intelligence, whereas childhood-onset schizophrenia is usually associated with normal-range IQ. *Presence of a formal thought disorder* is one of several core symptoms of schizophrenia, but is not characteristic of autistic disorder. *Family history of schizophrenia* is an important risk factor for childhood-onset schizophrenia but has not been shown to contribute to risk for autistic disorder.

53.4 The answer is D

Childhood-onset schizophrenia can be diagnosed in the absence of hallucinations: patients must have at least two of the following symptoms: hallucinations, delusions, grossly disorganized speech or behavior, and severe social withdrawal. These symptoms must cause a disturbance in the child's functioning, characterized by deterioration in function or failure to achieve developmental milestones, lasting at least six months. *Auditory hallucinations commonly occur in children with schizophrenia* and their content may be characterized by ongoing critical commentary or commands. *Visual hallucinations are also commonly experienced by children with schizophrenia* and often have frightening content. *Hallucinations, particularly auditory hallucinations, commonly occur in children with mood disorders*; these tend to be mood-congruent and also tend to be less bizarre than hallucinations occurring in schizophrenic children. *Both auditory and visual hallucinations may occur in children exposed to extreme stress* and do not necessarily indicate presence of a psychotic or mood disorder.

53.5 The answer is E (all)

There is a paucity of research examining schizophrenia in children, and methodological problems limit the generalizability of previous studies. However, because *schizophrenia in youth appears to be essentially the same heterogeneous disorder as in adults,* the adult literature can generally be applied to children and adolescents provided that developmental issues are taken into account. Early-onset schizophrenia has been defined as onset prior to age 18, and very-early-onset as onset prior to age 13. Despite limited reliable epidemiological studies, available date and clinical experience indicate that *onset prior to age 13 is very rare.* The *rate of onset increases sharply during adolescence*, with peak ages of onset occurring between 15 and 30. Schizophrenia with childhood onset occurs *more commonly in boys than in girls*; lifetime prevalence is equal among the genders, with significantly younger age of onset for men than women.

53.6 The answer is C

Children diagnosed with schizophrenia commonly have a history of premorbid behavioral disturbances, delayed motor milestones, and delayed language acquisition. Command auditory hallucinations, as well as other types of auditory hallucinations and visual hallucinations, commonly occur in children with schizophrenia. Rates of schizophrenia are more common (not less common) among parents of patients with childhood-onset schizophrenia as compared with parents of patients with adult-onset schizophrenia. Although antipsychotic medications, particularly second-generation or atypical antipsychotics, are indicated for the treatment of childhood-onset schizophrenia, *symptoms in these patients tend to respond less robustly (not more robustly) to these medications* than among patients with adult-onset schizophrenia. Epidemiological data indicate that *childhood-onset schizophrenic patients are usually not (rather than mildly to moderately) mentally retarded*, but rather function in the low-average to average range of intelligence.

53.7 The answer is B

Several factors are known to worsen prognosis of depression in children and adolescents, including *early onset, multiple recurrent episodes,* family history of significantly impairing depressive illness, and living in families with sustained and severe interpersonal conflict. *Depressive disorders are associated with short-term and long-term peer relationship difficulties, poor academic achievement, and low self-esteem*; additionally, there is a well-established *increase in risk of suicide among adolescents with major depression. Adolescents who have a major depressive episode are at significantly increased risk of going on to develop bipolar disorder* as compared with nondepressed teens.

54 Adolescent Substance Abuse

Adolescent substance use and abuse remain serious concerns regarding today's youth. Estimates of nearly 25 percent have been made of illicit drug use among adolescents from 12 to 17 years of age. Approximately one of five adolescents has used marijuana or hashish. Approximately one-third of adolescents have used cigarettes by age 17 years. Studies of alcohol use among adolescents in the United States have shown that by 13 years of age, one-third of boys and almost one fourth of girls have tried alcohol. By 18 years of age, 92 percent of males and 73 percent of females reported trying alcohol, and 4 percent reported using alcohol daily. Of high school seniors, 41 percent reported using marijuana; 2 percent reported using the drug daily. Emergency room visits for heroin use among 18- to 25-year-olds increased over 50 percent from 1997 to 2000.

Drinking among adolescents follows adult demographic drinking patterns: The highest proportion of alcohol use occurs among adolescents in the Northeast; whites are more likely to drink than are other groups; among whites, Roman Catholics are the least likely nondrinkers. The four most common causes of death in persons between the ages of 10 and 24 years are motor vehicle accidents (37 percent), homicide (14 percent), suicide (12 percent), and other injuries or accidents (12 percent). Of adolescents treated in pediatric trauma centers, more than one-third are treated for alcohol or drug use.

Studies considering alcohol and illicit drug use by adolescents as psychiatric disorders have demonstrated a greater prevalence of substance use, particularly alcoholism, among biological children of alcoholics than among adopted youngsters. This finding is supported by family studies of genetic contributions, by adoption studies, and by observing children of substance users reared outside the biological home.

During the past decade, several risk factors have been identified for adolescent substance abuse. These include high levels of family conflict, academic difficulties, comorbid psychiatric disorders such as conduct disorder and depression, parental and peer substance use, impulsivity, and early onset of cigarette smoking. The greater the number of risk factors, the more likely it is that an adolescent will be a substance user.

The student should study the questions and answers below for a useful review of these abuses.

HELPFUL HINTS

The student should be able to define the following terms.

- aerosols
- Al-Anon
- Alateen
- Alcoholics Anonymous (AA)
- Antabuse
- cocaine
- comorbidity
- demographic drinking patterns
- gateway drug
- genetic contributions and adoption studies
- glue
- high-risk behaviors
- inhalants
- marijuana
- Narcotics Anonymous (NA)
- polysubstance abuse
- severity-oriented rating scales
- substance abuse
- substance dependence
- substance intoxication
- substance withdrawal
- 12-step program

QUESTIONS

Directions

Each of the questions or incomplete statements below is followed by five responses or completions. Select the *one* that is *best* in each case.

54.1 Which of these substances is most commonly abused by adolescents?

A. Marijuana
B. Alcohol
C. Cocaine
D. Methylenedioxymethamphetamine (MDMA, "ecstasy")
E. Lysergic acid diethylamide (LSD)

54.2 Which of the following statements about adolescent substance abuse is *true*?

A. Substance use among adolescents does not differ between males and females.
B. White and Hispanic students are less likely than African-American students to report lifetime alcohol use and heavy episodic use.

C. White and Hispanic students are less likely than African-American students to report both lifetime and current marijuana use.
D. Students who are not college-bound have higher rates of alcohol, cigarette, and illicit drug use than college-bound youths.
E. None of the above

54.3 Which of these psychiatric disorders is most commonly associated with substance abuse in adolescents?

A. Conduct Disorder
B. Attention-Deficit/Hyperactivity Disorder (ADHD)
C. Schizophrenia
D. Generalized Anxiety Disorder
E. None of the above

54.4 Which of the following psychiatric symptoms commonly co-occur with adolescent substance use disorders?

A. Suicidal ideation and suicide attempts
B. Panic attacks
C. Reexperiencing, numbing, and avoidance
D. Bingeing and purging
E. All of the above

54.5 Which of the following statements regarding adolescent substance abuse is *true*?

A. Use of marijuana is the strongest predictor of future cocaine use.
B. Prevalence rates for cocaine use are currently lower among adolescents than among adolescents in the 1990s.
C. Children of alcohol abusers have a 25 percent chance of themselves developing alcohol abuse.
D. Inhalants are most commonly used by younger adolescents, and their use declines with age.
E. All of the above

54.6 Which of the following statements about adolescents and adults with substance use disorders is *true*?

A. Relapse in adults is primarily influenced by social pressure for use, whereas in adolescents situations involving negative affect more strongly contribute to relapse.
B. Compared with adults, adolescents have a lower level of return to substance use after treatment.
C. Adolescents are no likelier to experience noxious or adverse reactions to substances than more experienced adult users.
D. Comorbid conduct disorder in adolescents with substance use disorders predicts lower rates of treatment completion and future abstinence.
E. None of the above

54.7 Successful substance abuse prevention programs appear to be those that

A. target salient risk factors
B. teach skills
C. have follow-up
D. take into account the socioeconomic and cultural realities of targeted communities
E. All of the above

54.8 The treatments of choice for alcohol abuse in adolescents includes all of the following *except*

A. Drug-specific counseling
B. Self-help groups
C. Relapse prevention programs
D. Treatment with disulfiram and/or acamprosate
E. Individual psychotherapy

54.9 Risk factors for the development of adolescent substance abuse include all of the following *except*

A. Early onset of cigarette smoking
B. Diminished parental supervision
C. Pervasive developmental disorder
D. Parental substance abuse
E. Conduct disorder

54.10 The four leading causes of death among young people aged 15 to 24, all of which are correlated with substance abuse, include all of the following *except*

A. Motor vehicle accidents (MVA)
B. Cancer
C. Homicide
D. Suicide
E. Non-MVA accidents

Questions 54.11–54.15

A. Substance abuse
B. Substance dependence
C. Substance intoxication
D. Substance withdrawal

54.11 Only category in DSM-IV-TR in which caffeine is included.
54.12 A maladaptive pattern of substance use, causing clinically significant impairment or distress, manifested by tolerance, withdrawal, and inability to decrease use.
54.13 A reversible syndrome caused by a substance, involving behavioral or psychological changes.
54.14 A maladaptive pattern of substance use causing impairment manifested by diminished performance in school or work, recurrent use in hazardous situations, substance-related legal issues, and continued use despite recurrent social and interpersonal problems.
54.15 A substance-specific syndrome caused by the cessation or reduction in use of a substance causing distress and impairment.

ANSWERS

54.1 The answer is B

Alcohol is the most commonly abused substance by adolescents. According to the Monitoring the Future 2005 Survey, 75 percent of students report having tried more than a few sips of alcohol prior to finishing high school, and 41 percent have done so by 8th grade. Fifty-eight percent of 12th graders and 20 percent of 8th graders report having gotten drunk at least once. Seventeen percent of 8th graders, 33 percent of 10thgraders, and 47 percent of 12th graders reported using alcohol in the last 3 days in the 2005 study. Data indicate that alcohol use by adolescents leveled off in the early 2000s and may be declining slightly in recent years, but continues to be a significant issue for adolescent health.

After peaking in 1996, reported drug use among various adolescent age groups has declined—the annual prevalence of any illicit drug use among 8th graders declined by one-third among 8th graders, one-quarter among 10th graders, and 10 percent among 12th graders in 2005 as compared with 1996. The lifetime prevalence of illicit drug use among 8th, 10th, and 12th graders in 2005 was 21 percent, 38 percent and 50 percent, respectively. Although use of all illicit drugs appears to be holding steady or declining slightly in recent years, certain drugs appear to be increasing in rates of abuse, including inhalants and prescription analgesics and sedatives.

Marijuana is by far the most commonly used illicit drug among adolescents. In the 2005 survey, approximately 15 percent of 8th graders, 30 percent of 10th graders, and 35 percent of 12th graders reported using marijuana at least once in the year prior to the survey. Adolescents' use of other drugs has declined since the late 1990s, with the 2005 survey indicating annual prevalence of cocaine use of approximately 3 percent for 8th graders, 4 percent for 10th graders, and 5 percent for 12th graders; annual prevalence of MDMA use of less than 2 percent for 8th graders and approximately 3 percent for 10th and 12th graders; and annual prevalence of LSD use of approximately 2 percent for 8th, 10th, and 12th graders.

54.2 The answer is D

Male adolescents have higher reported rates of alcohol and drug use, and substantially higher rates of frequent use, than female adolescents. However, females, particularly in early adolescence, appear to be "catching up" with males in alcohol use. Cigarette smoking tends to occur at similar rates in both genders. Overall, *white and Hispanic youths are more likely (not less likely) than African-American students to report lifetime alcohol use and heavy episodic use, and are also more likely (not less likely) to report both lifetime and current marijuana use. Students who are not college-bound (a steadily decreasing proportion of the population) report higher rates of drinking, illicit drug use, and particularly cigarette smoking* than college-bound youths.

54.3 The answer is A

A number of psychiatric disorders are commonly comorbid with adolescent substance abuse, including conduct disorder, oppositional-defiant disorder, attention-deficit/hyperactivity disorder, dysthymia, major depressive disorder, bipolar disorder, posttraumatic stress disorder, social phobia, bulimia nervosa, and schizophrenia. Of these, *conduct disorder is most commonly associated with substance use disorders in adolescents*, with studies suggesting rates of conduct disorder ranging from 50 to 80 percent among adolescents with substance abuse or dependence. *Although ADHD is commonly observed in adolescents who abuse drugs and/or alcohol, the observed association is likely due to the high comorbidity between conduct disorder and ADHD.* Early onset of conduct disorder and comorbidity with ADHD likely increases risk for later substance abuse. *Generalized anxiety disorder* and *schizophrenia*, although less common than conduct disorder and ADHD in the adolescent population, are also associated with adolescent substance abuse.

54.4 The answer is E (all)

Substantial evidence supports the presence of substance use disorder as a risk factor for *adolescent suicidal ideation, suicide attempts, and completed suicides*. This relationship may in part be explained by the acute and chronic effects of substances; adolescents who attempt or complete suicide are often under the influence of substances when engaging in suicidal behavior. Acute effects of substances may include intensely dysphoric states, disinhibition, impaired judgment, increased impulsivity, and may exacerbate underlying anxiety, mood, or psychotic symptoms. Aggressive behaviors are also manifest in many adolescents with substance use disorders. Consumption of particular substances, such as alcohol, amphetamines, cocaine, and phencyclidine (PCP) may increase the likelihood of aggression. The direct pharmacological effects of these substances may be enhanced by preexisting psychopathology, mixing of substances, and relative inexperience of adolescent substance users.

Studies of clinical populations indicate high rates of anxiety disorders among adolescent substance abusers, with estimated rates ranging from 7 to 40 percent. The temporal relationship between anxiety symptoms and substance abuse varies; social phobia symptoms often precede substance use, whereas *panic attacks* may follow the onset of substance use. Adolescents with substance abuse are commonly found to have histories of traumatic exposure and symptoms such as *reexperiencing, emotional numbing, and avoidance*, underlining the relationship between substance use disorders and posttraumatic stress disorder. The *bingeing and purging* behaviors of bulimia nervosa are also common in teens with substance use disorders.

54.5 The answer is E

Marijuana is often referred to as a "gateway drug," as it is the most widely used illicit drug among adolescents, and marijuana use increases the likelihood of using additional drugs; for example, *marijuana use is the strongest predictor of future cocaine use*. The Monitoring the Future 2005 Survey indicates that *prevalence rates of cocaine use among adolescents remain at lower levels than were reported in the 1990s*. Unlike most other substances, *inhalants are most commonly used by younger adolescents, and their use declines with age.* Commonly used inhalants include glue, aerosols, and gasoline. Family transmission of risk for alcoholism is well established; *children of alcohol abusers have been reported to have a 25 percent chance of developing alcohol abuse themselves.*

54.6 The answer is D

Adolescents in substance abuse treatment programs as a group tend to have begun substance use at early ages, progress rapidly to use of "hard" drugs, and use multiple substances. Other clinical features of adolescents entering treatment often include high rates of comorbid psychiatric disorders, deviant behavior, school difficulties including truancy, family disruption, and substance abuse in family members.

Data indicate that many adolescents return to some level of alcohol or drug abuse following treatment. Specific predictors of outcome after treatment have been identified, including patient characteristics, social support system variables, and treatment program characteristics. Psychopathology that predated onset of substance abuse, particularly *conduct disorder, predicts lower rates of treatment completion and future abstinence.* Although factors such as severity of substance use may predict short-term treatment outcomes, longer-term outcomes may depend more on social and environmental factors. For example, studies suggest that *relapse in adolescence is frequently associated with social pressure to use, whereas in adults relapse is commonly tied to situations involving negative affect* (not vice versa). Attendance at support or aftercare groups, which can be sources of peer support as teens attempt abstinence, is associated with higher rates of abstinence and other measures of positive outcome among adolescents, as compared with youth who do not attend such groups.

Adolescents have higher rates of return to substance use after treatment than adults (not vice versa). Nevertheless, treatment has been demonstrated to have beneficial effects upon teens, with positive outcomes including decreased interpersonal conflict, improved academic achievement, and increased participation in social and occupational activities.

Adolescent substance users are more likely than adults to have minimal tolerance to substances, and thus *they may experience more noxious or adverse reactions to substances as compared with more experienced adult users.* Inexperienced teen users may not appreciate the extent of their intoxication, nor the deleterious effects of substance use on their overall functioning.

54.7 The answer is E (all)

Prevention efforts are based on theoretical models of the etiology of adolescent substance use and abuse. Most prevention interventions are based on social learning models: changing what young people see and learn in their environments produces behavioral changes. These interventions often include educational approaches, addressing three primary factors: (1) knowledge and attitude, (2) values and decision-making, and (3) social competency and skills. Family-based outreach (e.g., parent training), and community-based projects (advocacy groups, media campaigns, and regulatory changes) are also critical aspects of comprehensive prevention efforts. Successful prevention programs seem to be those that *target salient risk factors, teach skills, provide adequate follow-up, and take into account the socioeconomic and cultural realities of targeted communities.*

54.8 The answer is D

Treatment programs for adolescents with alcohol abuse contain a number of basic components, including *individual psychotherapy, a self-help group setting, drug-specific counseling, and relapse prevention efforts.* These may be combined in any of a number of inpatient or outpatient programs. *Disulfiram and acamprosate are not current treatments of choice for* adolescents with alcohol abuse.

54.9 The answer is C

Risk factors for the development of alcohol or drug abuse include *early onset of cigarette smoking, diminished parental supervision, parental substance abuse, and conduct disorder. Pervasive developmental disorder is not thought to be a risk factor* for substance abuse.

54.10 The answer is B

The leading causes of death among young people aged 15 to 24 are, in order, *MVA (37 percent), homicide (14 percent), suicide (12 percent), and non-MVA accidents (12 percent).* These events are frequently correlated with both the acute and chronic effects of alcohol and drug use among teenagers and young adults. Thirty percent of adolescents brought to a pediatric trauma center have evidence of involvement with drugs and alcohol. *Cancer is not one of the four leading causes of death in this age group* and does not commonly correlate with substance abuse in adolescents and young adults.

Answers 54.11–54.15

54.11 The answer is C

54.12 The answer is B

54.13 The answer is C

54.14 The answer is A

54.15 The answer is D

Substance dependence refers to a cluster of cognitive, behavioral, and sometimes physiological symptoms that accompany the continued heavy use of a substance. There is a pattern of repeated use that results in tolerance, withdrawal, and compulsive self-administration. *Substance abuse* refers to a maladaptive pattern of substance use leading to a clinically significant amount of distress within a 12-month period. The impairment may take the form of decreased performance in school or work, or it may lead to physical danger or legal problems. *Substance intoxication* is a reversible syndrome caused by use of a substance, in which clinically significant behavioral or psychological changes occur. The only DSM-IV-TR disorder that includes caffeine is substance intoxication. Substance withdrawal refers to a substance-specific syndrome caused by the cessation or reduction in use of a substance causing distress and impairment.

55 Child Psychiatry: Additional Conditions That May Be a Focus of Clinical Attention

This section covers borderline intellectual functioning, academic problem, antisocial behavior, and identity problem. Borderline intellectual functioning, according to the 4th edition of *Diagnostic and Statistical Manual of Mental Disorders* (DSM-IV-TR), is a category that can be used when the focus of clinical attention is on a child or adolescent's IQ in the 71 to 84 range. The intellectual functioning of children plays a major role in their adjustment to school, social relationships, and family function. Children who cannot quite understand class work and may also be slow in understanding rules of games and the "social" rules of their peer group are often bitterly rejected. Some children with borderline intellectual functioning can mingle socially better than they can keep up academically in class. In these cases, the strengths of these children may be peer relationships, especially if they excel at sports, but eventually, their academic struggles will take a toll on self-esteem if they are not appropriately remediated.

DSM-IV-TR refers to academic problem as a problem that is not caused by a mental disorder or, if caused by a mental disorder, is severe enough to warrant clinical attention. This diagnostic category is used when a child or adolescent is having significant academic difficulties that are not deemed to be due to a specific learning disorder or communication disorder or directly related to a psychiatric disorder. Nevertheless, intervention is necessary because the child's achievement in school is significantly impaired. Therefore, a child or adolescent who is of normal intelligence and is free of a learning disorder or a communication disorder but is failing in school or doing poorly falls into this category.

According to DSM-IV-TR, child or adolescent antisocial behavior refers to behavior that is not caused by a mental disorder and includes isolated antisocial acts, not a pattern of behavior. This category covers many acts by children and adolescents that violate the rights of others, such as overt acts of aggression and violence and covert acts of lying, stealing, truancy, and running away from home. Certain antisocial acts, such as fire setting, possession of a weapon, or a severe act of aggression toward another child, require intervention for even a single occurrence. Sometimes, children without a pattern of recurrent aggression or antisocial behavior become involved in occasional, less severe behavior that nevertheless require some intervention. The DSM-IV-TR definition of conduct disorder requires a repetitive pattern of at least three antisocial behaviors for at least 6 months, but childhood or adolescent antisocial behavior may consist of isolated events that do not constitute a mental disorder but do become the focus of clinical attention.

According to DSM-IV-TR, identity problem refers to uncertainty about issues such as goals, career choice, friendships, sexual behavior, moral values, and group loyalties. An identity problem can cause severe distress for a young person and can lead a person to seek psychotherapy or guidance. Identity problem is, however, not recognized as a mental disorder in DSM-IV-TR. It sometimes manifests in the context of such mental disorders as mood disorders, psychotic disorders, and borderline personality disorder.

The student should study the questions and answers below for a useful review of these conditions.

HELPFUL HINTS

The student should be able to define the following terms.

- abulia
- academic failure
- achievement tests
- adaptive function
- adolescent turmoil
- comorbid disorders
- dysfunctional family
- Erik Erikson
- hyperactivity and impulsivity
- identity formation
- irreconcilable conflicts
- juvenile delinquent
- learning disorder
- mental retardation
- parental criminality
- performance anxiety
- physical abuse
- role diffusion
- sense of self
- sexual orientation
- substance use
- superego
- tutoring
- underachievement
- "V" code
- violation of rights

QUESTIONS

Directions

The incomplete statement below is followed by five suggested completions. Select the *one* that is *best*.

55.1 Which of the following aspects of a child's peer relationships should be assessed when evaluating for identity problems?

A. Number of friends
B. Quality of friendships
C. Behavioral and emotional difficulties of friends
D. Friends' attitudes towards school and achievement
E. All of the above

Directions

Each group of questions below consists of lettered headings followed by a list of numbered phrases or statements. For each numbered phrase or statement, select the *one* lettered heading that is most closely associated with it. Each lettered heading may be selected once, more than once, or not at all.

Questions 55.2–55.4

A. Identity problem
B. Normal adolescence
C. Both
D. Neither

55.2 Deterioration in occupational, school, or social functioning
55.3 Subjective anxiety and confusion
55.4 Disturbances in thinking processes, such as flight of ideas or thought blocking

Questions 55.5–55.8

A. Academic problem
B. Childhood or adolescent antisocial behavior
C. Borderline intellectual functioning

55.5 Coded on Axis II in DSM-IV-TR nosology
55.6 Must be differentiated from conduct disorder
55.7 Consists of isolated events rather than a pattern of behavior
55.8 Normal intelligence and no learning disorder or communication disorder, but the child is failing in school

ANSWERS

55.1 The answer is E (all)

Numerous efforts have been made to describe the process of identity formation. Failure to negotiate an identity is described in the DSM-IV-TR as an "identity problem" in the section entitled, "Other Conditions That May Be a Focus of Clinical Attention," and describes a clinical situation, "when the focus of clinical attention is uncertainty about multiple issues relating to identity such as long-term goals, career choice, friendship patterns, sexual orientation and behavior, moral values, and group loyalties." Identity problem can cause significant stress for a young person, but it is not recognized as a mental disorder in DSM-IV-TR.

Four decades ago the syndrome of identity confusion was described by Erik Erikson in his classic paper, "The Problem of Ego Identity." Erikson described a group of adolescents who failed in the transition between childhood and adulthood. Adolescents who experienced difficulties with the formation of an identity shared clinical features with individuals with borderline personality disorder. Identity formation was described by Erikson as the central task of adolescence. Additionally, identity problems may appear as a prominent feature of a variety of psychopathologies during adolescence, such as mood disorders, borderline personality disorder, posttraumatic stress disorder, and schizophrenia.

Friends play an important role in forming a healthy identity, fostering a positive self-concept, and promoting healthy psychological functioning. A number of recent studies have demonstrated a positive correlation between healthy friendships and school success and effective problem-solving skills. Rejected children tend to fall into two groups: disruptive children with high levels of aggression, and socially withdrawn children who make easy targets for their peers. In both childhood and adolescence, friends tend to be similar to one another in abilities and outlook. Rejected children tend to become friends with other rejected children, and aggressive children with other acting-out children.

In evaluating possible identity problems in children, the following aspects of the child's relationships with friends should be considered: (1) *the number of friends*, (2) *the quality of friendships* (e.g., most girls show an increasing capacity for self-disclosure and intimacy in their friendships during the preadolescent years), (3) *the behavioral and emotional difficulties of friends* (a major predictor of antisocial behavior in adolescence is having a peer group composed of friends who smoke, drink, use drugs, or have a negative attitude toward education), and (4) *friends' attitudes toward school and achievement* (children who are attracted to friends with positive outlooks are more likely to develop positive school-related attitudes, career aspirations, and achievements).

Answers 55.2–55.4

55.2 The answer is A

55.3 The answer is C

55.4 The answer is D

Identity problem can be differentiated from the normal conflicts of adolescence and from adjustment disorders. *Normal adolescence is not associated with deterioration in occupational, school, or social functioning.* Adjustment disorders, by definition, occur due to a specific stressor and are time-limited. Although identity problems may coincide with stressors, concerns relating to identity issues such as career choice, gender identity, and group identification are less prominent in adjustment disorders than in identity problems.

Identity problem must be differentiated from identity concerns that may represent the prodromal manifestations of schizophrenia, schizoaffective disorder, schizophreniform disorder, and mood disorders. Psychotic symptoms, such as hallucinations, delusions, or *disturbances in thinking processes, such as thought blocking or flight of ideas, are not present in identity problem or in normal adolescence. Adolescents who are struggling with identity issues may have subjective anxiety and confusion, as do virtually all normal adolescents at various times.*

A particularly difficult differential diagnosis involves distinguishing identity problem from borderline personality disorder. Confusion regarding identity concerns may be present in both conditions. In borderline personality disorder, the dramatic clinical picture includes a much more complex set of diagnostic criteria, such as chaotic and unstable interpersonal and sexual relationships, alternating idealization and devaluation, intense anger, self-destructive behaviors, and chronic dysphoria. Borderline personality disorder does not resolve in several months to a year, as does identity problem, but rather persists well into adulthood, often with significant morbidity and mortality.

Answers 55.5–55.8

55.5 The answer is C

55.6 The answer is B

55.7 The answer is B

55.8 The answer is A

Borderline intellectual functioning is defined as having an intelligence quotient ranging from 71 to 84, with accompanying impairments in adaptive functioning leading to difficulties in academic, vocational, or social areas. *Borderline intellectual functioning is coded on Axis II.*

In DSM-IV-TR, academic problem describes a child or adolescent who has *normal intelligence and no learning disorder or communication disorder, but is failing or doing poorly in school.*

Childhood and adolescent antisocial behavior covers many acts that violate the rights of others, including acts of aggression, lying, stealing, truancy, and running away from home. *This condition consists of isolated events that become a focus of clinical attention, rather than a pattern of behavior*, thereby allowing childhood and adolescent antisocial behavior to be *distinguished from conduct disorder, which is defined as a repetitive pattern* of at least 3 antisocial acts over at least 6 months.

Isolated antisocial behavior and transgressions, first within families and then outside in the world, are one way in which children learn about societal rules and limitations. Although more serious instances of antisocial behavior are viewed as delinquent, they are also commonplace during adolescence. Up to one-quarter of youth are apprehended by police at some point in their lives, and the incidence of self-reported antisocial behavior is much higher than numbers of police arrests.

The relationship of antisocial behavior to psychopathology is complex. Not all antisocial behavior is pathological and therefore, may not require treatment. Although most forms of juvenile antisocial behavior do not progress to criminality, distinguishing youths with a good prognosis from those who will end up committing more severe criminal acts is very difficult. Careful differentiation of normative risk-taking behavior and isolated antisocial acts from syndromal clustering of behavior problems is crucial. Antisocial behavior must also be differentiated from behavior representative of more severe psychopathology, and behavioral disturbances may indicate psychiatric disturbance in many children and adolescents. As there appears to be a fairly consistent progression from certain antisocial behaviors to more severe forms of pathology, antisocial behavior that comes to the attention of the clinician should be regarded as a marker or risk factor for more severe problems, such as oppositional defiant disorder, conduct disorder, and antisocial personality disorder.

56 Psychiatric Treatment of Children and Adolescents

To approach a child therapeutically, one must have a sense of normal development for a child of a given age as well as an understanding of the life story of the particular child. Wide normal variation exists with respect to how facile children are at describing their emotions in words and the level of motivation with which they engage in this process. Individual psychotherapy with children focuses on improving children's adaptive skills in and outside the family setting. Treatment reflects an understanding of children's developmental levels and shows sensitivity toward families and environments in which children live. Most children do not seek psychiatric treatment; they are taken to a psychotherapist because of a disturbance noted by a family member, a schoolteacher, or a pediatrician. Children often believe that they are being taken for treatment because of their misbehavior or as a punishment for wrongdoing.

In individual psychotherapy, psychodynamic approaches are sometimes mixed with supportive and behavioral management techniques. Individual therapy is frequently associated with family therapy, group therapy, and, when indicated, pharmacotherapy. The goal of therapy is to help develop good coping and conflict-resolution skills in children who are having trouble achieving or resolving developmental tasks that can lead to difficulties fulfilling later developmental capacities.

An evaluation for the use of medication in children must include a thorough physical examination, an assessment of the child's caregivers' abilities to monitor medication compliance and risks, and a rigorous diagnostic evaluation. Often, the success of drug trials hinges on the physician being available on a daily basis, especially at the beginning. An understanding of childhood pharmacokinetics is essential. Children, compared to adults, have greater hepatic capacity, more glomerular filtration, and less fatty tissue. Thus, many drugs are eliminated more quickly in children than in adults, are less often stored in fat, and have shorter half-lives. The goals of pediatric psychopharmacology include decreasing maladaptive behaviors and increasing adaptive functioning in academic and social settings. Cognitive dulling must be avoided. Indications for the use of medications in children and adolescents include behavioral and emotional problems associated with mental retardation, learning disorders, autistic disorder, attention-deficit/hyperactivity disorder, conduct disorder, Tourette's disorder, enuresis, separation anxiety disorder, schizophrenia, mood and anxiety disorders, obsessive-compulsive disorder, eating disorders, and sleep disorders. Clinicians must be aware of the indications, side effects, and risk to benefit ratios associated with each of the medications used in treatment of children and adolescents. Electroconvulsive therapy (ECT) is not indicated in childhood or adolescence.

The student should study the questions and answers below for a useful review of these treatments.

HELPFUL HINTS

These terms should be known and defined by the student.

- acting out
- action-oriented defenses
- activity group therapy
- ADHD
- anticonvulsants
- atypical puberty
- autistic disorder
- behavioral contracting
- bell-and-pad conditioning
- biological therapies
- cardiovascular effects
- child guidance clinics
- child psychoanalysis
- classical and operant conditioning
- cognitive therapy
- combined therapy
- communication disorders
- compliance
- conduct disorder
- confidentiality
- conflict-resolution skills
- depressive equivalents
- developmental fluidity
- developmental lines
- developmental orientation
- dietary manipulation
- ECT
- enuresis
- externalization
- family systems theory
- filial therapy
- group living
- group selection criteria
- group therapy
- growth suppression
- haloperidol (Haldol)
- hospital treatment
- interview techniques
- learning-behavioral theories
- lithium

- liver to body-weight ratio
- MAOIs
- masked depression
- milieu therapy
- modeling theory
- mood disorders
- obsessive-compulsive disorder
- parent groups
- parental attitudes
- pharmacokinetics
- play group therapy
- playroom
- psychoanalytic theories
- psychoanalytically oriented therapy
- puberty and adolescence (differentiation)
- regression
- relationship therapy
- remedial and educational psychotherapy
- renal clearance
- residential and day treatment
- risk to benefit–ratio analysis
- same-sex groups
- schizophrenia
- self-observation
- sequential psychosocial capacities
- sleep terror disorder
- substance abuse
- suicide
- supportive therapy
- sympathomimetics
- tardive dyskinesia
- therapeutic interventions
- therapeutic playroom
- Tourette's disorder
- tricyclic drugs
- violence

QUESTIONS

Directions

Each of the questions or incomplete statements below is followed by five suggested responses or completions. Select the *one* that is *best* in each case.

56.1 Cognitive-behavioral therapy is useful in the treatment in which of the following disorders or situations?

A. Conduct disorder
B. Adolescent depression in a group setting
C. Obsessive-compulsive disorder
D. Socially rejected children
E. All of the above

56.2 In attention-deficit/hyperactivity disorder

A. Treatment with stimulant medication alone is maximally effective in older children and adolescents.
B. Stimulant medication equally improves the full range of symptoms of children with the disorder, including comorbid behavioral disturbances.
C. Treatment with stimulant medication alone tends to significantly improve outcomes for children with oppositional and aggressive behavior, academic underachievement, and poor peer relationships.
D. Presence of aggression in children and parents are strong predictors of poor outcome in treatment of ADHD.
E. All of the above

56.3 Parent–child conflict is a risk factor for

A. Depression
B. Poor treatment outcome in depression
C. Relapse after treatment for depression
D. Cognitive distortions that negatively bias perceptions
E. All of the above

56.4 The systems approach to family therapy

A. Places more emphasis on the meaning of a child's symptoms for the larger family than on the child's specific symptoms
B. Maintains that all things are interdependent and nothing changes without everything else changing
C. Sees symptoms as serving a purpose for the family system
D. Views each family member as acting in a way that opposes symptomatic improvement in the presenting patient
E. All of the above

56.5 With regard to adverse effects of medications in children and adolescents

A. Tardive dyskinesia has not been observed in this age group
B. Withdrawal dyskinesias do occur in this age group
C. Anticholinergic and cardiovascular side effects are rarely seen in this age group
D. There is less risk for adverse effects in this age group as compared with adults
E. None of the above

56.6 Which theorist described a series of "developmental pathways," for example a pathway that connects a child's capacity to play to the adult's capacity to work?

A. Sigmund Freud
B. Anna Freud
C. Donald Winnicott
D. Melanie Klein
E. Margaret Mahler

56.7 In terms of pharmacokinetics, as compared to adults, children have

A. Lower hepatic capacity
B. Lower glomerular filtration rates
C. More fatty tissue
D. Increased half-lives of medications
E. None of the above

Directions

Each group of questions below consists of lettered headings followed by a list of numbered phrases or statements. For each numbered phrase or statement, select the *one* lettered heading that is most closely associated with it. Each lettered heading may be selected once, more than once, or not at all.

Questions 56.8–56.15

A. Interpersonal, cognitive, and/or psychodynamic therapy plus fluoxetine
B. Response prevention plus sertraline
C. Guanfacine
D. Social skills group plus methylphenidate
E. Desmopressin (DDAVP) nasal spray plus behavioral conditioning
F. Family therapy
G. Partial hospital plus risperidone
H. Inpatient unit with psychodynamic, family, and behavioral interventions

56.8 A 12-year-old boy performs 3 hours of daily compulsive hand washing and has extreme difficulty going to school because of contamination fears

56.9 A 10-year-old girl became oppositional and defiant shortly after her mother married a man with three children

56.10 A 15-year-old girl has lost 25 percent of her body weight and cannot control her purging behaviors

56.11 A 17-year-old girl has recently been discharged from an inpatient unit after a suicide attempt in the midst of a severe depression

56.12 A 14-year-old girl has not been in school for several weeks because she has been bothered by derogatory auditory hallucinations; she is not suicidal or homicidal

56.13 An 8-year-old boy will not attend sleepover parties because of his bedwetting

56.14 A 7-year-old boy is about to be suspended from school because of his inability to sit in his seat and stay on task as well as his provocative behavior toward his classmates

56.15 A 9-year-old boy with chronic vocal and motor tics, as well as significant impulsivity and frequent aggressive behavior toward his peers at school and siblings; this patient's tics were severely exacerbated during a prior trial of methylphenidate.

ANSWERS

56.1 The answer is E (all)

Cognitive-behavioral therapy (CBT) is the most extensively, thoroughly researched therapy in use today for the treatment of psychological problems in children and adolescents. *CBT can be utilized in both individual and group settings.*

Children with conduct disorder may be impulsive, oppositional, defiant, moody, and angry. During assessment, the therapist gauges the child's thought processes in addressing a variety of situations. The child is then taught a step-by-step approach to solving problems. In this training, the child is guided to develop skills in appraising situations and making appropriate decisions for action. Dysfunctional thought processes are examined, and the therapist helps the child to generate alternative solutions to problems, focus on goals, see the consequences associated with their behaviors, and recognize the causes of others' behaviors. This technique may be adapted to accommodate children aged 4 years through young adulthood. The treatment uses structured tasks such as games, academic activities, and other age-appropriate tools. The therapist plays an active role in the treatment, encouraging modeling via practice and role-playing. Punishment or withdrawal of privileges is used when necessary.

Individual CBT has been demonstrated to be an effective treatment for depression in adolescents. Additionally, Peter Lewinsohn and colleagues developed the "Adolescents Coping with Depression Course," which consists of sixteen 2-hour sessions conducted over an 8-week period for groups of up to 10 adolescents. The program includes a psychoeducational component that aims to destigmatize depression, emphasize skills training to promote control over one's mood, and enhance adolescents' abilities to cope with problematic situations. The group activities include role-playing. Social skills training occurs throughout the treatment to facilitate and enhance communication, and includes teaching conversational techniques, planning social activities, and developing strategies for making friends. Sessions are designed to increase participation in pleasant activities, based on the assumption that depressed adolescents have few positively reinforcing activities in their lives. Relaxation training is provided to enhance comfort in social settings and to offset anxiety. Focus on changing depressogenic cognitions is provided by identifying, challenging, and changing negative thoughts and irrational beliefs. The teens are also taught negotiating and problem-solving techniques.

John March and colleagues developed the CBT treatment, "How I Ran OCD Off My Land," a manualized treatment for obsessive-compulsive disorder in children and adolescents. The treatment uses a variety of methods including exposure, response prevention, extinction, anxiety-management training, reinforcement, modeling and shaping, and habit reversal. After the initial assessment, the child and family are first educated about OCD, placing the disorder in a neurobiological framework that identifies OCD as a medical condition. Thereafter, the child learns to make OCD the "enemy" and is taught to "boss back" the OCD in order to gain a sense of agency in managing the anxiety that characterizes the disorder. The parameters of symptoms are "mapped" in order to fully identify obsessions, compulsions, triggers, and avoidance behaviors. The majority of subsequent sessions deal with anxiety-management techniques (such as relaxation, diaphragmatic breathing, and constructive self-talk) and exposure with response-prevention. Exposure involves therapist-assisted imaginal and in-vivo exposure, and response-prevention consists of exercises in session coupled with weekly homework assignments. Parents are trained to ally with the child to "boss back" OCD.

With regard to socially rejected children, Fred Frankel and colleagues developed the 12-session cognitive-behavioral treatment called "Parent Assisted Social Skills Training." First the child's social network is examined, taking into account family, home, school, and neighborhood to develop an integrated approach to treatment. Children are seen in groups where they learn rules of peer etiquette. They are also offered training skills to expand their peer networks, while parents and children are taught how to work together to promote more successful play dates and how to improve the child's competence with non-aggressive responses to teasing and conflict with other children and adults. Coached play is incorporated, and makes use of positive reinforcement and time-outs as feedback for behaviors. Child socialization homework is assigned, and didactic presentations are made to parents to inform them of their part in helping their children to gain peer acceptance, ensure that the parents adhere to assigned roles in the children's homework assignments, and provide supportive feedback for the principles being taught. Table 56.1 lists some of the techniques of CBT.

56.2 The answer is D

The best treatment of ADHD and its associated behavioral, academic, and social disruptions combines stimulant medication with cognitive-behavioral therapy. *Treatment with stimulant medication alone is effective, but may not be maximally effective for ADHD, particularly in older children and adolescents.* Many children experience a reduction in symptoms, but impairment persists at clinically significant levels. *Although many children improve substantially with pharmacotherapy, many do not achieve full remission of symptoms even with adequate doses and trials of medication.* More children achieve remission with combination therapy.

Stimulant medication may not equally affect the full range of symptoms of children with ADHD and associated behavioral disturbances. Although the primary symptoms of ADHD (inattention, impulsivity, and hyperactivity) may be greatly improved with medication, other primary or comorbid characteristics of the syndrome (e.g., oppositional and aggressive behavior, academic underachievement, and poor peer relationships) often do not respond to medication alone. *Because these associated features, together with family function, robustly predict long-term outcome of children with ADHD, treatment with stimulants alone may not significantly improve outcomes for these children.* These features are most effectively addressed with psychosocial interventions, particularly cognitive-behavioral therapy. Additionally, psychosocial treatments are sometimes the only therapies available to patients who don't respond to medications for primary symptoms of ADHD, who cannot tolerate medications due to side effects, or whose parents oppose the use of medications.

An additional limitation of stimulant treatment involves the complicating issue of home environment and home behavioral issues. Stimulants cover 6–12 hours of the day, typically the times when children are in school or other organized activities outside the home. This leaves parents on their own to manage impulsive, oppositional, and disruptive behaviors in the afternoons, evenings, weekends, and vacations. When no other treatment is made available to them, parents may develop coercive, hostile, and overly punitive approaches to dealing with their children's behaviors, which may in turn exacerbate the behavioral issues. *Child and parent aggression are among the best predictors of poor outcome in children with ADHD. For all of these reasons, CBT continues to be used and evaluated both alone and in combination with medications in the treatment of ADHD.*

Psychosocial treatment for ADHD optimally includes a behavioral approach that focuses on the child, parents, and school. Intervention with parents typically employs parent training designed to give parents tools to manage disruptive, impulsive, and oppositional behaviors at home and in the community. Intervention in the school involves direct consultation with teachers in order to establish behavioral-management strategies in the classroom.

56.3 The answer is E (all)

One-year incidence of major depression is estimated at 2 percent among school-age children, and rises to 15 percent among adolescents. The illness has significant impact upon academic and social functioning among children and teenagers, and additionally is highly correlated with risk for suicide, the third leading cause of death among teenagers in the United States. *Parent–child conflict is a risk factor for depression, poor treatment outcome in depression, relapse after treatment for depression, and cognitive distortions that negatively bias perceptions.* As a result, including a parent–child relational component in treatment for depression is well justified. Preliminary evidence suggests that addressing the parent–child relationship in treatment is more effective than treating the child alone. Parents can be taught contingency management procedures along with alternative effective methods for parenting and creating a positive family environment. Additionally, family interactions are targeted to shape and reinforce effective communication and to increase pleasant activities and positive affect in the home.

This parent–child treatment can be incorporated into cognitive-behavioral treatment of children and adolescents with depression, the psychotherapy modality most supported in the literature for treatment of this disorder. CBT for depression is a skill-based treatment centered around the assumption that depression is caused and maintained by inadequate cognitive skills for coping with stress. CBT posits that changes in behavior and cognition will lead to changes in emotions. Among the behavioral and cognitive skills deficits that may characterize depressed youths are low involvement in pleasant activities, poor problem-solving and assertion skills, cognitive distortions that negatively bias perceptions, negative automatic thoughts, negative views of self and future, and failure to attribute positive outcomes to internal causes. The therapist works with children or adolescents to help them reverse these patterns of thought and behavior. Treatment is designed to improve the patients' problem-solving ability when faced with stressful situations, including conflicts in their relationships with family members, particularly parents.

56.4 The answer is E (all)

The systems approach, a departure from so-called "linear theories," uses cybernetics and general systems theory. Cybernetics holds that systems maintain an equilibrium, while general systems theory describes all living systems as existing in tension between homeostasis and change. *All components of a family are interdependent and nothing changes without everything else changing accordingly.* In this approach to family problems, symptoms are seen not as residing within the child, but *rather as serving a purpose for the entire family system.* These symptoms provide systemic survival and maintain homeostasis. *Each family member is presumed to act in a way that opposes symptomatic improvement in the presenting patient.* Family-systems theorists attempt to counteract this hypothetical process in treatment—they believe that one must destabilize the family system to promote change. *The formulation for a family-systems therapist emphasizes the meaning that symptoms have for the family.* Problem-maintaining patterns are observed, and these patterns are interrupted.

56.5 The answer is B

Despite the fact that they may metabolize medications more rapidly than adults, children are at no less risk than adults for adverse effects of medications, and in some cases are at increased risk. The clinician must therefore know the adverse-effect

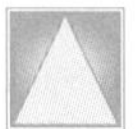

Table 56.1
Techniques of Cognitive-Behavioral Therapy

Term	Definition	Examples
Cognitive restructuring	Actively altering maladaptive thought patterns and replacing those negative thoughts with more constructive adaptive cognitions and beliefs	Challenging aberrant risk appraisal in the patient with panic disorder, or helplessness in the patient with depression
Contrived exposure	Exposure in which the patient seeks out and confronts anxiety-provoking situations or triggers	Intentionally touching a "contaminated" toilet seat
Differential reinforcement of appropriate behavior	Attending to and positively rewarding appropriate behavior, especially when incompatible with inappropriate behavior	Praising (and maybe paying) the child with obsessive-compulsive disorder who has contamination fears and washes the dinner dishes in a nonritualized fashion
Exposure	The exposure principle states that anxiety will decrease after prolonged contact with the phobic stimulus in the absence of real threat; exposure may be contrived (sought-out contact with feared stimuli) or uncontrived (unavoidable contact with feared stimuli)	A patient with fear of heights goes up a ladder; the first time it is scary; the tenth time it is boring
Extinction	By convention, extinction is usually defined as the elimination of problem behaviors through removal of parental positive reinforcement; technically, extinction often means removing the negative reinforcement effect of the problem behavior so that it no longer persists	Refusal to reassure the anxious patient Refusal by the mother to cave in to the oppositional child's tantruming by withdrawing a command
Generalization training	Moving the methods and success of problem-focused interventions to targets not specifically addressed in treatment	Exposure and response prevention for all toilets and sinks in the universe
Negative reinforcement	Self-reinforcing purposeful removal of an aversive stimulus; termination of an aversive stimulus, which when stopped, increases or stamps in the behavior that removed the aversive stimulus	Compulsions in obsessive-compulsive disorder provide short-term relief of obsessional anxiety via negative reinforcement blocking the negative reinforcement property of rituals is the job of response prevention
Positive reinforcement	Imposition of a pleasurable stimulus to increase a desirable behavior	Praise after successfully obeying a command
Prompting, guiding, and shaping	External commands and suggestions that increasingly direct the child toward more adaptive behavior that is then reinforced; typically, shaping procedures are rapidly faded in preference to generalization training	Gradually encouraging and helping the social phobic youngster to talk in class and with other children
Punishment	Imposition of an aversive stimulus to decrease an undesirable behavior	"Time out" because of unacceptable behavior or overcorrection (e.g., extra chores to make restitution for aggressive behavior)
Relapse prevention	Interventions designed to anticipate triggers for reemergence of symptoms; practicing skillful coping in advance	Imaginal exposure to a contamination fear followed by cognitive therapy and response prevention to resist the incursion of obsessive-compulsive disorder
Response cost	Removal of positive reinforcer as a consequence of undesirable behavior	Loss of points in a token economy
Response prevention	The response prevention principle states that adequate exposure is only possible in the absence of rituals or compulsions	Not doing an obsessive-compulsive disorder ritual (e.g., washing) after either contrived or uncontrived exposure (e.g., touching a toilet seat)
Restructure the environment	Changes in setting or stimuli that decrease problem behaviors, facilitate adaptive behavior, or both	Seating the child with attention-deficit hyperactivity disorder toward the front of the classroom
Stimulus hierarchy	A list of phobic stimuli ranked from least to most difficult to resist using fear thermometer rating scores	Unique list of obsessive-compulsive disorder specific contamination fears ranked by fear thermometer score; an individual patient may have one or more hierarchies, depending on the complexity of the disorder (e.g., a particular patient may have separate hierarchies for contamination fears and for touching and repeating rituals)
Token economy	A systematic set of contingencies that involve earning objects or symbols consequent on behaviors, which are then exchanged for meaningful positive reinforcers	A "star chart" linked to rewards that are meaningful to the child

profiles of all medications being prescribed, as well as how to manage adverse effects should they arise.

Many of the adverse effects of antipsychotic, antidepressant, and mood-stabilizing medications seen in adults are also seen in children and adolescents. Of particular concern are the anticholinergic and cardiovascular effects of the tricyclic medications, and the extrapyramidal effects of antipsychotics. *Withdrawal dyskinesias are more common than tardive dyskinesia among children and adolescents, though both have been observed in this age group.*

The best policy is usually to start with low dosage and titrate slowly upwards to therapeutic effect. Use of the lowest possible maintenance doses in the therapeutic range can minimize adverse effects. Monotherapy is preferable. Targeted combined pharmacotherapy may be necessary in children with multiple disorders, but should be utilized with caution in order to minimize adverse effects. Table 56.2 lists common adverse effects of medications.

56.6 The answer is B

Child psychotherapy began with Sigmund Freud's case of Little Hans, a 5-year old boy with phobia. Published in 1909, the case was the first description of the psychotherapeutic treatment of a child. The therapy in the case was actually rendered by Hans's father, who reported to Freud and received guidance from him. Significant interest in the mental and emotional lives of children was generated by Freud's theory of psychosexual development, which posited that symptoms in adulthood could be traced to conflicts arising at earlier stages of development.

Decades later, Anna Freud and Melanie Klein developed the field of child psychoanalysis. Klein understood play to be the childhood equivalent of free association in adults. She explored early object relations; the role of primitive defenses such as projection, projective identification, and omnipotent control; the process of early identifications; and the role of envy and guilt in these early relationships. *Anna Freud looked at play from a psychoanalytic perspective and learned about the child from the play, but did not view play as a substitute for free association. Her work concerned the development of the ego, the evolution of defenses, and the developmental pathway of various ego functions. In one example of a developmental pathway, she described a continuity from the child's capacity to play to the adult's capacity to work.*

There were several other major early contributors to the field. Donald Winnicott emphasized the importance of the mother-infant relationship. His understanding of the transitional object, for instance, as playing a role in the child's ability to separate from the maternal figure, instilled a new appreciation of the meaning of commonly observed childhood behaviors. Margaret Mahler observed mother-toddler interactions in a systemized way and described the evolution of early object relations from the perspective of separation and individuation. August Aichorn first extended psychoanalytic work to delinquent adolescents. Jean Piaget focused on children's cognitive development.

56.7 The answer is E (none)

Pharmacokinetics in children differ from those in adults because children have greater (not lower) hepatic capacity, greater (not lower) glomerular filtration rates (GFR), less (not more) fatty tissue, and decreased (not increased) half-lives of many medications. As a result of differences in hepatic capacity, GFR, and fatty tissue content, children tend to eliminate medications more rapidly than adults and to store less drug in fat. Meanwhile, for many medications, there is little evidence that blood level corresponds in any predictable way to drug effect. As a result, medications have to be dosed carefully in children, and dosing patterns and predicted responses in adults often do not apply to children and adolescents.

Answers 56.8–56.15

56.8 The answer is B

56.9 The answer is F

56.10 The answer is H

56.11 The answer is A

56.12 The answer is G

56.13 The answer is E

56.14 The answer is D

56.15 The answer is C

The majority of children who present for psychiatric treatment are brought in by family members who are concerned about the child's functioning, or who have followed up on suggestions from teachers or pediatricians. Often, children do not express a desire for treatment, nor do they understand the degree to which they have caused concern in others. Occasionally, an adolescent will ask a parent for help, but more often distress in this age group is manifested by troubling behaviors. To synthesize a useful treatment approach, it is generally necessary to understand the views of both the child and the parents. In most cases, treatment consists of multiple modalities through which to manipulate the child's environment positively as well as to influence the feelings and behaviors of the child. The brief vignettes that follow exemplify the combined approach to addressing children's and adolescents' psychiatric needs.

A boy of 12 who presents with impairment due to compulsive hand washing and obsessions regarding fears of contamination is a candidate for combined treatment with medication and behavioral therapy. *Several drugs from the SSRI class of medications, including sertraline, have established efficacy in reducing obsessions and compulsions in children and adolescents with OCD.* The benefit of medication is enhanced when combined with *response prevention*, a form of behavioral therapy that diminishes compulsive behaviors by challenging the patient to tolerate the feared situation (e.g., fear that his hands are dirty) without carrying out the compulsion (e.g., washing). In this way, the child learns that the exposure to the situation will not have the feared negative effects, and anxiety thereby diminishes.

A 10-year-old girl who responds to a new family constellation with oppositional and defiant behaviors is expressing her discomfort about a major change in the family's functioning. *Family therapy is a useful modality to understand the triggers, responses, and meanings of these behaviors to the family and to the child.* It is likely that when the child is given a forum in which to express her discomfort, the behaviors will diminish.

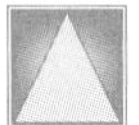

Table 56.2
Adverse Effects and Their Management in Children and Adolescents

Drug Category	Common Adverse Effects	Clinical Management
Antipsychotics (dopamine receptor antagonists and serotonin-dopamine antagonists)	**Short term**	
	Autonomic nervous system	
	Dry mouth	In general, lower dosage if possible or switch drug if persistent, child may equilibrate after several weeks
	Urinary retention	Bethanechol (Urecholine) only if severe and persistent
	Constipation	Dioctyl sodium sulfosuccinate (Colace) tablets or bisacodyl (Dulcolax) suppositories
	Orthostatic hypotension	Avoid sudden postural changes; dosage reduction if severe
	Extrapyramidal	
	Acute dystonia	Diphenhydramine (Benadryl) or benztropine (Cogentin) intramuscularly, then switch to oral form
	Parkinsonism	Anticholinergic or antiparkinsonian medication p.r.n.
	Akathisia	Lower dosage; sometimes an anticholinergic agent can help
	Other	
	Hypersensitivity or rash	Discontinue use
	Drowsiness	Child usually becomes tolerant; if persistent switch to less sedating class
	Photosensitivity	Avoid sun exposure
	LFTs	May not have clinical significance; follow-up indicated
	Blood dyscrasias	
	Long term	
	Weight gain	Lower dosage; consider switch to another class
	Dyskinesias (tardive and withdrawal)	Prevention is best; use lowest possible dose for maintenance
Psychosympathomimetics stimulants	**Short term**	
	Anorexia, nausea, abdominal pain	Reduce dose; give most of dosage in the AM; consider switch
	Insomnia	Move PM dose to earlier in the day; reduce dosage then reintroduce
	Dysphoria	Consider another stimulant if persistent or tricyclic drug
	Long term	
	Weight loss	Supplement diet, institute drug holidays or change drug
	Tics	Discontinue, if stimulant is effective consider rechallenge; consider tricyclic drug
Tricyclic drugs	Autonomic nervous system	See antipsychotic agents
	Cardiovascular (blood pressure, HR, PR, T-wave changes, ↑ QTc, and arrhythmias)	Monitor ECGs serially; most changes have little clinical significance in healthy child
	CNS (seizures)	Discontinue medication gradually, EEG; may need anticonvulsant
Anxiolytics and sedative-hypnotic agents		
Antihistamines	Oversedation	Decrease total dosage; administer most at bedtime
	Rash	Discontinue medication
Benzodiazepines	Disinhibition	Discontinue medication
	Cognitive decrements	Reduce dosage or discontinue
Lithium	Gastrointestinal: nausea, vomiting, abdominal pain, diarrhea, metallic taste	Consider dose reduction if persistent
	CNS: tremor, memory lapses, fatigue	Consider dose reduction if persistent
	Endocrine: goiter	Discontinue medication and follow with laboratory studies
	Renal: polyuria/polydipsia	Monitor BUN, creatinine, electrolytes, and urinalysis on a regular basis (every 2–3 months)
	Hematological: leukocytosis	Monitor; may not be of clinical significance

LFTs, liver function tests; TCA, tricyclic antidepressant; ECG, electrocardiogram; CNS, central nervous system; EEG, electroencephalogram; BUN, blood urea nitrogen.

A 15-year-old girl who has lost 25 percent of her body weight and cannot control her purging behaviors generally requires an *inpatient setting* in which to initiate treatment, to establish refeeding, and to observe her continuously to prevent purging. Given the complex effects of starvation, a malnourished adolescent is not a good candidate for outpatient treatment. The treatment approaches for the restricting and purging type of anorexia nervosa are multimodal. A behavioral component is necessary to systematically address nutritional needs and to prevent behaviors that further increase malnutrition. *A family approach is needed to probe the family's role in the disorder. A psychodynamic approach may be beneficial* in order to work with adolescent in identifying the meaning of the disorder and the psychological forces that drive the behaviors. Medications are sometimes used to treat concurrent anxiety and depression and to ameliorate bingeing and purging.

A 17-year-old girl who has been discharged from an inpatient unit presumably is stable, not posing an imminent danger to herself, and is ready to engage in outpatient treatment. There is evidence from several double blind, placebo-controlled trials that *fluoxetine is effective in the treatment of major depression in adolescents*. Several studies also indicate that medications are most effective when combined with psychotherapy; particularly following the potentially jarring effects of a suicide attempt and hospitalizations, *psychotherapy (interpersonal, cognitive-behavioral, and/or psychodynamic) is certainly indicated in this case*.

A 14-year-old girl who has recently stopped attending school because of an increase in auditory hallucinations is in crisis. *Since she is not suicidal, she may not need the containment of an inpatient unit, but she would be a good candidate for a partial hospitalization program, in which she can receive daily monitoring of antipsychotic medication as well as daily support and therapy from staff.* A return to an appropriate school setting would be a primary goal of the treatment.

Enuresis (in this case, in an 8-year-old boy) is much more common in boys than girls, and may cause psychological distress and social difficulties for children who continue to have this problem into the school-age years. Approximately 7 percent of 5-year olds have enuresis on a regular basis, and 3 percent of 10 year olds have the condition. *Desmopressin (DDAVP) nasal spray is effective in some children with enuresis, and may be useful in the short-term. The most effective treatment, however, is a behavioral approach using methods such as the bell-and-pad conditioning treatment.*

A 7-year-old boy who cannot stay on task and who is hyperactive and socially provocative is exhibiting typical symptoms of attention-deficit/hyperactivity disorder. *The treatment for the core symptoms is a stimulant medication such as methylphenidate. Most children with ADHD also have social difficulties and may be rejected by peers. Thus it is often beneficial to include social skills groups as an additional therapeutic intervention.*

A 9-year-old boy with both motor and vocal tics lasting over a year meets criteria for Tourette's Disorder; this diagnosis is very commonly comorbid with ADHD, which likely also exists in this patient, as evidenced by his hyperactive, impulsive, and aggressive behavior. Treatment of comorbid ADHD and Tourette's is complicated by the fact that stimulant treatment can exacerbate tics in these patients. While recent data suggests that stimulants are safe and effective in the majority of patients with these two diagnoses, some patients are unable to tolerate stimulants due to effects on their tics. *In these patients, alpha-2 agonists, such as guanfacine, are indicated for their effectiveness in both reducing tics and in treating some symptoms of ADHD, particularly impulsivity, hyperactivity, and associated aggression.*

57 Forensic Issues in Child and Adolescent Psychiatry

Child and adolescent psychiatrists are increasingly sought out by patients and attorneys for evaluations and expert opinions related to child custody and criminal behaviors perpetrated by minors, and to evaluate the relations between traumatic life events and the emergence of psychiatric symptoms in children and adolescents. In medicine, ethics historically has alluded to moral obligations as well as to the accepted behavior that physicians follow; on the broadest scale, the Hippocratic oath summarizes ethical values in medicine. During the past few decades, however, new ethical and moral dilemmas have arisen with the growth of medical knowledge and technology. The traditional ethical tenet that physicians must consider each patient above all else has often been challenged. For example, a patient may be kept alive for long periods while in a coma or a pregnant woman's life may be saved by aborting her fetus.

Society's view of children and their rights has evolved dramatically in the 20th century. The institution of a juvenile court system about 100 years ago was an acknowledgment that children must be protected and provided for differently than adults. In 1980, the American Academy of Child and Adolescent Psychiatry published a code of ethics that was developed to publicly endorse the ethical standards of this discipline. The code is based on the assumption that children are vulnerable and unable to take adequate care of themselves, but as they mature, their capacity to make judgments of, and choices about, their well-being develop as well. The code has several caveats: from the standpoint of child and adolescent psychiatrists, issues of consent, confidentiality, and professional responsibility must be seen in the context of overlapping and potentially conflicting rights of children, parents, and society.

Students should study the questions and answers below for a useful review of basic issues.

HELPFUL HINTS

These terms should be known and defined by the student.

- adjudicated delinquent
- adjudication
- "best interests of the child"
- breach of confidentiality
- child custody evaluation
- confidentiality
- delinquent act
- disposition
- intake
- joint custody
- juvenile court
- mediation
- proof beyond a reasonable doubt
- rehabilitation
- status offenses
- "tender-years" doctrine
- waiver of confidentiality

QUESTIONS

Directions

The incomplete statement below is followed by five suggested completions. Select the *one* that is *best*.

57.1 Breach of confidentiality by a psychiatrist is required in all of the following situations *except*

A. A suicidal adolescent patient
B. A homicidal adolescent patient
C. Disclosure of sexual abuse by a patient
D. A child custody evaluation
E. Drug or alcohol use by an adolescent patient

Directions

Each set of lettered headings below is followed by a list of numbered statements. For each numbered statement, select

A. if the item is associated with A only
B. if the item is associated with B only
C. if the item is associated with both A and B
D. if the item is associated with neither A nor B

Questions 57.2–57.7

A. Juvenile court system
B. Adult court system

57.2 Rights to legal counsel, Fifth Amendment privilege, and notice of charges
57.3 Pretrial hearing, trial, sentencing
57.4 Trial by jury
57.5 Intake, adjudication, disposition
57.6 Disposition occurs immediately after confession
57.7 Trial only by judge, without a jury

Questions 57.8–57.10

A. "Tender-years" doctrine
B. "Best interests of the child" doctrine

57.8 Young children are usually better off with their mothers.
57.9 Current law in the United States.
57.10 There may be a situation in which custody should reside with a non-parent.

Directions

The group of questions below consists of lettered headings followed by a list of numbered phrases or statements. For each numbered phrase or statement, select the *one* lettered heading that is most closely associated with it. Each lettered heading may be selected once, more than once, or not at all.

Questions 57.11–57.14

A. "In re Gault" case
B. "In re Winship" case
C. Tarasoff I and Tarasoff II rulings
D. Education for All Handicapped Children Act of 1975

57.11 Specified that the standard "beyond a reasonable doubt" must be followed in delinquency hearings
57.12 Specified that juveniles have the right to confront witnesses in delinquency trials
57.13 Identified clinicians' duties to warn third parties of imminent danger
57.14 Determined that all handicapped children should be provided a free and appropriate public education in the least restrictive environment

ANSWERS

57.1 The answer is E

Breaches of confidentiality occur in situations of danger to the life of a patient or information disclosure leading the clinician to believe that the patient poses a threat to the life of another individual. Patients who are *suicidal or homicidal* and cases of *sexual abuse* automatically require breaches of confidentiality. *Child custody evaluations are also exempt from confidentiality*, as is established via a written waiver of confidentiality at the outset of the custody evaluation. *Disclosure by an adolescent patient of drug or alcohol use does not necessarily fall into the category of required breach of confidentiality*. The specific nature and situation of use, and the substance used, indicate to the clinician whether such behaviors constitute an imminent danger to the life of the patient. If so, the clinician is obliged to override the confidentiality.

Answers 57.2–57.7

57.2 The answer is C

57.3 The answer is B

57.4 The answer is B

57.5 The answer is A

57.6 The answer is A

57.7 The answer is A

Both the juvenile court and the adult court systems must conform to the same rights of due process, which include the right to notice of charges, right to legal counsel, the Fifth Amendment privilege against self-incrimination, and the right to confront witnesses. The *adult court system uses the following process: pretrial hearing, trial, and sentencing*. The *juvenile court differs, and includes intake, adjudication, and disposition*. If a *juvenile makes a confession, disposition may proceed without the trial. The adult court system uses both trial by jury and trial by judge* without a jury in its decision making, whereas *in juvenile court all trials are decided by a judge.*

Answers 57.8–57.10

57.8 The answer is A

57.9 The answer is B

57.10 The answer is B

Child custody disputes throughout recorded history have reflected a society's view of the child in the family. The practice of courts becoming involved in private family affairs is fairly recent. The history of these issues traces a change from seeing children as essentially owned by their parents, to considering what is likely to be in the child's best interests. Judicial decisions have been informed by various doctrines, including the "tender-years" and the "best interests of the child" doctrines. *The "tender-years" doctrine existed well into the 20th century and held that young children (from birth to about age 7) were usually better off with their mothers,* who were presumed to be best able to raise and nurture their offspring. With this doctrine in mind, most custody decisions were made in the mother's favor. This presumption was replaced in the last third of the 20th century by the "*best interests of the child" doctrine, which is the current law in the United States.* This doctrine holds that the focus of a child custody case should be the child, and that courts ought not to lean toward one parent or the other based exclusively on gender. Considerations of the optimal parent for the child expanded beyond mother-child relationship and included assessing issues of emotional climate, safety, and educational and social opportunities for the children. *There may be situations in which "best interest of the child" dictates that custody should reside with a non-parent rather than a parent.*

Answers 57.11–57.14

57.11 The answer is B

57.12 The answer is A

57.13 The answer is C

57.14 The answer is D

Knowledge of the juvenile court system and its strengths and weaknesses is essential for forensic child and adolescent psychiatrists. The clinician must also appreciate the indications for waiver hearings and the grounds for judicial determination that a minor be tried as an adult. Although the juvenile court system operated for decades as supposedly child oriented and protective, the United States Supreme Court, in the landmark case "In re Gault," determined that the system sometimes does not accord juveniles rights equal to those of adults. This decision held that in delinquency cases, juveniles must be accorded basic due process rights: the right to notice of charges, the right to legal counsel, the Fifth Amendment privilege against self-incrimination, and *the right to confront witnesses*. Another important Supreme Court case, "In re Winship," held that that standard *"beyond a reasonable doubt" must be followed in delinquency hearings.*

Child and adolescent psychiatrists may be involved in forensic evaluations outside the more common venues of the family or criminal court. For example, they may be called upon to make certain recommendations for a student with special needs under the landmark *Education for All Handicapped Children Act of 1975. This law requires that all handicapped children, regardless of the severity of their condition, be provided a free and appropriate public education in the least restrictive environment*. Handicapped children are defined as those who are mentally retarded, learning disabled, physically disabled, or emotionally disturbed. A treating or evaluating child psychiatrist may be asked to testify at various hearings required under the law. Knowledge of the law's implications as well as of the particular child will be critical to performing a proper evaluation.

Most clinicians working with children and adolescents spell out the limits of confidentiality to the families they work with at the outset of treatment and also clarify how communications with parents are to be handled; they may particularly need to review limits of confidentiality with respect to insurance plans. Additional limits to confidentiality include behavior harmful to self or others. When disclosures need to be made to parents, the patient may be given the option of telling them himself or herself, or of having the discussion together with the parents and the patient. Other exceptions to confidentiality include a law on reporting child abuse, which is mandatory in all states. A physician who fails to report suspicion of abuse may be liable for civil as well as criminal sanction. If an abuse report needs to be filed, parents should be informed. In some states, *physicians have a duty to protect third parties, as specified under Tarasoff I and Tarasoff II*, the 1976 and 1982 rulings of the California Supreme Court in the two cases of Tarasoff v. Regents of University of California.

58

Geriatric Psychiatry

Geriatric psychiatry is concerned with preventing, diagnosing, and treating psychological disorders in older adults. It is also concerned with promoting longevity; persons with a healthy mental adaptation to life are likely to live longer than those stressed with emotional problems. Mental disorders in the elderly often differ in clinical manifestations, pathogenesis, and pathophysiology from disorders of younger adults and do not always match the categories in the text revision of the 4th edition of *Diagnostic and Statistical Manual of Mental Disorders* (DSM-IV-TR). Diagnosing and treating older adults can present more difficulties than treating younger persons because older persons may have coexisting chronic medical diseases and disabilities, may take many medications, and may show cognitive impairments.

Prevalence data for mental disorders in elderly persons vary widely, but a conservatively estimated 25 percent have significant psychiatric symptoms. The number of mentally ill elderly persons is expected to rise to 20 million by the middle of the century. The American Board of Psychiatry and Neurology established geropsychiatry (from the Greek *geros* ["old age"] and *iatros* ["physical"]) as a subspecialty in 1991, and today geriatric psychiatry is one of the fastest growing fields in psychiatry.

Predisposing psychosocial risk factors for mental disorders in the elderly include many losses, such as those of social roles, autonomy and independence, family and friends, health, and finances. There is a high prevalence of cognitive disorders in older people, ranging from what are considered minor age-related memory impairments, termed benign senescent forgetfulness, to full-blown dementias, such as Alzheimer's disease. Dementia is the second most common cause of disability in people over 65 years of age, after arthritis. In the United States, about 5 percent of people over 65 years of age have severe dementia, and about 15 percent have mild dementia. Over the age of 80 years, about 20 percent have severe dementia.

The student should study the questions and answers below for a useful review of these issues in this field.

HELPFUL HINTS

Each of the following terms relating to geriatric issues should be defined.

- adaptational capacity
- advocacy
- agedness
- agitation and aggression
- akathisia
- alcohol- and other substance-use disorders
- Alzheimer's disease
- anoxic confusion
- anxiety disorder
- benign senescent forgetfulness
- benzodiazepines
- cerebral anoxia
- code of ethics
- cognitive functioning
- consent for disclosure of information
- conversion disorder
- delirium
- dementia
- dementing disorder
- depression
- developmental phases
- diabetes
- disorders of awareness
- drug blood level
- elder abuse
- hypochondriasis
- hypomanic disorder
- ideational paucity
- insomnia
- L-dopa (Larodopa)
- late-onset schizophrenia
- LH
- lithium
- loss of mastery
- manic disorder
- MMSE (Mini-Mental Status Examination)
- mood disorder
- neurosis
- norepinephrine
- nutritional deficiencies
- obsessive-compulsive disorder
- organic mental disorder
- orientation
- overt behavior
- paradoxical reaction
- paraphrenia
- presbyopia
- psychopharmacology
- psychotropic danger
- ranitidine (Zantac)

QUESTIONS

Directions

Each of the questions or incomplete statements below is followed by five suggested responses or completions. Select the *one* that is *best* in each case.

58.1 Which of the following is *true*?

A. The prevalence of dementia is higher in institutionalized patients than in patients in the community.
B. The prevalence of Alzheimer's disease is higher in African Americans compared to Caucasians.

C. Approximately 60 percent of dementias in Asian populations are of the vascular type.
D. Depression is a risk factor for dementia.
E. All of the above

58.2 Anxiety disorders in the elderly

A. are uncommon
B. are more common in men
C. most commonly present as phobic disorder
D. most commonly present as panic disorder
E. increase in prevalence with increasing age

58.3 Which of the following statements about the biology of aging is *false*?

A. Each cell of the body has a genetically determined life span.
B. The optic lens thins.
C. The T-cell response to antigens is altered.
D. A decrease in melanin occurs.
E. Brain weight decreases.

58.4 Which of the following statements about learning and memory in the elderly is *false*?

A. Complete learning of new material still occurs.
B. On multiple choice tests, recognition of correct answers persists.
C. Simple recall remains intact.
D. IQ remains stable until age 80 years.
E. Memory-encoding ability diminishes.

58.5 In the physical assessment of the aged, which of the following statements is *false*?

A. Toxins of bacterial origin are common.
B. The most common metabolic intoxication causing mental symptoms is uremia.
C. Cerebral anoxia often precipitates mental syndromes.
D. Severe vitamin deficiencies are common.
E. Nutritional deficiencies may cause mental symptoms.

58.6 In a neuropsychological evaluation

A. verbal memory is measured by reading patients a list of words and then having them repeat the words recalled
B. information processing speed is measured by having patients rapidly complete rote tasks
C. word retrieval is measured by having patients provide precise names for pictured objects
D. visual perception is measured by having patients identify missing parts of pictured objects
E. all of the above

58.7 Creutzfeld Jakob disease is

A. not an inherited disease
B. associated with agnosia
C. infectious
D. another name for Kuru
E. associated with tau-containing intra-neuronal inclusion bodies

58.8 Elderly persons taking antipsychotics are especially susceptible to the following side effects *except*

A. tardive dyskinesia
B. akathisia
C. a toxic confusional state
D. paresthesias
E. dry mouth

58.9 Abnormalities of cognitive functioning in the aged are most often due to

A. depressive disturbances
B. schizophrenia
C. medication
D. cerebral dysfunctioning or deterioration
E. hypochondriasis

58.10 Neuro-imaging of brains in Alzheimer's disease

A. reveals T2 hyper-intensities on MRI
B. reveals reductions in the entorhinal cortex on volumetric MRI
C. reveals reductions in the cerebral metabolic rate for glucose (CMRgl)
D. all of the above
E. none of the above

58.11 Which of the following is *true*?

A. The prevalence of major depression is higher in the elderly than in younger patients.
B. Older adults experience sadness more than younger people.
C. Aging results in a decreased ability to inhibit negative emotions.
D. Emotional distress increases with age.
E. In general, elderly African Americans are less distressed than elderly Caucasians.

58.12 Which of the following statements about the pharmacological treatment of the elderly is *false*?

A. The elderly use more medications than any other age group.
B. 25 percent of prescriptions are for those over age 65 years.
C. In the United States, 250,000 people a year are hospitalized because of adverse reactions to medications.
D. About 25 percent of hypnotics dispensed in the United States each year are to those over age 65 years.
E. About 70 percent of the elderly use over-the-counter (OTC) medications.

58.13 All of the following risk factors for dementia of the Alzheimer's type are regarded as confirmed *except*

A. apolipoprotein E genotype
B. Down's syndrome
C. family history
D. aluminum
E. age

58.14 Possible protective factors against dementia include

A. anti-inflammatory drugs
B. estrogen replacement therapy
C. red wine
D. education
E. all of the above

58.15 Sleep changes associated with normal aging include

A. reduction in stage 4 sleep
B. increased fragmentation of sleep
C. reduction in REM sleep
D. disruption of the circadian sleep–wake rhythm
E. all of the above

ANSWERS

58.1 The answer is E (all)

The overall prevalence estimates of dementia in people over age 65 ranges from approximately 1 to 20 percent. *The prevalence of dementia in institutional samples is higher than that reported in community samples.* Some geographic and ethnic differences in prevalence by subtype have been noted. *The prevalence of Alzheimer's disease is higher among African Americans compared to Caucasians.* Among Caucasians, the vast majority of the dementias are of the Alzheimer's type, whereas, in *Asian populations, approximately 60 percent of the dementias are of the vascular type. A history of depression has been identified as a risk factor for dementia.* Depression may be the result of an awareness of early cognitive decline. Depression and dementia may also share common risk factors. Cognitive decline has also been shown to be a risk factor for the onset of depression.

58.2 The answer is C

While epidemiological studies show that anxiety disorders are less prevalent in older adults compared to younger adults, the prevalence of anxiety disorders in this older age group is high when compared to that of other disorders. Indeed, anxiety disorders are the most prevalent psychiatric disorders, excluding the dementias, in people over age 65. *The most prevalent anxiety disorder among older adults is phobic disorder. Panic disorder is the least common anxiety disorder in this age group.* Across all age groups, *anxiety disorders are move prevalent in women than in men. The prevalence of anxiety disorders decreases with increasing age.*

58.3 The answer is B

As a person ages, *the optic lens thickens (not thins)* in association with an inability to accommodate (presbyopia), and hearing loss is progressive, particularly at the high frequencies. The process of aging, known as senescence, results from a complex interaction of genetic, metabolic, hormonal, immunological, and structural factors acting on molecular, cellular, histological, and organ levels. The most commonly held theory is that *each cell of the body has a genetically determined life span* during which replication occurs a limited number of times before the cell dies. One study found 50 such replications in human cells. Structural changes in cells take place with age. In the central nervous system (CNS), for example, age-related cell changes occur in neurons, which show signs of degeneration.

Changes in the structure of deoxyribonucleic acid (DNA) and ribonucleic acid (RNA) are also found in aging cells; the cause has been attributed to genotypic programming, X-rays, chemicals, and food products, among others. Aging probably has no single cause. All areas of the body are affected to some degree, and changes vary from person to person.

A progressive decline in many bodily functions includes a *decrease in melanin* and decreases in cardiac output and stroke volume, glomerular filtration rate, oxygen consumption, cerebral blood flow, and vital capacity. Many immune mechanisms are altered, with *impaired T-cell response to antigens* and an increase in the formation of autoimmune antibodies. These altered immune responses probably play a role in aged persons' susceptibility to infection and possibly even to neoplastic disease. Some neoplasms, most notably cancers of the colon, prostate, stomach, and skin, show a steadily increasing incidence with age.

Variable changes in endocrine function are seen. For example, postmenopausal estrogen levels decrease, producing breast tissue involution and vaginal epithelial atrophy. Testosterone levels begin to decline in the 6th decade; however, follicle-stimulating hormone and luteinizing hormone increase. In the central nervous system, there is a *decrease in brain weight,* ventricular enlargement, and neuronal loss of approximately 50,000 a day, with some reduction in cerebral blood flow and oxygenation.

58.4 The answer is C

In the elderly, *simple recall* becomes difficult *(does not remain intact)* and *memory-encoding ability diminishes.* Those functions decline with age. However, many cognitive abilities are retained in old age. Although the elderly take longer than young persons to learn new material, *complete learning of new material still occurs.* Old adults maintain their verbal abilities, and their *IQs remain stable until approximately age 80 years. On multiple-choice tests, recognition of correct answers persists.*

58.5 The answer is D

Severe vitamin deficiencies in the aged are *rare (rather than common).* However, a number of conditions and deficiencies are typical and should be considered in the physical assessment of the aged. *Toxins of bacterial origin* and metabolic origin are common in old age. Bacterial toxins usually originate in occult or inconspicuous foci of infection, such as suspected pneumonic conditions and urinary infections. In the aged, the most common metabolic intoxication causing mental symptoms is *uremia,* which is an excess of urea and other nitrogenous waste products in the blood. Mild diabetes, hepatic failure, and gout are also known to cause mental symptoms in the aged and may easily be missed unless they are actively investigated. Alcohol and drug misuse may cause many mental disturbances in late life. These abuses, with their characteristic effects, are usually determined by taking a history.

Cerebral anoxia often precipitates mental symptoms as a result of cardiac insufficiency or emphysema. Anoxic confusion may follow surgery, a cardiac infarct, gastrointestinal bleeding, or occlusion or stenosis of the carotid arteries. *Nutritional deficiencies may cause mental symptoms* or may be a symptom of a mental disorder.

58.6 The answer is E (all)

A neuropsychological evaluation involves standardized paper and pencil testing of a broad range of cognitive functions, including memory and learning, language, visual-spatial skills, executive/problem-solving skills, motor dexterity, attention, information processing speed, and overall intelligence. Memory testing usually involves measurement of the ability to learn both verbal and nonverbal information. *Verbal memory*, an ability primarily tied to the left temporal lobe, *is typically measured by reading patients a list of words and then having them repeat the words recalled*. Basic attention is typically assessed by having patients repeat spoken numbers both in forward and reverse order. *Information processing speed can be measured by having patients rapidly complete rote tasks*, such as drawing lines between numbers in sequential order, copying names from a template, or naming words. Language skills are tied to the functions of the left hemisphere. The typical language skills assessed in a neuropsychological evaluation include word retrieval, word generation, and vocabulary range. *Word retrieval is measured by having patients provide precise names for pictured objects*, and word generation is quantified by having them generate words beginning with particular letters or in specific categories within a circumscribed time period. Visual-perceptual and constructional abilities are skills primarily associated with right posterior cerebral functioning. *Visual perception can be sampled by having patients identify missing parts of pictured objects*.

58.7 The answer is C

Creutzfeldt-Jakob disease (CJD) is one of the transmissible spongiform encephalopathies. *These diseases are both inherited and infectious. Kuru, another* of the spongiform encephalopathies, first came to the attention of Western medicine in the 1950s when it was reported as endemic to the Fore people of the eastern Highlands of Papua, New Guinea. It was named for its hallmark "shivering" or "trembling." *CJD is characterized by progressive dementia and ataxia, not agnosia*. A unique infectious protein termed a *prion* (for proteinaceous infectious particle that lacks nuclecic acid) has been isolated from the brains of people with transmissible spongiform encephalopathies. *Tau-containing intra-neuronal inclusion bodies (Pick bodies) is associated with Pick's disease*, a progressive dementia characterized by prominent behavioral and language deficits, atrophy of the fronto-temporal region of the brain and ballooned neurons.

58.8 The answer is D

Paresthesias, which are spontaneous tingling sensations, are not typically a side effect of antipsychotics. Elderly persons, particularly if they have organic brain disease, are especially susceptible to the side effects of antipsychotics, which include *dry mouth, tardive dyskinesia, akathisia,* and a *toxic confusional state.* Tardive dyskinesia is characterized by disfiguring and involuntary buccal and lingual masticatory movements; akathisia is a restlessness marked by a compelling need for constant motion. Choreiform body movements, which are spasmodic and involuntary movements of the limbs and the face, and rhythmic extension and flexion movements of the fingers may also be noticeable. Examination of the patient's protruded tongue for fine tremors and vermicular (worm-like) movements is a useful diagnostic procedure. A toxic confusional state, also called a central anticholinergic syndrome, is characterized by a marked disturbance in short-term memory, impaired attention, disorientation, anxiety, visual and auditory hallucinations, increased psychotic thinking, and peripheral anticholinergic side effects.

58.9 The answer is D

Abnormalities of cognitive functioning in the elderly are *most often due to some cerebral dysfunction or deterioration,* although they may also be the result of *depressive disturbances, schizophrenia,* or the effects of *medication.* In many instances, intellectual difficulties are not obvious, and a searching evaluation is necessary to detect them. The elderly are sensitive to the effects of medication; in some instances, cognitive impairment may result from overmedication. *Hypochondriasis,* the fear that one has a disease or preoccupation with one's health, is not the cause of an abnormality of cognitive functioning.

58.10 The answer is D (all)

MRI studies in Alzheimer's disease *show an increased number of T2 hyper-intensities, as well as an increased number of hyper-intensities in peri-ventricular regions. PET studies find abnormalities in the cerebral metabolic rate for glucose (CMRgl).* Volumetric MRI studies find *reductions in the volume of medial temporal lobe structures*, namely the hippocampus and entorhinal cortex, which are correlated with the severity of cognitive impairment, and increased rates of atrophy in medial temporal structures and the whole brain in patients with Alzheimer's disease.

58.11 The answer is E

Interesting racial differences have been noted between elderly African American and Caucasian people when measuring psychological distress. *Elderly African Americans have been noted to be less distressed than elderly Caucasians.* It has been suggested that elderly African Americans may be afforded higher status and stay more engaged within their communities than elderly Caucasians. With the exception of dementing disorders and delirium, *mental disorders are no more common in the elderly as compared to younger age groups. Prevalence estimates of common disorders such as major depression are lower for those over the age of 65 than they are in younger cohorts.* Older adults report experiencing *less negative emotions* such as sadness, anger, and fear than younger adults, and aging is associated with an *increased ability to inhibit negative emotional states and maintain positive emotional states.*

58.12 The answer is D

Psychotropic drugs are among those most commonly prescribed for the elderly; *40 percent (not 25 percent) of all hypnotics* dispensed in the United States each year are to those over age 65 years. *The elderly use more medications than any other age group.* Indeed, *25 percent of all prescriptions are written for those over age 65 years.* Many old persons have adverse drug reactions, as evidenced by the fact that, *in the United States, 250,000 people a year are hospitalized because of adverse medication reactions.* The physician must remember that about *70 percent of the elderly use over-the-counter* (OTC) *medications.* These preparations can interact with prescribed drugs and lead to dangerous side effects. The physician should include the use of OTC medications when taking a patient's drug history.

58.13 The answer is D

The power of individual case-control studies of dementia of the Alzheimer's type has been greatly enhanced by an initiative undertaken by the European Consortium on Dementia (EURODEM) established by the European community. They carried out a collaborative reanalysis of 11 case-controlled studies, six from the United States and one each from Australia, Finland, Italy, Japan, and the Netherlands. That analysis revealed risk factors that had hitherto been only speculative. From this and other sources, only four risk factors can now be regarded as confirmed.

As for dementia in general, the incidence rises steeply with *age*, making it the strongest of all risk factors.

Having a parent or sibling with dementia of the Alzheimer's type increases the risk of developing the disease about 3.5 times. The risk is greater for relatives of early-onset patients than later-onset patients. In interpreting the epidemiological data for individual patients, however, the clinician needs to emphasize that the risk conferred by a positive family history depends on how long that person lives. Those who do not reach old age have a low risk. Even for relatives who live to age 90 years, the probability that they themselves will develop the disease is only about 50 percent.

The much rarer, early-onset dementia of the Alzheimer's type is caused by single genes, such as a mutation of the amyloid precursor gene on chromosome 21 or the presenilin genes on chromosomes 1 and 14. But in most cases of dementia of the Alzheimer's type, onset is not until the 70s or 80s. In this group, of much greater public health importance, there are multiple genetic and environmental influences. One of the most exciting discoveries is that the apolipoprotein E $\varepsilon4$ allele on chromosome 19 affects the risk of developing the disease. The $\varepsilon4$ allele of this gene increases risk; the $\varepsilon2$ allele may reduce it. Although early research with clinical samples showed a very strong relationship between *apolipoprotein E $\varepsilon4$ genotype* and dementia of the Alzheimer's type, more recent studies with general population samples show a weaker relationship. Currently, much interest exists in preliminary findings that a combination of having the $\varepsilon4$ allele and being infected with the herpes simplex type 1 virus confers a very high risk. It is now clear that although all individuals with the $\varepsilon4$ allele are at increased risk, even homozygotes can live to age 90 years with only a 50 percent chance of developing a dementia. An interesting proposal is that the apolipoprotein E genotype predicts when (not whether) a person is predisposed to develop this dementia. These epidemiological findings may in time lead to the development of pharmacological methods to slow the deposition of β-amyloid.

Persons with *Down's syndrome* may develop the brain changes of dementia of the Alzheimer's type before age 40 years. This is believed to be related to their having an extra copy of the amyloid precursor gene on chromosome 21.

Because *aluminum*, known to be neurotoxic, occurs in neuritic plaques, evidence has been sought for an association between exposure to this metal and the development of dementia of the Alzheimer's type. Aluminum is ingested in food, drinking water, antacids, and toothpaste. It is used in kitchen utensils and it is applied to the body in antiperspirants. The widespread use of aluminum as a flocculent in water supplies has led to public concern, although drinking water provides only a tiny percentage of dietary aluminum. The amount absorbed depends on its bioavailability, and considerable uncertainty exists about its subsequent deposition in the brain. From the epidemiological evidence, involvement of aluminum from drinking water or other sources in causing dementia of the Alzheimer's type remains unproven.

58.14 The answer is E (all)

A recurrent finding in field surveys is that rates for dementia and cognitive impairment are higher in elderly persons who have had little *education*. This may be partly due to bias in ascertainment, whereby the tests are done better by persons who are more literate. Although such bias may be present in the detection of mild impairment in surveys, it is much less likely to influence the diagnosis of a fully developed dementia. There may indeed be a true gradient in the incidence of dementia, including dementia of the Alzheimer's type, across educational levels. In this way, lack of education could be seen as an exposure that may confer increased risk. One interpretation is that education may delay the point at which a developing dementia becomes clinically manifest. In interpreting results of a large survey in Shanghai, the authors raised the possibility that having no education may lower brain reserve, allowing the earlier appearance of symptoms of dementia. It is also possible that education is a proxy for other beneficial factors, as in diet or lifestyle. But a recent longitudinal study of American nuns suggests that education and intelligence may actually protect against the neuropathological processes in dementia of the Alzheimer's type. This means that exposure to education in childhood may conceivably have some protective effect many decades later.

Since an inverse association between rheumatoid arthritis and dementia of the Alzheimer's type was first observed, over 20 publications have examined the possibility that persons who have taken steroids, aspirin, or other nonsteroidal *anti-inflammatory drugs* (NSAIDs) over long periods have a lower risk of dementia or have slower cognitive decline in late life. Some of these studies have reported a protective effect, but many have deficient designs, and there may be publication bias (i.e., papers with negative evidence for such an effect are less likely to be submitted and accepted for publication). Yet comprehensive and balanced information on the topic is needed. The most recent information is that anti-inflammatory drugs probably do prevent or attenuate the symptoms of dementia of the Alzheimer's type. This effect is biologically plausible in terms of the action of these drugs to inhibit the immune and chronic inflammatory pathology suspected to apply in dementia of the Alzheimer's type. But it is premature for physicians to prescribe anti-inflammatory drugs for dementia of the Alzheimer's type before their effect is established in a randomized controlled trial and the findings balanced with their risks.

Case-controlled studies suggest possible protection against dementia of the Alzheimer's type afforded to women who take *estrogen*. But since these women also tend to be better educated and to differ in other lifestyle factors, this finding could be misleading. The use of estrogen replacement therapy is currently controversial.

A large population-based prospective study in Bordeaux, France has found evidence that *moderate consumption of red wine* protects against the onset of dementia.

58.15 The answer is E (all)

Age-related changes in the amount and pattern of the various stages of sleep and wakefulness are well described. Elderly people spend more time in bed and less time asleep and are more easily aroused from sleep than are young people. The most striking changes include a *reduction in slow-wave sleep (particularly stage 4 sleep)*, increased nighttime wakefulness, and *increased fragmentation of sleep* by periods of wakefulness. Less striking age-related changes such as *reductions in rapid eye movement (REM) sleep* and total nighttime sleep also occur. The age-related impairments in sleep depth and maintenance seem to be accompanied by an age-related increase in sensitivity to environmental stimuli that disturb sleep; for example, elderly people are more easily aroused from nighttime sleep by auditory stimuli than are young people.

Many age-related changes in sleep patterns suggest that aging may *disrupt the circadian sleep–wake rhythm.* Increased nighttime wakefulness in elderly persons is mirrored by more daytime fatigue, more daytime napping, and a greater likelihood of falling asleep during the day. Advancing age has also been associated with a tendency to fall asleep and awaken earlier than in earlier years, and older people are less tolerant of phase shifts of the sleep–wake schedule, such as those caused by shift work and transmeridian flight (jet lag). Because these changes are also observed in healthy seniors, they are attributed to normal, age-related neuronal alterations in brain areas controlling sleep physiology rather than to pathological processes.

59 End-of-Life Care and Palliative Medicine

End of life refers to all those issues involved in caring for the terminally ill. It begins when curative therapy ceases and encompasses the following areas: (1) communication of prognosis to family and patient, and defining the patient's understanding of his or her illness; (2) advance directives about life-sustaining treatment; (3) the need for hospitalization and hospice care; (4) legal and ethical matters; (5) bereavement support and psychiatric care; and finally (6) palliative care to relieve pain and suffering. The hospice movement began in the early 1960s, and provides a place (it may be an institution or a home) where a multidisciplinary team provides round-the-clock coverage to the terminal patient.

The control of pain is a primary goal, and narcotics are provided without fear of addiction. Effective pain management is critical, and physicians must use narcotics as liberally as they are needed and tolerated. This aspect of care is difficult for many doctors, who have been trained to use narcotics sparingly, if at all, out of fear of creating addictions, and who may also have become desensitized to or skeptical of expressions of pain in their patients. Hospice care's essential goal is to allow dying patients and their families to conduct their final interactions with as much dignity and control as possible.

A living will is a legal document in which patients provide instructions to their doctors about what life-support measures they will and will not accept. The American Medical Association (AMA) states that doctors can withhold all life-support treatment, including food and water, from patients in irreversible comas, as long as the diagnosis is confirmed adequately. In these cases, a physician does not intentionally cause the person's death (euthanasia) but rather, in consultation with the patient's family or guardian, lets the patient die. Euthanasia, or physician-assisted suicide, is defined as the doctor's deliberate act to kill a patient by directly administering a lethal dose of some drug or other agent. The ethical issues surrounding euthanasia are profound.

The student should study the questions and answers below for a useful review of this field.

HELPFUL HINTS

The student should know and define the following terms.

- advance directives
- DNI
- DNR
- end-of-life symptoms
- euthanasia (active, passive, involuntary, voluntary)
- health care proxies
- hospice
- hydromorphone
- living wills
- maintenance versus prn analgesics
- mercy killing
- morphine
- neonatal and child end-of-life decisions
- neuropathic pain
- opioids
- pain suppression pathways
- palliative versus curative treatment
- Patients Self-Determination Act
- physician-assisted suicide
- psychogenic pain
- psychotoxicity
- somatic pain
- Uniform Rights of the Terminally Ill Act
- visceral pain

QUESTIONS

Directions

Each of the questions or incomplete statements below is followed by five suggested responses or completions. Select the *one* that is *best* in each case.

59.1 A risk factor for the development of aversive reactions in physicians is when

A. the physician identifies the patient with someone in his or her own life
B. the physician is dealing with a sick family member
C. the physician feels professionally insecure

D. the physician is fearful of death and disability
E. all of the above

59.2 The most common cause of undertreatment in patients is

A. lack of knowledge or resources
B. lack of communication between the doctor and patient
C. patients with high pain threshold
D. when inexperienced doctors are overanxious
E. noncompliance

59.3 Of the following drugs, the *least* likely to cause psychotoxicity is

A. morphine
B. levorphanol (Levo-Dromoran)
C. methadone (Dolophine)
D. hydromorphone (Dilaudid)
E. none of the above

59.4 Which of the following is *not* true regarding patients with strong religious beliefs?

A. Patients with strong religious beliefs are often better able to deal with end of life issues.
B. Patients with strong religious beliefs may explain illness as a test of their faith.
C. Patients with strong religious beliefs may see suffering as having redemptive values.
D. Patients with strong religious beliefs have a higher pain threshold.
E. Patients with strong religious may be strengthened by their illness.

59.5 Advance directives

A. are legally binding in all 50 states
B. include living wills
C. include health care proxies
D. include DNR and DNI
E. all of the above

59.6 When communicating with a severely ill child, all of the following are true *except*

A. The doctor must let the ill child know they will never be abandoned.
B. Parents may tell the child about their illness.
C. The physician may tell the child that he or she is going to die.
D. A doctor may sedate the child to limit anxiety about bad news.
E. The physician must clarify what the child already knows about their illness.

59.7 Which of the following limits anxiety in terminally ill children?

A. Adequate relief of physical symptoms
B. Consistent contact with parents
C. Child-friendly hospital environment
D. Avoiding prolonged separation
E. All of the above

59.8 What percentage of cancer patients are said to suffer from excruciating pain if left untreated?

A. 10 percent
B. 20 percent
C. 50 percent
D. 75 percent
E. 90 percent

59.9 Adequate palliative pain control should be sought in all of the following conditions *except*

A. AIDS
B. Advanced multiple sclerosis
C. Pancreatic cancer
D. Coma
E. Metastatic melanoma

59.10 Which of the following statements regarding pain control is *true*?

A. Providing patients with medications as needed (PRN) is the best option.
B. Rescue doses of medications should not be made available.
C. Around the clock medication administration does not provide the best pain control.
D. Faster pain control is achieved with PRN doses.
E. Maintenance pain dosing allows for an early and preemptive response.

59.11 All of the following statements regarding pain and psychiatric illness are true *except*

A. Patients with a history of substance abuse should never be given opioids.
B. Treatment of pain can improve mental illness.
C. Treatment of mental illness can improve pain.
D. Patients with pain have higher incidences of depression.
E. Psychiatric patients' pain is often dismissed.

59.12 Mr. S is a 50-year-old male with newly diagnosed metastatic small cell lung cancer. He was noted by his family to be anxious, to the point of having panic symptoms when his wife would leave his bedside to attend to chores. He would start hyperventilating; would feel short of breath; would become restless and unable to concentrate on anything; and would be overwhelmed with morbid ruminations about his future. He was upset and felt guilty at having become overly dependent on his wife.

All of the following interventions would help this patient *except*

A. Relaxation and breathing exercises
B. Clonazepam
C. Psychoanalysis
D. Meditation
E. Fluoxetine

59.13 A psychiatric consultation was sought to evaluate depression in a 56-year-old male with pancreatic cancer. His severe back pain was being well-treated with morphine. The patient was noted by the inpatient staff to be more withdrawn, disengaged, and quiet, making poor eye contact and sleeping most of the day. On examination, the psychiatric consultant found the man to be difficult to arouse and to be mildly confused and disoriented. His speech was slow and his thought process disorganized. He admitted to intermittently experiencing visual hallucinations that he had been too embarrassed to report earlier to the nursing staff. The man was diagnosed with a hypoactive delirium secondary to opioid medications.

Which of the following is the most appropriate next step in his management?

A. Decrease dose of morphine
B. Decrease frequency of morphine
C. Discontinue morphine
D. Add an antipsychotic
E. Do nothing

59.14 When should the transition to palliative care be made?

A. At diagnosis of illness
B. At realization illness is not curable
C. When nearness of death is acknowledged
D. When the physician has no more options to consider
E. None of the above

59.15 Which of the following is a legitimate reason to withhold PCA opioid pain medications from children?

A. Possibility of addiction
B. Sedation
C. Injudicious use/Overmedication
D. Non-terminal disease
E. None of the above

Directions

Each group of questions below consists of lettered headings followed by a list of numbered phrases or statements. For each numbered phrase or statement, select the *one* lettered heading that is most closely associated with it. Each lettered heading may be selected once, more than once, or not at all.

Questions 59.16–59.21

A. Delusions
B. Fatigue or weakness
C. Dysphagia
D. Incontinence
E. Dyspnea or cough

59.16 Occurs in 80 percent of terminal lung cancer patients
59.17 May follow pelvic radiation
59.18 Common in end-state multiple sclerosis
59.19 Most common occurrence in terminal illness
59.20 Occurs in the majority of all terminal patients
59.21 Opioids may be of use

Questions 56.22–56.26

A. Euthanasia
B. Physician-assisted suicide
C. Both
D. Neither

59.22 Mercy killing
59.23 Physician withholds artificial life-sustaining measures
59.24 Physician deliberately intends to kill a patient to alleviate or prevent suffering
59.25 Imparting of information or means that enable a person to take his or her own life
59.26 Palliative care designed to alleviate the suffering of a dying patient

Questions 59.27–59.30

A. Somatic pain
B. Visceral pain
C. Neuropathic pain
D. Psychogenic pain
E. None of the above

59.27 Sense of pain in a limb that has been amputated
59.28 Diaphragmatic pain referred to the shoulder
59.29 Bone metastases
59.30 Somatization disorder

ANSWERS

59.1 The answer is E

All people are equal in the face of death, yet physicians are expected to put aside their personal reactions and to remain attentively focused on the care of any dying patient. There is evidence that doctors have more death anxiety than other professionals and may have become physicians to conquer that fear. In addition, long exposure to disease and death breeds anxiety, despite the appearance of familiarity. The practice of medicine requires and reinforces intellectual coping skills, teaches that disease must be conquered, and expects that doctors function effectively under any circumstance. However, confrontation with death arouses threatening emotions, the deepest being an inchoate fear that is so rapidly submerged that it is barely experienced, much less explored. Beyond that, *all health professionals are at risk for feeling frustrated, helpless, or defeated.* Lowered self-assurance is transmuted into rescue fantasies, cynicism, or anger. Hardest of all is the grief when a *familiar patient* dies, a pain they repeatedly steel themselves to control. Table 59.1 lists risk factors for the development of aversive reactions in physicians.

59.2 The answer is A

The most concrete causes of undertreatment are *lack of knowledge or resources.* Patients in pain require aggressive use of analgesics and doctors should not be intimidated by criticism about addicting patients. *Lack of communication between the doctor and patient, a patient with a high threshold for pain* and *overanxious doctors* are not concrete causes of undertreatment in patients. *Noncompliance* can be a source of undertreatment but not to the extent that lack of resources account for this phenomenon.

59.3 The answer is D

Opioids commonly cause delirium and hallucinosis. A frequent mechanism of psychotoxicity is the accumulation of drugs or

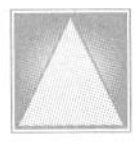

Table 59.1
Risk Factors for the Development of Aversive Reactions in Physicians

The physician:
- Identifies with the patient: looks, profession, age, character, etc.
- Identifies the patient with someone in his or her own life.
- Is currently dealing with a sick family member.
- Is recently bereaved or dealing with unresolved loss or grief issues.
- Feels professionally insecure.
- Is fearful of death and disability.
- Is unconsciously reflecting feelings felt or expressed by the patient or family.
- Cannot tolerate high and protracted levels of ambiguity or uncertainty.
- Carries a psychiatric diagnosis, such as depression or substance abuse.

Adapted from Meier DE, Back AL, Morris RS. The inner life of physicians and care of the seriously ill. *JAMA*. 2001;286:3007–3014.

metabolites whose duration of analgesia is shorter than their plasma half-lives (*morphine*, *levorphanol [Levo-Dromoran]*, and *methadone [Dolophine]*). Use of drugs like *hydromorphone (Dilaudid)*, with half-lives closer to their analgesic duration, can relieve the problem without loss of pain control. Cross-tolerance is incomplete between opiates; hence, several may be tried in any patient, with the dosage lowered when switching drugs. Table 59.2 lists opioid analgesics used in the management of pain.

59.4 The answer is D

Patients with a well-elaborated faith, especially one that includes a reunion with God in the afterlife, *tend to do better at the end.* Some patients *may experience illness as a test of their faith*, *may view suffering as having redemptive value*, and others *gain strength from the belief* that God will not send them more than they can handle. However, they also often ask "why me?" and struggle with anger, a sense of betrayal or abandonment, disappointment, self-imposed guilt, and a loss of faith that leaves them truly desolate. Patients with strong religious beliefs *do not have a higher pain threshold.*

59.5 The answer is E (all)

Advance directives are wishes and choices about medical intervention when the patient's condition is considered to be terminal. *Advance directives are legally binding in all 50 states.* There are three types:

1. *Living Will.* A patient who is mentally competent gives specific instructions that doctors must follow when he or she is unable to communicate with them because of illness. They may include rejection of (1) feeding tubes, (2) artificial airways, or (3) any other measures to prolong life.
2. *Health Care Proxy.* Also known as durable power of attorney, the health care proxy gives another person the power to make medical decisions if the patient is unable to do so. That person, also known as the surrogate, is empowered to make

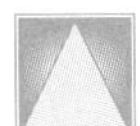

Table 59.2
Opioid Analgesics for Management of Pain

Drug and Equianalgesic Dose Relative Potency	Dose (mg IM or oral)	Plasma Half-Life (hr)[a]	Starting Oral Dose[b] (mg)	Available Commercial Preparations
Morphine	10 IM 60 oral	3–4	30–60	Oral: tablet, liquid, slow-release tablet Rectal: 5–30 mg Injectable: SC, IM, IV, epidural, intrathecal
Hydromorphone	1.5 IM 7.5 oral	2–3	2–18	Oral: tablets: 1, 2, 4 mg Injectable: SC, IM, IV 2 mg/mL, 3 mg/mL, and 10 mg/mL
Methadone	10 IM 20 oral	12–24	5–10	Oral: tablets, liquid Injectable: SC, IM, IV
Levorphanol	2 IM 4 oral	12–16	2–4	Oral: tablets Injectable: SC, IM, IV
Oxymorphone	1 IM	2–3	NA	Rectal: 10 mg Injectable: SC, IM, IV
Heroin	5 IM 60 oral	3–4	NA	NA
Meperidine	75 IM 300 oral	3–4 (normeperidine 12–16)	75	Oral: tablets Injectable: SC, IM, IV
Codeine	130 oral 200 oral	3–4	60	Oral: tablets and combination with acetylsalicylic acid, acetaminophen, liquid
Oxycodone[c]	15 oral 30 oral	—	5	Oral: tablets, liquid, oral formulation in combination with acetaminophen (tablet and liquid) and aspirin (tablet)

[a]The time of peak analgesia in nontolerant patients ranges from ½ hour to 1 hour, and the duration from 4 to 6 hours. The peak analgesic effect is delayed and the duration is prolonged after oral administration.
[b]Recommended starting IM doses; the optimal dose for each patient is determined by titration, and the maximal dose is limited by adverse effects.
[c]A long-acting sustained-release form of oxycodone (Oxycontin) has been abused by drug addicts and its use has been criticized because of this: however, it is a very useful preparation available in 10-, 20-, 40-, and 160-mg doses that need to be taken once every 12 hours. It is used as a maintenance therapy for severe persistent pain.
Adapted from Foley K. Management of cancer pain. In: DeVita VT, Hellman S, Rosenberg SA, eds. *Cancer: Principles and Practice of Oncology*. 4th ed. Philadelphia: JB Lippincott: 1993;936.

all decisions about terminal care based upon what he or she thinks the patient would have wanted.

3. *DNR and DNI.* These are orders that prohibit doctors from attempting to resuscitate—do not resuscitate (DNR)—or intubate—do not intubate (DNI)—the patient who is in extremis. DNR and DNI orders are made by the patient who is competent to do so. They can be made part of the living will or expressed by the health care proxy.

59.6 The answer is D

The basis for effective communication with a child is a trusting relationship with the physician and other caregivers. Children quickly learn in whom they can trust and confide. Whether or not a particular child should be told about his or her prognosis is not a simple matter. Parental wishes must be considered. Some parents do not want the child to be told that he or she is going to die, whereas other families do. It is useful to discuss with parents how they would respond if the child asked them about possibly dying. If the family has decided that they want their child to be fully informed, one individual should be selected to talk to the child, and all other caregivers, including parents, physicians, and nursing staff, should be instructed to give the same message. Inconsistent explanations can be confusing and even emotionally crippling to a child.

Some families want the physician to give the child the news, so as to protect the parent–child dynamic by not bearing bad news. When the child asks a question about his or her death, it is *important to clarify what the child already knows* and the reasons behind the question, because they are often different from what the adults expect. Some children are responding to the anxiety and grief projected by the parents; others are preoccupied with pain, discomfort, mutilation, abandonment, and loneliness. The child should be given ample time and opportunity to express his or her concerns, and any frightening misconceptions should be clarified. Even when the child is told that the illness is fatal, he or she should be comforted and reassured that the physicians will do everything possible to keep him or her comfortable and that *he or she will always be loved and cared for and never abandoned. Sedation* is not used when communicating with a child about his or her illness.

59.7 The answer is E (all)

Anxiety in the face of death is ubiquitous. It may stem from physiological issues such as intractable pain, compromised respiratory state, or medications, as well as from psychological issues such as separation from parents, unfamiliarity of the hospital environment, and fear of death itself. Generally, interventions aimed at the etiology of the anxiety are most effective. Adequate relief of physical symptoms, especially pain and respiratory distress, can significantly allay anxiety. *Ensuring consistent contact with parents, avoiding prolonged separation, addressing the emotional states of caregivers, and making the hospital milieu more child-friendly* goes a long way toward reducing the child's fears and anxieties.

59.8 The answer is B

Pain is common in dying patients. In cancer, the overall incidence of 51 percent of patients who experience pain rises to 74 percent in advanced disease, of which 40 to 50 percent is said to be moderate to severe, *and 20 to 30 percent* is said to be excruciating if untreated. In the hands of a skilled physician, adequate relief should be obtainable in the majority of cases, but the significant side effects often associated with pain control should also be considered. Many of them can be corrected or minimized, but patient and physician must decide together what symptom or side effect is most acceptable.

59.9 The answer is D

Adequate pain control is an important component of palliative care. Pain is a component of all of the following conditions: *AIDS, advanced multiple sclerosis, pancreatic cancer,* and, *metastatic melanoma.* Pain is not a component in *patients who slip into coma.* People in coma may well react to pain by moving, or even groaning, but most often have no memory of pain. In *cancer,* the overall pain incidence of 51 percent rises to 74 percent in advanced disease. Pain is also frequent in *acquired immune deficiency syndrome (AIDS)* and *advanced multiple sclerosis (MS)* and can be expected in almost any advancing illness. Because there are side effects associated with pain medications, patient and physician must decide together what symptom or side effect is most acceptable. The psychiatrist has a special role to play, because psychological symptoms are intimately connected to the experience of pain.

59.10 The answer is E

The need for regular by-the-clock administration of pain medications, as opposed to as needed (PRN) administration, cannot be overemphasized. It may be counterintuitive, but a *maintenance schedule achieves faster and better pain control* with a smaller total dose. *PRN orders do not allow for an early or preemptive response.* Patients often wait until pain is significant before calling for medication and then wait again for it to be given, during which time increasing pain is worsened by anxiety and growing resentment. Patients ring repeatedly, often annoying genuinely overburdened nurses. *Rescue doses should be available for breakthrough pain,* and their repeated use should signal the need to raise the maintenance dose.

59.11 The answer is A

Patients with pain have a significantly higher incidence of depression and anxiety. It has been suggested that (1) chronic pain may be a depressive equivalent, (2) pain may cause psychiatric syndromes, and (3) pain may coexist with psychopathology in vulnerable subjects. *Because emotional reactions are a consequence of and a contribution to pain, treatment of one improves the other.* In the face of advanced disease, the role of personality factors, affective states, and environment becomes less significant, so the psychiatric consultant should avoid psychiatric diagnoses that may minimize the patient's complaints in the eyes of others. Patients with psychopathology are more difficult to evaluate, and *their complaints are more easily dismissed*; hence, the consultant must help the staff to treat their pain as aggressively as that of other patients. The use of opiates in chronic pain is still controversial, *even with patients who have a history of substance abuse.* With or without controversy, there is no justification for withholding them in a patient with a predictably limited future, even one that may extend over many months.

59.12 The answer is C

Anxious patients are often helped by supportive therapy, cognitive-behavioral techniques, and complementary modalities, such as *deep relaxation, meditation, and adapted yoga.* There are several classes of effective antianxiety medications that can and should be used even in the presence of hepatic or renal impairment, given careful drug selection, dosage adaptation, and ongoing monitoring. *Benzodiazepines (such as clonazepam)* are effective anxiolytics. Their action is immediate and, with careful dosage titration, can almost always be of benefit. They must be chosen with the patient's hepatic function in mind. Habituation can require dosage escalation of all benzodiazepines, but this is acceptable if the drug is improving the patient's quality of life. Several antidepressants, such as *fluoxetine* (Prozac), are also known to have antianxiety effects, although these are less immediate in action. Antipsychotics are also frequently used, because mild confusional states are common, and they are associated with anxiety. *Psychoanalysis would not be useful for the relief of this man's symptoms in the short-term.*

59.13 The answer is D

Patients frequently experience some disorientation, impaired memory, and concentration loss as they become increasingly ill. *Hypoactive delirium* is a subcategory of delirium with a clinical picture that is different from the recognized hyperactive, hallucinatory state. The patient is hypoactive and withdrawn, with varying levels of somnolence and unresponsiveness. These quiet, undemanding patients do not present any management problems; hence, the diagnosis of a reversible condition is often overlooked, and it goes untreated. Hypoactive delirium should be diagnosed and treated as aggressively as hyperactive delirium. Antipsychotics alone can be effective in controlling symptoms when cognitive impairment and early delirium are present. The weight gain and type II diabetes seen in chronic psychiatric patients treated with antipsychotics are not a problem here, but dyskinesias, akathisia, tremors, parkinsonian rigidity, and, rarely, tardive dyskinesia occur. Benzodiazepines, given alone, worsen delirium and are contraindicated, but they are useful adjuncts to antipsychotic drugs, in which cases they provide sedation for persistently agitated patients. *Adding an antipsychotic is the best option in this case*, as this accomplishes treatment of his delirium without needing to decrease his much needed pain medications.

59.14 The answer is C

The transition to palliative care is not always clear. As soon as a diagnosis of an incurable disease is made, cure is no longer the goal of care. However, if death is distant, or even if some life extension can still be obtained, patient and family focus on this positive goal. The physician is under no illusion about the future but has the delicate task of promoting short-term gains without obliterating the awareness of what lies ahead. Only when the *nearness of death is acknowledged* can thoughtful decisions be made about palliative care.

59.15 The answer is E

Pain assessment in children is more complicated than in adults. Children who lack verbal skills may not be able to communicate pain to caregivers. Yet, with the use of appropriate rating scales, children can be reliable reporters. Most parents recognize their child's pain and are eager to see it relieved. But some parents worry about *addiction*, and others do not like the *sedation and especially the loss of relatedness* that may result from the use of opiates. Some may resist the use of patient-controlled analgesia (PCA) because they fear the child will *overmedicate* him- or herself. Yet, one study of patient-controlled epidural analgesia versus continuous epidural analgesia in children old enough to understand the technique showed significantly diminished use of opioids with the PCA. Family education around these issues is important, but often a consultant must ease the parents into a realization of how much their reactions are a way of avoiding the truth of their child's condition. Optimal pain management should never be withheld from a child due to *non-terminal disease*, just as in adult pain management.

Answers 59.16–56.21

59.16 The answer is E

59.17 The answer is D

59.18 The answer is C

59.19 The answer is B

59.20 The answer is A

59.21 The answer is E

Symptom management is an area of high priority in palliative care. Patients are often more concerned about the day-to-day distress of their symptoms than they are about their impending death, which may not be as real to them. Table 59.3 lists common end-of-life symptoms. A comprehensive approach to palliation involves attending to end-of-life symptoms as well as to pain. Sources of distress include psychiatric symptoms (e.g., severe anxiety) and physical symptoms (e.g., nausea). *Dyspnea or cough* can occur in 80 percent of terminal lung cancer patients and may be responsive to opioid treatment. *Incontinence* not uncommonly follows pelvic radiation. *Dysphagia* is common in end-state multiple sclerosis, while *fatigue or weakness* is the most common occurrence in all terminal illness. Psychiatric symptoms are frequent in terminal patients, in particular *delusions* of various types.

Answers 59.22–59.26

56.22 The answer is A

56.23 The answer is A

56.24 The answer is A

56.25 The answer is B

56.26 The answer is D

Euthanasia is defined as a physician's deliberate act to cause a patient's death by directly administering a lethal dose of medication or another agent. Because such patients are deemed by

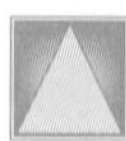

Table 59.3
Common End-of-Life Symptoms/Signs

Symptom/Sign	Comments
Delusions	Occur in 90% of all terminal patients; can be reversed if cause is treatable, e.g., pain, medication; respond to antipsychotic medication
Fatigue or weakness	Most common occurrence in terminal illness; psychostimulants can be used for short-term relief
Dysphagia	Common in neurological disease end states, e.g., multiple sclerosis, amyotrophic lateral sclerosis
Incontinence	May follow pelvic radiation, which can produce fistulas; use indwelling or condom catheter
Dyspnea or cough	Produces severe anxiety with fear of suffocation; occurs in 80% of terminal lung cancer patients; opioids, bronchodilators of use
Nausea or vomiting	Adverse effect of radiation and chemotherapy; antiemetics, e.g., metoclopramide, prochlorperazine, of use; marijuana cigarettes of use in selected patients
Anorexia	All terminal disease states are associated with cachexia secondary to anorexia and dehydration; feeding tubes do not prevent aspiration
Loss of skin integrity	Decubiti most common on weight-bearing areas, e.g., hips, sacrum, outer ankle; important to turn body frequently; elbow and hip pads of use
Anxiety or depression	Psychological factors, e.g., fear of death, abandonment; physiological factors, e.g., pain, hypoxia; antianxiety and antidepressant medication of use; opioids have strong antianxiety effects

From Mitka M. Suggestions for help when the end is near. *JAMA* 2000; 284:2441; adapted from National Coalition on Health Care (NCHC) and the Institute for Health Care Improvement (IHI). *Promises to Keep: Changing the Way We Provide Care at the End of Life,* release, October 12, 2000, with permission.

the treating physician to be hopelessly ill or injured, euthanasia has been called *mercy killing.*

On the basis of the doctor's action and the patient's condition, several types of euthanasia have been described: *active euthanasia,* in which *a physician deliberately intends to kill a patient to alleviate or prevent uncontrollable suffering; passive euthanasia,* in which *a physician withholds artificial life-sustaining measures; voluntary euthanasia,* in which the person who is to die is competent to give consent and does so; *and involuntary euthanasia,* in which the person who is to die is incompetent or incapable of giving consent.

Suicide is a deliberate taking of a person's own life. *Assisted suicide* is the *imparting of information or means that enable such an act* to take place. When the assistance is provided by a physician, the suicide is physician assisted. Assisted suicide and euthanasia should not be confused with *palliative care designed to alleviate the suffering of dying patients.* Palliative care includes giving pain relief and emotional, social, and spiritual support, as well as psychiatric care, if indicated. The intent of palliative care is to relieve pain and suffering, not to end a patient's life, even though death may result from palliative care.

In a survey of physicians in Oregon (the only U.S. state at the time of this writing where assisted suicide is legal), 5 percent of 2,649 physicians reported that they had received one or more requests for lethal prescriptions between late 1997 and early 1999. Most patients in question had cancer and a life expectancy of less than 6 months.

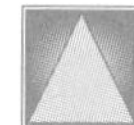

Table 59.4
Types of Pain

Somatic pain	Usually, but not always, constant, aching, gnawing, and well localized: for example, bone metastases
Visceral pain	Usually, but not always, constant, deep, squeezing, and poorly localized, with possible cutaneous referral: for example, pleural effusion leading to (1) deep chest pain and (2) diaphragmatic irritation referred to shoulder
Neuropathic pain	Burning dysesthetic pain with shock-like paroxysms associated with direct damage to peripheral receptors, afferent fibers, or the central nervous system leading to loss of central inhibitory modulation and spontaneous firing: for example, phantom limb pain; can involve sympathetic somatic afferents
Psychogenic pain	Variable characteristics, secondary to psychological factors in the absence of medical factors: vanishingly rare as a pure phenomenon in patients with advanced conditions, in which pain is often present, but often is an additional factor in the presence of organic pain

Answers 59.27–59.30

59.27 The answer is C

59.28 The answer is B

59.29 The answer is A

59.30 The answer is D

Dying patients are subject to several different kinds of pain, summarized in Table 59.4. The distinctions are important because they call for different treatment strategies. Phantom limb syndrome (*pain in an amputated limb*) is an example of *neuropathic pain. Diaphragmatic pain referred to the shoulder* is an example of *visceral pain. Somatic pain* is exemplified by the pain of *bone metastases. Psychogenic pain* is experienced in *somatization disorder.*

60 Forensic Psychiatry

Forensic psychiatry is the branch of medicine that deals with disorders of the mind and their relation to legal principles. The word forensic means belonging to the courts of law. At various stages in their historical development, psychiatry and the law have converged. Today, the two disciplines often intersect, especially when dealing with the criminal who, by violating the rules of society secondary to mental disorder, adversely affects the functioning of the community. Traditionally, the psychiatrist's efforts help explain the causes and, through prevention and treatment, reduce the self-destructive elements of harmful behavior. The lawyer, as the agent of society, is concerned that the social deviant is a potential threat to the safety and security of other persons. Both psychiatry and the law seek to implement their respective goals through the application of pragmatic techniques based on empirical observations.

Psychiatrists can act as either witnesses of fact or expert witnesses. As a witness of fact, a psychiatrist is acting as an ordinary witness, someone who has observed something and is being called to describe it in open court. This can include simply reading portions of a medical record into the legal record, but does not include expressing opinions or reporting others' statements. An expert witness is one who is accepted by the court and by advocates of both sides of the case as qualified to perform expert functions, and whose qualifications may include education, publications, and board certifications. Expert witnesses may render opinions, for example, that a patient meets the legal criteria for a guardian appointment. Psychiatrists often act as expert witnesses and may be hired by the defense or prosecution to provide opinions. This may lead to the common situation in which two psychiatrists representing two different sides provide diametrically opposed opinions about the case under dispute. The result can be confusion both on the parts of juries and the public about the value of psychiatric testimony, as well as cynicism and disillusionment. Many experts in forensic psychiatry believe that this problem could be minimized if the testifying psychiatrists were appointed by, and reported only to, the court.

The student should study the questions and answers below for a useful review of all of these topics.

HELPFUL HINTS

The student should be able to define each of these terms and know each of these cases.

- abandonment
- *actus reus*
- alliance threat
- antisocial behavior
- battery
- Judge David Bazelon
- civil commitment
- classical tort
- competence to inform
- competency
- confidentiality
- consent form
- conservator
- court-mandated evaluation
- credibility of witnesses
- culpability
- custody
- disclose to safeguard
- discriminate disclosure
- documentation
- Durham rule
- duty to warn
- emancipated minor
- emergency exception
- forced confinement
- the four Ds
- Gault decision
- going the extra mile
- *habeas corpus*
- hearsay
- informal admission
- informed consent
- insanity defense
- involuntary admission
- irresistible impulse
- judgment
- leading questions
- malpractice
- mature minor rule
- medical expert
- *mens rea*
- mental-health information service
- M'Naghten rule
- model penal code
- *O'Connor v Donaldson*
- *parens patriae*
- peonage
- plea bargaining
- pretrial conference
- probationary status
- right to treatment
- right-wrong test
- rules of evidence
- seclusion and restraint
- state training school standards
- Thomas Szasz
- *Tarasoff v Regents of University of California* (I and II)
- task-specific competence
- temporary admission
- testamentary capacity
- testator
- testimonial privilege
- voluntary admission
- *Wyatt v Stickney*

QUESTIONS

Directions

Each of the questions or incomplete statements below is followed by five suggested responses or completions. Select the *one* that is *best* in each case.

60.1 A tort is a

A. wrongdoing
B. writ
C. subpoena
D. judgment
E. good deed

60.2 An example of a tort is when a doctor

A. hugs a patient
B. dates a family member of a former patient
C. tells a patient that sex with him or her is therapeutic
D. maintains confidentiality in the face of a subpoena
E. lists the adverse effects of drugs when prescribing

60.3 Psychiatrists can be sued for

A. battery
B. invasion of privacy
C. misrepresentation
D. false imprisonment
E. all of the above

60.4 The most frequent issue involving lawsuits against psychiatrists is

A. suicide
B. improper use of restraints
C. sexual involvement
D. drug reactions
E. violence

60.5 Durable Power of Attorney

A. is an attorney whose main expertise is psychiatric malpractice cases
B. is power which permits the patient to have visitation rights
C. is a document that permits the doctor to breach confidentiality
D. is a document that permits persons to make provisions for their decision-making capacity
E. has a limited duration of time

60.6 Involuntary termination of treatment of a patient by a therapist

A. may result in a malpractice claim of abandonment
B. cannot be done during a patient emergency
C. requires careful documentation
D. should include transfer of services to others
E. all of the above

60.7 A person considered competent to be executed

A. must be aware of the punishment
B. must know its purpose
C. may come to whatever peace is appropriate with religious beliefs
D. might recall forgotten details of the events
E. all of the above

60.8 Pick the best answer regarding *Dusky v United States*:

A. Harmless mental patients cannot be confined against their wills without treatment if they can survive outside.
B. An involuntary patient who is not receiving treatment has a constitutional right to be discharged.
C. A test of competence was approved to see if a criminal defendant can rationally consult with a lawyer and has a factual (and rational) understanding of the proceedings against him or her.
D. Civilly committed persons have a constitutional right to adequate treatment.
E. A clinician must notify the intended victim(s) when there is an imminent threat posed by his or her patient.

60.9 In a child-custody dispute, which of the following is *not true*?

A. A natural parent has the inherent right to be named custodial parent.
B. The best interest of the mother may be served by naming her as the custodial parent.
C. More fathers are asserting custodial claims.
D. Courts presume that a child is best served by maternal custody when the mother is a good and fit parent.
E. In 5 percent of all cases, fathers are named the custodians.

60.10 Confidential communications can be shared with which of the following *without* the patient's consent?

A. A medical or psychiatric consultant
B. The patient's family
C. The patient's attorney
D. The patient's previous therapist
E. An insurer of the patient

60.11 Product rule is concerned with

A. testimonial privilege
B. involuntary admission
C. criminal responsibility
D. competency to stand trial
E. all of the above

60.12 Negligent prescription practices may include

A. prescribing the wrong dosages
B. unreasonable mixing of drugs
C. failure to disclose side effects

D. poor hand writing
E. all of the above

60.13 The Gault decision applies to

A. minors
B. *habeas corpus*
C. informed consent
D. battery
E. none of the above

60.14 Situations in which there is an obligation on the part of the physician to report to authorities information that may be confidential include

A. suspected child abuse
B. the case of a patient who will probably commit murder and can only be stopped by notification of police
C. the case of a patient who will probably commit suicide and can only be stopped by notification of police
D. the case of a patient who has potentially life-threatening responsibilities (for example, airline pilot) and who shows marked impairment of judgment
E. all of the above

60.15 Of the following, which is the *least* common cause of malpractice claims against psychiatrists by patients?

A. suicide attempts
B. improper use of restraints
C. failure to treat psychosis
D. sexual involvement
E. substance dependence

60.16 Which of the following is *not* one of the basic elements of the insanity defense?

A. Presence of a mental disorder
B. Presence of a defect of reason
C. Finding of incompetence to stand trial
D. Lack of knowledge of the nature of the act
E. Incapacity to refrain from the act

60.17 A 43-year-old prisoner is found to have major depressive disorder. The correctional psychiatrist wants to start him on antidepressant therapy due to the severity of his disease. He was very often in solitary confinement for violent behavior with correctional staff. The prisoner refuses to take any medications, stating he doesn't want to complicate his life any more by having to take drugs everyday. Correctional officers tell you it would be a security risk to have this prisoner out of his cell every day for treatment anyway.

What is the most appropriate next step in his management?

A. Don't give the prisoner antidepressants, as he has the right to refuse.
B. Don't give the prisoner antidepressants, as it is a security risk.
C. Don't give the prisoner antidepressants, as it is not a medical emergency.
D. Give the prisoner antidepressants, as he does not have the right to refuse.
E. Do nothing, and observe the prisoner for worsening symptoms.

60.18 Which of the following statements regarding juvenile detention centers is *true*?

A. Suicide in juvenile detention centers occur 4 times as often as in the general population.
B. Suicide prevention guidelines are strictly enforced in juvenile detention centers.
C. Prevalence of mental illness in detention centers is extensively researched.
D. Juvenile detention centers are long-term facilities for juveniles convicted of a crime.
E. More than 80 percent of incarcerated boys meet the criteria for PTSD.

60.19 A 30-year-old white woman was admitted to a local hospital because of cocaine abuse and major depression with suicidal ideation. She had been referred to the hospital after being arrested for cocaine use. She had a history of bipolar disorder since childhood.

Which of the following is the most appropriate discharge plan for this patient?

A. Discharge to local jail
B. Discharge to home
C. Discharge to care of her family
D. Discharge to psychiatric ward within a correctional facility
E. Discharge to substance abuse detoxification center

60.20 In the case above, the patient cut her wrists four days later. The most appropriate next step is

A. Dismiss this act as it is manipulative
B. Treat her as she has documented mental illness
C. Continue to withhold psychiatric medications
D. Continue one-on-one suicidal watch
E. Complete examination by a mental health professional

60.21 In the case above, two days later, her family succeeded in obtaining a court order for the patient to get medication for her psychiatric illness. Which medication should this patient be given at this time?

A. Haloperidol
B. Imipramine
C. Lorazepam
D. Carbamazepine
E. Lithium

60.22 A 42-year-old, single, male patient committed suicide while on a 4-hour therapeutic pass from the hospital before anticipated discharge. The patient was hospitalized with a diagnosis of major depression, single episode, and suicidal ideation. The patient steadfastly denied suicidal thoughts or impulses after admission. He experienced moderate to severe depression, anhedonia, global insomnia, hopelessness, agitation, and loss of appetite. The patient signed a suicide prevention contract, promising to inform the psychiatrist immediately of any suicidal ideation or impulses. After antidepressant treatment was started, the patient's energy level improved. The man's family sued the psychiatrist for wrongful death. The expert found no evidence in the psychiatric record that a formal suicide risk assessment was conducted before the pass was issued. During the trial, the psychiatrist testified that he did a formal suicide risk assessment, but that it was an oversight that he did not record it.

Which of the following is the most likely outcome of a trial under these circumstances?

A. The psychiatrist is not liable as a formal assessment of suicide risk was done.
B. The psychiatrist is not liable as adequate medical treatment was started.
C. The psychiatrist is not liable as the patient contracted for safety.
D. The psychiatrist is liable since a formal assessment of suicide risk was not documented.
E. The psychiatrist is liable as antidepressant therapy is known to increase risk for suicide.

60.23 A 45-year-old male has a documented history of paranoid schizophrenia. Upon returning home from work one day, he finds his wife in bed with another man. He immediately grabs a butcher knife and kills both his wife and her lover. He then systematically attempts to dispose of the bodies, but is caught in the act.

What is the most likely outcome of a trial under these circumstances?

A. Guilty charge
B. Not guilty by reason of insanity
C. Guilty by mens rea
D. Guilty by actus reus
E. Not guilty by reason of diminished capacity

60.24 In the case above, which of the following is the most appropriate placement for this man?

A. Prison
B. Mental hospital
C. Home confinement
D. Jail facility
E. Local lockup

60.25 A 34-year-old mentally retarded woman is arrested for killing her mother. At her trial, neither the defense nor the prosecution puts the woman on the stand as her communication skills are poor, and she is never fully evaluated by a psychiatrist before or during the trial. She is found guilty of murdering her mother and is sent to prison. Her father, although devastated, tells a lawyer his daughter is severely mentally retarded and can not possibly be held responsible for the murder.

Which of the following is the lawyer most likely to claim to appeal the decision?

A. Automatism defense
B. Testimonial privilege
C. Habeas corpus
D. Parens patriae
E. Respondeat superior

60.26 If a patient threatens to harm another person

A. Psychiatrists in all states are required by law to perform some intervention to prevent the harm from occurring
B. Psychiatrists in all states are permitted by law to perform some intervention to prevent the harm from occurring
C. The duty to protect patients and endangered third parties should be considered a professional obligation and only secondarily a legal issue
D. The Tarasoff duty applies only in state in which there is a duty to warn and to protect
E. Psychiatrists cannot intervene as they must protect the confidentiality privilege

60.27 Incompetence

A. is determined by a clinician
B. is a global assessment of mental function
C. can be presumed if a patient is psychiatrically institutionalized
D. is rendered by virtue of a patient having a mental disability
E. refers to a court adjudication

Directions

Each group of questions below consists of lettered headings followed by a list of numbered phrases or statements. For each numbered phrase or statement, select the *one* lettered heading that is most closely associated with it. Each lettered heading may be selected once, more than once, or not at all.

Questions 60.28–60.31

A. Indications for seclusion and restraint
B. Contraindications to seclusion and restraint

60.28 Patient voluntarily requests
60.29 Prevent significant disruption to treatment program
60.30 Part of ongoing behavior therapy
60.31 For punishment

Questions 60.32–60.36

A. Irresistible impulse
B. M'Naghten rule
C. Model penal code
D. Durham rule
E. Diminished capacity

60.32 Known commonly as the right-wrong test

60.33 A person charged with a criminal offense is not responsible for an act if the act was committed under circumstances that the person was unable to resist because of mental disease

60.34 An accused is not criminally responsible if his or her unlawful act was the product of mental disease or mental defect.

60.35 As a result of mental disease or defect, the defendant lacked substantial capacity either to appreciate the criminality of his or her conduct or to conform the conduct to the requirement of the law.

60.36 The defendant suffered some impairment (usually but not always because of mental illness) sufficient to interfere with the ability to formulate a specific element of the particular crime charged.

Questions 60.37–60.41

A. *Rouse v Cameron*
B. *Wyatt v Stickney*
C. *O'Connor v Donaldson*
D. *The Myth of Mental Illness*
E. None of the above

60.37 Harmless mental patients cannot be confined against their wills.

60.38 Standards were established for staffing, nutrition, physical facilities, and treatment.

60.39 The purpose of involuntary hospitalization is treatment.

60.40 A patient who is not receiving treatment has a constitutional right to be discharged.

60.41 All forced confinements because of mental illness are unjust.

ANSWERS

60.1 The answer is A

A tort is any *wrongdoing* for which an action for damages may be brought.

A writ is a written court order directing a person to perform or refrain from performing a specific act.

A subpoena is a writ commanding a designated person upon whom it has been served to appear (as in court or before a congressional committee) under a penalty (as a charge of contempt) for failure to comply.

A judgment is a formal decision or determination on a matter or case by a court.

A good deed is obviously not a tort.

60.2 The answer is C

In a tort, wrongdoers are motivated by the intent to harm another person or should have realized that such harm is likely to result from their actions. For example, *telling a patient that sex with the therapist is therapeutic* perpetrates a fraud.

While *hugging a patient* and *dating a patient's family member* are both unethical, they are examples of boundary violations and not a tort. Various criminal law statutes have been used against psychiatrists who violate this ethical principle.

Privilege is the right to *maintain confidentiality in the face of a subpoena*. Privileged communications are statements made by certain persons within a relationship—such as husband–wife, priest–penitent, or doctor–patient—that the law protects from forced disclosure on the witness stand. *Listing the adverse effects of drugs when prescribing drugs* is an example of good medical practice and is not a tort.

60.3 The answer is E (all)

Psychiatrists, like other people, can be sued for anything. This includes *battery*, defined as the unlawful and unwanted touching or striking of one person by another, with the intention of bringing about a harmful or offensive contact. *Invasion of privacy*, defined as the intrusion into the personal life of another, without just cause, and can give the person whose privacy has been invaded a right to bring a lawsuit for damages against the person or entity that intruded. *Misrepresentation*, defined as a statement made by a party to a contract, that a thing relating to it is in fact in a particular way, when he knows it is not so. *False imprisonment*, defined as restraining another person without having the legal right to do so, is a misdemeanor and a tort.

60.4 The answer is A

Suicide and suicide attempts are the most frequent causes for lawsuits against psychiatrists; 50 percent of suicides lead to malpractice actions by relatives. The greatest degree of supervision (inpatient setting) is associated with the most culpability. The *use of restraints, drug reactions*, and *patients committing violence* are all potential causes of malpractice that can be forestalled with proper documentation of clinical decision making and informed consent. *Sexual involvement* with a patient is both illegal and unethical.

60.5 The answer is D

A modern development that *permits persons to make provisions for their own anticipated loss of decision-making capacity* is called a durable power of attorney. The document permits the advance selection of a substitute decision maker who can act without the necessity of court proceedings when the signatory becomes incompetent through illness, progressive dementia, or perhaps a relapse of bipolar I disorder. The term *durable* means that it continues forever and does *not have a limited duration of time*.

60.6 The answer is E (all)

A potential pitfall of involuntary discharge or termination is the *charge of abandonment*. Malpractice litigation is often associated with situations in which there are bad feelings and a bad outcome. Consultation and *careful documentation* are important safeguards. Charges of abandonment can be avoided by referring the patient to another hospital or therapist. Some *authorities recommend giving a patient three names* of therapists, clinics, or hospitals. *A patient's treatment cannot be terminated while in a state of emergency.* The emergency must be resolved (for example, by hospitalization in cases of dangerousness) before treatment can be terminated and the patient transferred.

60.7 The answer is E (all)

The requirement for competence to be executed rests on a few general principles. A person's awareness of what is happening is supposed to heighten the retributive element of the punishment. Punishment is meaningless unless the person *is aware* of it and *knows the punishment's purpose.* A competent person who is about to be executed is believed to be in the best position to *make whatever peace is appropriate with religious beliefs*, including confession and absolution. A competent person who is about to be executed preserves, until the end, the possibility (admittedly slight) of *recalling a forgotten detail* of the events or the crime which may prove exonerating.

60.8 The answer is C

The Supreme Court, in *Dusky v United States* (1960), approved a test of competence that seeks to *ascertain whether a criminal defendant "has sufficient present ability to consult with his lawyer* with a reasonable degree of rational understanding and whether he has a rational as well as factual understanding of the proceedings against him." According to the 1976 case of *O'Connor v Donaldson*, the Supreme Court ruled that *harmless mental patients cannot be confined against their wills without treatment* if they can survive outside. In 1966, the District of Columbia Court of Appeals ruled in *Rouse v Cameron* that an involuntary inpatient who is not receiving treatment has a constitutional *right to be discharged.* According to this decision, the purpose of involuntary hospitalization is treatment.

In *Wyatt v Stickney* (1971), it was decided that civilly committed patients have a constitutional right to receive *adequate treatment.* In Tarasoff I (the case of *Tarasoff v Regents of the University of California* in 1974), it was ruled that *a psychotherapist or physician who has reason to believe that a patient may injure or kill someone must notify* the potential victim, the patient's relatives or friends, or the authorities.

60.9 The answer is A

The action of a court in a child-custody dispute is now predicated on the child's best interests. The maxim reflects the idea that *a natural parent does not have an inherent right to be named a custodial parent*, but the presumption, although a bit eroded, remains in favor of the mother in the case of young children. As a rule, courts presume that the welfare of a child of tender years generally is best served by *maternal custody when the mother is a good and fit parent. The best interest of the mother may be served by naming her as the custodial parent*, because a mother may never resolve the effects of the loss of a child, but her best interest is not to be equated ipso facto with the best interest of the child.

More fathers are asserting custodial claims. In *about 5 percent of all cases, fathers are named custodians.* The movement supporting women's rights also is enhancing the chances of paternal custody. With more women going to work outside the home, the traditional rationale for maternal custody has less force today then it did in the past.

60.10 The answer is A

Confidentiality pertains to the premise that all information imparted to the physician by the patient should be held secret. However, sharing information with other staff members treating the patient, clinical supervisors, and *a medical or psychiatric consultant* does not require the patient's permission. Sharing patient information with the *patient's family*, the *patient's attorney*, the *patient's previous therapist*, or *an insurer of the patient* does require the patient's permission. Courts may compel disclosure of confidential material *(subpoena duces tecum).* In emergencies, limited information may be released, but after the emergency, the clinician should inform the patient.

60.11 The answer is C

In 1954, in the case of *Durham v United States,* a decision was made by Judge David Bazelon, a pioneering jurist in forensic psychiatry in the District of Columbia Court of Appeals, that resulted in the *product rule of criminal responsibility.* An accused is not criminally responsible if his or her unlawful act was the product of mental disease or defect. Judge Bazelon stated that the purpose of the rule was to get good and complete psychiatric testimony. He sought to break the criminal law out of the theoretical straitjacket of the M'Naghten test.

Testimonial privilege is the right to maintain secrecy or confidentiality in the face of a subpoena. The privilege belongs to the patient, not to the physician, and it is waivable by the patient. *Involuntary admission* involves the question of whether or not the patient is a danger to self or others, such as in the suicidal or homicidal patient. Because those individuals do not recognize their need for hospital care, application for admission to a hospital may be made by a relative or friend and is involuntary. *Competency to stand trial* refers to defendants being able to comprehend the nature and the object of the proceedings against them in order to consult with counsel as well as to assist in preparing the defense.

60.12 The answer is E (all)

Negligent prescription practices usually include *exceeding recommended dosages* and then failing to adjust the medication level to therapeutic levels, *unreasonable mixing of drugs, prescribing medication that is not indicated, prescribing too many drugs at one time*, and then failing to disclose medication effects. Although exceeding the recommended dosage may be considered negligent, if it must be done, it should be documented in the patients chart. Multiple psychotropic medications must be prescribed with special care because of the possible harmful interactions and adverse effects. Psychiatrists must explain the diagnosis, risks, and benefits of the drug. Informed consent should be obtained each time a medication is changed and a new drug is introduced. If patients are injured because they were not properly informed of the risks and consequences of taking a medication, sufficient grounds may exist for a malpractice action. Finally, *poor handwriting* and the misreading of the prescription by nurses or pharmacists is a major source of error.

60.13 The answer is A

The Gault decision applies to minors, those under the care of a parent or guardian and usually under age 18. In the case of minors, the parent or guardian is the person legally empowered to give consent to medical treatment. However, most states by statute list specific diseases or conditions that a minor may consent to have treated, such as venereal diseases, pregnancy, substance-related disorders, and contagious diseases. In an emergency, a physician may treat a minor without parental consent. The trend is to adopt the mature minor rule, allowing minors to consent to treatment under ordinary circumstances. As a result of the Gault decision, the juvenile must now be represented by counsel, be able to confront witnesses, and be given proper notice of any charges. Emancipated minors have the rights of adults when it can be demonstrated that they are living as adults with control over their own lives.

A writ of *habeas corpus* may be proclaimed on behalf of anyone who claims he or she is being deprived of liberty illegally. The legal procedure asks a court to decide whether hospitalization has been accomplished without due process of the law, and the petition must be heard by a court at once, regardless of the manner or form in which it is filed. Hospitals are obligated to submit those petitions to the court immediately. *Informed consent* is knowledge of the risks and alternatives of a treatment method and formal acceptance of treatment.

Under classical tort (a tort is a wrongful act) theory, an intentional touching to which one has given no consent is a *battery*. Thus, the administration of electroconvulsive therapy or chemotherapy, although it may be therapeutic, is a battery when done without consent. Indeed, any unauthorized touching outside of conventional social intercourse constitutes a battery. It is an offense to the dignity of the person, an invasion of the right of self-determination, for which punitive and actual damages may be imposed.

60.14 The answer is E (all)

In some situations—such as *suspected child abuse*—the physician must report to the authorities, as specifically required by law. According to the American Psychiatric Association (APA), confidentiality may be broken when the patient will *probably commit murder* and the act can only be stopped by notification of police, when the patient will *probably commit suicide* and the act can only be stopped by notification of police, or when a patient who has *potentially life-threatening responsibilities* (for example, an airline pilot) shows marked impairment of judgment.

60.15 The answer is D

Sexual involvement with patients accounts for 6 percent of malpractice claims against psychiatrists and is the *least common cause of malpractice litigation*. This fact does not, however, minimize its importance as a problem. (It should be noted that the short statute of limitations for this particular offense may well discourage patients from pursuing litigation because they have not had sufficient time to reach a point of emotional readiness.) Sexual intimacy with a patient is both illegal and unethical. There are also serious legal and ethical questions about a psychotherapist's dating or marrying a patient even after discharging the patient from therapy. Most psychiatrists believe in the adage "Once a patient, always a patient."

For other malpractice claims, the following figures are given: *failure to manage suicide attempts*, 21 percent; *improper use of restraints*, 7 percent; and *failure to treat psychosis*, 14 percent. *Substance dependence* accounts for about 10 percent of claims and refers to the patient's having developed a substance-related disorder as a result of a psychiatrist's not monitoring carefully the prescribing of potentially addicting drugs.

60.16 The answer is C

No precise, generally accepted definition of *legal insanity* exists. Tests of insanity have always been controversial and have undergone much modification and refinement over the years. The insanity defense standard has four basic elements:

1. Presence of a mental disorder
2. Presence of a defect of reason
3. A lack of knowledge of the nature or wrongfulness of the act
4. An incapacity to refrain from the act

The insanity defense is one of the most controversial issues in American jurisprudence. The presence of a mental disorder has remained the consistent core of the insanity defense; the other elements have varied in importance over time. *The finding of incompetence to stand trial* is unrelated to this defense. Defendants with mental impairments who are found competent to stand trial may still seek acquittal on the claim of insanity, alleging that they were not criminally responsible for their actions at the time the offense was committed. The term *insanity* is a legal construct, not a psychiatric diagnosis.

60.17 The answer is D

The law and ethical analysis of informed consent and refusal inside corrections are complicated. The legal rule is that inmates have the right to consent to care but do not necessarily have equally extensive rights to refuse care. Complicating this issue is the reality that distinguishing between a refusal of care and a possible denial of care is often difficult. An additional complication is the fact that other correctional staff may not want to offer appropriate psychiatric treatment for a variety of reasons (e.g., security risks, cost, deservedness). Simultaneously, inmates can be insistent and manipulative and sometimes seek care for inappropriate reasons. Despite these pressures from opposite poles, correctional psychiatric personnel *must ensure that patients get appropriate care*. Medical autonomy means that nonmedical personnel cannot overrule the professional judgment of correctional psychiatrists regarding their patients' needs. Medical autonomy means that only legitimate clinical decisions direct patient care, not patient wishes. Correctional psychiatrists should be neutral in nonmedical matters. Aligning with security staff costs them their rapport with their patients. Alternatively, being inmate advocates for non–health-related issues would cost them their rapport with their correctional coworkers.

60.18 The answer is A

Youth suicides in juvenile detention and correctional facilities have been shown to occur four times more often than youth suicide in the general population. Yet, 75 percent of the nation's confined juveniles are in facilities that *fail to conform to even the most basic suicide prevention guidelines*. Several studies note that *one-fourth (not 80 percent) of incarcerated boys and one-half of the incarcerated girls meet criteria for PTSD*. Juvenile detention centers *are short-term facilities that confine juveniles who are awaiting trial*, while juvenile confinement facilities are long-term facilities (such as residential treatment centers and training schools) for the confinement of juveniles convicted of a crime. *Mental illness in detention centers has not been extensively researched.*

60.19 The answer is D

The most appropriate placement for this patient is in a *psychiatric facility within a correctional facility*. Because she was arrested for cocaine use prior to her hospital referral, she still has charges pending against her and cannot be released to home or the care of her family. Although a substance abuse detoxification center may be helpful in the future, she first must have her legal situation dealt with. Discharge to a local jail is inappropriate in this case as well, as the local jail will not be able to adequately address her mental illness (major depression).

60.20 The answer is E

Because self-mutilation is hard to control, it is a serious challenge for correctional officials and psychiatric staff. When self-mutilation is not the product of a mental disorder, mental health professionals often deny admission to the mental health unit. This confuses correctional authorities who view such behavior as a sign of mental instability. It is essential to have clear protocols for self-mutilation when it is (1) a psychiatric symptom, (2) a manipulative gesture to escape a dangerous situation, and (3) an effort to manipulate the system for personal gain. This woman's documented history of major depressive disorder should alert correctional staff to the likelihood that cutting her wrists is a true suicide attempt. She should have a *complete evaluation by a psychiatrist* to determine the extent of her current symptoms. If this woman is indeed having an exacerbation of her symptoms of major depression, continuing to withhold medications and simply putting her on a one-on-one suicidal watch may not be enough and is neglectful. However, a thorough evaluation should precede any treatment.

60.21 The answer is A

Haloperidol is an appropriate treatment for this psychotic patient who is hearing voices telling her to cut her wrists. Acute psychosis, with significant risk for impulsive behavior such as suicide attempts, is effectively treated with Haldol. *Imipramine*, a tricyclic antidepressant, is lethal in overdose and should be prescribed carefully and not at all in high doses to actively suicidal patients. In a patient with a history of substance abuse, benzodiazepines such as *lorazepam* should be carefully prescribed. Benzodiazepines also work only by sedating, without addressing this patient's psychosis. *Carbamazepine* and *lithium* are mood stabilizers indicated for patients with bipolar disorder, not major depression.

60.22 The answer is D

The failure to adequately document events in the written clinical record is a major reason for lack of credibility to legal testimony. The psychiatrist in this case testified that he completed a formal assessment of suicide risk, but there is no way to prove this is true with no documentation. Although the patient was at a greater risk of suicide after administration of an antidepressant drug, the psychiatrist cannot be held liable for starting treatment with an antidepressant, the standard of care. It is also arguable that the psychiatrist had not placed total reliance on the suicide prevention contract but had used it appropriately to assess the working alliance with the patient, that is, the patient's willingness to work towards getting better. *There is an adage in legal circles that if it is not documented it was not done.*

60.23 The answer is A

To be found *not guilty by reason of insanity*, the defendant, as a result of a severe mental disease or defect, must be unable to appreciate the nature and quality or the wrongfulness of his acts. In making an insanity determination, the threshold issue is not the existence of a mental disease or defect per se but the lack of substantial capacity caused by it. In this case, the fact that the man tried to dispose of the bodies shows he was aware of the criminal act, negating any insanity plea. For conviction of any crime, a criminal state of mind (*mens rea*) must be accompanied by the commission of a prohibited act (*actus reus*). Both must be present for a guilty verdict, and neither has to do with mental illness. The physical act must be conscious and volitional for a person to be found guilty. The law also recognizes shades of mental impairment that can affect mens rea, but not necessarily to the extent of completely nullifying it. The concept of *diminished capacity* allows the defendant to introduce medical and psychological evidence that relates directly to the mens rea for the crime charged, without having to assert a defense of insanity. For example, in the crime of assault with the intent to kill, psychiatric testimony may be permitted to address whether the offender acted with the purpose of committing homicide at the time of the assault. Mental illness per se is not a defense and nothing in the case indicates this man did not intend to kill his wife and her lover.

60.24 The answer is B

What happens to a defendant after a judge or jury returns a finding of insanity depends on the crime committed, and on the state in which the trial takes place. Usually, those found "not guilty by reason of insanity" are confined for treatment in a *special hospital for severely mentally ill persons who have committed crimes*. After a period of time, the person may request a hearing to determine if he or she is no longer a danger to self or others or no longer mentally ill, and is therefore eligible to be released. Studies show that persons found not guilty by reason of insanity, on average, are held at least as long as—and often longer than—persons found guilty and sent to prison for similar crimes.

Jails are correctional facilities that confine individuals involved in the criminal justice system who are awaiting trial or serving short sentences for misdemeanors.

A *local lockup* may be a police precinct cell, a sheriff's office, or any other place including a correctional facility used to detain an arrested individual pending arraignment.

60.25 The answer is C

A writ of *habeas corpus* (literally, "you must have the body") is a legal procedure that asks a court to decide whether a patient has been hospitalized or imprisoned without due process of law. The writ tests only whether a prisoner has been accorded due process, not whether he is guilty. The *automatism* (or unconscious) defense recognizes that some criminal acts may be committed involuntarily. *Testimonial privilege* is the right of the patient to maintain secrecy or confidentiality in the face of a subpoena. *Parens patriae* is the doctrine that allows the state to intervene and act as a surrogate for those who are unable to care for themselves or may harm themselves. *Respondeat superior* is Latin for "let the master answer for the deed of the servant." This states a person high in the chain of command is responsible for the actions of those under his or her supervision.

60.26 The answer is C

The duty to protect patients and endangered third parties *should be considered primarily a professional and moral obligation, and only secondarily, a legal duty*. Most psychiatrists acted to protect their patients and threatened others from violence long before Tarasoff. *Psychiatrists should consider the Tarasoff duty to be a national standard of care, even if they practice in states that do not have a duty to warn and protect*. Indeed, not all states have duty to warn statutes, and so *there is no legal obligation necessarily in all states that permits or requires psychiatrists to prevent the harm from occurring. If a patient gives the psychiatrist sufficient reason to believe that a warning should be issued to the endangered third party, the confidentiality of the communication that gave rise to the warning may be lost.*

60.27 The answer is E

Incompetence is a broad concept that encompasses many different legal issues and contexts. *It refers to a court adjudication*, whereas incapacity indicates a functional inability determined by a clinician. It is a legal term that is applied to people who are considered by law not to be mentally capable of performing a particular act or assuming a particular role. Its adjudication is issue specific, if someone judged to be incompetent to do one thing is not automatically incompetent to do other things. *A lack of competency cannot be presumed from a person's treatment for mental illness or from institutionalization. Mental disability does not necessarily render a person incompetent or incompetent in all areas of functioning.*

Answers 60.28–60.31

60.28 The answer is A

60.29 The answer is A

60.30 The answer is A

60.31 The answer is B

Most states have enacted statutes that regulate the use of restraints, often specifying the circumstances in which restraints can be used—usually when a risk of harm to self or danger to others is imminent. Statutory regulation of the use of seclusion is much less common. About one-half of states have laws governing seclusion. Most states with laws regarding seclusion and restraint require some type of documentation of the usage. A number of courts and state statutes outline certain due-process procedures that must be followed before restraint or seclusion can be used for nonclinically indicated, disciplinary purposes. These include some form of notice, a hearing, and involvement of an impartial decision-maker.

The APA Task Force on the Psychiatric Uses of Seclusion and Restraint has developed guidelines for the appropriate use of seclusion and restraints, and the Joint Commission on Accreditation of Healthcare Organizations (JCAHO) has promulgated guidelines for hospitals regarding seclusion and restraint requirements. Professional opinion concerning the clinical uses of physical restraints and seclusion varies considerably among psychiatrists. Seclusion can be justified on both clinical and legal grounds for a variety of uses, unless precluded by state freedom from restraint and seclusion statutes.

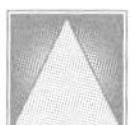

Table 60.1
Indications for Seclusion and Restraint

1. Prevent clear, imminent harm to the patient or others
2. *Prevent significant disruption to treatment program* or physical surroundings
3. Assist in treatment as *part of ongoing behavior therapy*
4. Decrease sensory overstimulation[a]
5. At *patient's voluntary reasonable request*

[a]Seclusion only.
Reprinted with permission from Simon RI. *Concise Guide to Psychiatry and the Law for Clinicians*. 2nd ed. Washington, DC: American Psychiatric Press; 1998.

Seclusion and restraint raise complex psychiatric legal issues and *have both indications and contraindications* (Tables 60.1 and 60.2). Further, seclusion and restraint have become increasingly regulated over the past decade.

Legal challenges to the use of restraints and seclusion have been brought on behalf of institutionalized mentally ill and mentally retarded persons. Typically, these lawsuits do not stand alone but are part of a challenge to a wide range of alleged abuses.

Generally, courts hold, or consent decrees provide, that restraints and seclusion be implemented only when a patient creates a risk of harm to self or others and no less-restrictive alternative is available. Additional restrictions include the following:

1. Restraint and seclusion can only be implemented by a written order from an appropriate medical official.
2. Orders are to be confined to specific, time-limited periods.
3. A patient's condition must be reviewed regularly and documented.
4. Any extension of an original order must be reviewed and reauthorized.

Answers 60.32–60.36

60.32 The answer is B

60.33 The answer is A

60.34 The answer is D

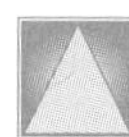

Table 60.2
Contraindications to Seclusion and Restraint

1. Extremely unstable medical and psychiatric conditions
2. Delirious or demented patients unable to tolerate decreased stimulation
3. Overtly suicidal patients
4. Patients with severe drug reactions, overdoses, or requiring close monitoring of drug dosages
5. *For punishment* or convenience of staff

60.35 The answer is C

60.36 The answer is E

The precedent for determining legal responsibility was established in the British courts in 1843. The *M'Naghten rule* is known commonly as the right-wrong test because the alleged perpetrator is not guilty, by reason of insanity, if he or she is unable to tell right from wrong due to a mental disease. In 1922, jurists in England reexamined the M'Naghten rule and suggested broadening the concept of insanity in criminal cases to include the concept of the *irresistible impulse*—that is, a person charged with a criminal offense is not responsible for an act if the act was committed under circumstances that the person was unable to resist because of mental disease. To most psychiatrists the law is unsatisfactory because it covers only a small group of those who are mentally ill. However, it was used successfully in Virginia in the 1994 case of *Virginia v Bobbitt*, in which the defendant was acquitted of malicious wounding. The wife had cut off her husband's penis after apparently enduring a prolonged period of sexual, physical, and emotional abuse.

In 1954 in the case of *Durham v United States*, a decision resulted in the product rule of criminal responsibility, or the *Durham rule*, which states that an accused is not criminally responsible if his or her unlawful act was the product of mental disease or mental defect. Judge Bazelon stated that the purpose of the rule was to get good and complete psychiatric testimony. In 1972, the Court of Appeals for the District of Columbia in *United States v Brawner* discarded the rule in favor of the American Law Institute's 1962 model penal code test of criminal responsibility.

In its *model penal code*, the American Law Institute (ALI) recommended the following test of criminal responsibility: (1) Persons are not responsible for criminal conduct if at the time of such conduct, as the result of mental disease or defect, they lacked substantial capacity either to appreciate the criminality of their conduct or to conform their conduct to the requirement of the law, and (2) the term "mental disease or defect" in this test does not include an abnormality manifested only by repeated criminal or otherwise antisocial conduct.

Other attempts at reform have included the defense of *diminished capacity*, which is based on the claim that the defendant suffered some impairment (usually but not always because of mental illness) sufficient to interfere with the ability to formulate a specific element of the particular crime charged. Hence, the defense finds its most common use with so-called specific-intent crimes, such as first-degree murder.

Answers 60.37–60.41

60.37 The answer is C

60.38 The answer is B

60.39 The answer is A

60.40 The answer is A

60.41 The answer is D

Various landmark legal cases have affected psychiatry and the law over the years. In the 1976 case of *O'Connor v Donaldson*, the U.S. Supreme Court ruled that *harmless mental patients cannot be confined against their will* without treatment if they can survive outside. According to the Court, a finding of mental illness alone cannot justify a state's confining persons in a hospital against their will; such patients must be considered dangerous to themselves or others before they are confined.

In 1971, in *Wyatt v Stickney* in Alabama Federal District Court, it was decided that persons civilly committed to a mental institution have a constitutional right to receive adequate care, and *standards were established for staffing, nutrition, physical facilities, and treatment*. In 1966, the District of Columbia Court of Appeals in *Rouse v Cameron* ruled that *the purpose of involuntary hospitalization is treatment* and that *a patient who is not receiving treatment has a constitutional right to be discharged* from the hospital.

In *The Myth of Mental Illness*, Thomas Szasz argued that the various psychiatric diagnoses are totally devoid of significance and that therefore *all forced confinements because of mental illness are unjust*. Szasz contended that psychiatrists have no place in the courts of law.

61 Ethics in Psychiatry

Ethics in psychiatry refers to the principles of conduct that govern the behavior of psychiatrists as well as other mental health professionals. Ethics as a discipline deals with what is good and what is bad, what is right and what is wrong, and moral duties, obligations, and responsibilities.

Psychiatrists routinely confront basic ethical issues, in particular through the imposing of involuntary treatments on patients against their wills. These issues highlight the profound ethical dilemmas between autonomy and beneficence that psychiatrists and their patients deal with continually. In other words, it is the potential—and common—conflict between the right of patients to self-determination and the duty of psychiatrists to act in the best interest of their patients. Beneficence refers to "the duty to do no harm," and autonomy to a patient's right to choose. It is easy to see how in psychiatry these concepts can be highly complex, leading to conflicting interpretations and opinions about appropriate care. Psychiatry has a less-than-illustrious history with regard to adequately safeguarding the rights of mentally ill patients, and this history has led to an extensive involvement of the legal system in all aspects of psychiatric involuntary care and decision making.

Major ethical theories underlie most of the ethical questions routinely faced by psychiatrists, and clinicians need to be aware of how these theories conceptualize the issues. These theories include utilitarian theory, which postulates that a fundamental obligation in decision making is to produce the greatest possible benefit to the greatest number of people. Utilitarian theory is most often the basis of large societal decisions about the allocation of services and resources. Autonomy theory postulates that the patient–doctor relationship is one between two equal parties, and that patients are self-governing, with a fundamental right to self-determination in medical and psychiatric decision making. Truth telling, confidentiality, informed consent, the right to refuse treatment, the right to die, limitations on the right of psychiatrists to involuntarily treat and hospitalize people, and sexual contact with patients are all examples of ethical concerns addressed by ethical theory.

The student should study the questions and answers below for a useful review of this topic.

HELPFUL HINTS

The student should be able to define each of these terms and know each of these cases.

- autonomy theory
- best-interests principle
- confidentiality
- *Cruzan v Missouri*
- decisional capacity
- duty of beneficence
- duty to protect
- individual paternalism
- informed consent
- *Planned Parenthood v Casey*
- *Principles of Medical Ethics,* with annotations
- especially applicable to psychiatry
- professional standards
- right to die
- right to health care
- *Roe v Wade*
- state paternalism
- substituted-judgment principle
- surrogate decision making
- *Tarasoff I and II*
- utilitarian theory

QUESTIONS

Directions

Each of the questions or incomplete statements below is followed by five suggested responses or completions. Select the *one* that is *best* in each case.

61.1 An autonomous choice is

A. made with informed consent of the patient
B. made by the family of the patient
C. made by the patient after coercion
D. made by the patient who is confused
E. None of the above

61.2 A boundary violation occurs in all of the following situations *except*

A. When the doctor accepts tickets to a football game
B. When the doctor hugs the patient after a session
C. When confidentiality is breached
D. When the doctor's needs are gratified at the expense of the patient

E. When the doctor has sexual relations with a former patient

61.3 Which of the following about confidentiality is *true*?

A. Confidentiality does not need to be maintained after that patient is deceased.
B. Confidentiality prevents the psychiatrist from releasing information about a patient to an insurance company.
C. Video-taped segments of a therapy session cannot be used at a workshop for professionals.
D. A physician is obligated to report a suspicion of child abuse in a state that requires such reporting.
E. Informing ones spouse of the identity of one's patient violates the ethical principle of confidentiality.

61.4 Choose the best answer about *Cruzan v Missouri Board of Health*:

A. All patients hold the right to have life support withdrawn.
B. Early-stage fetuses have no legal standing.
C. Only conscious patients can have life-sustaining treatment withdrawn.
D. All competent patients can refuse medical care.
E. None of the above

61.5 In the *Tarasoff* case

A. The principle of beneficence outweighed the principle of justice.
B. The principle of beneficence outweighed the principle of nonmaleficence.
C. The principle of justice outweighed the principle of nonmaleficence.
D. The principle of nonmaleficence outweighed the principle of justice.
E. None of the above

61.6 *Tarasoff II*

A. requires that therapists report a patient's fantasies of homicide
B. reinforces that a therapist has only the duty to warn
C. expands on the earlier ruling to include the duty to protect
D. states that usually the patient must be a danger both to a person and property
E. none of the above

Directions

The set of lettered headings below is followed by a list of numbered words or statements. For each numbered word or statement, select the *one* lettered heading most closely associated with it. Each lettered heading may be selected once, more than once, or not at all.

Questions 61.7–61.12

A. Yes
B. No

61.7 Sexual relations with a family member of a patient.
61.8 Discussing cases with spouse.
61.9 Confidentiality must be maintained after the death of a patient.
61.10 The psychiatrist can make a determination of suicide as a result of mental illness for insurance purposes solely from reading the patient's records.
61.11 Dating a patient 1 year after discharge is ethical.
61.12 The psychiatrist may divulge information about the patient if the patient desires.

Directions

The group of lettered headings below is followed by a list of numbered phrases. For each numbered phrase, select

A. if the item is associated with A only
B. if the item is associated with B only
C. if the item is associated with both A and B
D. if the item is associated with neither A nor B

Questions 61.13–61.17

A. Ethical dilemma
B. Ethical conflict

61.13 Preserving patient confidentiality versus protecting endangered third parties.
61.14 Patient–therapist sexual relations.
61.15 Choice between two ethically legitimate alternatives.
61.16 Compromise of an ethical principle, usually because of self-interest.
61.17 American Psychiatric Association (APA) may expel or suspend members from the organization.

Directions

The set of lettered headings below is followed by a list of numbered words or statements. For each numbered word or statement, select the *one* lettered heading most closely associated with it. Each lettered heading may be selected once, more than once, or not at all.

Questions 61.18–61.21

A. Nonmaleficence
B. Autonomy
C. Beneficence
D. Justice

61.18 The right of the patient to self-determination.
61.19 The duty of the physician to act in the best interest of the patient.
61.20 The duty of the physician to inflict no harm on the patient.
61.21 Refers to the changing social, political, religious and legal mores of the moment.

ANSWERS

61.1 The answer is A

The principle of patient autonomy has central importance and, conceptually, is in many ways coextensive with the legal concept of competence. A patient makes an autonomous choice by *giving informed consent* when that choice is (1) *intentional*, (2) *free of undue outside influence, and* (3) *made with rational understanding.* Usually, when patients respond to a choice by saying "yes," the desire to comply is assumed. However, that assumption may not be valid with a highly confused patient.

61.2 The answer is C

A *boundary* can be considered as crossing a line beyond which the patient is exploited. *It gratifies the doctor's needs at the expense of the patient.* The doctor is responsible for preserving the boundary and for ensuring that boundary crossings are held to a minimum and that exploitation does not occur.

The issue of whether sexual relations between an ex-patient and a therapist violate an ethical principle remains controversial. Proponents of the view "Once a patient always a patient" insist that any involvement with an ex-patient—even one that leads to marriage—should be prohibited. According to the American Medical Association's *Principles of Medical Ethics with Annotations Especially Applicable to Psychiatry*, *"Sexual activity with a current or former patient is unethical."* Because of that, *hugging a patient at the end of a session* would most likely fall into that category. Similarly, *accepting football tickets from a patient might be considered exploitative.* However, when confidentiality is breached it is not considered a boundary violation because it involves the direct relationship between the doctor and the patient, whereas confidentiality being breached involves a third party.

61.3 The answer is E

The medical profession overall is bound by rules of confidentiality, but these rules seem to apply especially to the field of psychiatry. Psychiatrists should never discuss their patients outside the office. Patients assume what they tell the psychiatrist stays inside the consulting room. *Merely informing a spouse of the identity of one's patient violates the ethical principles. Confidentiality survives even the death of one's patient* and is subsequently owned by the executor, not the psychiatrist. A confidence cannot be broken just because a patient died. *A psychiatrist can break a confidence to give information to an insurance company*, as long as it is limited to only that which is needed to process the insurance claim. *If informed, uncoerced consent has been obtained by the patient for segments of videotaped sessions to be used in conferences, these can be used.* Anonymity must be maintained and the patient must know the purpose of the videotape. *The suspicion of child abuse does not warrant a break of confidentiality.* The psychiatrist must make several assessments before deciding whether to report suspected abuse. One must consider if the abuse is ongoing, whether abuse is responsive to treatment, and whether reporting will causes potential harm. The safety of potential victims must be the top priority.

61.4 The answer is D

In *Cruzan v Missouri Board of Health*, the U.S. Supreme Court upheld *the right of a competent person* to have "a constitutionally protected liberty interest *in refusing* unwanted *medical treatment." The Court applied this principle to all patients, conscious or unconscious, who have made their wishes clearly known,* whether or not they ever regain consciousness. *Life support can be refused or withdrawn provided that the patient made his or her wishes known.* The *legal standing of fetuses relates to Roe v Wade,* not *Cruzan v Missouri.* Cruzan applies to both conscious and unconscious patients, provided that the latter have already made their wishes known. The U.S. Supreme Court permits each state to decide the standards it wishes to apply when asked to withhold or withdraw treatment from a person in a persistent vegetative state who has not previously stated his or her wishes on the subject.

61.5 The answer is E (none)

The Tarasoff case is an example of the legal system's attempt to solve a social problem—the need to safeguard life—by creating an ethical dilemma for the psychiatrist. This case, which began as a civil lawsuit, ended up with the California Supreme Court ruling that a psychotherapist has a duty to warn and protect a potential victim of a potentially dangerous patient. *The court proclaimed that the principles of justice and nonmaleficence outweighed the principle of beneficence.* Most states have agreed with the Tarasoff court and have enacted laws requiring psychotherapists to warn potential victims or to warn the police when an identified person is threatened.

Nonmaleficence is the duty of the psychiatrist to avoid either inflicting physical and emotional harm on the patient or increasing the risk of such harm. That principle is captured by *primum non nocere*, "first, do no harm."

Like the principles of autonomy, nonmaleficence, and beneficence, the principle of justice in psychiatry does not operate in a vacuum but is responsive to the ever-changing social, political, religious, and legal mores of the moment.

Does establishment of a patient–therapist relationship oblige the therapist to care for the safety of not only the patient but also others? This issue was raised in 1976 in the case of *Tarasoff v Regents of University of California* (now known as *Tarasoff I*). In this case, Prosenjit Poddar, a student and voluntary outpatient at the mental health clinic of the University of California, told his therapist that he intended to kill a student readily identified as Tatiana Tarasoff. Realizing the seriousness of the intention, the therapist, with concurrence of a colleague, concluded that Poddar should be committed for observation under a 72-hour emergency psychiatric detention provision of the California commitment law. The therapist notified the campus police both orally and in writing that Poddar was dangerous and should be committed.

Concerned about the breach of confidentiality, the therapist's supervisor vetoed the recommendation and ordered all records relating to Poddar's treatment destroyed. At the same time, the campus police temporarily detained Poddar but released him on his assurance that he would "stay away from that girl." Poddar stopped going to the clinic when he learned from the police about his therapist's recommendation to commit him. Two months later, he carried out his threat to kill Tatiana. The young woman's parents then sued the university for negligence.

The California Supreme Court deliberated the case for the unprecedented time of about 14 months and ruled that a physician or a psychotherapist who has reason to believe that a patient may injure or kill someone must notify the potential victim, the victim's relatives or friends, or the authorities.

61.6 The answer is C

The *Tarasoff I* ruling *does not require that therapists report a patient's fantasies of homicide;* instead, it requires therapists to report an intended homicide; further, it is the therapist's duty to exercise good judgment.

In 1982, the California Supreme Court issued a second ruling in the case of *Tarasoff v Regents of University of California (now known as Tarasoff II), which broadened (rather than merely reinforced) its earlier ruling, the duty to warn, to include the duty to protect.*

The *Tarasoff II* ruling has stimulated intense debates in the medicolegal field. Lawyers, judges, and expert witnesses argue the definition of protection, the nature of the relationship between the therapist and the patient, and the balance between public safety and individual privacy. Clinicians argue that the duty to protect hinders treatment because a patient may not trust a doctor if confidentiality is not maintained. Furthermore, because it is not easy to determine whether a patient is dangerous enough to justify long-term incarceration, unnecessary involuntary hospitalization may occur because of a therapist's defensive practices.

As a result of such heated debates in the field since 1976, the state courts have not made a uniform interpretation of the *Tarasoff II* ruling (the duty to protect). Generally, clinicians should note whether a specific identifiable victim seems to be in imminent and probable danger from the threat of an action contemplated by a mentally ill patient; the harm, in addition to being imminent, should be potentially serious or severe. *Usually the patient must be a danger to another person, not to property*, and the therapist should take clinically reasonable actions.

In a few cases (none successful so far) claims have already been advanced that a *Tarasoff*-like duty applies to potential infection of partners with human immunodeficiency virus (HIV) by patients under mental health treatment. The breach of confidentiality in *Tarasoff* cases is justified only by the threat of violence. Laws vary confusingly by jurisdiction. Perhaps the ideal solution is to persuade patients to make the disclosure to and report the matter to public health authorities.

Answers 61.7–61.12

61.7 The answer is B (no)

61.8 The answer is B (no)

61.9 The answer is A (yes)

61.10 The answer is A (yes)

61.11 The answer is B (no)

61.12 The answer is A (yes)

Sexual relations with a patient's family member are unethical. This is most important when the psychiatrist is treating a child or adolescent. Most training programs in child and adolescent psychiatry emphasize that the parents are patients too and that the ethical and legal proscriptions apply to parents (or parent surrogates) as well as to the child.

Psychiatrists should never discuss their patients outside the office. Some psychiatrists feel that it is all right to discuss cases at the dinner table with their spouse. "After all," they say, "I trust my spouse." However, trust is beside the point. Patients assume that what they tell the psychiatrist stays inside the consulting room. Merely informing a spouse of the identity of one's patient violates the ethical principles.

Ethically, confidences survive a patient's death. Exceptions include proper legal compulsions and protecting others from imminent harm.

It is *ethical to make a diagnosis of suicide secondary to mental illness* on the basis of reviewing the patient's records. Sometimes called a psychological autopsy, interviews with friends, family, and others who knew the deceased may also be useful.

Proponents of the view "Once a patient, always a patient" insist that any involvement with an ex-patient—even a date or one that leads to marriage—should be prohibited. They maintain that a transferential reaction always exists between the patient and the therapist and that it prevents a rational decision about their emotional or sexual union. Some psychiatrists maintain that a reasonable time should elapse before any such liaison. The length to the "reasonable" period remains controversial: Some have suggested 2 years, not 1 year.

The Principles of Medical Ethics with Annotations Especially Applicable to Psychiatry, however, states: "Sexual activity with a current or former patient is unethical."

The patient has the right (known as privilege) of insisting that information about his or her case be divulged to those who request it. Psychiatrists are allowed to contest that right if they believe that the patient will be harmed by revealing such information. Psychiatrists may stipulate that a report sent to a third party not be shown to the patient; however, in complex cases proper disposition of records may have to be adjudicated.

Answers 61.13–61.17

61.13 The answer is A

61.14 The answer is B

61.15 The answer is A

61.16 The answer is B

61.17 The answer is B

The term *ethics* is usually reserved for the moral principles restricted to certain groups, such as those in a profession. That role-bound morality can consist of internal or external standards of ethical conduct. For the psychiatric profession, *The Principles of Medical Ethics with Annotations Especially for Psychiatry,* developed by the American Psychiatric Association (APA), is an example of an internal standard used by the profession's major organization to regulate the behavior of its members. Judicial, legislative, or executive bodies may impose external standards as well.

Distinguishing between an ethical dilemma and an ethical violation or conflict is important. One is faced with an *ethical dilemma when asked to choose between two ethically legitimate alternatives,* such as *preserving patient confidentiality or protecting endangered third parties.* An *ethical conflict* involves the *compromise of an ethical principle, usually because of self-interest,* such as *patient–therapist sexual relations.*

For ethical violations the *APA may expel members* from the organization *or*, for less severe violations , *suspend membership for a time.* During that time a member may be required to undergo supervision or extra training. For still less severe violations a member may be reprimanded or admonished, with no effect on membership status. Expulsion or suspension from the APA is publicly reported. Further, such actions must be reported to the National Practitioners Data Bank.

Answers 61.18–61.21

61.18 The answer is B

61.19 The answer is C

61.20 The answer is A

61.21 The answer is D

The above principles are basic to all ethical questions. Nonmaleficence is the duty of the psychiatrist to avoid inflicting physical and emotional harm on the patient. It is captured by *prumim non nocere*, "first do no harm." The principle of patient autonomy revolves around a patient's right to self-determination. A patient makes autonomous choices by giving informed consent when that choice is intentional, free of undue outside influence, and made with rational understanding.

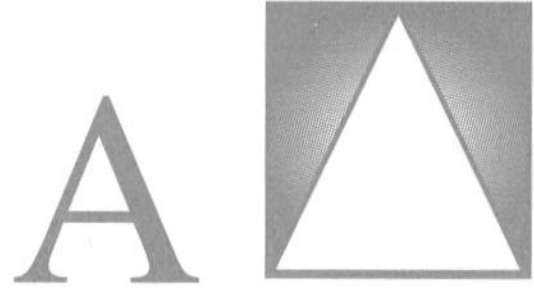

Objective Examinations in Psychiatry

There is a wide variety of objective multiple-choice question formats. They range from case histories followed by a series of questions relating to diagnosis, laboratory findings, treatment complications, and prognosis to the most widely used form, known as the one-best-response type, wherein a question or incomplete statement is followed by four or five suggested answers or completions, with the examinee being directed to select the one best answer. The multiple-choice questions are described as objective because the correct response is predetermined by a group of experts who compose the items, eliminating the observer bias seen in ratings of essay questions. The responses are entered on an answer sheet, which is scored by machine, giving a high degree of reliability. Two basic item types are used with the greatest frequency, one-best-response type (type A) and matching type (type B), which are detailed in Table A.1.

The case history or situation type of item consists of an introductory statement that may be an abbreviated history, with or without the results of the physical examination or laboratory tests, followed by a series of questions, usually of the A type. In similar fashion, charts, electroencephalograms, pictures of gross or microscopic slides, or even patients' graphs may be presented, again followed by the one-best-response type or matching type.

Present testing procedures using objective multiple-choice items are highly effective in regard to reliability and validity in measuring the examinee's knowledge and its application. Experienced test constructors are able to develop items based on a given content and to word the answers in a neutral fashion. Thus, correct and incorrect responses are similar in style, length, and phrasing. However, no matter how well constructed a test is, with a high degree of reliability and validity for a large group of examinees, it is subject to inaccuracies about individual testees. Some examinees underscore, and others overscore, depending on their experience and test-taking skills, known as testmanship. In the final analysis, there is no substitute for knowledge, understanding, and clinical competence when a physician is being evaluated. However, some suggestions and clues inevitably appear in the most carefully composed and edited multiple-choice test. To improve one's testmanship, one should consider the following:

1. There is no penalty for a wrong response in the objective-type multiple-choice question. The testee has a 20 percent chance of guessing correctly when there are five options. Therefore, no question should be left unanswered.
2. In medicine it is rare for anything to be universally correct or wrong. Thus, options that imply "always" or "never" are more likely to be incorrect than otherwise.
3. Especially in psychiatry, many words are often needed to include the exceptions or qualifications in a correct statement. Thus, the longest option is likely to be the correct response. Test constructors who are also aware of this fact often try to lengthen the shorter incorrect responses by adding unnecessary phrases, but that tactic can readily be detected by experienced test takers.
4. The use of a word like "possibly," or "may," or "sometimes" in an option often suggests a true statement, whereas choices with universal negative or positive statements tend to be false.
5. Each distractor that can be ruled out increases the percentage chance of guessing correctly. In a five-choice situation, being able to discard three options increases the percentage from 20 percent to 50 percent and enables the examinee to focus on only the two remaining choices.
6. With questions in which one cannot rule out any of the distractors and these suggestions do not apply, the testee should always select the same lettered option. The examination constructors try to distribute the correct answers among the five options. In some tests the middle, or C, response is correct more often than the others.

Examinations are constructed for the most part by persons from the cultural background in which the test originates. Therefore, those who have been trained abroad and whose native languages are not English are often slower in reading the items and have less time to reflect on the options.

A significant contribution to the evaluation of clinical competence is the development of patient management–problem tests. Those tests try to simulate an actual clinical situation, with emphasis on a functional problem-solving, patient-oriented approach. From thousands of reported examples of outstandingly good or poor clinical performance, test designers defined the major areas of performance, such as history taking, physical examination, use of diagnostic procedures, laboratory tests, treatment, judgment, and continuing care. Armed with that information, the test designers evolved a type of test known as programmed testing. The test provides feedback of information to the examinee, who can use these data in the solution of additional problems about the same patient.

The format starts with general patient information, which gives historical data. The section may be followed by a

Table A.1
Types of Items Used in Multiple Choice Questions

Type A: One-best-response type

Each item consists of an introductory statement or question, known as the stem, followed by four or five suggested responses. The incorrect options are known as distractors, as differentiated from the correct response. Some of the distractors may be true in part, but the one *best* response of those offered must be selected to receive full credit.

DIRECTIONS: Each of the statements or questions below is followed by five suggested responses or completions. Select the one that is best in each case.

1. A2year old boy occasionally plays with his older sister's doll, imitating her activities. Thisi mplies	Stem	
A. pathological problems with sibling rivalry B. undue identification with his mother C. future problems with heterosexual orientation D. development of problems with gender identity	Distractors	Choices or Options
E. natural xploration of his environment	Correct Response	
2. Children in the fourth grade in urban area schools who cannot read are most commonly	Stem	
A. isolated from peers B. mentally retarded	Distractors	Choices or Options
C. culturally disadvantaged disadvantaged	Correct Responses	
D. brain damaged E. handicapped by a major perceptual deficiency deficiency	Distractor	

Type B: Matching type

DIRECTIONS: Each group of questions consists of five lettered headings, followed by a list of numbered words or phrases. For each numbered word or statement, select the one lettered heading or component that is most closely associated with it.

Questions 3–8

A. Mood disorder
B. Psychotic disorder
C. Chromosomalab normality
D. Cognitive disorder
E. None of the above

	Correct responses
3. Delusional disorder	B
4. Conversion disorder	E
5. Down's syndrome	C
6. Bipolarl disorder	A
7. Obsessivecompulsive disorder	E
8. Wernicke's syndrome	D

The use of "None of the above" in a type A or B question of ten makes the item more difficult and tends to lower the percentage of candidates giving correct responses. It should also be noted that the same response may be used more than once.

Type C:

A modified form of the matching type (type C) is also used. It necessitates the ability to compare and contrast two entities, such as diagnostic procedures, treatment modalities, or causes. The association is on an allornone basis. For instance, even if a treatment is only occasionally used or associated with a given disorder ,it is to bei ncluded as a correct response.

DIRECTIONS: Each set of lettered headings below is followed by a list of numbered words or phrases. For each of the numbered words or phrases select

A. if the item is associated with *A only*
B. if the item is associated with *A only*
C. if the item is associated with *both A and B*
D. if the item is associated with *neither A nor B*

Questions 9–13

A. Down's syndrome (mongolism)
B. Tuberous sclerosis (epiloia)
C. Both
D. Neither

	Correct responses
9. Mental deficiency	C
10. Nodular type of skin rash	B
11. Higher than chance association withl eukemia	A
12. Chromosomal nondisjunction	A
13. Specific disorder of amino acid metabolism	D

Adapted from Small SM. Role of examinations in psychiatry. In: Kaplan HI, Sadock BJ, eds. *Comprehensive Textbook of Psychiatry.* 6th ed. Baltimore: Williams & Wilkins; 1995:2734.

summary of the physical examination and positive elements in the psychiatric status. Then the testees are presented with a series of problems, each with a variable number of options. If the examinees select an option, they receive the results of the laboratory test they requested, the patients' reaction to the medication they ordered, or just a confirmation of the order. The examinees may select as few or as many options as befits good clinical judgment. The testees lose both credit and informational feedback if they do not select an important and necessary option. They may also lose credit by selecting unnecessary or dangerous options.

Having completed problem 1 about a patient, the testee is usually given some additional follow-up information, and the procedure is repeated for problems 2, 3, and so on. An oversimplified and much abbreviated example is as follows:

A young college student has been hyperactive, has slept poorly, and has lost weight during the past month. He has been known to use cannabis and possibly other substances on many occasions. Last night he became excited, thought he was going insane, and complained of a rapid pounding sensation over his heart. He was taken to the emergency room by his roommate. No history of prior psychiatric difficulty was obtained. Physical examination reveals a temperature of 99.5°F, pulse rate of 108 per minute, respiration rate of 22 per minute, and a blood pressure of 142/80 mm Hg. His pupils are dilated but react to light, his mouth is dry, and the rest of the examination is noncontributory except for a generalized hyperreflexia. On psychiatric examination he is irritable, restless, and very suspicious. He states that people are after him and wish to harm him. He is well oriented.

1. At this time you would

   A. order morphine sulfate, 30 mg, intramuscularly
   B. inquire about drug usage
   C. order an electrocardiogram
   D. tell the patient that no one wants to harm him and that it is all his imagination
   E. arrange for hospitalization plus many additional options

   Of the choices given, the feedback on B could be "Roommate states patient was taking amphetamines." D feedback: "Patient becomes excited and refuses to answer questions." E feedback: "Arrangements made."

2. The following morning, after a restless sleep, the patient continues to express fears of being harmed. You would now order

   F. chlorpromazine, 100 mg, three times daily
   G. urine screen for drugs
   H. projective psychological tests
   I. imipramine, 50 mg, four times daily and other options

The feedback on F might be "Patient quieter after a few hours." G feedback: "Ordered." H feedback: "Patient uncooperative." I feedback: "Order noted."

Although programmed testing differs from the real-life situation—in which the physician has to originate his orders or recommendations, rather than selecting them from a given set of options—it does simulate the clinical situation to a great extent. Examinees like this type of test and readily appreciate its clinical significance and relevance.

Various modifications of patient management problems have been introduced. It seems that the format, coupled with other forms of testing, is a favorable development in approaching the goal of a standardized, reliable, and valid means of evaluating some major components of clinical competence.

New methods of testing using computer-based systems for objective evaluation of clinical competence are being developed and tested. They are useful in patient management problems because they provide extensive and instantaneous feedback. They also provide contemporaneous scoring, so the testee knows the result of the test upon completion.

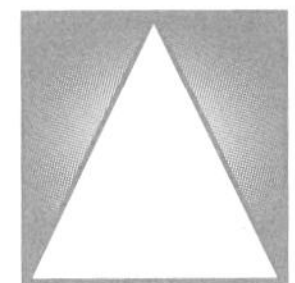

Index

Page numbers followed by *f* indicate figures; page numbers followed by *t* indicate tables.